AF683469

Atlas of Oncology Imaging

For further volumes:
http://www.springer.com/series/8759

Ariadne M. Bach • Jingbo Zhang
Editors

Atlas of Genitourinary Oncological Imaging

Springer

Editors
Ariadne M. Bach, M.D.
Department of Radiology
Memorial Sloan-Kettering Cancer Center
New York
USA

Jingbo Zhang, M.D.
Department of Radiology
Memorial Sloan-Kettering Cancer Center
New York
USA

ISBN 978-1-4614-4871-6 ISBN 978-1-4614-4872-3 (eBook)
DOI 10.1007/978-1-4614-4872-3
Springer New York Heidelberg Dordrecht London

Library of Congress Control Number: 2013932450

© Springer Science+Business Media New York 2013
This work is subject to copyright. All rights are reserved by the Publisher, whether the whole or part of the material is concerned, specifically the rights of translation, reprinting, reuse of illustrations, recitation, broadcasting, reproduction on microfilms or in any other physical way, and transmission or information storage and retrieval, electronic adaptation, computer software, or by similar or dissimilar methodology now known or hereafter developed. Exempted from this legal reservation are brief excerpts in connection with reviews or scholarly analysis or material supplied specifically for the purpose of being entered and executed on a computer system, for exclusive use by the purchaser of the work. Duplication of this publication or parts thereof is permitted only under the provisions of the Copyright Law of the Publisher's location, in its current version, and permission for use must always be obtained from Springer. Permissions for use may be obtained through RightsLink at the Copyright Clearance Center. Violations are liable to prosecution under the respective Copyright Law.
The use of general descriptive names, registered names, trademarks, service marks, etc. in this publication does not imply, even in the absence of a specific statement, that such names are exempt from the relevant protective laws and regulations and therefore free for general use.
While the advice and information in this book are believed to be true and accurate at the date of publication, neither the authors nor the editors nor the publisher can accept any legal responsibility for any errors or omissions that may be made. The publisher makes no warranty, express or implied, with respect to the material contained herein.

Printed on acid-free paper

Springer is part of Springer Science+Business Media (www.springer.com)

To my husband Mark and children Christina and Matthew for their constant love and support. I thank them for all I have learned from them and how they have made me a better doctor and person. To my parents who have taught me to do the best I can.

Ariadne M. Bach

Preface

The *Atlas of Genitourinary Oncological Imaging* presents a comprehensive visual review of appearances for normal anatomy and oncological diseases in the genitourinary system through extensive radiological images and illustrations. This book also presents current imaging techniques and discusses the role of imaging in pretreatment staging and post-treatment follow-up. This atlas is the product of hard work of the radiologists at Memorial Sloan-Kettering Cancer Center. Most of the authors are part of the genitourinary disease management team, which is dedicated to patient care and service. Memorial Sloan-Kettering Cancer Center is one of the premier cancer centers in the world with cutting edge technology and patient care. The disease management team encompasses diagnostic radiologists, surgeons, oncologists, and radiation oncologists in this particular case of genitourinary malignancies. The team members are able to uniquely add to the care of the individual patient. Authors have been selected for their expertise in a particular disease process.

Diseases discussed include kidney, adrenal glands, upper tracts, bladder, prostate, testes, and pediatric malignancies. Nuclear medicine and interventional medicine are in separate chapters. The chapter on chemotherapy toxicities discusses drugs reactions to treatment therapies that are unique to the genitourinary system. The chapters include normal anatomy, imaging techniques, and pathology of the particular cancer. The staging of the particular malignancy and what to include in the radiology reports are discussed. Expected and complicated postoperative and post-treatment findings and recurrence are presented.

This book is geared to both radiology and urology trainees seeking a review of the basics and to practicing radiologists looking for answers to challenging cases confronted in daily practice.

Acknowledgement

Ariadne M. Bach would like to express her appreciation to her authors and colleagues for their contributions and sharing their expertise.

Contents

Contributors

Sara J. Abramson, M.D., FACR Department of Radiology, Memorial Sloan-Kettering Cancer Center, New York, NY, USA

Asim A. Afaq, M.B.B.S., FRCR Department of Radiology, Memorial Sloan-Kettering Cancer Center, New York, NY, USA

Oguz Akin, M.D. Department of Radiology, Memorial Sloan-Kettering Cancer Center, New York, NY, USA

Ariadne M. Bach, M.D. Department of Radiology, Memorial Sloan-Kettering Cancer Center, New York, NY, USA

Vandan Caur, M.D. Wirral University Teaching Hospitals NHS Foundation Trust, Wirral, UK

Joshua Chaim, D.O. Department of Radiology, Memorial Sloan-Kettering Cancer Center, New York, NY, USA

Mark Dunphy, D.O. Department of Radiology, Memorial Sloan-Kettering Cancer Center, New York, NY, USA

Scott Gerst, M.D. Department of Radiology, Memorial Sloan-Kettering Cancer Center, New York, NY, USA

Nathalie Ibrahim, M.D. Department of Radiology, McGill University Health Center, Montreal, QC, Canada

Tunc A. Iyriboz, M.D. Department of Radiology, Memorial Sloan-Kettering Cancer Center, New York, NY, USA

Yulia Lakhman, M.D. Department of Radiology, Memorial Sloan-Kettering Cancer Center, New York, NY, USA

Robert A. Lefkowitz, M.D. Department of Radiology, Memorial Sloan-Kettering Cancer Center, New York, NY, USA

Harpreet K. Pannu, M.D. Department of Radiology, Memorial Sloan-Kettering Cancer Center, New York, NY, USA

Anita P. Price, M.D. Department of Radiology, Memorial Sloan-Kettering Cancer Center, New York, NY, USA

Bradley B. Pua, M.D. Department of Interventional Radiology, New York—Presbyterian Hospital/Weill Cornell Medical Center, New York, NY, USA

Michael J. Sohn Department of Radiology, Breast and Imaging Center, Memorial Sloan-Kettering Cancer Center, New York, NY, USA

Stephen B. Solomon, M.D. Department of Radiology,
Memorial Sloan-Kettering Cancer Center, New York, NY, USA

Jerrold B. Teitcher, M.D. Department of Radiology,
Memorial Sloan-Kettering Cancer Center, New York, NY, USA

Jean M. Torrisi, M.D. Department of Radiology,
Memorial Sloan Kettering Cancer Center, Basking Ridge, NJ, USA

Hebert Alberto Vargas, M.D. Department of Radiology,
Memorial Sloan-Kettering Cancer Center, New York, NY, USA

Han Xiao, M.D. Department of Medicine,
Memorial Sloan-Kettering Cancer Center at Basking Ridge, Basking Ridge, NJ, USA

Jingbo Zhang, M.D. Department of Radiology,
Memorial Sloan-Kettering Cancer Center, New York, NY, USA

1 Renal Parenchymal Tumor Imaging

Robert A. Lefkowitz and Jingbo Zhang

The kidney is a retroperitoneal structure surrounded by perirenal fat and the renal (Gerota's) fascia. Most renal tumors arise from the renal parenchyma (renal cell tumors, renal cortical tumors, or renal parenchymal tumors), with a much smaller number arising from the urothelium of the renal pelvis (urothelial carcinoma or transitional cell carcinoma) or the mesenchyma (e.g., angiomyolipoma, leiomyoma, liposarcoma).

Historically, malignant renal cell tumors have been described as a single entity, renal cell carcinoma (RCC). Per the Heidelberg classification, malignant renal parenchymal tumors are further categorized as clear cell type (approximately 75 % of renal neoplasms in surgical series); papillary type (approximately 10 %); chromophobe type (approximately 5 %); collecting duct (Bellini duct) carcinoma (approximately 1 %); and a small number of unclassified tumors [1]. Medullary carcinoma of the kidney is a variant of collecting duct carcinoma initially described in patients who were sickle-cell-trait positive. Benign renal parenchymal tumors include renal oncocytoma (approximately 5 %) and the rarer metanephric adenoma, metanephric adenofibroma, and papillary renal cell adenoma.

It is now understood that different subtypes of renal cell tumors are associated with different disease progression and metastatic potential. For example, the overall 5-year survival rates for papillary and chromophobe subtypes (80–90 %) are much higher than those for conventional RCC (50–60 %). Among these three most common types of malignant renal cortical tumors, the chromophobe type is associated with the least metastatic potential and best prognosis.

This chapter focuses on renal parenchymal tumors, with a brief discussion of renal mesenchymal tumors. Urothelial carcinoma of the kidneys is discussed in a subsequent chapter.

R.A. Lefkowitz, M.D. (✉) • J. Zhang, M.D.
Department of Radiology, Memorial Sloan-Kettering Cancer Center, 1275 York Avenue, New York, NY, 10065, USA
e-mail: lefkowir@mskcc.org; zhangj12@mskcc.org

Imaging Techniques

The most commonly used imaging modalities for the evaluation of renal parenchymal tumor are computed tomography (CT), magnetic resonance (MR), and ultrasonography (US). Among these diagnostic tools, CT is considered the modality of choice for detection, diagnosis, and staging of renal cortical tumors, with MR and US frequently applied as problem-solving tools or reserved for patients with contraindications to the iodinated contrast used in CT.

Pathology

Another important concept in the evaluation of potential renal cystic lesions on CT is the spurious elevation of Hounsfield unit measurements due to two distinct entities: volume averaging and pseudoenhancement. Volume averaging is encountered with lesions that are nearly as small or smaller than the thickness of the imaging slice, such that the resultant attenuation measurement will lie part way between that of the lesion in question and that of the surrounding tissue. Pseudoenhancement, on the other hand, is related to the beam-hardening artifact caused by the very high density of contrast within enhancing renal parenchyma. CT scanners use an algorithm that compensates for these beam-hardening effects, causing an apparent increase in attenuation that can range from 1 to 33 HU greater than the measurement obtained on the precontrast images, leading one to the erroneous conclusion that the lesion is enhancing when in reality it is not—hence, the term "pseudoenhancement" [10]. Pseudoenhancement is seen with both simple cysts (<20HU) and hyperdense cysts (>20HU), and is more pronounced with smaller lesions, with intraparenchymal versus exophytic lesions, with more intensely enhancing surrounding renal parenchyma, and with a larger number of detectors for multidetector CT [11, 12].

A.M. Bach, J. Zhang (eds.), *Atlas of Genitourinary Oncological Imaging*, Atlas of Oncology Imaging,
DOI 10.1007/978-1-4614-4872-3_1, © Springer Science+Business Media New York 2013

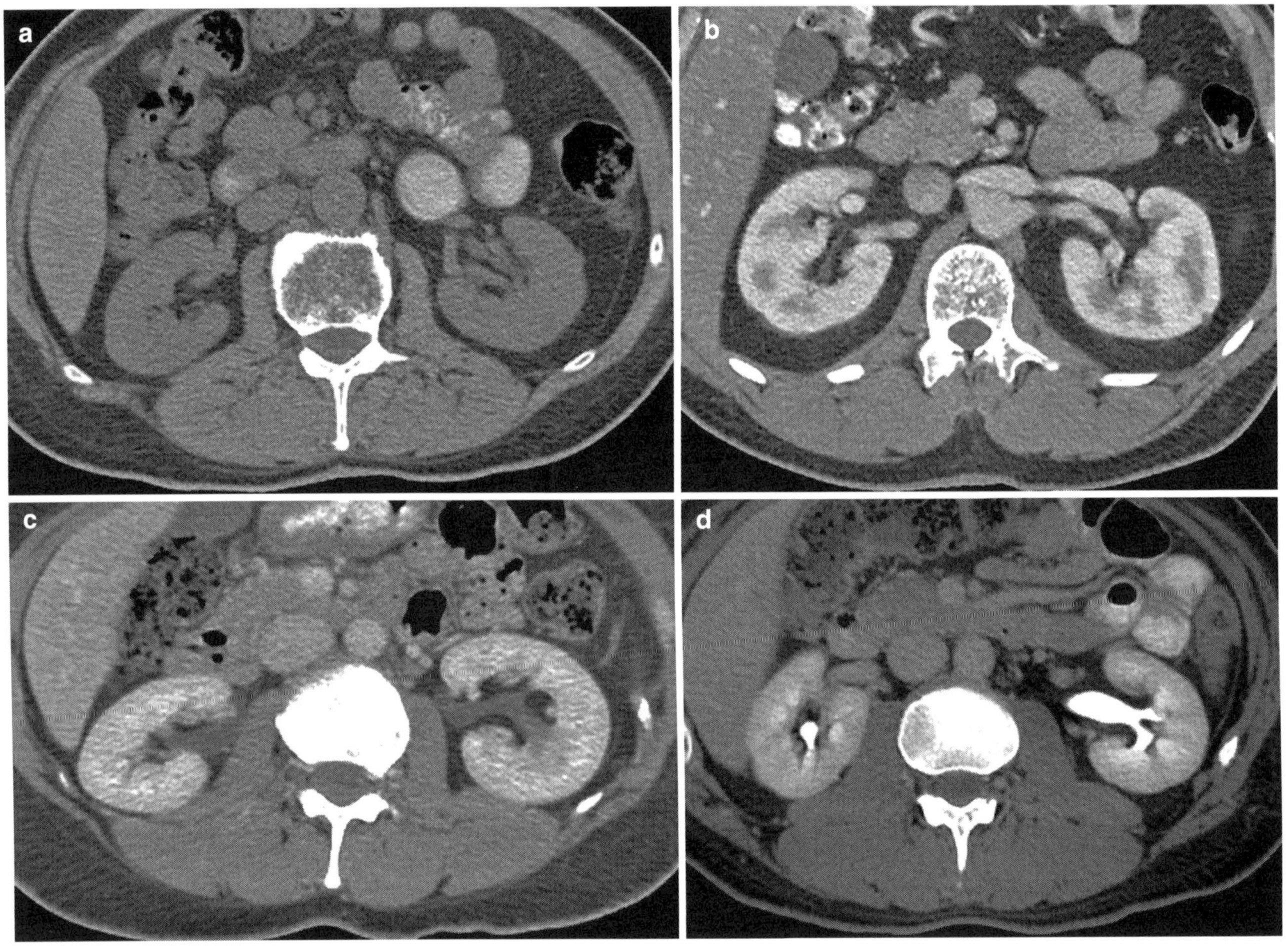

Fig. 1.1 A dedicated imaging protocol is needed for optimized evaluation of the renal mass by CT. At our institution, a CT scan dedicated for evaluation of a renal mass typically consists of three imaging series performed during breath-hold: precontrast, corticomedullary phase, and late nephrographic/early excretory phase. (**a**) Precontrast images are essential for evaluation of the presence of calcifications and/or hemorrhagic components. They also provide a baseline density measurement for evaluating the presence, degree, and pattern of enhancement in cystic or solid renal masses. (**b**) Corticomedullary images (typical scan delay 25–30 s after injection) are superior in lesion characterization and anatomic assessment. (**c**) The nephrographic (approximately 90 s after injection) phase can facilitate the detection of renal masses, especially those of smaller size, due to the homogeneous nephrogram on these images. (**d**) In addition, excretory phase images (these can typically be achieved with a scan delay of 3 min) are helpful for delineation of the renal collecting system. High accuracy (sensitivity up to 100 %; specificity up to 95 %) has been reported in the detection of renal masses when proper technique is applied

Staging

Currently, the most commonly used staging system is the TNM (tumor, node, metastasis) system of the American Joint Committee on Cancer (AJCC) (*see* Table 2.4). The radiology report should include pertinent staging information such as size of tumor, extension to adjacent structures including the adrenal gland, Gerota's fascia and vessels, as well as presence or absence of adenopathy or metastatic disease (most commonly to the lung, bone, brain, liver, and mediastinum).

Post-treatment Imaging Follow-Up

For many years, radical nephrectomy (removal of entire kidney, adrenal gland, and lymph nodes) has been the standard treatment for surgically resectable renal cortical neoplasms. More recently, in an effort to preserve maximum renal function, partial nephrectomy (removal of only a portion of the kidney) has become the treatment of choice for certain renal cancers. Initially reserved for patients with diminished renal function, a solitary kidney (either congenital or from prior

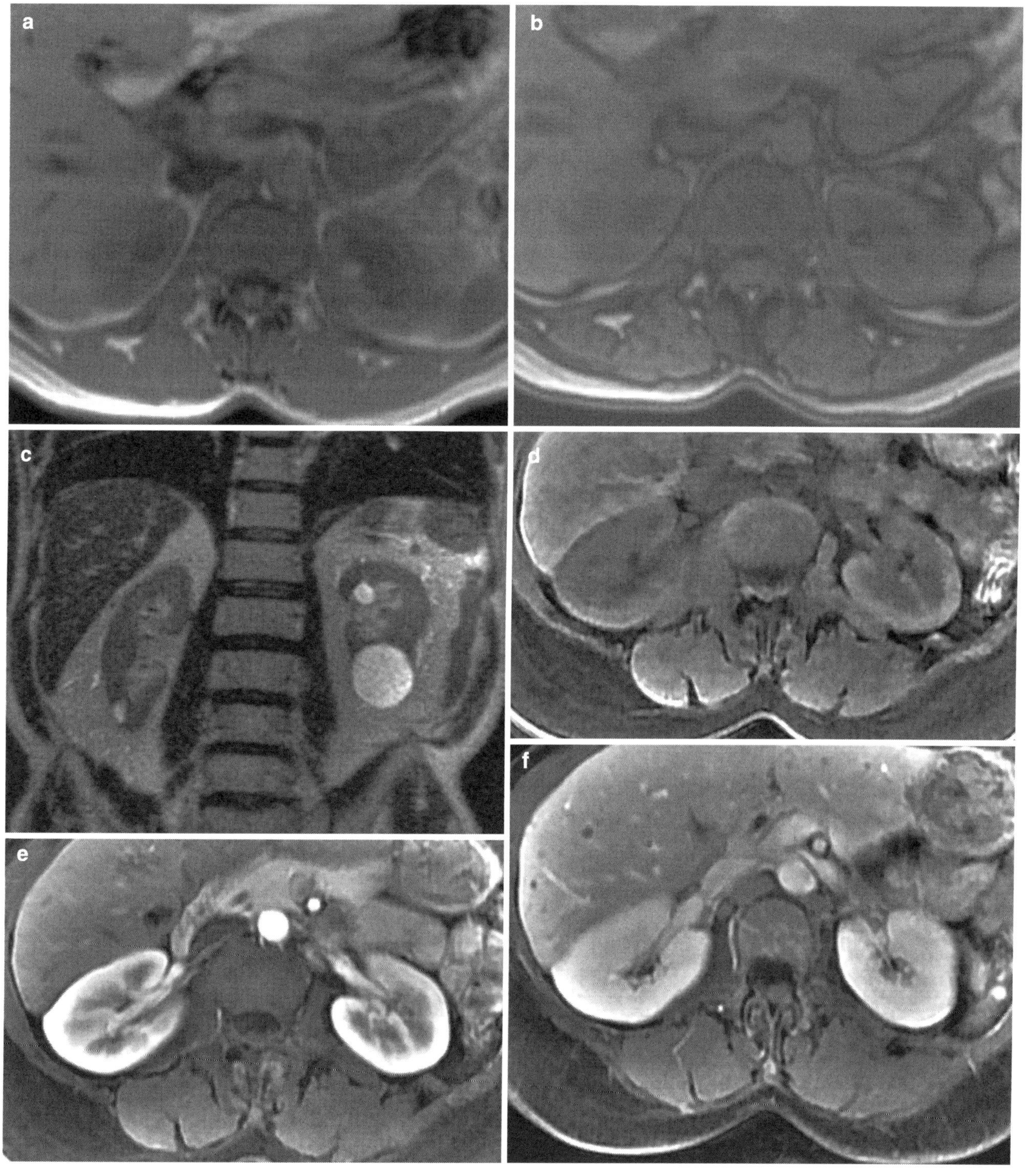

Fig. 1.2 The advantages of MR imaging include its intrinsic high soft-tissue contrast, direct multiplanar imaging capabilities, and lack of radiation exposure. MR imaging of renal masses commonly includes the following breath-hold sequences: (1) axial T1-weighted image (T1WI) in (**a**) and out of phase (**b**) gradient echo sequence, which is helpful in identification of both macroscopic and microscopic fat in a renal tumor; (2) T2-weighted half-Fourier single-shot fast spin-echo sequence in axial and/or coronal planes (**c**), which is useful for evaluating the overall anatomy, renal collecting system, and the complexity of a cystic renal lesion; and (3) a dynamic contrast-enhanced T1-weighted fat-suppressed sequence. For the dynamic contrast-enhanced images, 3D fast spoiled gradient echo sequences are typically performed before (**d**) and after contrast administration during the arterial, corticomedullary (**e**), nephrographic (**f**), and excretory phases for evaluation of the presence and pattern of enhancement in a renal mass. Multiplanar reconstruction may be performed if necessary to better delineate the spatial relationship of the renal mass to adjacent anatomic structures. If necessary, a dedicated magnetic resonance angiography (MRA) sequence during the arterial phase may be performed for better visualization of accessory renal vessels and facilitation of surgical planning. Coronal images may also be obtained during the excretory phase with administration of diuretics, from which maximum intensity projection (MIP) images can then be obtained to produce intravenous pyelogram (IVP)–like images

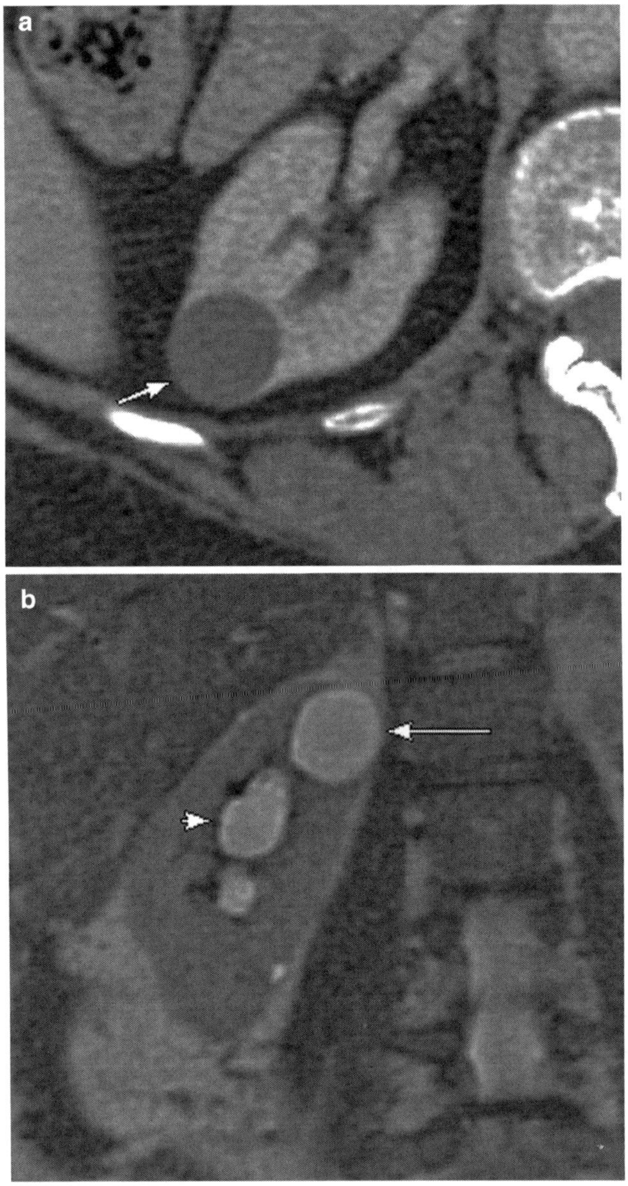

Fig. 1.3 Simple renal cyst. One of the most basic principles of cross-sectional imaging in the evaluation of a renal mass is to determine whether a renal lesion is cystic or solid, and if cystic, whether it represents a benign cystic lesion (nonsurgical lesion) or a potentially malignant one (surgical lesion). (**a**) This contrast-enhanced CT demonstrates a fluid attenuation lesion with a thin imperceptible wall (*arrow*) arising from the right kidney consistent with a simple cyst. A simple cyst is defined as a homogenous density lesion measuring between −20 and 20 HU (on noncontrast and contrast-enhanced studies) and containing a thin imperceptible wall without septations or calcifications. A simple cyst should have a sharp interface with the adjacent renal parenchyma [2]. (**b**) This coronal T2WI demonstrates a very high T2 signal lesion with a thin, imperceptible wall (*long arrow*), arising from the upper pole of the right kidney, consistent with a cyst. Incidentally noted is partially imaged hydronephrosis (*short arrow*). On MRI, the signal intensity of a simple cyst is equivalent to fluid on all sequences (very high T2 signal, low T1 signal without enhancement) is uniform in signal and lacks septations or wall thickening

nephrectomy), or bilateral renal tumors, partial nephrectomy is now the treatment of choice for early stage tumors [75]. Tumors best suited for partial nephrectomy include those that measure less than 4 cm, are peripheral in location, do not involve the renal sinus fat or renal collecting system, and do not invade the renal vein or IVC [75, 76]. Some more recent reports demonstrate that partial nephrectomy can safely be performed in tumors measuring up to 7 cm.

CT is the modality of choice for following patients after treatment. CT can detect postoperative complications, the most common of which are hematoma, urinoma or urinary fistula, pseudoaneurysm, arterial thrombosis, and abscess. CT is also used to restage patients after surgery and/or chemotherapy and to detect local recurrence or distant metastases. In patients with contraindications to iodinated contrast, MRI can be performed in place of CT for imaging follow-up.

Fig. 1.4 (**a**) This contrast-enhanced CT of the left kidney in a patient with adult polycystic kidney disease, demonstrate numerous simple cysts, and one additional lesion posteriorly (*arrow*), which is clearly higher than fluid in attenuation, measuring 65 HU (*measurement not shown*). Based on this sequence alone, one should consider the possibility that this lesion represents a solid enhancing mass. (**b**) However, noncontrast images were also performed in this case, demonstrating that the lesion (*arrow*) is clearly higher in attenuation than the adjacent solid renal parenchyma and actually measured 62 HU (*not shown*). Because the attenuation difference between the pre- and postcontrast images is less than 10 HU, this is consistent with a hyperdense cyst rather than an enhancing neoplasm. A cyst that contains sufficient hemorrhagic or proteinaceous content will measure more than 20 HU on both noncontrast and contrast-enhanced CT images, and thus cannot be called a simple cyst. If both pre- and postcontrast images are available and the attenuation difference of the lesion on these two sequences is less than 10 HU (an attenuation difference of at least 10 HU is required before a lesion is considered "enhancing"), then the lesion is consistent with a hyperdense cyst. These T1-weighted precontrast (**c**) and nephrographic-phase (**d**) MR images both demonstrate a high signal lesion arising from the left kidney (*arrows*). (**e**) This subtraction image (precontrast image **c** subtracted from postcontrast image **d**) shows that the lesion (*arrow*) is now dark, therefore not enhancing, which confirms the diagnosis of a hemorrhagic or proteinaceous cyst. On both CT and MRI, these minimally complex cysts demonstrate lack of enhancement; the presence of enhancement is the hallmark of a solid lesion. Note the small focus of apparent enhancement in (**e**) (*arrowhead*), actually representing misregistration artifact and not enhancement (*arrow* on remainder of cyst which subtracts out indicating lack of enhancement). Protein and methemoglobin, the latter of which is present in hemorrhagic cysts (methemoglobin forms from oxidized hemoglobin and is paramagnetic), cause T1 shortening, resulting in high signal intensity on T1WI [3]. (**f**) In the same patient, this T2WI demonstrates that the hemorrhagic cyst is low in signal intensity (*arrow*). Hemorrhagic cysts can have high- or low-signal intensity on T2WI depending on the age and concentration of various blood products

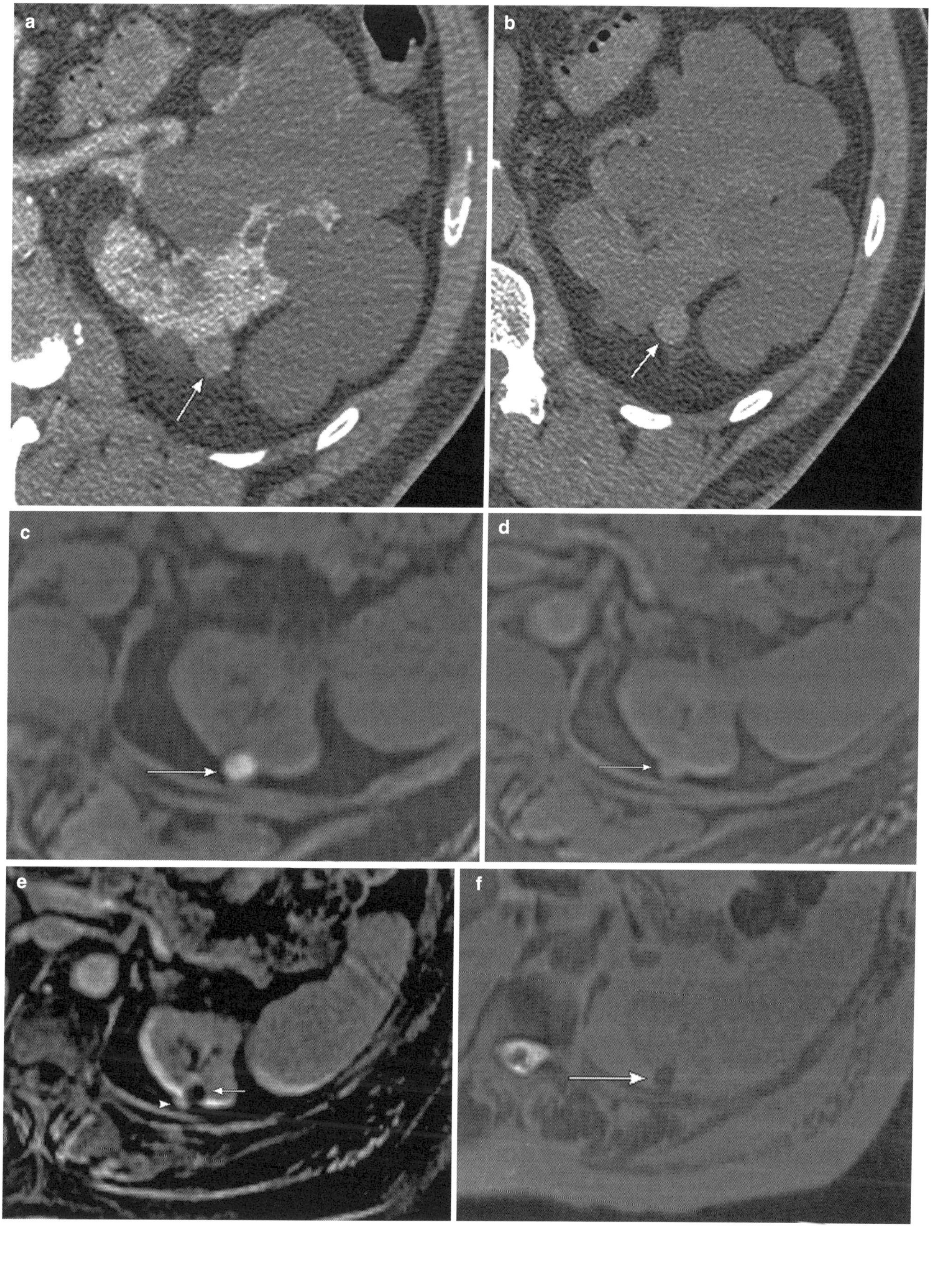

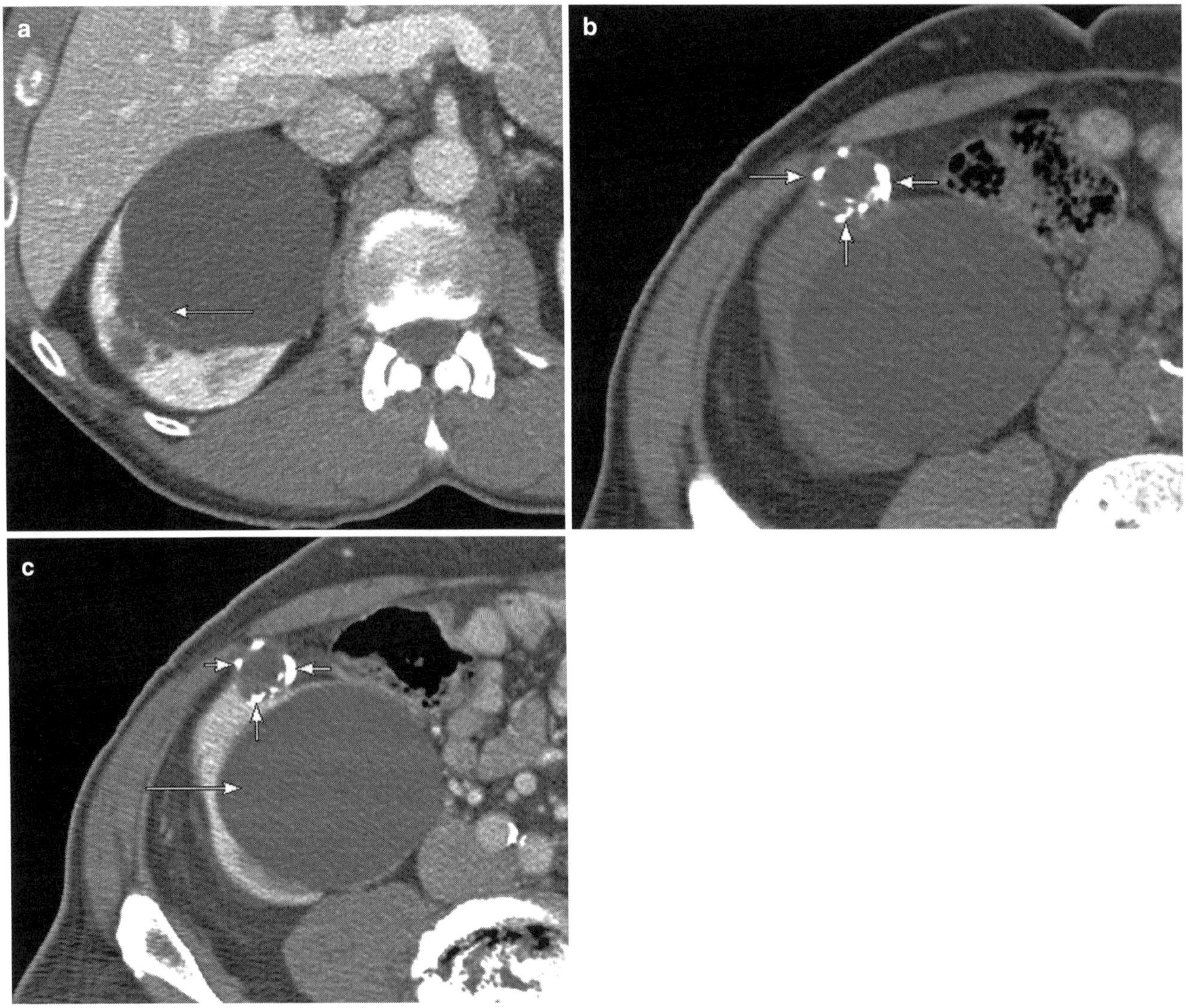

Fig. 1.5 Renal cystic lesions: septations, calcification, and mural nodules. (**a**) This contrast-enhanced CT demonstrates a large right upper pole renal cyst, which contains a thin, approximately 1 mm enhancing septation (*arrow*). This lesion remained stable for at least 9 years. (**b**, **c**) Pre- and postcontrast CT images, respectively, of a complex right lower pole renal cyst at the same level. (**b**) Thick calcifications are seen in the wall of this cyst (*arrows*), but there is no evidence of any solid enhancing mural nodule. This lesion subsequently remained stable for at least 8 years. Incidentally seen on the image is hydronephrosis due to a longstanding ureteropelvic junction obstruction (*long arrow in* **c**). Radiologically benign complex cysts can contain up to a few septations measuring 1 mm or less in thickness and/or mural calcifications. Thin septations are better seen on MRI and ultrasound than on CT, whereas calcifications are best evaluated on noncontrast CT. However, the presence of thickened enhancing septations or an enhancing solid nodule indicates a potentially malignant lesion that is generally managed surgically. In the early days of CT, the presence of thick and irregular calcifications in a cyst was indicative of a surgical lesion because such lesions occasionally harbor malignancy [2, 4]. However, with improved CT imaging techniques, it has subsequently been shown that the presence of a calcification alone, even if thick or irregular, is not indicative of malignancy in the absence of a thickened or nodular enhancing septation or cyst wall [5]. Benign calcifications are frequently caused by old hemorrhage or infection within a cyst [6]. Such lesions are currently classified as 2F lesions in the Bosniak Renal Cyst Classification System [6] and require follow-up imaging; if enhancing soft tissue becomes evident on follow-up CT, then the lesion becomes a potential surgical lesion (Bosniak III). Follow-up imaging (generally 3–6 month at first and then annually for several years [7]) should be performed on all complex cysts that fall into the "2F" category, which includes cystic renal lesions with a few thin septations, a thickened septation without nodularity, thick and nodular calcifications without associated enhancing soft tissue, and hyperdense cysts larger than 3 cm [8]. Due to its superior contrast resolution, MRI can be more sensitive than CT in detecting small amounts of enhancing soft tissue, especially when subtraction techniques are utilized (*see* Fig. 1.4e), and particularly in calcified cystic lesions (calcification is much less apparent on MR, thus, potentially "unmasking" underlying enhancement that can be otherwise be obscured on CT) [7]

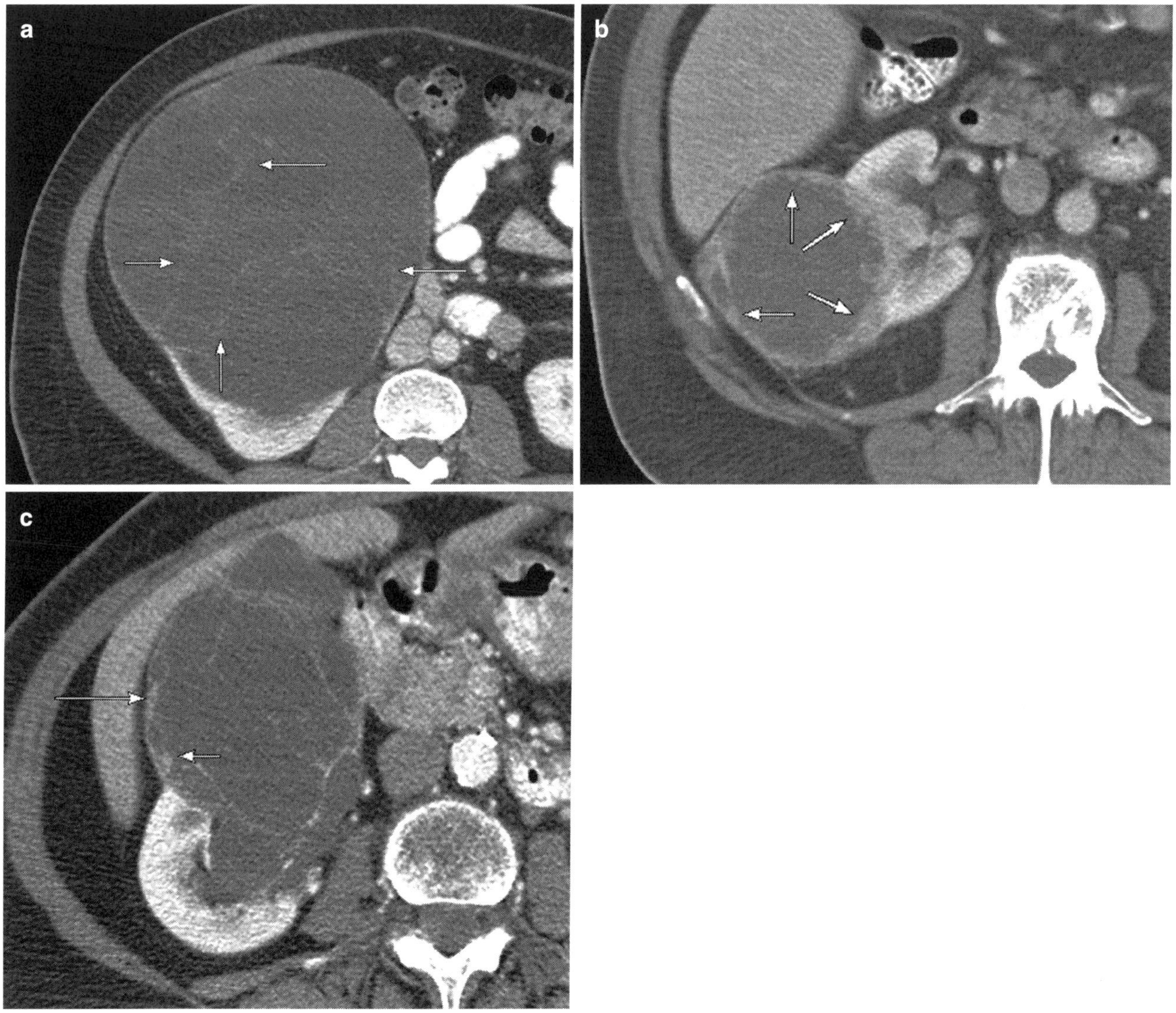

Fig. 1.6 Multiloculated cystic masses. (**a**) This contrast-enhanced CT scan in a middle-aged woman demonstrates a 16 cm cystic mass with multiple thin enhancing septations (*arrows*). Although the septations are relatively thin and without solid nodules, the multiplicity of the septations prompted surgical resection. At pathology, the mass proved to be a cystic nephroma (also known as multilocular cystic nephroma), which is a multiloculated cystic mass with numerous fibrous septae, typically seen in middle-aged women. The vast majority of these lesions are benign (a radiographically indistinguishable lesion known as cystic nephroblastoma is generally seen in boys up to 2 years old) [9]. (**b**) This contrast-enhanced CT demonstrates a large cystic mass with a thick enhancing wall and multiple enhancing mural nodules (*arrows*) (noncontrast images not shown), consistent with a cystic renal neoplasm. At pathology, this lesion proved to be a clear cell carcinoma with prominent cystic changes. Cystic nephroma and RCC are the two most common causes of multilocular cysts in adults. These lesions cannot be reliably distinguished from each other, but RCC, unlike cystic nephroma, can contain hemorrhagic components, have relatively large solid components, and can demonstrate additional signs of malignancy such as renal vein invasion [7]. (**c**) A CT scan of this multiloculated cystic right renal mass demonstrates multiple thin enhancing septations with areas of mural thickening (*long arrow*) and several enhancing nodules along the septations (one shown; *short arrow*). This lesion was subsequently resected and proved to be a cystic renal cell carcinoma

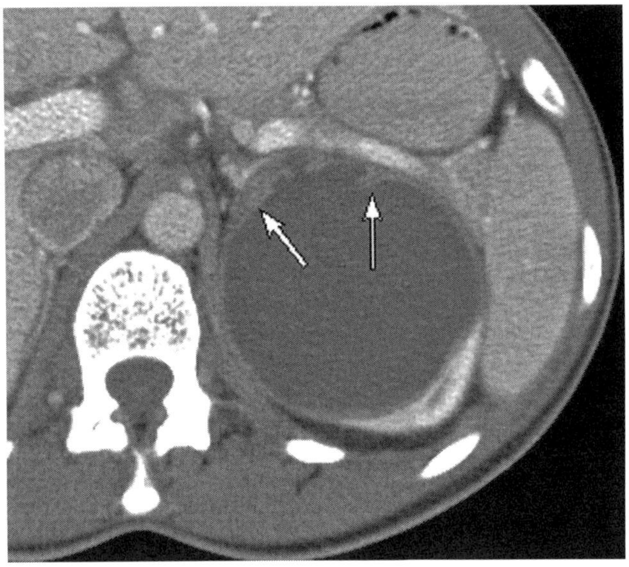

Fig. 1.7 This contrast-enhanced CT demonstrates a left renal cystic mass with a thickened, nodular wall (*arrows*), suspicious for a cystic renal neoplasm. However, at pathology, this lesion turned out to be a chronically inflamed cyst, which was not suspected preoperatively because the patient did not present with signs of infection. Mural thickening with enhancement due to granulation can be seen in infected or hemorrhagic cysts, abscesses, and organizing hematomas, and thus, these lesions are usually difficult to distinguish from cystic RCC radiologically. Although clinical symptoms can occasionally suggest a benign etiology, such lesions are usually surgically excised for diagnostic purposes [7]. If a renal abscess is suspected preoperatively, the lesion should be biopsied before attempting resection and then drained if pus is found [6]

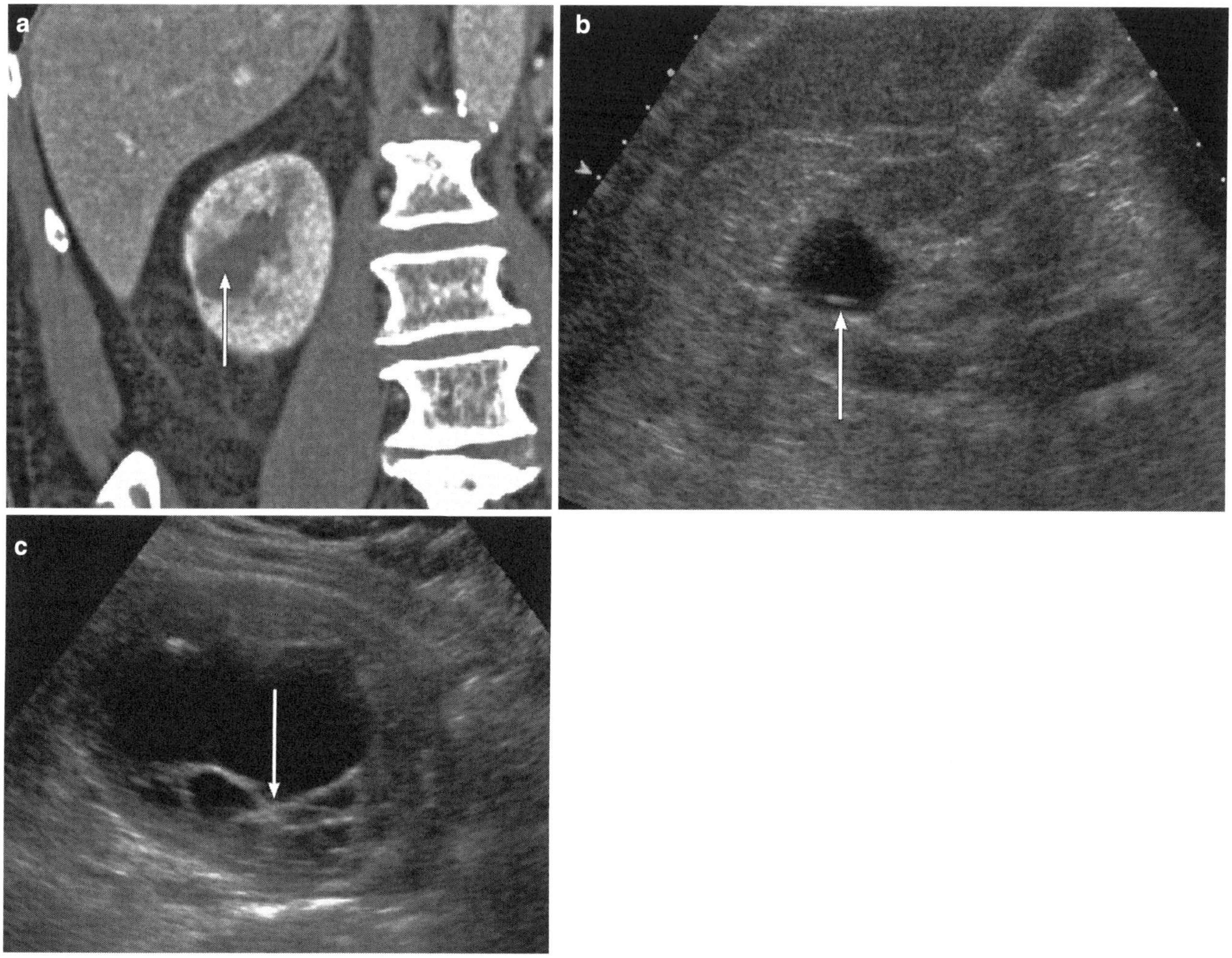

Fig. 1.8 Ultrasound evaluation of cystic renal lesions. (**a**) This contrast-enhanced CT demonstrates a right renal cyst that contains a very thin, enhancing septation (*arrow*). (**b**) An ultrasound of the right kidney demonstrates the same lesion seen in *A*. Note that the same septation (*arrow*) is much easier to appreciate on ultrasound than CT. (**c**) This ultrasound of the right kidney demonstrates a multilocular cystic mass with thickened septations and at least one small solid nodule (*arrow*). This lesion proved to be a cystic RCC at histology. Ultrasound is commonly used to distinguish cystic from solid renal lesions, to further assess complex cysts detected on other imaging tests, and to follow-up known complex cystic lesions. Compared with CT, ultrasound is more cost-effective, does not expose the patient to ionizing radiation, and does not require intravenous contrast. On ultrasound, simple renal cysts are spherical or ovoid, anechoic structures; contain a smooth, thin, sharp back wall; and demonstrate increased through transmission [7]. If a cyst is hemorrhagic or proteinaceous, low-level echoes or layered echoes can be seen within the cyst [7]. Septations within cysts are echogenic and can create reverberation artifacts within the cyst; thus, septations are much more obvious on ultrasound than on CT [7]. Calcification within a cyst wall or septation appears as an echogenic focus that causes posterior acoustic shadowing. Due to shadowing and reverberation artifact, calcifications in renal cysts are better seen on noncontrast CT than ultrasound. Solid components in a cystic renal neoplasm are typically echogenic and fail to show posterior acoustic enhancement. Even small nodules within a cyst can be quite conspicuous on ultrasound due to the acoustic window of the cyst fluid [7]. Doppler imaging frequently demonstrates flow within these solid components [7]

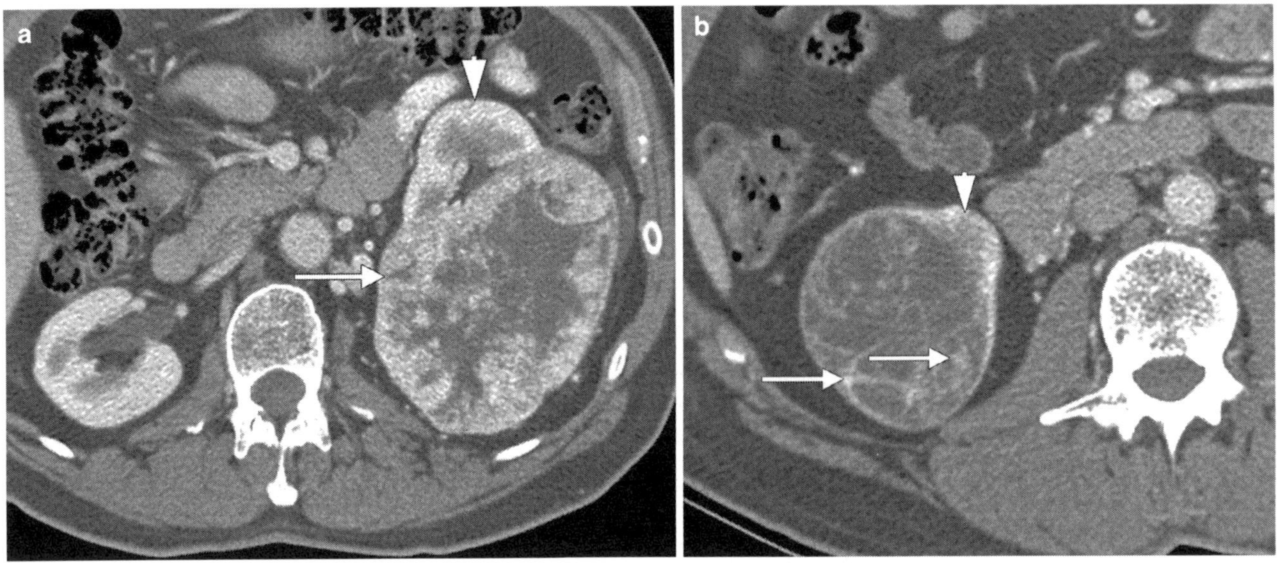

Fig. 1.9 Clear cell carcinoma: CT. (**a**) This contrast-enhanced CT scan demonstrates a large, hypervascular left renal mass with central areas (*arrow*) of cystic change or necrosis. Note that the hypervascular peripheral areas (*arrow*) enhance to nearly the same degree as adjacent renal cortex (*short arrow*). Clear cell carcinoma is the most vascular of the malignant renal cortical neoplasms, demonstrating the greatest degree of enhancement after contrast administration, usually similar to, or slightly less than that of adjacent renal cortex [13–15]. In addition, clear cell carcinomas usually contain prominent areas of cystic change and/or necrosis, manifesting as areas of low attenuation on CT. In a study by Zhang et al. [15], a mixed pattern of hypervascularity with prominent areas of cystic change/necrosis, was most predictive of clear cell carcinoma. Peritumoral vascularity, or the presence of prominent, often irregular collateral feeding arteries and draining veins around the affected kidney confined within Gerotas fascia, are more often seen with clear cell carcinomas than with other types of renal tumors, and are more common with larger tumors. These collateral feeding arteries and draining veins are more likely to be seen with larger tumors [16]. In this example, note that the small vascular structures surrounding the left kidney (*arrows*) are absent on the right side. (**b**) In a different patient, this right lower pole renal mass, also a clear cell carcinoma, demonstrates extensive cystic change, although multiple small areas within the tumor (*arrows*) still enhance similar to adjacent renal cortex (*arrowhead*), indicating hypervascular nature of this tumor

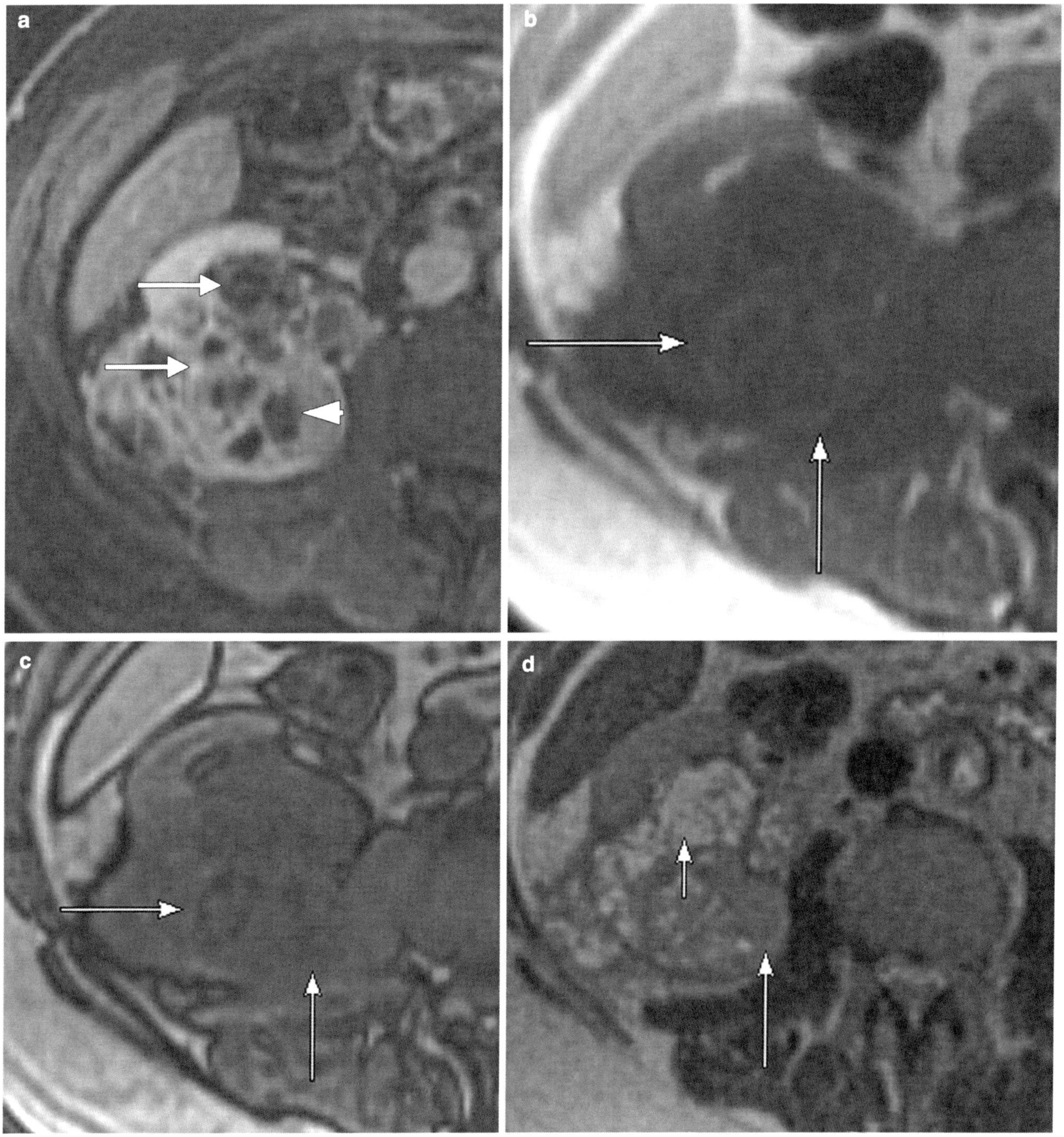

Fig. 1.10 Clear cell carcinoma: MRI. (**a**) This postcontrast nephrographic phase image of a clear cell carcinoma demonstrates a heterogeneously hypervascular mass invading into the renal sinus (*top arrow*). This is a classic appearance for clear cell carcinoma on postcontrast MR images, as in CT, containing a mixed pattern of hypervascular (*lower arrow*) and hypovascular, necrotic or cystic areas (*arrowhead*) [15]. (**b**) Some clear cell carcinomas contain small amounts of intracellular lipid, which are variably hyperintense on T1 in-phase images (*arrows*). (**c**) These same areas demonstrate signal loss on opposed-phase images (*arrows*), indicating the presence of intracellular lipid [17, 18]. The presence of microscopic fat in a renal mass does not necessarily indicate an angiomyolipoma, which usually contains gross fat (*see* Figs. 1.16, 1.17, 1.18, 1.21, 1.22, and 1.23) [18]. (**d**) This T2WI of the same lesion demonstrates that the solid viable portions of the tumor are mildly T2 hyperintense (*long arrow*) whereas the cystic components are markedly T2 hyperintense (*short arrow*). Clear cell carcinoma is typically isointense to normal renal parenchyma on T1WI and so- to mildly hyperintense on T2WI. Heterogenous areas of central necrosis, which are commonly seen in clear cell carcinoma, demonstrate greater T2 signal hyperintensity and T1 signal hypointensity than the adjacent solid areas of tumor; these central necrotic/cystic areas demonstrate no enhancement in contrast to the rest of the tumor [19]. Clear cell carcinoma can contain intratumoral hemorrhage that manifests as high T1 and T2 signal in the subacute to chronic stage and low T1 and T2 signal in the longstanding chronic phase due to the predominance of hemosiderin [19, 20]

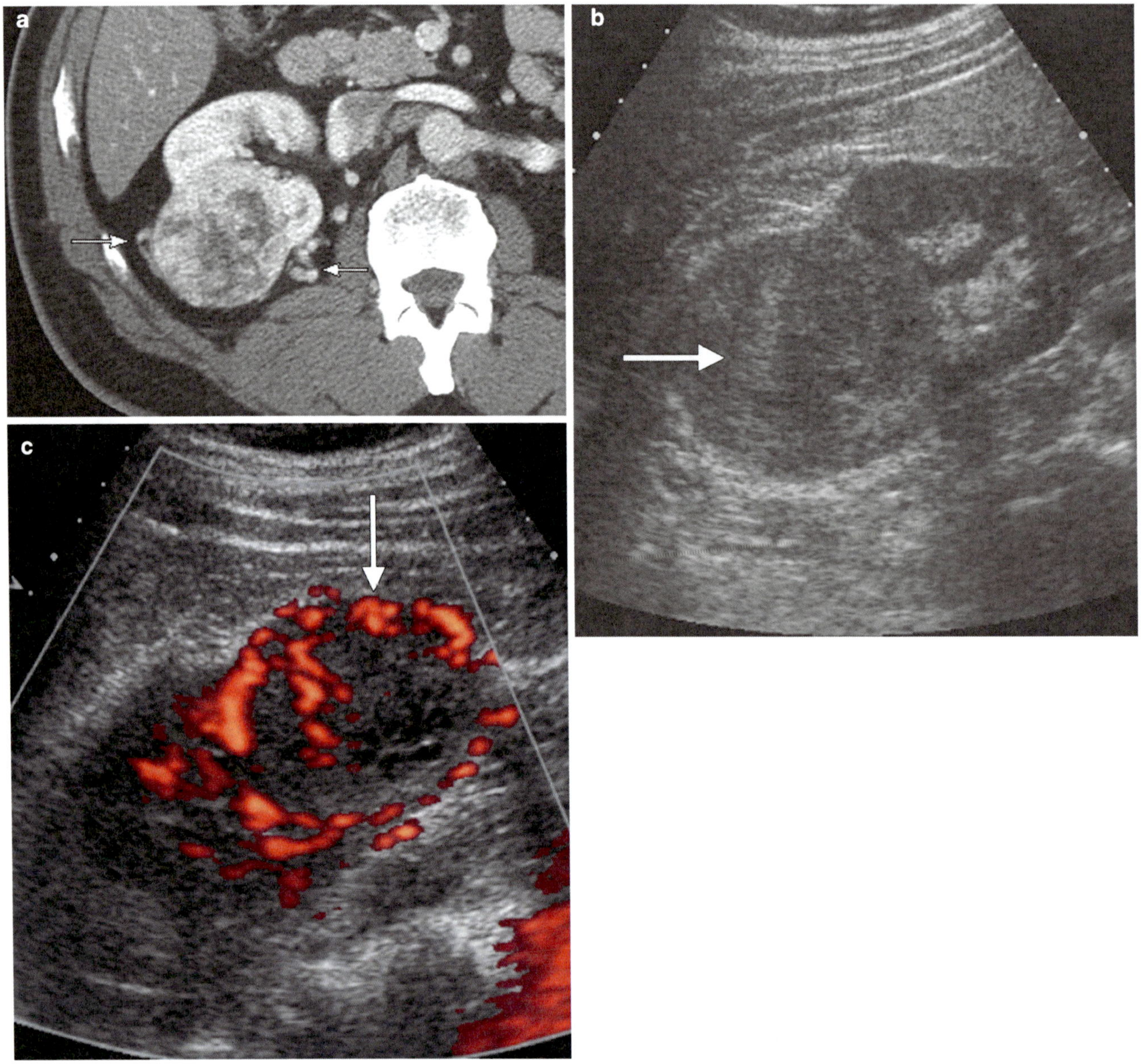

Fig. 1.11 Clear cell carcinoma: ultrasound. (**a**) This contrast-enhanced CT demonstrates a 7 cm heterogeneously hypervascular right interpolar renal mass consistent with clear cell carcinoma. Note the prominent peritumoral vascularity (*arrows*). (**b**) A longitudinal ultrasound on the same patient demonstrates that the mass (*arrow*) is solid and slightly hyperechoic relative to adjacent renal parenchyma. The mass involves the renal sinus fat. (**c**) Power Doppler imaging demonstrates marked vascularity, especially along the periphery of the mass (*arrow*), consistent with a renal cortical neoplasm. The ultrasound findings correlate well with the findings on CT (mass with prominent peritumoral vascularity with some areas of central necrosis). Renal carcinomas, including clear cell, are variable in their appearance on ultrasound, and can be hypo-, iso-, or hyperechoic relative to renal parenchyma [21]. However, prominent vascularity on Doppler imaging can help suggest the diagnosis of clear cell carcinoma. In a study by Raj et al. [22] vascularity was more likely to be associated with clear cell carcinoma than any other subtype of renal cortical neoplasm, although there was overlap with other subtypes

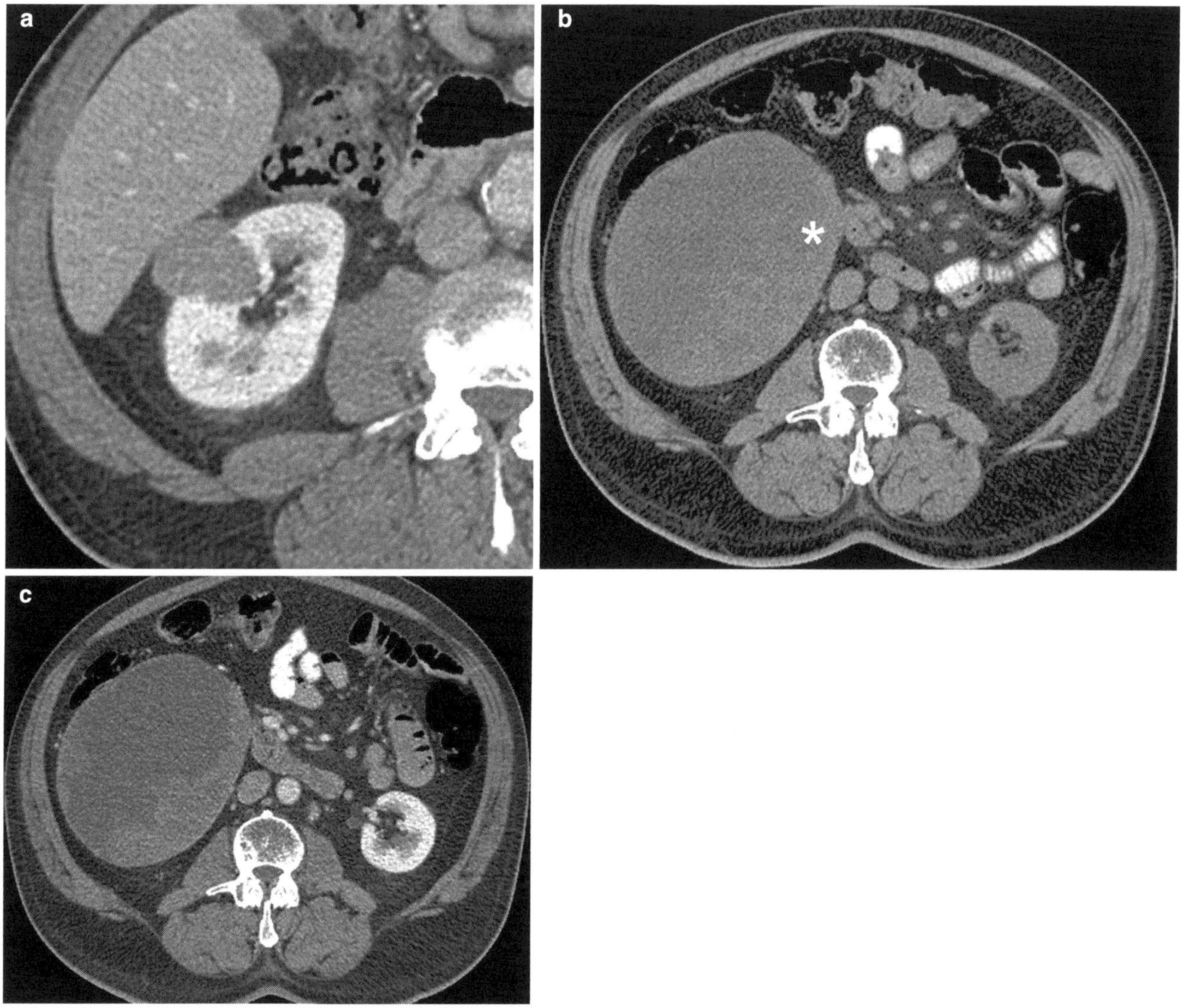

Fig. 1.12 Papillary carcinoma: CT. (**a**) This contrast-enhanced CT scan demonstrates a very homogenous right renal mass, which enhances much less than the adjacent renal parenchyma; these imaging features are most consistent with papillary subtype of renal carcinoma. Renal papillary carcinomas are usually low-grade malignant neoplasms with a favorable prognosis. These tumors are relatively hypovascular compared to renal parenchyma on CT, are usually homogenous in attenuation when they are small (<3 cm) and frequently demonstrate calcifications [15, 23]. They are more likely to be multiple and bilateral than renal neoplasms in general and can be hereditary [23]. (**b**) Noncontrast CT image from a different patient with papillary renal carcinoma demonstrates a large right renal mass with solid tissue in the periphery (*asterisk*) and a central lower attenuation area consistent with cystic change (measuring <20 HU). (**c**) After IV contrast administration, the tumor demonstrates mild enhancement in the solid peripheral region, whereas the central region remains fluid in attenuation. This is a typical imaging appearance for a large papillary carcinoma. Although homogenous when small, papillary carcinoma may demonstrate heterogeneity due to hemorrhage and necrosis when greater than 3 cm [21, 23, 24]. Some papillary carcinomas can manifest as cystic masses with mural nodules or peripheral enhancement as seen in (**b** and **c**). These tumors can be inherently cystic or can become this way due to cystic degeneration and necrosis [21]. Cystic degeneration is almost as common in papillary RCC as it is in clear cell RCC [25]. However, these entities can usually be distinguished by analyzing the solid component, which is much more vascular with clear cell carcinoma [15, 21]. In addition, the cystic component in papillary RCC is usually unilocular whereas in clear cell RCC it is usually multilocular [21]. It should be noted that papillary carcinomas are further classified into type 1 and type 2 subtypes; the former are more common and quite indolent in behavior whereas the latter can be quite aggressive and have a poorer prognosis [26, 27]. The imaging features of both tumors show substantial overlap, including similar degrees of enhancement (both being hypovascular); however, type 2 tumors are more likely to have indistinct margins, infiltrative growth pattern, heterogenous attenuation, and an advanced stage at diagnosis (including renal vein invasion), all of which reflect the more aggressive nature of this tumor [27]

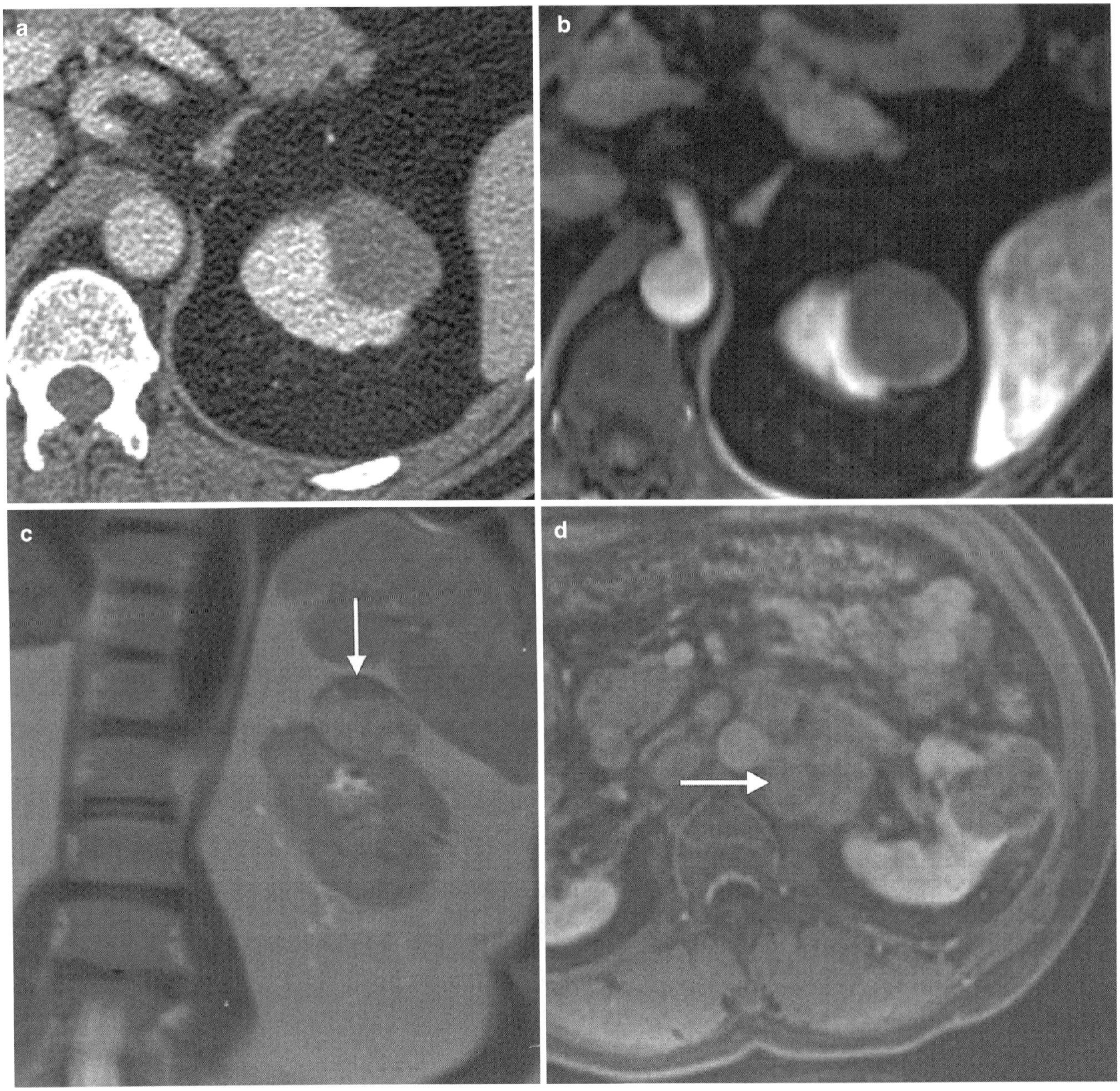

Fig. 1.13 Papillary carcinoma: MRI. (**a**) This contrast-enhanced CT demonstrates a papillary carcinoma with typical imaging feature for a small papillary tumor: homogenous and relatively hypovascular. (**b**) This T1WI with fat saturation in the corticomedullary postcontrast phase demonstrates the same feature seen on the CT image: homogeneity and hypovascularity. Just as in CT, one must compare the precontrast and postcontrast images to determine if the lesion actually enhances, in order to distinguish it from a complex cyst. Although absolute numbers cannot be used to quantify enhancement as with CT (>20 HU), subtraction images can be utilized to subjectively determine the presence or absence of enhancement (pre- and postcontrast images must have identical calibration) [21]. (**c**) This coronal single-shot fast spin-echo (SSFSE) image demonstrates a left upper pole renal mass that contains areas of both T2 hyperintensity and T2 hypointensity. Note the low T2 signal pseudocapsule (*arrow*), a feature which is frequently seen in papillary RCC [21, 28]. (**d**) Nephrographic phase imaging in a different patient with papillary carcinoma demonstrates a mildly enhancing but unusually aggressive papillary carcinoma with retroperitoneal adenopathy (*arrow*). (**e**) SSFSE sequence in the same patient demonstrates a very low T2 signal mass (*long arrow*) compared to adjacent renal parenchyma (*short arrow*). The retroperitoneal adenopathy is also low in T2 signal (*arrowhead*). Papillary RCC is typically low signal on T1 and T2WI, mostly due to the presence of hemosiderin. Other contributing factors include the presence of a fibrous stalk in the papillary architecture and, to a lesser degree, the presence of calcium [28–32]. (**f**) This contrast-enhanced CT of a large papillary RCC demonstrates a mass with cystic change and mildly enhancing peripheral soft tissue, typical of this tumor type. (**g**) T1WI of the same mass shows that the central cystic portion of this tumor is very high in signal consistent with hemorrhagic necrosis. (**h**) SSFSE sequence of same lesion demonstrates that the central cystic portion is high in T2 signal whereas the solid portion is low in T2 signal. Note the small cyst in the adjacent renal parenchyma (*arrow*)

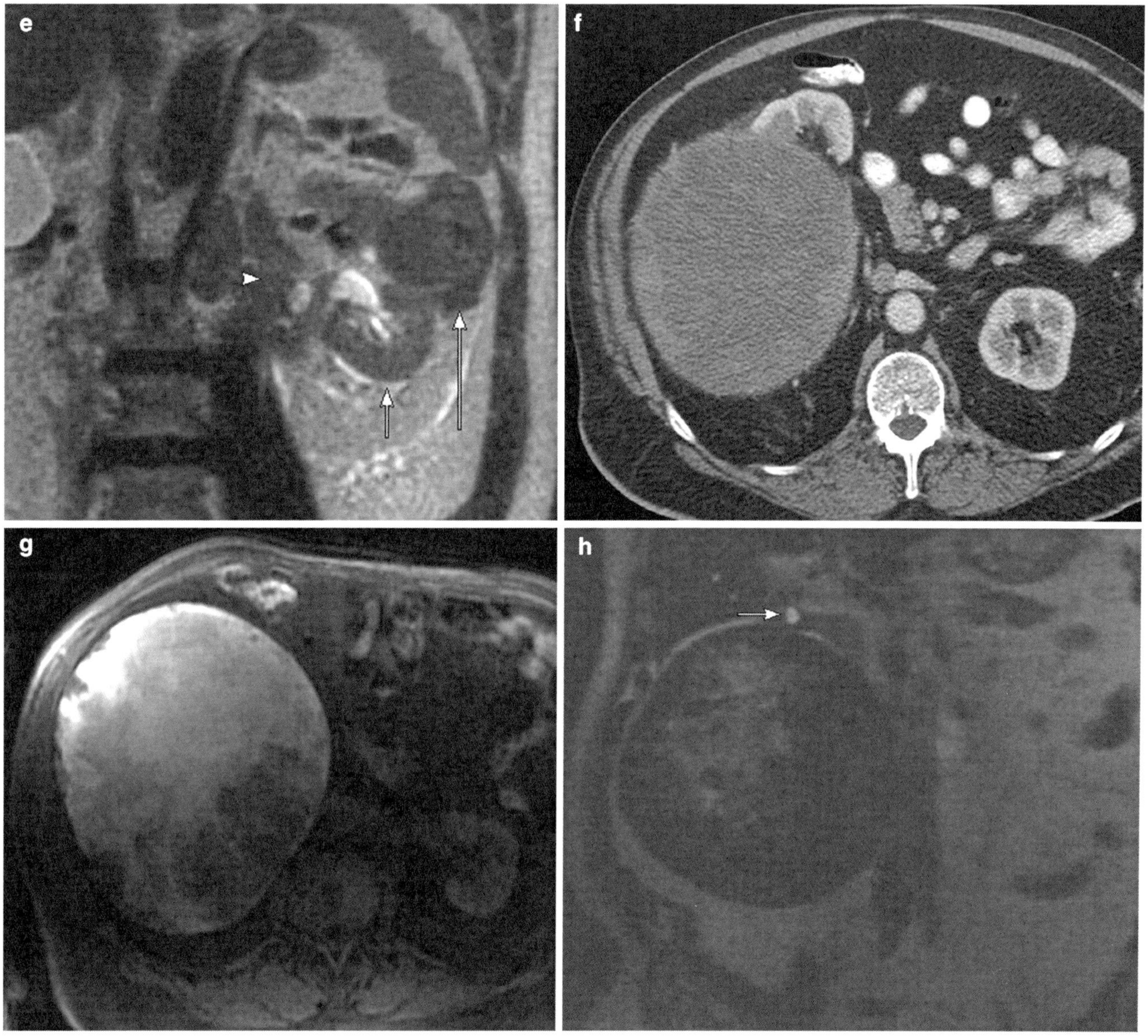

Fig. 1.13 (continued)

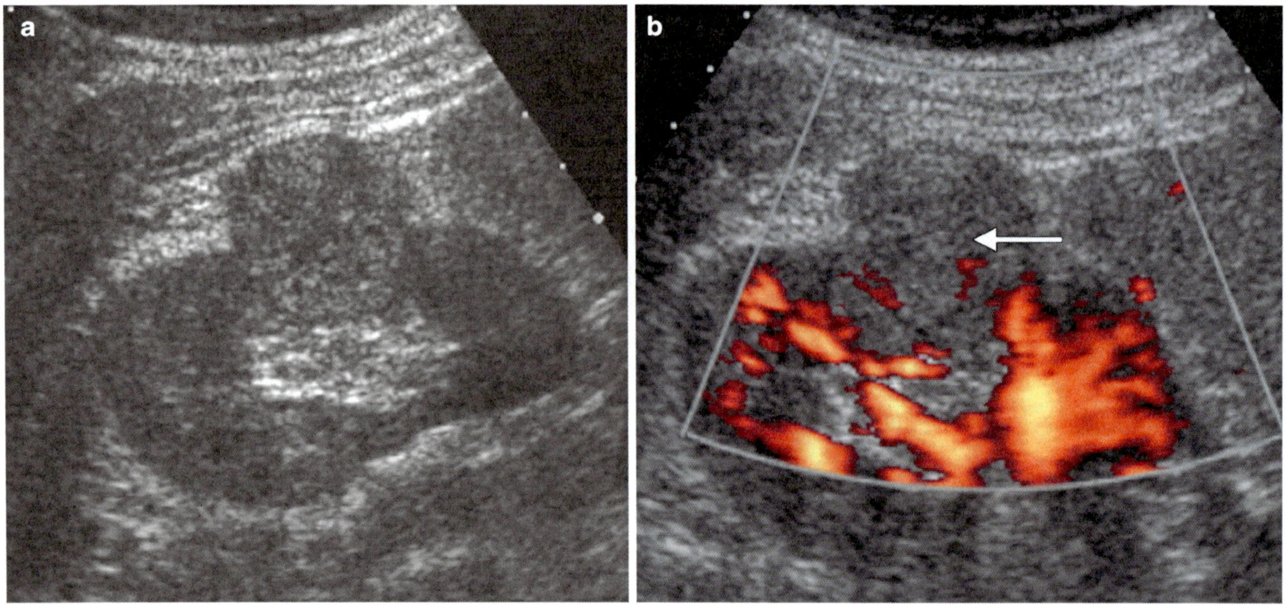

Fig. 1.14 Papillary carcinoma: ultrasound. (**a**) A renal ultrasound on the same patient in Fig. 1.12a demonstrates a mildly hyperechoic, homogenous, exophytic renal mass, which does not involve the renal sinus fat. Currently, there is no technique that has been shown to be accurate in differentiating different subtypes of RCC on ultrasound. In addition, CT and MRI have largely replaced US as the preferred techniques for diagnosing and staging renal cancer [21]. However, ultrasound still has a valuable adjunct role in its ability to distinguish cystic from solid masses, especially for those lesions, particularly papillary carcinoma, which demonstrate only borderline enhancement at CT [21]. On CT hypovascular lesions, especially small ones, can demonstrate very small increases in attenuation from pre- to postcontrast images, which can difficult to distinguish from pseudoenhancement and/or volume averaging (see discussion following Fig. 1.7). In such cases, ultrasound can be more reliable in distinguishing solid from cystic lesions. (**b**) Power Doppler imaging shows a hypovascular lesion (*arrow*). In a study by Raj et al. [22], papillary carcinomas were the least likely of all the RCC subtypes to show vascularity. Thus, the demonstration of a hypovascular mass on Doppler ultrasound can further support the diagnosis of papillary carcinoma but with low specificity

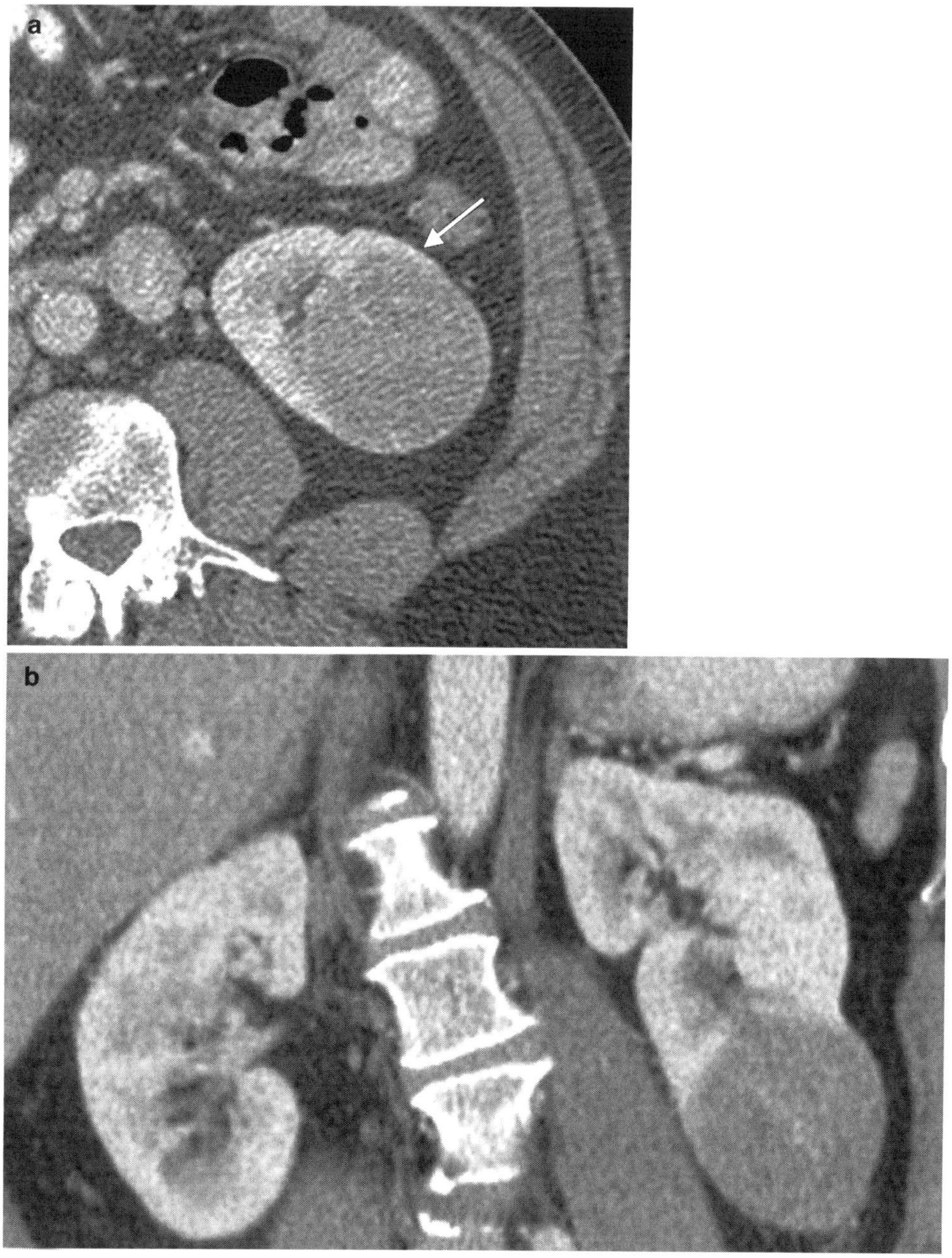

Fig. 1.15 Chromophobe carcinoma: CT. (**a**, **b**) These contrast-enhanced axial (**a**) and (**b**) coronal CT images in the nephrographic phase demonstrate a homogenous, moderately vascular mass arising from the lower pole of the left kidney. Pathology demonstrated a chromophobe carcinoma. Chromophobe carcinoma is generally less vascular than clear cell carcinoma and oncocytoma but more vascular than papillary carcinoma [15]. These tumors tend to be uniform in attenuation, lacking the high degree of necrosis and cystic change characteristic of clear cell carcinoma. Even when large, chromophobe carcinomas tend to lack cystic changes, unlike papillary carcinomas, which are often heterogenous when greater than 3 cm [14]

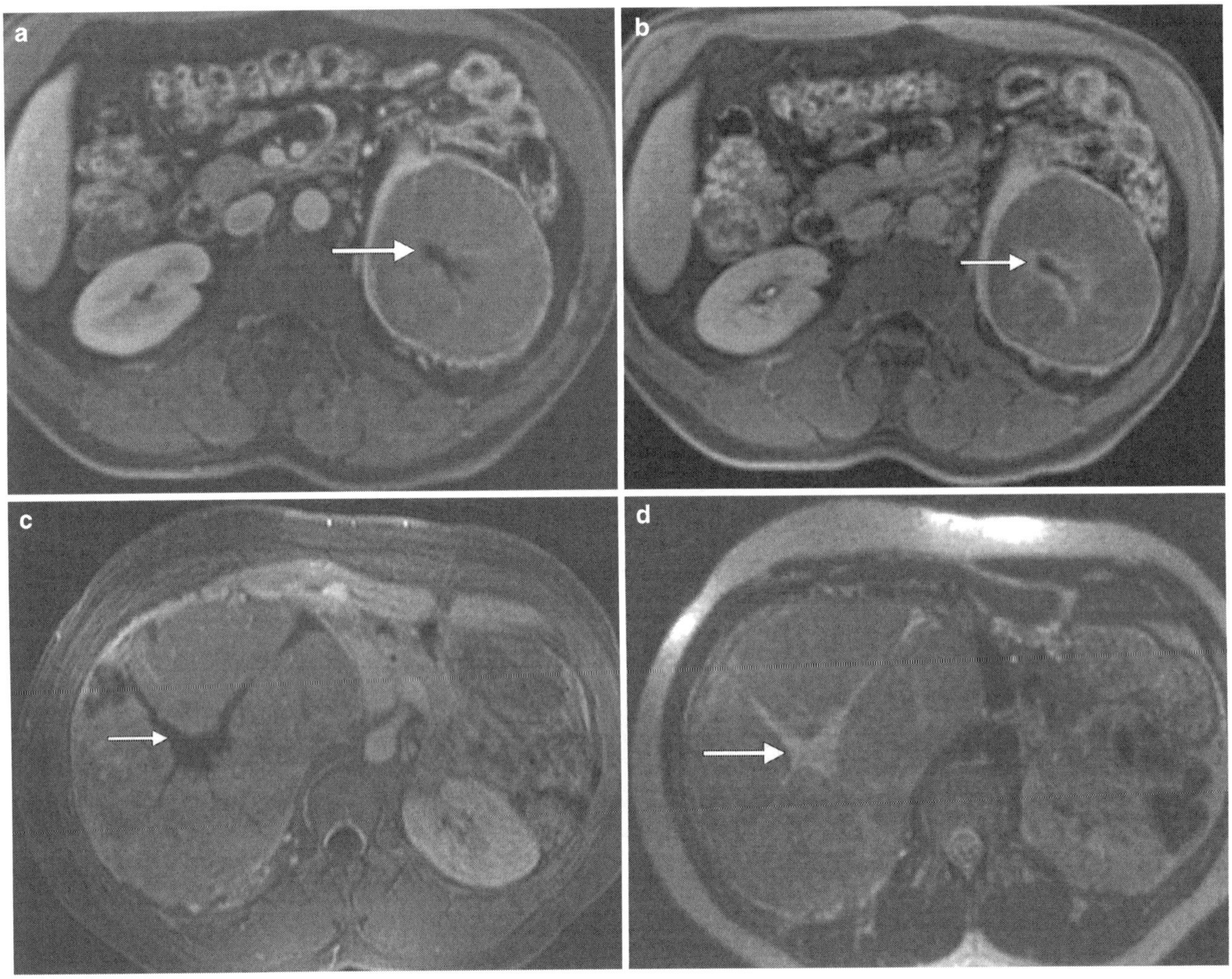

Fig. 1.16 Chromophobe carcinoma: MRI. (**a**) This contrast-enhanced MR image in the nephrographic phase demonstrates a left lower pole renal chromophobe carcinoma, which is relatively homogenous in signal, except for a central scar (*arrow*), which is relatively hypovascular in this phase. Just as on CT, chromophobe carcinomas demonstrate an intermediate degree of enhancement in both the corticomedullary and nephrographic phases, greater than that seen with papillary carcinoma but less than that of clear cell carcinoma [33]. Cochand-Priollet et al. [34] observed that a central fibrous scar is present 23 % of cases of chromophobe carcinoma at histologic analysis (the same study also showed the presence of a central scar in 45 % of oncocytomas, highlighting their similar morphologic, histologic, immunohistochemical, and ultrastructural features) [34, 35]. (**b**) In this excretory phase image at the same location, the central scar is now hypervascularity (*arrow*) relative to the rest of the tumor, which demonstrates washout from the nephrographic phase. Kim et al. [36] described a phenomenon seen in renal oncocytomas called *segmental enhancement inversion* in which the peripheral portion of the lesion is hypervascular on corticomedullary phase images with a relatively hypovascular central lesion, while the pattern reverses in the early excretory phase. Rosenkrantz et al. [35] observed this phenomenon in chromophobe carcinomas and with equal frequency to oncocytomas. (**c**) This is a different chromophobe carcinoma on postcontrast MRI demonstrating moderate vascularity and a large central hypovascular scar (*arrow*). (**d**) The same lesion on this SSFSE image is intermediate in signal with a hyperintense central scar (*arrow*)

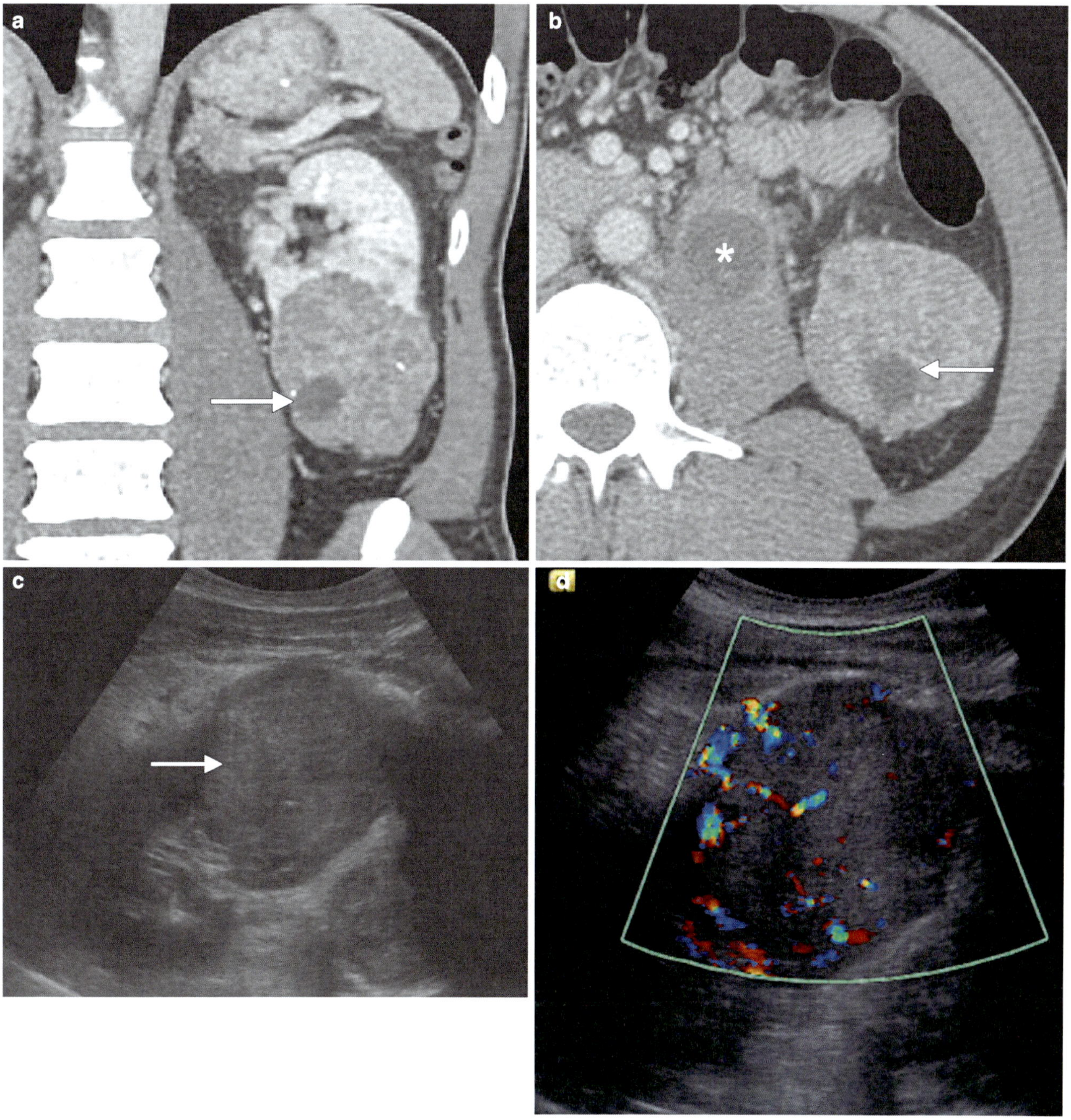

Fig. 1.17 Chromophobe carcinoma: US. (**a**, **b**) Coronal and axial images from a contrast-enhanced CT show a large, relatively homogenous, moderately vascular mass in the lower pole of the left kidney consistent with a chromophobe RCC. The mass contains a few punctate calcifications and only small foci of cystic change (*arrows*). Also note metastatic retroperitoneal adenopathy (*asterisk* in **b**). (**c**) Ultrasound of the same lesion shows a homogenous, relatively hyperechoic, solid mass (*arrow*). (**d**) Prominent vascularity is seen within the mass on Doppler imaging. Although the sonographic imaging features in this case are not specific for chromophobe carcinoma, the homogenous appearance and moderate vascularity correlate well with the imaging features on CT

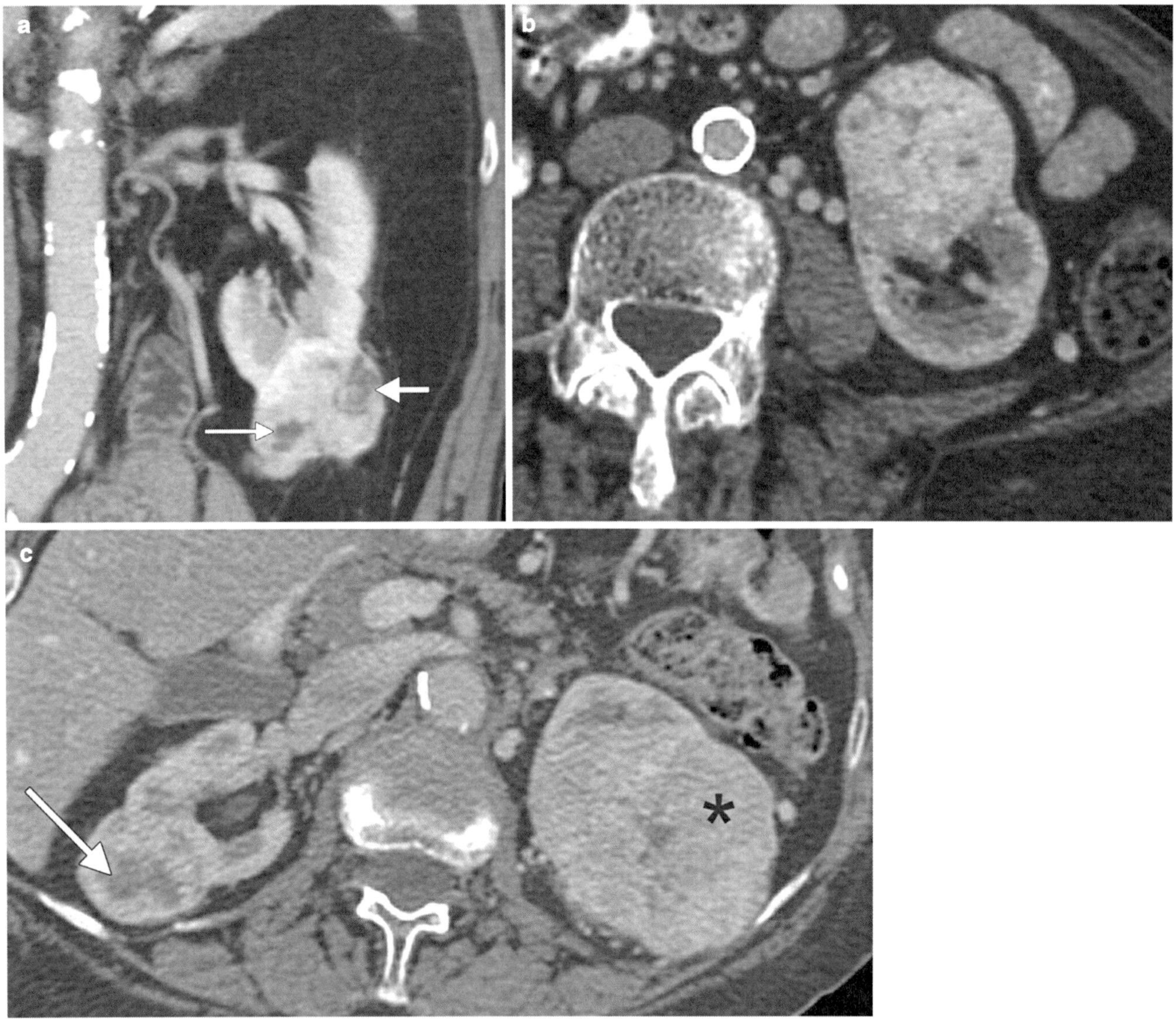

Fig. 1.18 Oncocytoma: CT. (**a**) This coronal reconstructed image in the late corticomedullary or early nephrographic phase demonstrates a hypervascular mass, with attenuation only slightly lower than that of adjacent renal cortex, which proved to be an oncocytoma after surgical resection. Note that there are small areas of low attenuation (*arrows*), but otherwise, the tumor is relatively homogenous. Renal oncocytomas are hypervascular tumors that demonstrate a similar degree of enhancement as clear cell carcinomas, which is similar to or slightly less than that of adjacent renal cortex on nephrographic phase images [15]. In general, oncocytomas tend to be more homogenous in attenuation than clear cell carcinomas, which typically demonstrate prominent cystic change and necrosis as previously discussed. In some oncocytomas, a well-defined central stellate scar can be identified in an otherwise homogenous mass [37, 38]. One study by Kim et al. [36] demonstrated the presence of segmental enhancement inversion in small oncocytomas on biphasic CT, in which areas of higher attenuation in the tumor on the corticomedullary phase became lower in attenuation than adjacent areas on the nephrographic phase. In another study by McGahan et al. [39], on biphasic CT, the most common feature of oncocytoma was a mass, which was slightly heterogenous on corticomedullary phase that became homogenous on the nephrographic phase. However, there is significant overlap in the imaging appearances of oncocytomas and clear cell carcinomas, and, thus, they cannot be reliably distinguished on cross-sectional imaging [37, 38]. (**b**, **c**) These axial CT images in the corticomedullary phase demonstrate multiple bilateral renal oncocytomas. (**b**) The left renal mass is almost completely homogenous and isoattenuating to the renal cortex, with only small foci of low attenuation. (**c**) This image at a different level demonstrates a large, uniformly hypervascular oncocytoma on the left (*asterisk*) and a smaller yet more heterogenous hypervascular mass on the right, also an oncocytoma (*arrow*). Note the prominent vessels surrounding the mass on the left. Prominent peritumoral vascularity is often seen with vascular renal neoplasms, especially when these tumors are large [16]

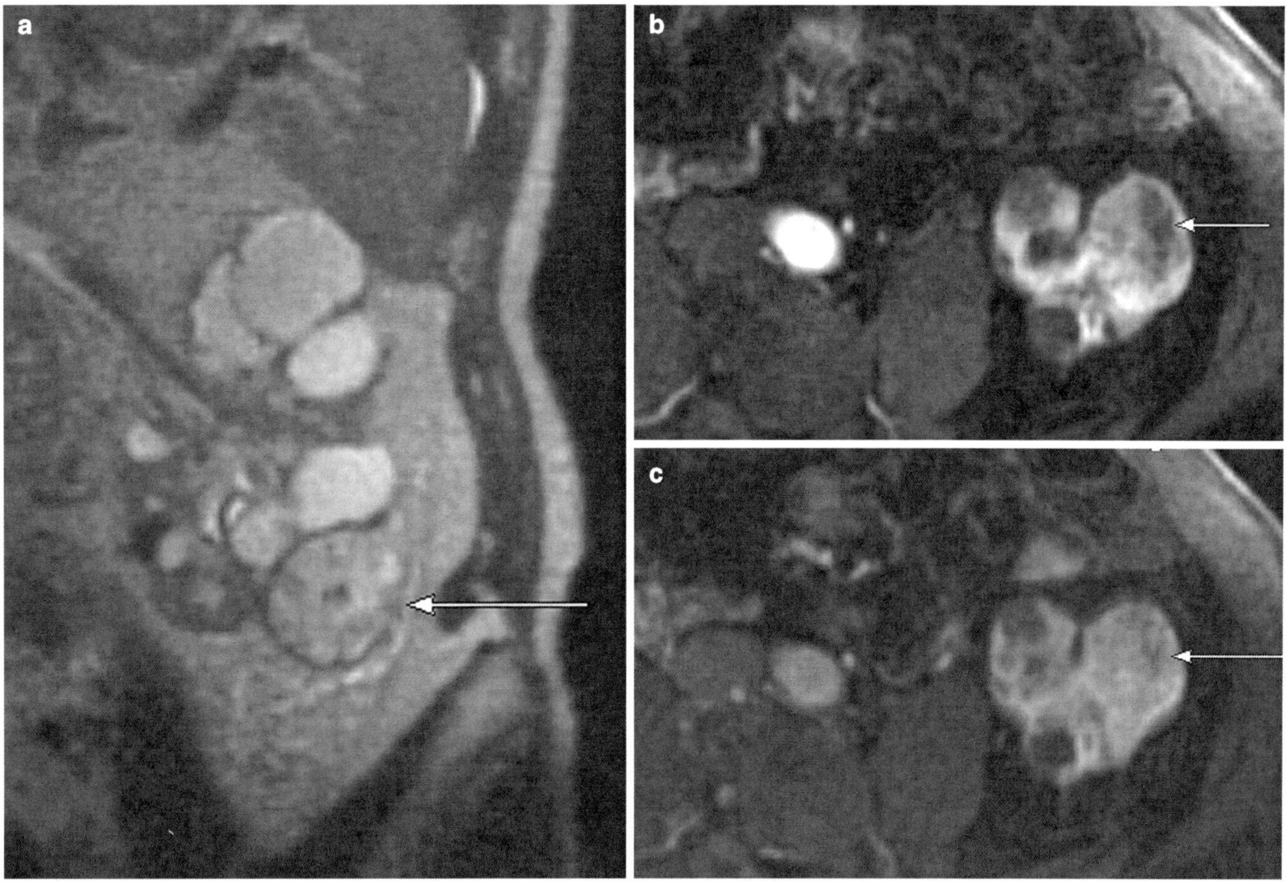

Fig. 1.19 Oncocytoma: MRI. (**a**) A left lower pole renal oncocytoma on this SSFSE coronal sequence demonstrates a predominantly high T2 signal mass (*arrow*). Although the mass is higher in signal than renal parenchyma, it is clearly lower in signal than the multiple renal cysts also shown in this image. (**b**) On corticomedullary phase imaging, this same mass is hypervascular although quite heterogenous (*arrow*). (**c**) On the nephrographic phase image, this oncocytoma has become almost completely homogenous (*arrow*). On MRI, like CT, oncocytomas are hypervascular masses, demonstrating a similar degree of enhancement as clear cell carcinoma. Oncocytomas are generally spherical, well-circumscribed, relatively homogenously enhancing lesions, often becoming more homogenous in the nephrographic phase versus the corticomedullary phase. Occasionally, the central scar may show delayed enhancement [19]. Approximately two thirds of oncocytomas are hypointense to renal parenchyma on T1WI and hyperintense on T2WI [19, 40]. Subacute hemorrhage (high T1 signal), hemosiderin (low T1 and T2 signal), and microscopic lipid (signal loss on opposed phase images) are very rarely seen in oncocytoma, and when seen in a hypervascular renal mass, should favor the diagnosis of clear cell carcinoma over oncocytoma [34, 35]

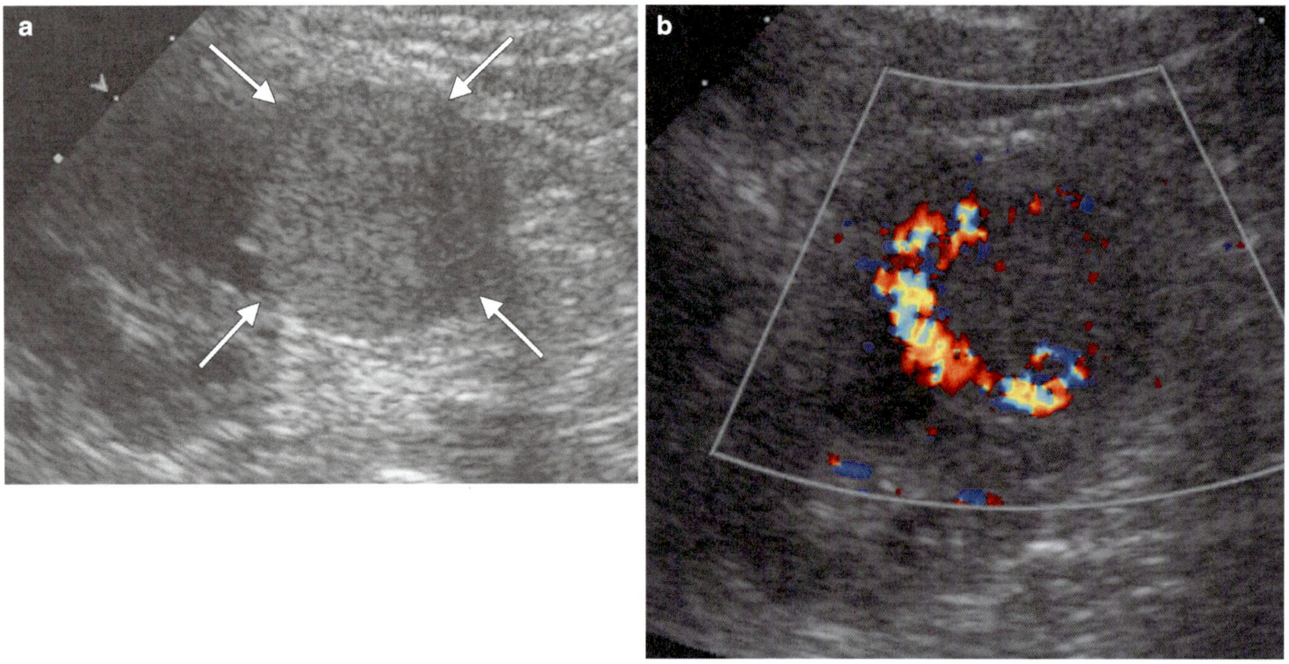

Fig. 1.20 Oncocytoma: ultrasound. (**a**, **b**) Ultrasound of an oncocytoma demonstrates a homogenous mildly hyperechoic mass (*arrows*) with significant vascularity on color Doppler imaging. Although the imaging features are nonspecific for oncocytoma, these tumors are more likely to demonstrate vascularity on Doppler imaging than all other renal cortical tumors except clear cell carcinoma [22]. In addition, the homogenous appearance and prominent vascularity correlate well with the features of oncocytoma typically seen on CT and MR

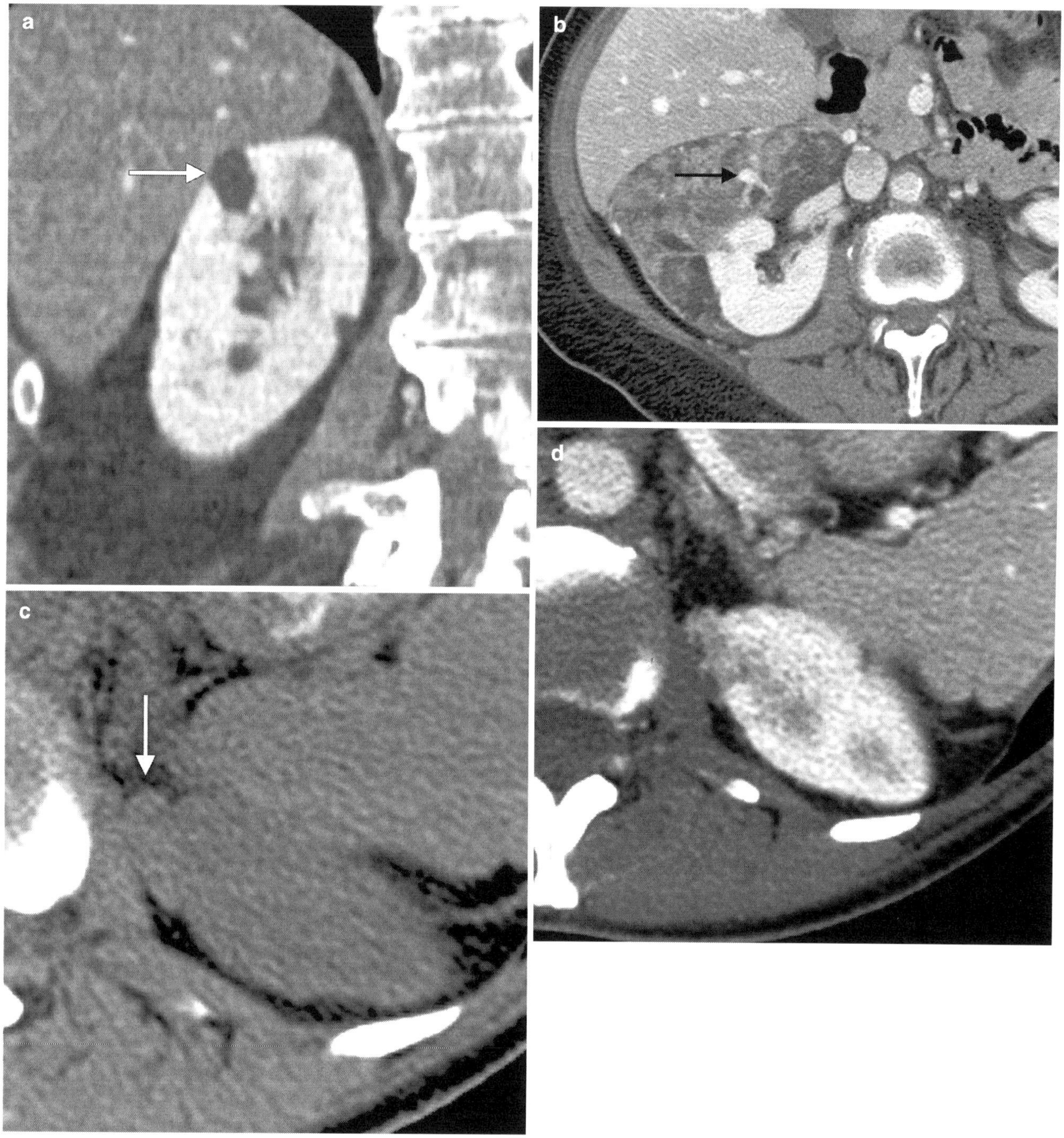

Fig. 1.21 Angiomyolipoma: CT. (**a**) This coronal image from a contrast-enhanced CT demonstrates a small lesion (*arrow*) in the upper pole of the right kidney. This lesion, which measures −75 HU, appears similar in attenuation to adjacent retroperitoneal fat, and is, thus, diagnostic of a renal angiomyolipoma (AML). AML is a type of renal hamartoma that, as the name implies, contains variable amounts of blood vessels, smooth muscle, and fat [41]. The lesion in this example is predominantly fatty in attenuation, which is a common appearance for small AML. (**b**) This contrast-enhanced CT demonstrates a 10 cm mass arising from and partially surrounding the right kidney. The mass contains areas of gross fat, along with heterogenous areas of soft tissue and prominent, irregularly shaped blood vessels (*arrow*), which is consistent with AML. Prominent tumor vascularity is a common feature of AML, as seen in this patient. These tumor vessels are characteristically tortuous, lack normal vessel tapering, and due to an incomplete elastic layer in the wall are predisposed to aneurysm formation (*arrow*) and hemorrhage after minimal or no trauma [41]. (**c**, **d**) Noncontrast and contrast-enhanced CT scans, respectively, demonstrating a small exophytic lesion (*arrow* in **c**) arising from the upper pole of the left kidney. The lesion is slightly hyperattenuating to renal parenchyma on the noncontrast images (lesion measures 45 HU compared with 30 HU for renal parenchyma), and no gross fat is detectable in this lesion. Subsequent partial nephrectomy revealed a smooth-muscle predominant AML with minimal fat. Approximately 3–4 % of AMLs contain insufficient fat to be detected on cross-sectional imaging [42], and in one study nearly 7 % of patients undergoing partial nephrectomy for suspected RCC had pathologically confirmed AML [43]. A study performed by Jinzaki et al. [44], demonstrated that AMLs composed mostly of smooth muscle, with minimal fat, tend to be high in attenuation on noncontrast CT, often protrude from renal parenchyma without the "beak sign" or "claw sign" (acute angle of renal parenchymal at edge of lesion usually seen with renal carcinoma [*arrowhead* in Fig. 1.10a]). The absence of the beak sign with some AMLs suggests a capsular or subcapsular origin of the lesion

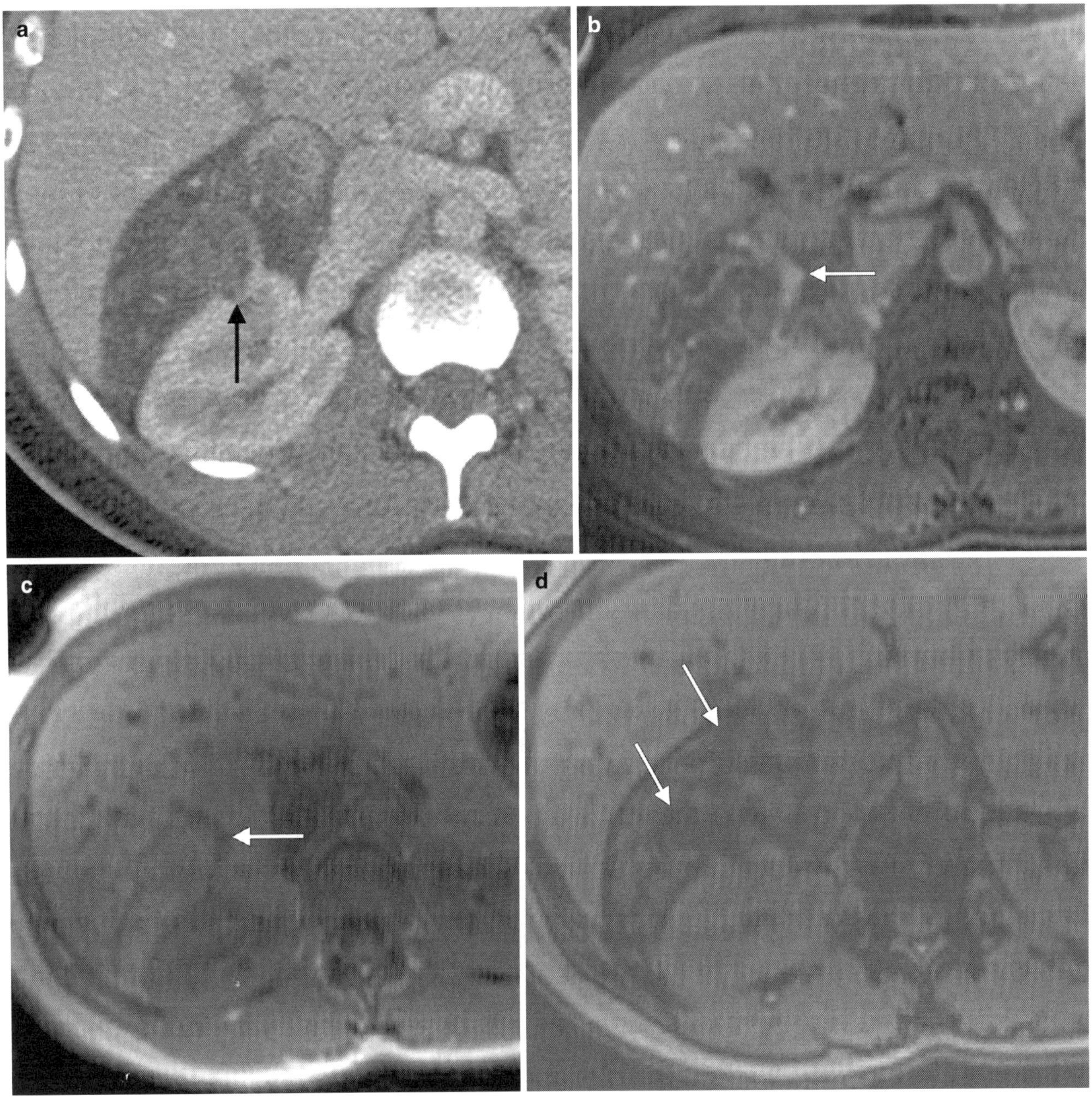

Fig. 1.22 Angiomyolipoma: MRI. (**a**) This contrast-enhanced CT of the right kidney demonstrates a predominantly fatty mass with small soft tissue components and small vascular structures, consistent with an AML. Note, that there is a small defect in the renal parenchyma (*arrow*), indicating the origin of the tumor from the renal parenchyma. The presence of such a defect is the most important feature for distinguishing large exophytic AMLs from retroperitoneal liposarcomas, which do not contain such a notch because they do not arise from the kidney itself [45]. (**b**) This nephrographic phase, fat-saturated, MR image of the same patient in *A* demonstrates, a predominantly fatty mass (low in signal due to fat saturation), with numerous small vessels and one large vessel (*arrow*) emphasizing the vascular nature of these tumors. (**c**) This T1-weighted in-phase image without fat saturation or contrast demonstrates that the lesion is predominantly high in signal (fat) with prominent curvilinear foci of low signal (*arrow*) consistent with vessels. (**d**) This T1-weighted out-of-phase image at the same location as in *C* demonstrates marked signal loss in the lesion (*arrows*) at voxels that contain both lipid and water protons. Dual-echo chemical shift imaging can reliably distinguish AMLs with minimal fat from other renal cortical neoplasms because even the small amount of fat present in the types of AML is sufficient to cause signal loss on the out-of-phase images in contrast to other renal cortical neoplasms that do not contain fat [24]. In rare cases, clear cell carcinomas and oncocytomas have been shown to contain microscopic lipid, but in general, the amount of fat in these tumors is less than that in minimal fat AMLs (follow-up should still be obtained to confirm stability when a minimal-fat AML is diagnosed) [24]. (**e**) T1 fat-suppressed sequence without contrast in same patient shows marked signal loss of predominantly fatty AML. (**f**) In another patient with an angiomyolipoma (*see* CT in Fig. 1.24a of same patient), this T2WI without fat saturation demonstrates that the central fatty component is high in signal intensity (*short arrow*) whereas the lipid-poor portion is diffusely low in signal intensity (*long arrow*). On T2WI, angiomyolipomas with minimal fat generally demonstrate homogenous low signal intensity relative to adjacent renal parenchyma reflecting their high smooth muscle content [17]

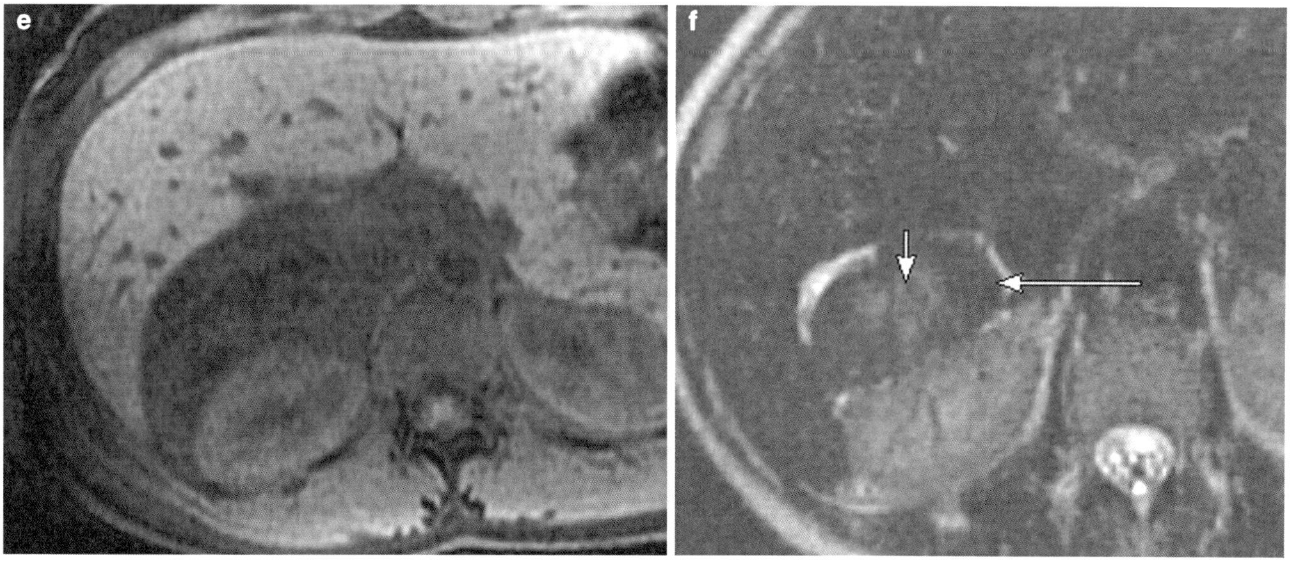

Fig. 1.22 (continued)

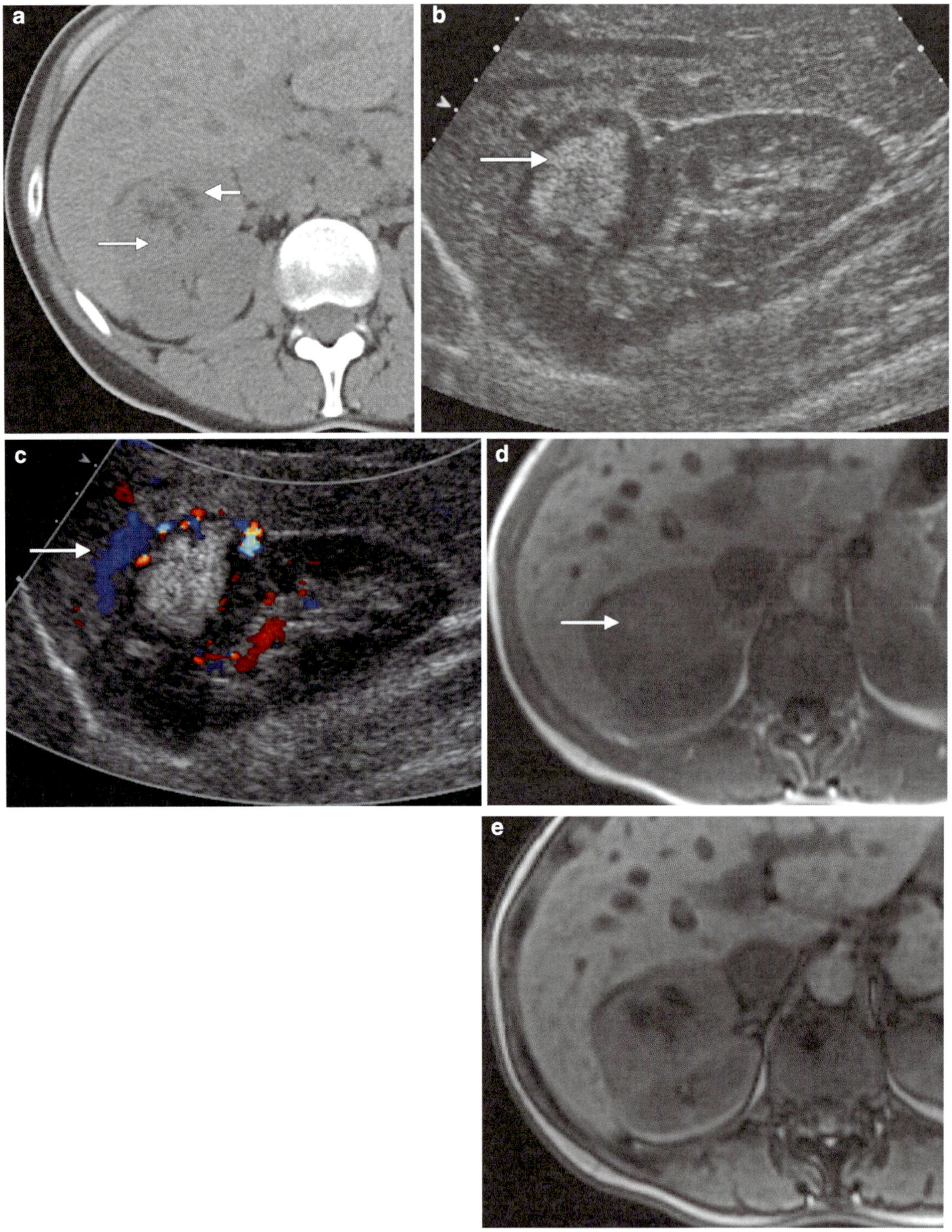

Fig. 1.23 Angiomyolipoma: ultrasound. (**a**) This noncontrast CT shows a right anterior renal mass containing areas of soft tissue (*long arrow*) and fat (*short arrow*) consistent with an AML. (**b**) An ultrasound of this lesion demonstrates marked echogenicity within the central portion of this mass (*arrow*) due to the presence of gross fat. The vast majority of AML are hyperechoic relative to adjacent renal parenchyma and most are markedly hyperechoic, approximating the echogenicity of renal sinus fat [46]. The marked hyperechogenicity in these lesions is largely due to the presence of significant quantities of fat; however, even AMLs with little or no fat are frequently echogenic, indicating that their hyperechogenicity is not necessarily due to the presence of fat alone [20]. Although most hyperechoic renal masses, especially those that are homogenously hyperechoic, turn out to be AML, up to 12 % of all RCC and as many as 33 % of RCC smaller than 3 cm have been shown to be hyperechoic [46]. Thus, noncalcified hyperechoic lesions detected on ultrasound should be further characterized with CT or MR to confirm the presence or absence of gross fat. Calcified hyperechoic solid masses, on the other hand, are theoretically surgical lesions even without further work-up because AMLs rarely calcify [20]. (**c**) Color Doppler imaging of the lesions demonstrates hypervascularity in the periphery of the mass (*arrow*). AMLs frequently demonstrate vascularity on Doppler imaging [22]. Corresponding T1-weighted MR image of the same lesion without fat saturation (**d**) shows high signal intensity centrally (*arrow*), which subsequently loses signal intensity on T1WI with fat saturation (**e**), consistent with bulk fat

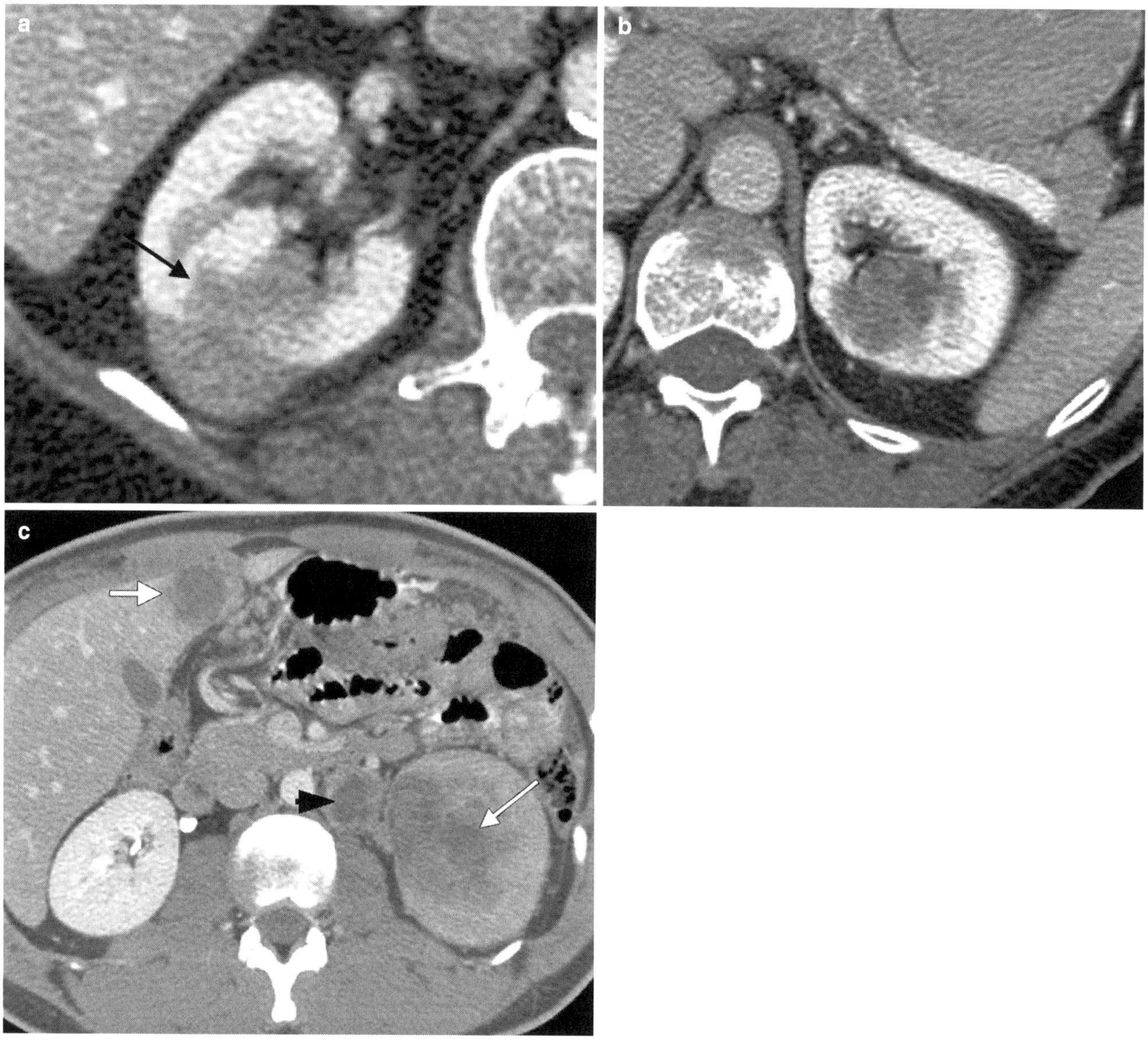

Fig. 1.24 Malignant neoplasms of renal medulla: collecting duct and medullary carcinomas. (**a**) This contrast-enhanced CT demonstrates a mildly enhancing mass with both exophytic and intraparenchymal components. The central component of this lesion, which involves the medullary pyramid, is infiltrative and poorly defined (*arrow*), unlike the more common renal parenchymal tumors described previously, which are well-defined. This lesion proved to be a collecting duct carcinoma at histology. (**b**) This contrast-enhanced CT scan in a different patient demonstrates a centrally located, infiltrative, mildly enhancing tumor invading the renal sinus fat, which also proved to be a collecting duct carcinoma at histology. Collecting duct carcinoma accounts for 1 % of all malignant renal tumors in adults [47]. Collecting duct carcinoma is a very aggressive neoplasm: 40 % of patients have metastatic disease at the time of presentation; the mean survival from time of diagnosis is 12 months [47, 48]. On imaging, collecting duct carcinomas are typically centered around the medulla, can grow in either an infiltrative or expansile fashion (or both), and are hypovascular, demonstrating only mild enhancement with contrast. Further, 25 % demonstrate calcifications and cystic changes can be seen occasionally [47, 49]. On ultrasound, these lesions can be either hyperechoic or hypoechoic, although the former is more characteristic, and they are frequently hypointense on T2-weighted MR images [47, 49]. (**c**) This contrast-enhanced CT scan in a 20-year-old man with sickle cell trait demonstrates a poorly defined, infiltrative, centrally located, partially necrotic mass (*long arrow*) in the left kidney consistent with medullary carcinoma. The left nephrogram is abnormal due to a combination of urinary obstruction and pyelonephritis (*not shown*). This image also demonstrates a heterogenous left para-aortic mass consistent with adenopathy (*arrowhead*) and a mass in the left hepatic lobe consistent with metastatic disease (*short arrow*). In addition, this patient had pulmonary metastases (*not shown*). Renal medullary carcinoma is an extremely aggressive tumor with a male predominance that is seen almost exclusively in young patients (11–39 year) with sickle cell trait [47, 50]. The prognosis is extremely poor, with a mean survival of 15 weeks from the time of diagnosis [47]. Metastases occur most commonly in lymph nodes, followed by lung, adrenal gland, and liver [50]. Cross-sectional imaging demonstrates poorly defined, infiltrative masses that arise in the renal medulla and invade the renal sinus. A typical finding is caliectasis without pelviectasis due to obstruction at the level of the pelvis and infundibulum [47, 51]

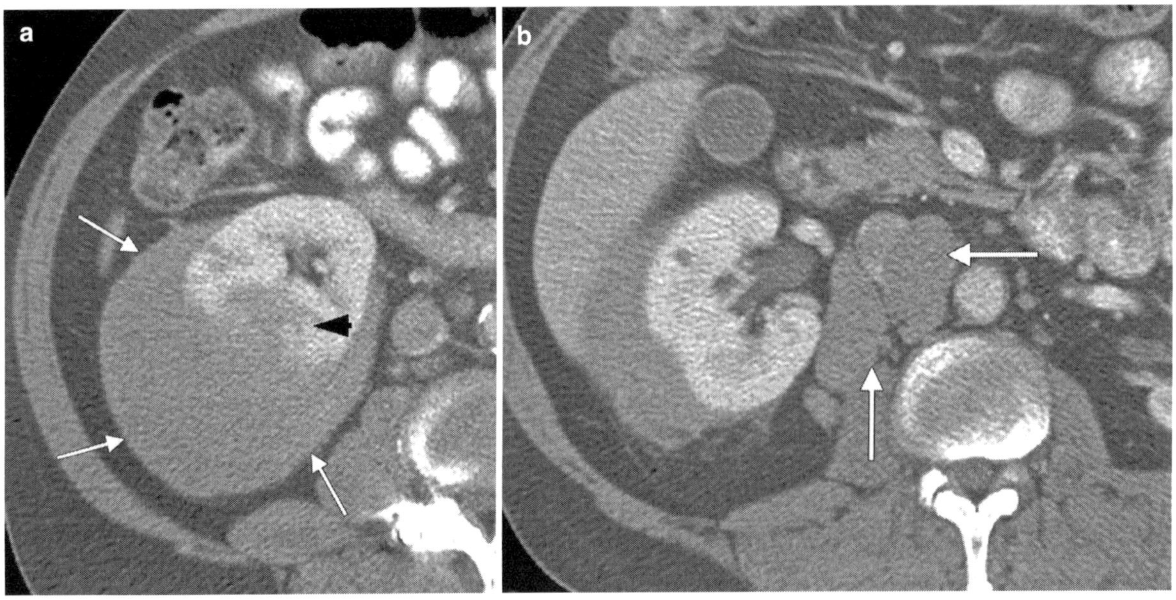

Fig. 1.25 Renal lymphoma. (**a**) This contrast-enhanced CT demonstrates a large, yet strikingly homogenous, mildly enhancing mass involving the right kidney. This mass is also atypical compared to other renal neoplasms in that it extends around the renal capsule (*arrows*) in a crescentic fashion, causing little, if any mass upon the adjacent parenchyma. An additional component within the renal parenchyma itself (*arrowhead*) demonstrates a poorly defined, infiltrate growth pattern. These imaging features are characteristic of renal lymphoma, which is typically very homogenous in attenuation (even when large) and enhances much less than adjacent renal parenchyma. Lymphoma tends to cause very little mass effect upon the renal capsule, collecting system or vessels [52–54]. Several patterns of renal involvement have been described on cross-sectional imaging, the most common of which is multiple soft tissue masses in one or both kidneys. Less frequent patterns include a solitary renal mass, a mass that infiltrates through the perirenal space without significant parenchymal involvement, invasion of renal sinus and hilum directly from the retroperitoneum, or diffuse infiltration of the entire kidney. A characteristic feature of renal lymphoma is that the reniform shape of the kidney is usually preserved as the tumor enlarges, even the entire kidney is involved [54–56]. (**b**) This image is from the same patient as in (**a**), a few centimeters cranially. The mass is again noted to infiltrate around the renal capsule within Gerota's fascia. In addition, there is significant retroperitoneal adenopathy, which is also homogenous in attenuation (*arrows*). Most patients with renal lymphoma have concomitant retroperitoneal adenopathy. Often, lymphoma can secondarily involve the kidney via direct spread from retroperitoneal adenopathy [55]. In fact, the presence of retroperitoneal adenopathy, which is homogenous in attenuation in combination with a homogenous, infiltrative, relatively hypovascular renal mass, is highly suggestive of renal lymphoma. (**c**) This maximum-intensity projection (MIP) image from a positron emission tomography scan on the same patient as in (**a, b**) demonstrates intense uptake from the right renal mass (*arrow*) and the retroperitoneal adenopathy (*arrowhead*). (**d**) In a different patient, this contrast-enhanced CT scan shows at least two relatively hypovascular, homogenous renal masses (*arrows*) consistent with lymphoma. (**e**) In the same patient, this nephrographic phase post-contrast MR sequence demonstrates numerous small solid renal lesions (*arrows*) consistent with multifocal lymphoma. Many of these small lesions were not visible on the CT, which was performed in the corticomedullary phase on the same day as the MRI. (**f**) This is a contrast-enhanced CT scan from a different patient with bilateral renal lymphoma. Note how the tumor infiltrates the renal sinuses, encasing the vessels (*arrows*) without narrowing and the renal collecting systems without associated hydronephrosis. Lymphoma lacks the desmoplastic reaction/fibrosis typically seen with carcinomas, and thus, does not typically cause obstruction (bowel, renal, or vascular) even when they are large [52–54]

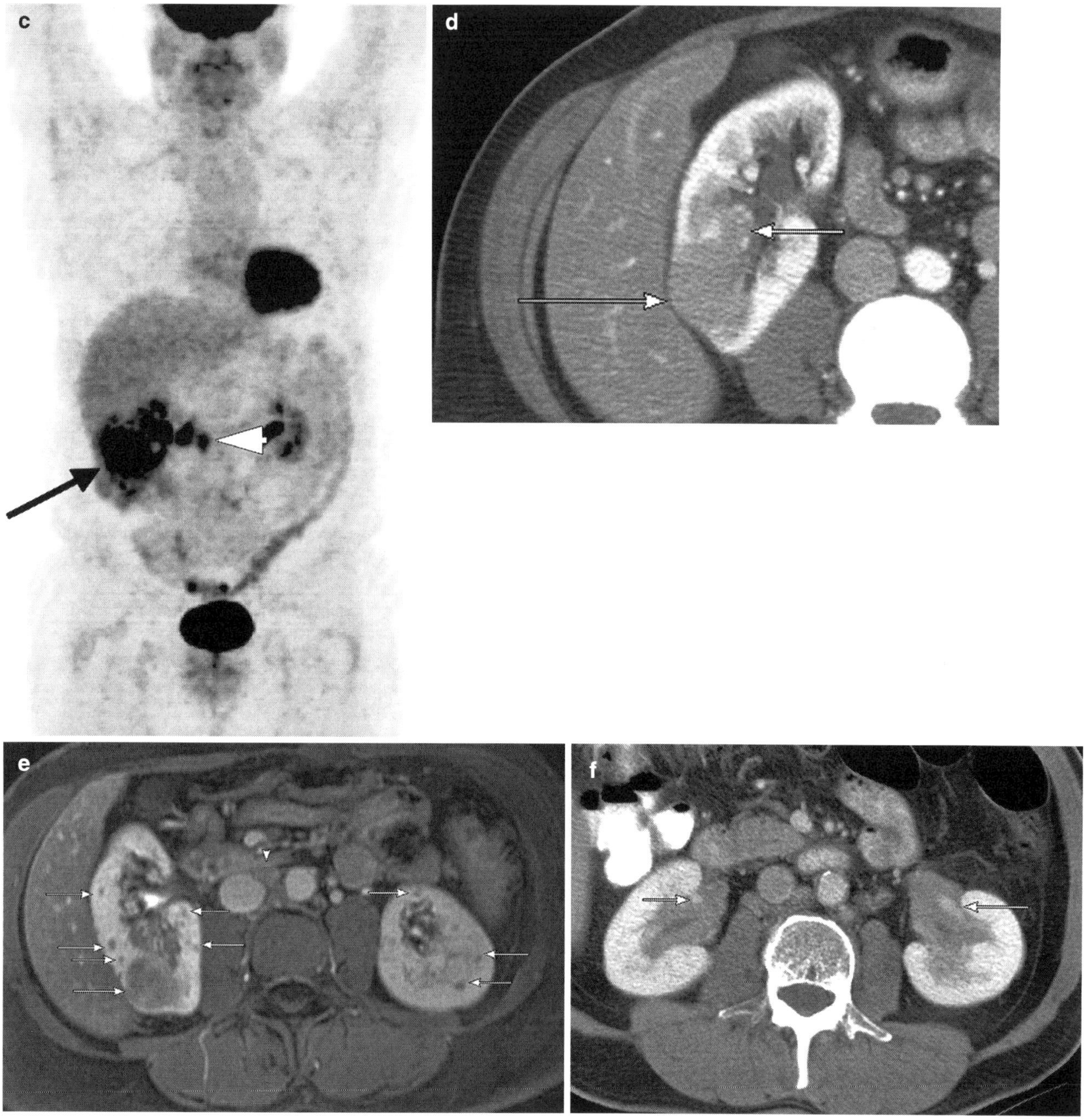

Fig. 1.25 (continued)

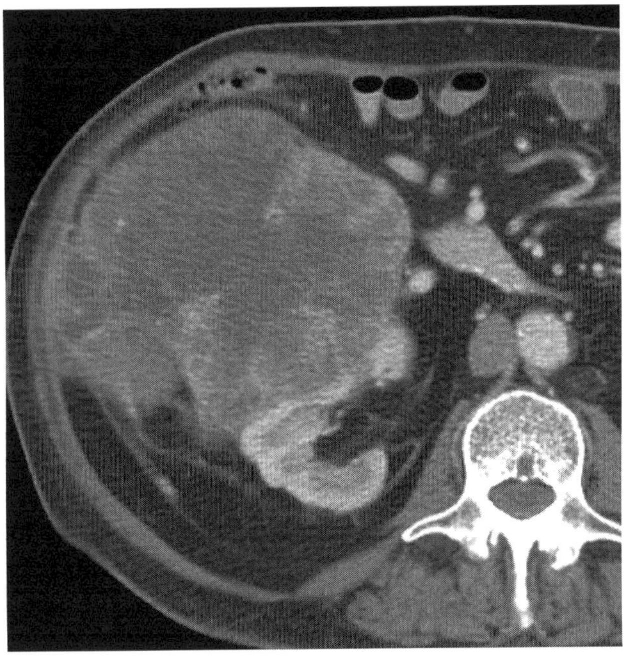

Fig. 1.26 Renal sarcoma. This contrast-enhanced CT scan demonstrates a large, heterogenous renal mass representing a malignant fibrous histiocytoma arising from the renal capsule. Note how the tumor is extremely exophytic and mostly compresses the renal parenchyma with only mild invasion. Renal sarcomas are rare tumors, accounting for less than 1 % of all renal neoplasms. Most patients are between 40 and 70 years old [57, 58]. The most common histologic subtype is leiomyosarcoma, followed by liposarcoma and fibrosarcoma. Less common histologies include malignant fibrous histiocytoma, angiosarcoma, chondrosarcoma, osteosarcoma, rhabdomyosarcoma, clear cell sarcoma, and malignant peripheral nerve sheath tumor [57–59]. Renal sarcomas typically arise from the renal capsule or renal sinus. As a result, these tumors tend to be extremely exophytic on cross-sectional imaging, often displacing and compressing, rather than invading, the renal parenchyma [57–59]. On CT and MR, they are usually large, heterogenous masses with areas of necrosis. Only occasionally can specific diagnoses be made on imaging (i.e., fat in liposarcoma, osteoid matrix in osteosarcoma) [57]

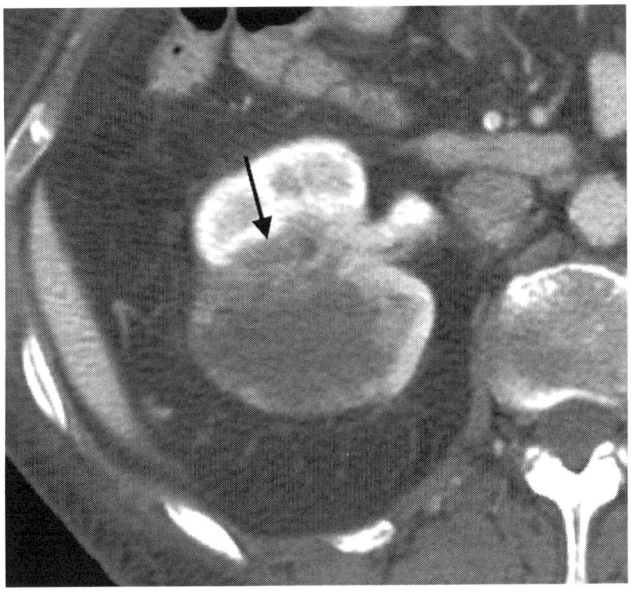

Fig. 1.27 Metastasis to kidney. This contrast-enhanced CT scan demonstrates a relatively hypovascular mass in the right kidney with central necrosis and a somewhat poorly defined interface (*arrow*) with the normal, hypervascular renal parenchyma. Although uncommon, solid tumors do occasionally metastasize to the kidneys but these patients generally have metastases in other locations, as well. In patients with known metastatic disease, an incidentally detected renal mass is more likely to represent metastatic disease than a primary renal tumor [54, 60]. However, in the absence of metastatic disease to other organs, an incidental solitary renal mass in a patient with known malignancy is more likely to be a primary renal neoplasm [61]. The most common tumors to metastasize to the kidneys are lung, breast, stomach, and contralateral kidney [62, 63]. Renal metastases are frequently multiple and bilateral [60]. Although the imaging features are nonspecific, metastases tend to be more infiltrative than primary renal cortical neoplasms and less vascular, especially compared to clear cell carcinoma and oncocytoma. However, the imaging features do overlap, and a biopsy is usually necessary to distinguish these entities given their differences in management [63]

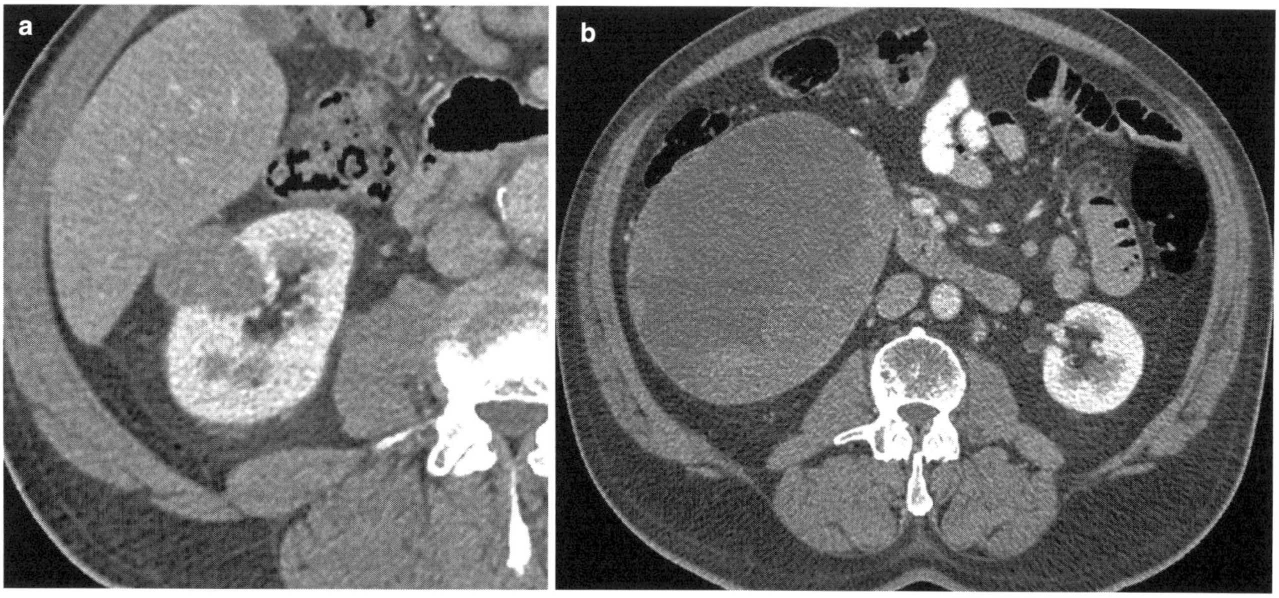

Fig. 1.28 Stage T1 and T2 renal carcinoma. (**a**) This CT image (same as Fig. 1.10a) demonstrates a 5 cm exophytic right renal mass that was pathologically proven to be a stage T1b (pT1b) (>4 cm, ≤7 cm, confined to kidney) renal papillary carcinoma. The tumor is grossly confined within the renal capsule (not easily visible on imaging) and does not extend into the renal sinus fat. (**b**) This mass on CT, a papillary carcinoma measuring 17 cm, proved to be a stage T2 lesion at pathology, measuring more than 7 cm and remaining confined to the renal capsule (*not shown*). Under- and overstaging of renal tumors through the capsule into the perinephric fat, also known as perinephric invasion, are the most common staging errors at CT [64–66]. However, the distinction of T1 and T2 tumors from T3a tumors is not critical on CT because all are amenable to both radical and partial nephrectomy. The distinction does have prognostic implications but this can be accurately determined at histologic analysis [64]. Although the finding of a separate tumor nodule within the perinephric fat is a specific sign of T3 disease, the sensitivity of this sign is low [65, 66]. Perinephric stranding is a more sensitive sign for the detecting of T3 disease, although much less specific as it is seen in approximately half of patients with T1 and T2 tumors due to edema, vascular engorgement, or previous inflammation [64]. Accurate staging is important for surgical planning. Nephron-sparing surgery, or partial nephrectomy, is now a commonly used procedure. Traditionally used in patients with a solitary functioning kidney, compromised renal function, or multiple bilateral tumors [64], it is now commonly used to preserve as much renal function as possible even in patients with solitary tumors and with two normally functioning kidneys. The lesions most amenable to partial nephrectomy include those that are smaller than 4 cm, cortical in location, located away from the renal hilum and collecting system, and are in a polar location [64]

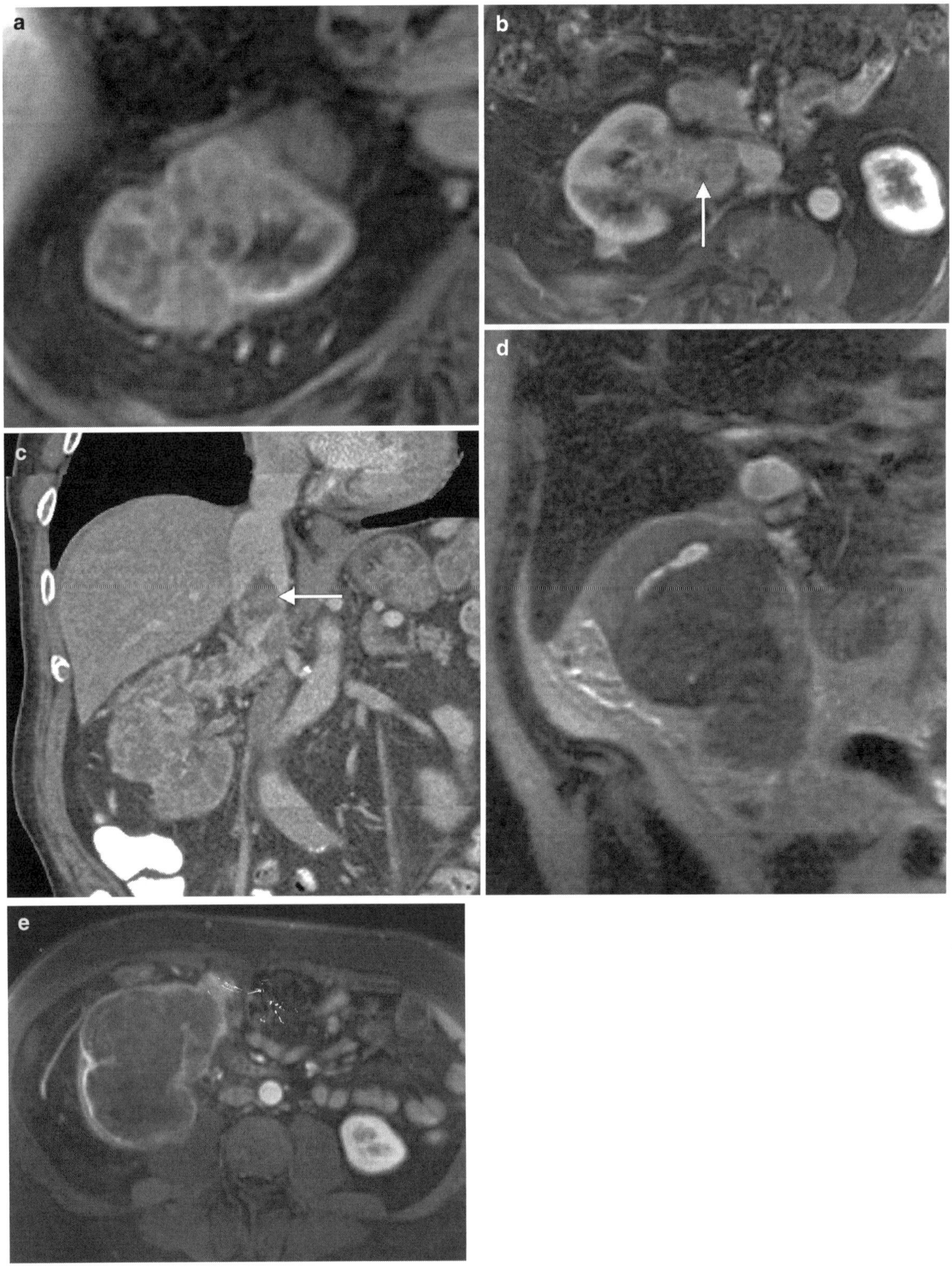

Fig. 1.29 T3 renal carcinoma. (**a**, **b**) These nephrographic phase axial MR images of a right renal clear cell carcinoma demonstrate a heterogeneously hypervascular mass (**a**) that extends into the renal vein, consistent with a T3b lesion. (**b**) Note the expanded right renal vein (*arrow*) that enhances in a pattern identical to that of the primary lesion itself. (**c**) This coronal reconstructed CT image in another patient demonstrates a clear cell carcinoma extensively involving the right renal vein, as well as the infradiaphragmatic inferior vena cava (IVC) (*arrow*). Twenty-three percent of renal carcinomas demonstrate renal vein invasion and 4–10 % demonstrate IVC invasion, which is more common with right-sided tumors due to the shorter right renal vein [67–69]. Patients with renal vein and IVC extension actually have a good prognosis if the thrombus does not invade the vessel wall and can be entirely resected. It is important to denote the level of tumor extension within the IVC (infrahepatic, intrahepatic, supradiaphragmatic) because the surgical approach varies at different levels [64]. Renal vein expansion alone is not adequate to make the diagnosis of tumor thrombus because increased blood flow from the tumor itself can result in renal vein expansion [70]. Heterogenous enhancement within the vessel, indicative tumor neovascularity, and contiguity with the primary lesion are more convincing signs of tumor thrombus [71]. (**d**, **e**) SSFSE and postcontrast MR images, respectively, demonstrate a large renal mass that grossly extends into the renal sinus fat, consistent with a T3a lesion

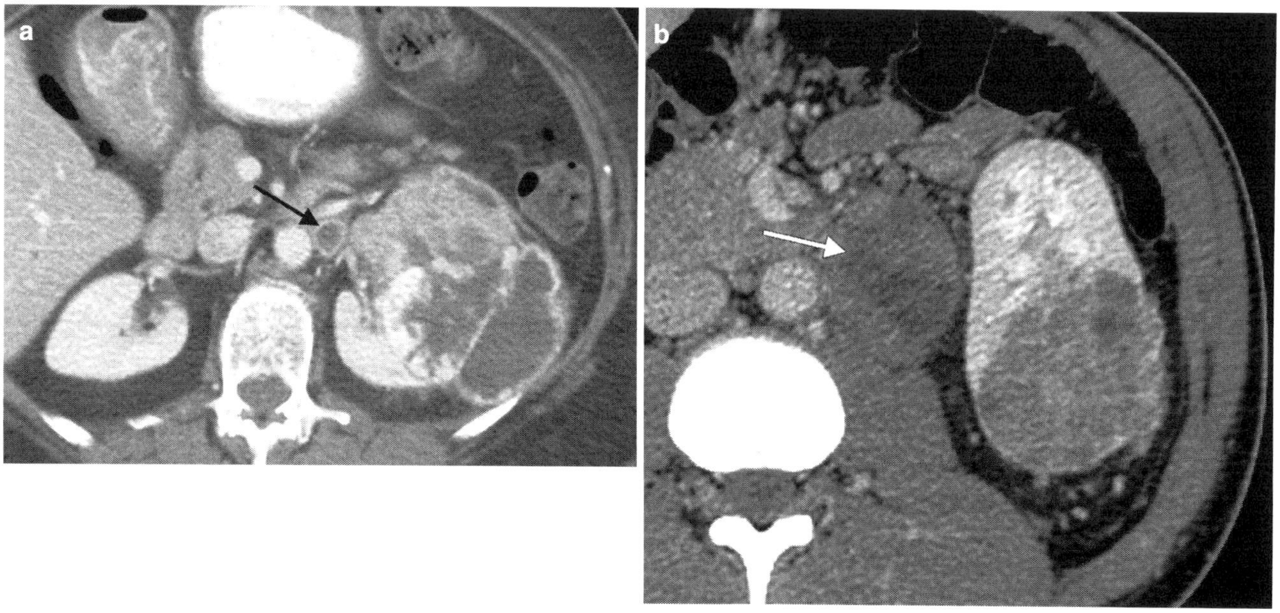

Fig. 1.30 Nodal metastases. (**a**) This nephrographic-phase CT image demonstrates a clear cell carcinoma extensively involving the left kidney, including the renal sinus. Note the small round cystic, peripherally enhancing lesion (*arrow*) just to the left of the aorta. This lesion shows an enhancement pattern identical to the primary tumor and is consistent with a para-aortic nodal metastasis. (**b**) This nephrographic-phase CT image shows a chromophobe carcinoma posteriorly in the left kidney. The mass adjacent to the aorta (*arrow*) demonstrates similar morphology to the primary tumor itself, consistent with a para-aortic nodal metastasis. The presence of regional (retroperitoneal), nodal metastases adversely affects prognosis and automatically advances a patient from stage I or II disease to stage III disease. Using 1 cm (short-axis) as the cutoff for determining the presence of nodal disease, results in a sensitivity of 83 % and specificity of 88 % [66]. Reactive lymph nodes, more commonly seen in the presence of necrotic tumors or tumors that involve the renal vein, cause positive results whereas micrometastases in normal size nodes cause false negatives [72]. Metastatic lymph nodes are also more likely to enhance in a pattern similar to the primary tumor, as seen in the two examples above [64]

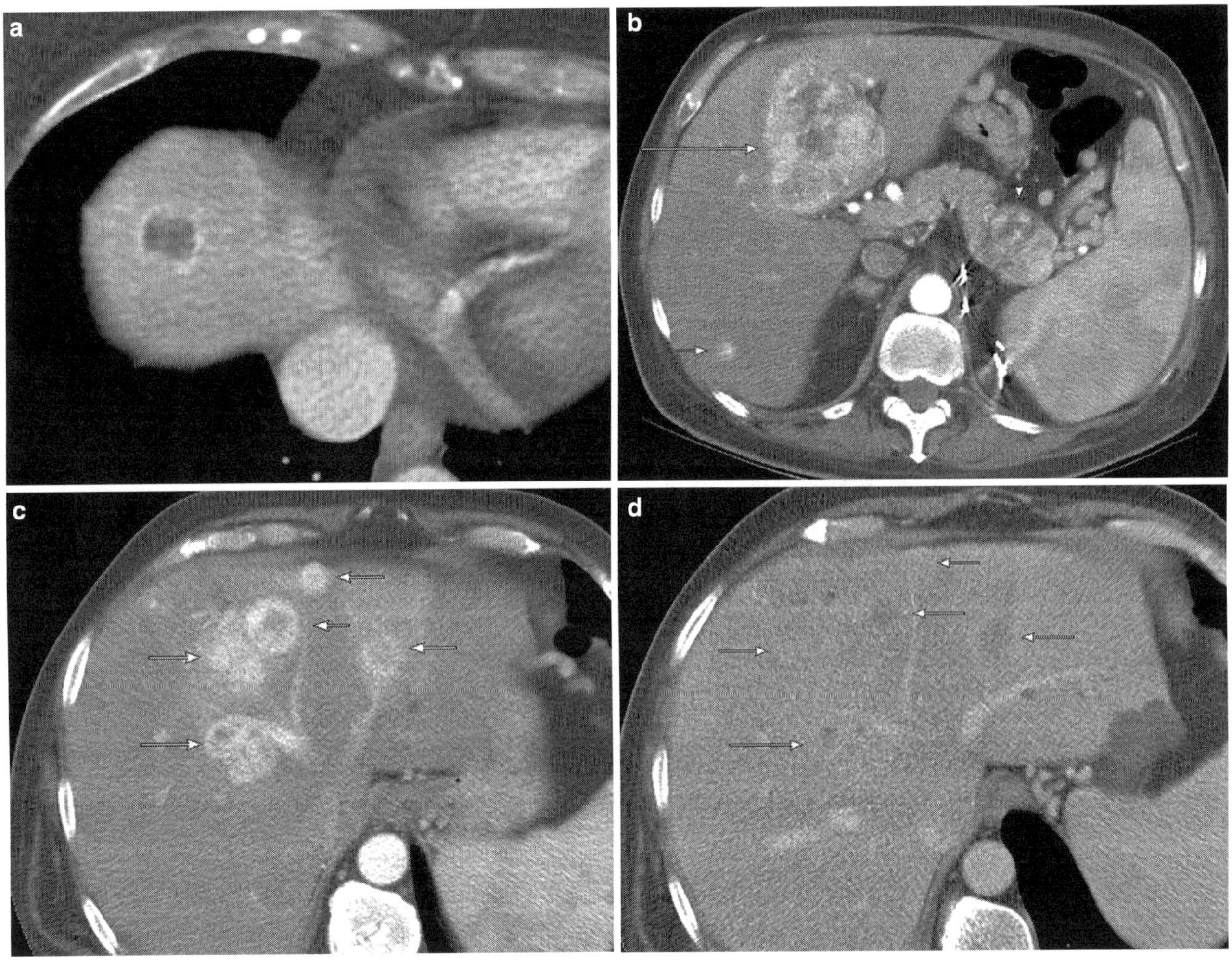

Fig. 1.31 Distant metastases. (**a**) This contrast-enhanced CT scan in the same patient as Fig. 1.30a with clear cell carcinoma demonstrates a hypervascular, partially necrotic lesion at the hepatic dome consistent with metastatic disease. (**b**) In a different patient with clear cell carcinoma, this late arterial phase image demonstrates a large hypervascular metastasis in the left hepatic lobe (*long arrow*) and a very small hypervascular metastasis in the right lobe (*short arrow*); the smaller lesion is not visible on the portal venous phase images (*not shown*) because it becomes isodense to liver. Note that there is also a hypervascular metastatic lesion in the pancreatic tail. Surgical clips are present in the left nephrectomy bed. (**c, d**) In this same patient, note additional hypervascular metastases (*arrows*) more superiorly in the liver on the arterial phase images (**c**). In the portal venous phase (**d**), these lesions become nearly isodense to hepatic parenchyma and are much more difficult to detect (*arrows*). (**e**) In a different patient with clear cell carcinoma, this contrast-enhanced CT scan shows multiple bilateral hypervascular pulmonary metastases. (**f**) In yet another patient with clear cell carcinoma, a CT scan shows a hypervascular metastasis to a mediastinal lymph node (*arrow*). (**g, h**) The radiograph (**g**) demonstrates a purely lytic metastasis in the subtrochanteric right femur, which is mostly photopenic on the posterior projection of this bone scan (*arrow*) (**h**). (**i**) CT scan showing a hypervascular, lytic left anterior rib metastasis (*arrow*). The most common site of hematogenous metastases for renal carcinoma is the lungs, followed by the mediastinum, bones, and liver; less common sites include the contralateral kidney, adrenal gland, brain, pancreas, mesentery, and abdominal wall [73, 74]. Metastatic lesions tend to be hypervascular, like the primary tumor (most often clear cell carcinoma). Thus, hepatic metastases are better seen on scans obtained during the hepatic arterial phase because they may become isodense to the liver parenchyma during the portal venous phase (**b, c**) [64]

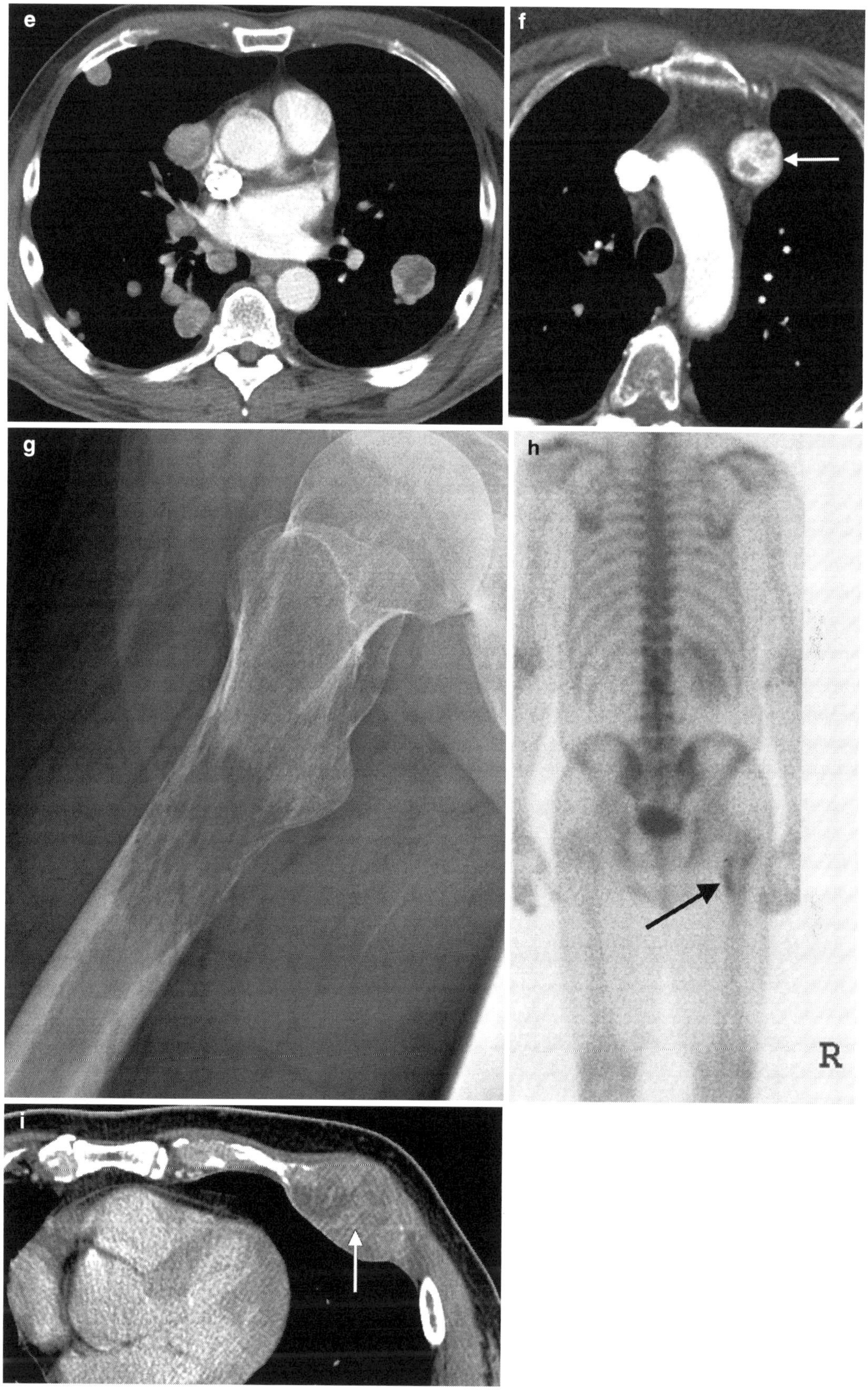

Fig. 1.31 (continued)

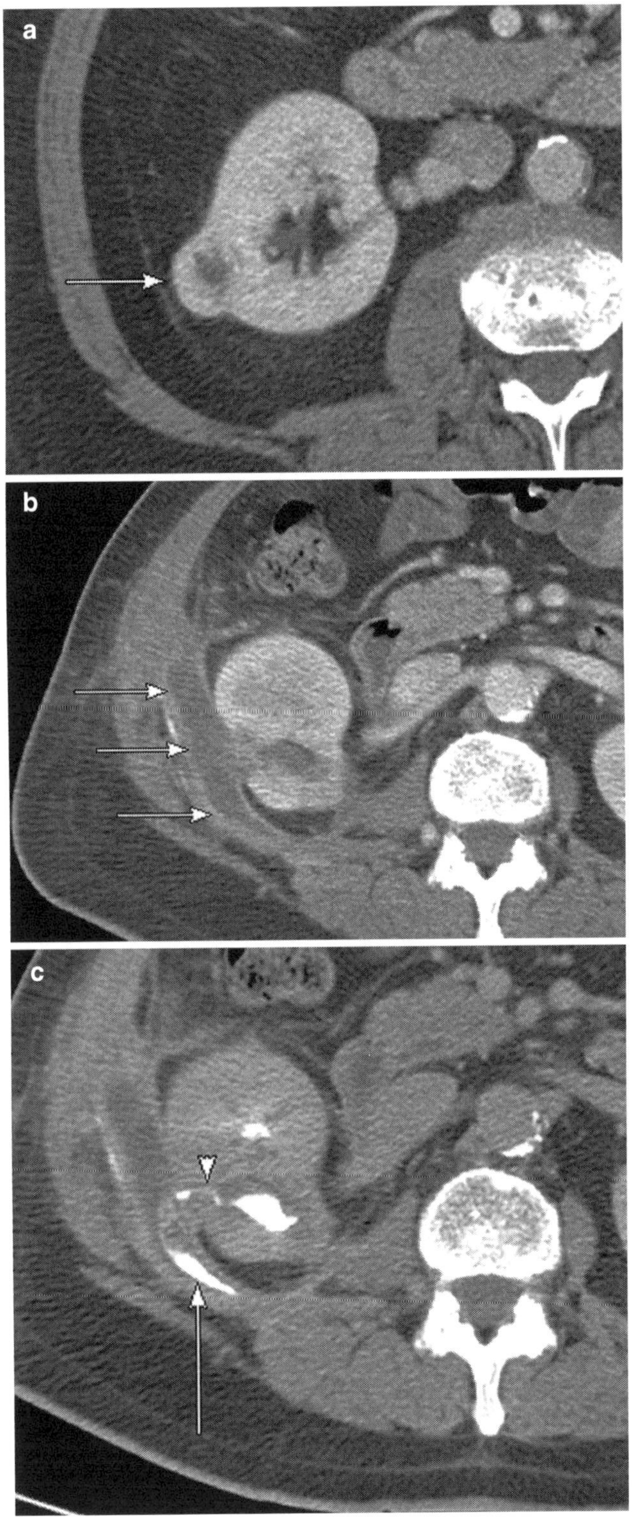

Fig. 1.32 Partial nephrectomy complications: urinoma. (**a**) Nephrographic phase CT show a hypervascular right interpolar renal mass that proved to represent clear cell carcinoma (*arrow*). (**a**, **b**) nephrographic phase CT performed 2 months after partial nephrectomy demonstrates a lentiform postoperative fluid collection (*arrows*) in the surgical bed, extending along the posterior pararenal space. (**c**) Fifteen-minute delayed image on same examination in (**b**) now demonstrates IV contrast extending into the fluid collection confirming the presence of an urinoma (*arrow*). The actual site of communication between the renal calyx and the collection is visible on this image (*arrowhead*). During partial nephrectomy for deep tumors, it is often necessary to resect a small portion of the adjacent renal calyx to ensure adequate resection margins. If calyceal repair is not watertight, it is possible for urine to leak into the surgical bed [77]. Usually simple fluid is seen within these collections on CT (<20 HU) or MRI, but occasionally they can contain hemorrhage and appear more complex [78]. If one suspects that a perirenal fluid collection is of urinary tract origin, delayed post-contrast images should be performed (excretory phase or later). If contrast from the collecting system leaks into the fluid collection on the delayed images, then the presence of a urinary leak is confirmed. Postoperative urine leaks usually resolve spontaneously or with placement of a nephrostomy tube or ureteral stent [77]. However, in a minority of cases, the leak persists, and becomes a urinoma, which is defined as a fluid collection with a fibrous rim that persistently communicates with the urinary tract

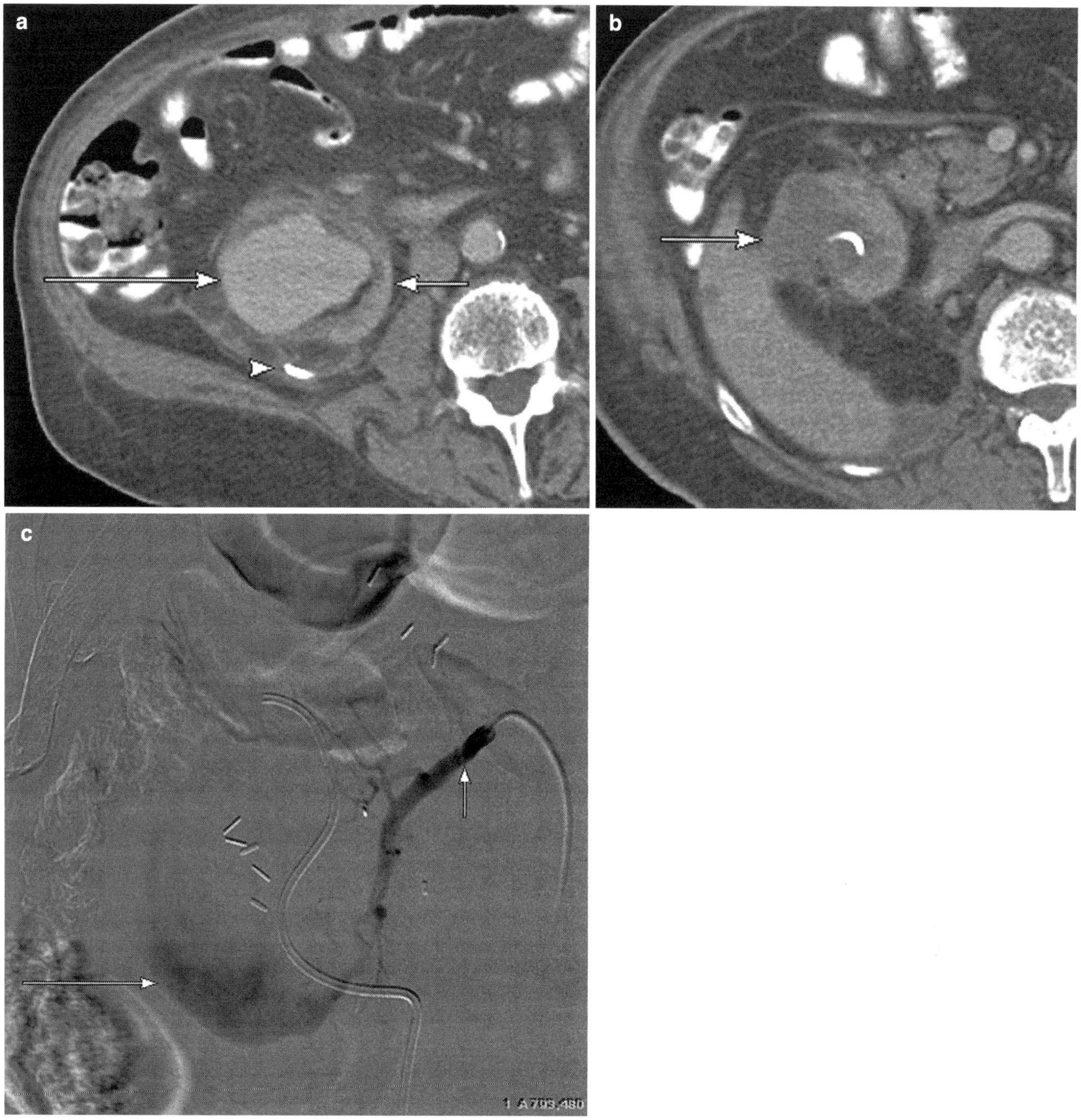

Fig. 1.33 Partial nephrectomy complications: pseudoaneurysm with hematoma. (**a**) A contrast-enhanced CT was performed on this patient 1 month after partial nephrectomy for a 19 cm, exophytic, right lower pole papillary carcinoma. There is a 7 cm homogenous, very high density collection (*long arrow*) in the renal sinus suspicious for a large pseudoaneurysm. Note the residual renal parenchyma (*short arrow*) and a ureteral stent (*arrowhead*). (**b**) More superiorly on the same examination, there is a mildly hyperdense (45 HU), less well-circumscribed fluid collection mostly confined within the renal capsule consistent with subcapsular hematoma (*arrow*). (**c**) An angiogram with injection (*long arrow*) into the right renal artery (*short arrow*) demonstrates contrast pooling in the large cavity seen in (**a**) confirming the diagnosis of a pseudoaneurysm arising from a lower pole branch of the renal artery. The patient was successfully treated with coil embolization of the lower pole arterial branch. Major hemorrhage, which can result if a transected vessel during surgery is inadequately sutured, is the most common complication of partial nephrectomy during the early postoperative period, with a reported incidence ranging from 0 to 5.26 % [77, 79]. Vascular injury often results in perinephric hematoma [79]. A smaller percentage of arterial injuries can result in pseudoaneurysm if the bleeding is contained by the renal parenchyma. Due to the more central location and higher pressure of pseudoaneurysms compared with perinephric hematomas in general, they are prone to erode into the renal collecting system (resulting in massive hematuria) or into a vein with resultant arteriovenous fistula [79, 80]. Superselective percutaneous embolization of the feeding arteries at the bleeding site is the treatment of choice versus surgical repair, which often requires total nephrectomy [79]

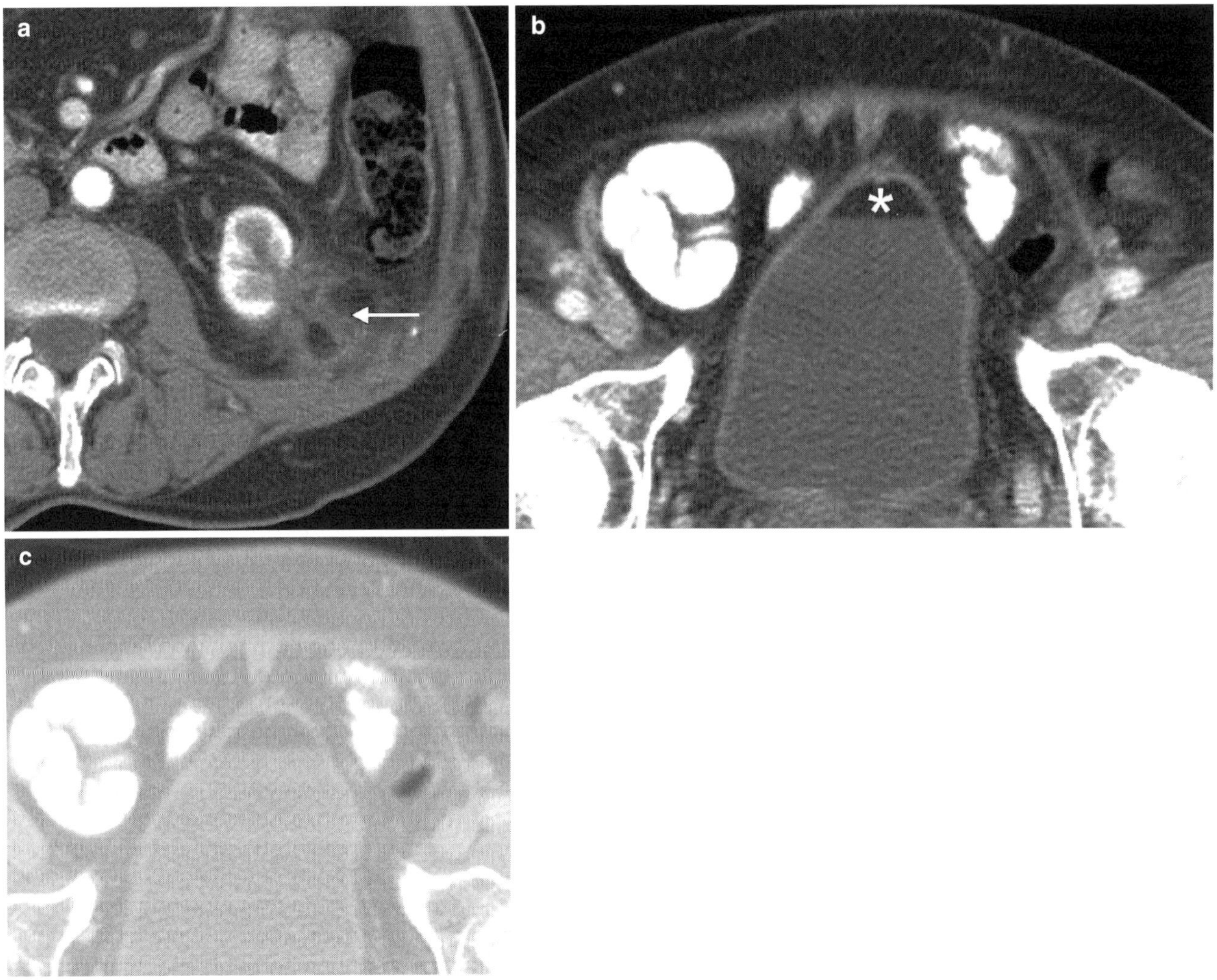

Fig. 1.34 Partial nephrectomy complications: chyluria. (**a**) 1 month after partial left nephrectomy for oncocytoma with typical postoperative changes in resection bed (*arrow*). (**b**) Images through the pelvis on the same examination demonstrate a fat-fluid level within the bladder, with the low attenuation region in the nondependent portion of the bladder lumen measuring −85 HU (*asterisk*). (**c**)The same image as (**b**) with lung windows visually confirms that the abnormality represents fat, rather than air, within the bladder. Lymphatic vessels normally surround the renal pelvis and fornices. Surgical trauma can result in the rupture of dilated lymphatics into the renal collecting system, thus decompressing the vessels and causing a lymphatic–forniceal fistula [81–83]. Chyle subsequently drains into the collecting system and accumulates in the bladder. In one study of 125 patients who had undergone CT of the pelvis after partial nephrectomy, four patients had evidence of chyluria [82]. It is believed that chyluria is more common in partial than radical nephrectomy because unlike radical nephrectomy, partial nephrectomy leaves behind components of both the lymphatics and the collecting system, allowing the communication to develop at either the microscopic or macroscopic level [82]. Chyluria may be asymptomatic or present with "milky" urine, which is the most common symptom [82]. Patients with chronic chyluria may occasionally develop hypoproteinemia, hypolipidemia, and decreased immune function. These patients can be treated surgically with an excellent outcome [82, 84]

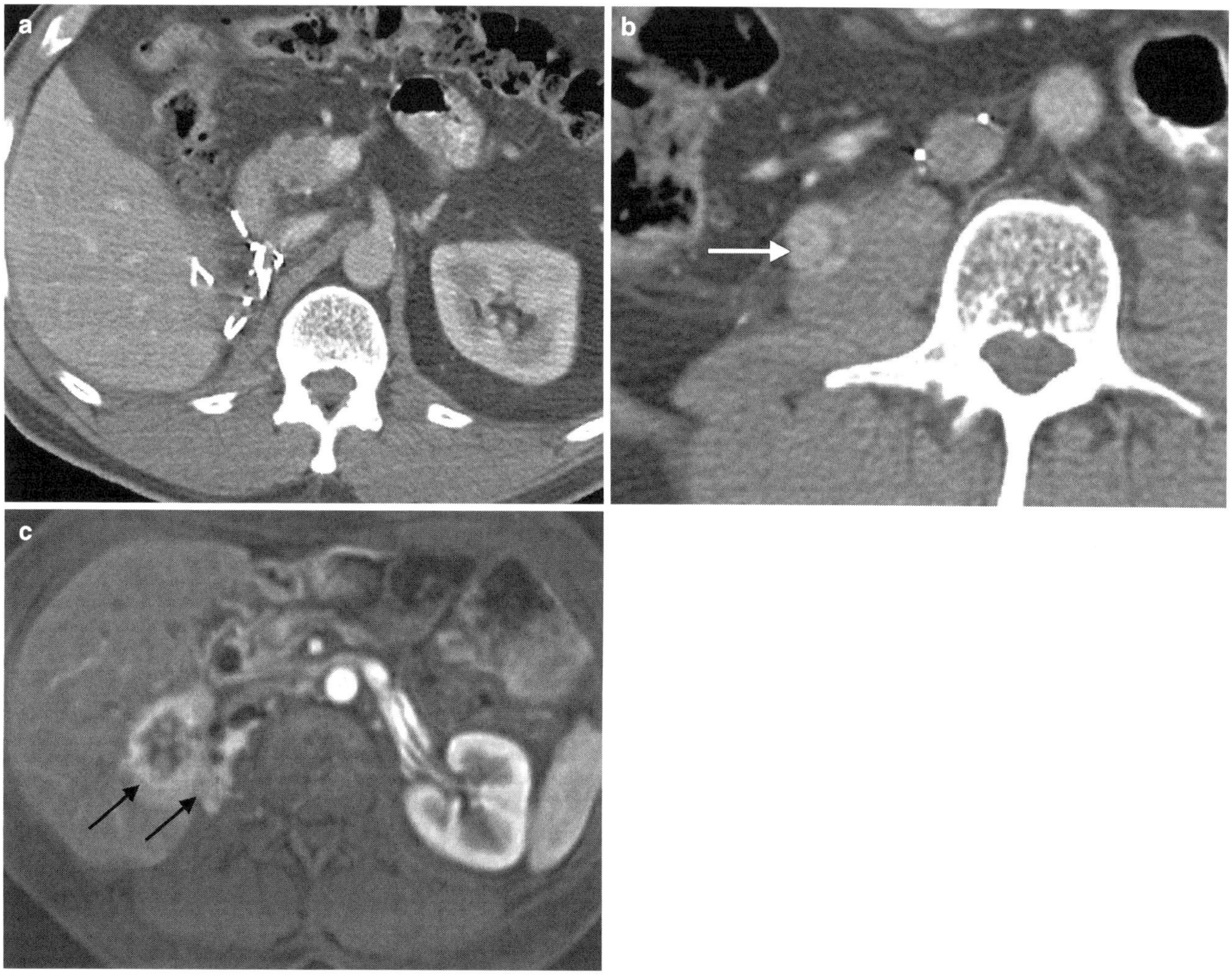

Fig. 1.35 Radical nephrectomy complications: local tumor recurrence. (**a**) A contrast-enhanced CT scan 3.5 years after right radical nephrectomy for clear cell carcinoma demonstrates surgical clips in the right nephrectomy bed. (**b**) More inferiorly on the same study, there is an enhancing nodule along the right psoas muscle (*arrow*) consistent with local tumor recurrence within the nephrectomy bed. (**c**) This corticomedullary phase MR image in the same patient demonstrates a 4 cm hypervascular mass in the nephrectomy bed (*arrows*), with invasion of the hepatic parenchyma, consistent with an additional site of local tumor. In renal carcinoma, the local tumor recurrence rate in the nephrectomy bed is approximately 20–40 %. These recurrences usually occur within the first 5 years after nephrectomy and most of these occur within the first 2 years. Patients with positive surgical margins are at greatest risk [85–87]. Local tumor recurrence is also more likely in tumors that are larger than 5 cm at resection, those that are higher grade, and those that are at a more advanced stage at presentation [64]. On cross-sectional imaging, local tumor recurrence manifests as an enhancing nodule, usually similar in appearance to the original tumor, within the surgical bed, which extends from the crus of the diaphragm, along the adrenal gland (if not resected) inferiorly toward the pelvic inlet along the psoas and quadratus lumborum muscles, and along the right hepatic lobe, right colon, and IVC for right-sided tumors and the pancreatic tail, left colon, and aorta for left-sided tumors

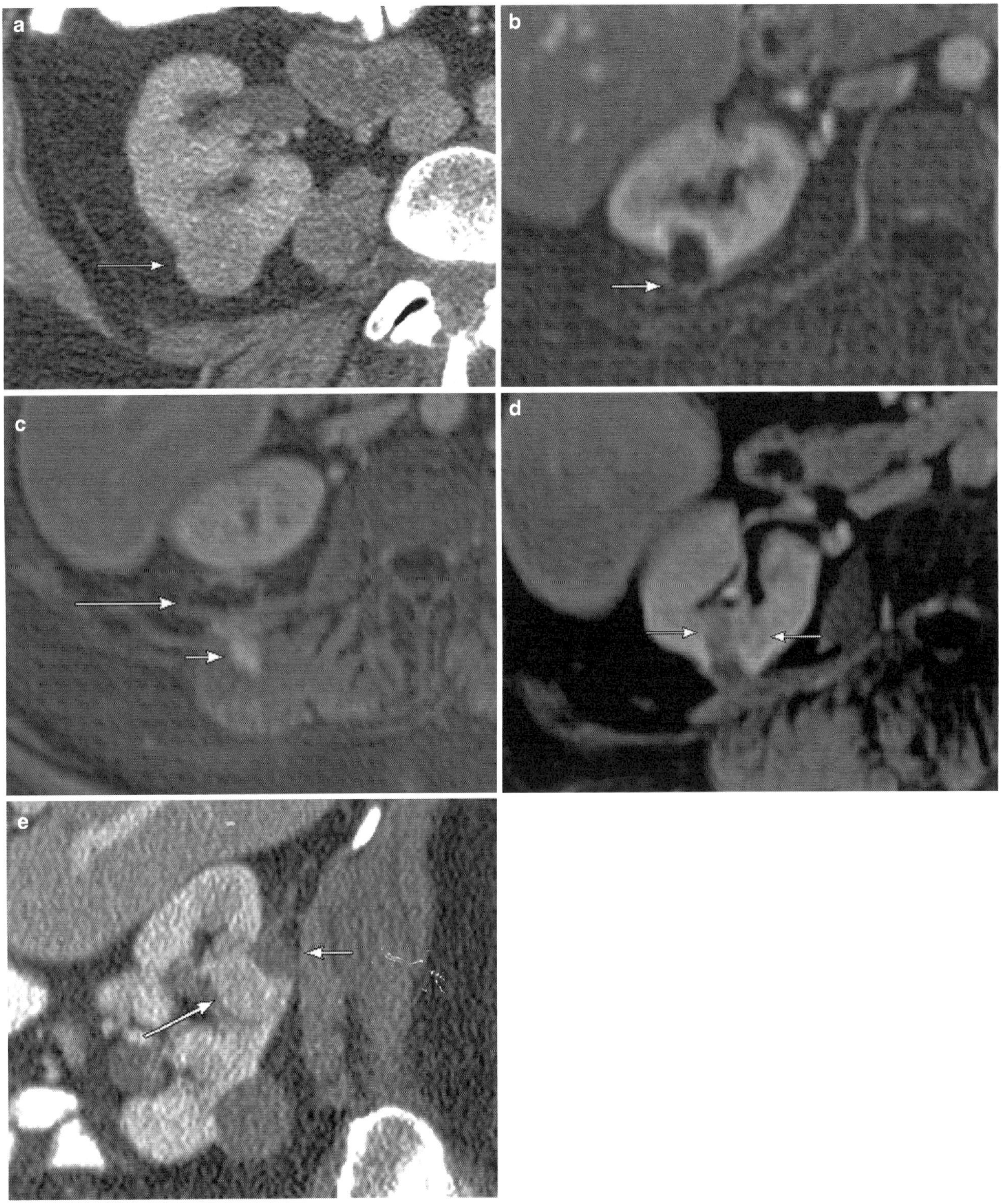

Fig. 1.36 Radiofrequency ablation (RFA) with local recurrence. (**a**) This contrast-enhanced CT shows a hypervascular clear cell carcinoma in a 76-year-old patient who is a poor surgical candidate due to coronary artery disease. Although the mass (*arrow*) has a significant exophytic component, it also extends deep into the renal parenchyma, close to the renal sinus. The patient subsequently chose to undergo RFA at another institution (*images unavailable*). (**b**) These postcontrast subtraction MR images 4 months after RFA demonstrate a nonenhancing defect at the site of the previous tumor consistent with successful tumor ablation. Note that there is only a thick enhancing rim (*arrow*) surrounding the ablation defect, but no nodular enhancement within the defect. (**c**) This nephrographic-phase image from the same examination demonstrates fat necrosis with thin rim of enhancement in the perinephric space (*long arrow*) and enhancement in the adjacent paraspinal muscles (*short arrow*), which are expected changes following ablation in the soft tissues immediately surrounding the tumor. In recent years, RFA and cryoablation have been developed as minimally invasive alternatives to surgery in patients with small renal tumors, particularly in patients who are poor surgical candidates. Although the procedure can be performed at surgery, percutaneous ablation with CT or MR guidance has become more common in recent years [88]. Patients treated with ablation should be followed with CT or MRI to assess for tumor recurrence. On CT, the ablated tumor appears as a mass that is usually slightly larger than the original lesion immediately after treatment because a small margin of normal tissue must be included in the ablation zone. This ablation zone generally decreases in size over time [88]. Axial MR (**d**) and coronal CT postcontrast images (**e**) in the same patient approximately 1 year after post-ablation demonstrate a focal area of nodular enhancement (*arrows*) within the ablation zone consistent with local tumor recurrence. Pre- and postcontrast images should be performed to assess for recurrence. The noncontrast images may show a mass that is mildly hyperdense due to hemorrhage. Following contrast administration, no significant enhancement should be seen in the central portion of the ablation zone, which consists of coagulative necrosis [88, 89]. An enhancing "halo" representing a reactive zone of sublethal injury to surrounding tissue and hemorrhage is typically seen in the adjacent perinephric fat [90]. However, the presence of nodular enhancement within or an increase in size of the ablation zone should be considered suspicious for recurrent tumor [88, 90]. The imaging findings of cryoablation and RFA are similar on CT, except that the cryoablated lesions often decrease in size faster than those treated with RFA [89]. MRI, similar to CT, depicts a nonenhancing zone of ablation, with a surrounding halo, that decreases in size over time. The ablated tumor is usually hyperintense to renal parenchyma on T1WI at least partially due to hemorrhage, and hypointense on T2WI (in contrast to residual or recurrent tumor, which is relatively hyperintense) [88, 91]. Postcontrast subtraction images are helpful in evaluating for local recurrence because enhancing tumor can be obscured by the underlying high signal from hemorrhage on the T1WI [88]

References

1. Kovacs G, Akhtar M, Beckwith BJ, et al. The Heidelberg classification of renal cell tumours. J Pathol. 1997;183:131–3.
2. Bosniak MA. The current radiological approach to renal cysts. Radiology. 1986;158:1–10.
3. Hilpert PL, Friedman AC, Radecki PD, et al. MRI of hemorrhagic renal cysts in polycystic kidney disease. AJR Am J Roentgenol. 1986;146:1167–72.
4. Israel GM, Bosniak MA. Calcification in cystic renal masses: is it important in diagnosis? Radiology. 2003;226:47–52.
5. Israel GM, Bosniak MA. Follow-up CT of moderately complex cystic lesions of the kidney (Bosniak category IIF). AJR Am J Roentgenol. 2003;181:627–33.
6. Israel GM, Bosniak MA. How I do it: evaluating renal masses. Radiology. 2005;236:441–50.
7. Hartman DS, Choyke PL, Hartman MS. A practical approach to the cystic renal mass. Radiographics. 2004;24:S101–15.
8. Bosniak MA. Problems in the radiologic diagnosis of renal parenchymal tumors. Urol Clin North Am. 1993;20:217–30.
9. Hopkins JK, Giles Jr HW, Wyatt-Ashmead J, Bigler SA. Best cases from the AFIP: cystic nephroma. Radiographics. 2004;24:589–93.1.
10. Abdulla C, Kaira MK, Saini S, et al. Pseudoenhancement of simulated renal cysts in a phantom using different multidetector CT scanners. AJR Am J Roentgenol. 2002;179:1473–6.
11. Birnbaum BA, Hindman N, Lee J, Babb JS. Renal cyst pseudoenhancement: influence of multidetector CT reconstruction algorithm and scanner type in phantom model. Radiology. 2007;244:767–75.
12. Tappouni R, Kissane J, Sarwani N, Lehman EB. Pseudoenhancement of renal cysts: influence of lesion size, lesion location, slice thickness, and number of MDCT detectors. AJR Am J Roentgenol. 2012;198:133–7.
13. Jinzaki M, Tanimoto A, Mukai M, et al. Double-phase helical CT of small renal parenchymal neoplasms: correlation with pathologic findings and tumor angiogenesis. J Comput Assist Tomogr. 2000;24:835–42.
14. Kim JK, Kim TK, Ahn HJ, et al. Differentiation of subtypes of renal cell carcinoma on helical CT scans. AJR Am J Roentgenol. 2002;178:1499–506.
15. Zhang J, Lefkowitz RA, Ishill NM, et al. Solid renal cortical tumors: differentiation with CT. Radiology. 2007;244:494–504.
16. Zhang J, Lefkowitz RA, Wang L, et al. Significance of peritumoral vascularity on CT in evaluation of renal cortical tumor. J Comput Assist Tomogr. 2007;31:717–23.
17. Pedrosa I, Chou MT, Ngo L, et al. MR classification of renal masses with pathologic correlation. Eur Radiol. 2008;18:365–75.
18. Outwater EK, Bhatia M, Siegelman ES, et al. Lipid in renal clear cell carcinoma: detection on opposed-phase gradient-echo MR images. Radiology. 1997;205:103–7.
19. Pedrosa I, Sun MR, Spencer M, et al. MR imaging of renal masses: correlation with findings at surgery and pathologic analysis. Radiographics. 2008;28:985–1003.
20. Wagner BJ. The kidney: radiologic-pathologic correlation. Magn Reson Imaging Clin N Am. 1997;5:13–28.
21. Vikram R, Ng CS, Tamboli P, et al. Papillary renal cell carcinoma: radiologic-pathologic correlation and spectrum of disease. Radiographics. 2009;29:741–54.
22. Raj GV, Bach AM, Iasonos A, et al. Predicting the histology of renal masses using preoperative Doppler ultrasonography. J Urol. 2007;177:53–8.
23. Herts BR, Coll DM, Novick AC, et al. Enhancement characteristics of papillary renal neoplasms revealed on triphasic helical CT of the kidneys. AJR Am J Roentgenol. 2002;178:367–72.

24. Kim JK, Kim SH, Jang YJ, et al. Renal angiomyolipoma with minimal fat: differentiation from other neoplasms at double-echo chemical shift FLASH MR imaging. Radiology. 2006;239:174–80.
25. Brinker DA, Amin MB, de Peralta-Venturina M, et al. Extensively necrotic cystic renal cell carcinoma: a clinicopathologic study with comparison to other cystic and necrotic renal cancers. Am J Surg Pathol. 2000;24:988–95.
26. Delahunt B, Eble JN. Papillary renal cell carcinoma: a clinicopathologic and immunohistochemical study of 105 tumors. Mod Pathol. 1997;10:537–44.
27. Yamada T, Endo M, Tsuboi M, et al. Differentiation of pathologic subtypes of papillary renal cell carcinoma on CT. AJR Am J Roentgenol. 2008;191:1559–63.
28. Roy C, Sauer B, Lindner V, et al. MR imaging of papillary renal neoplasms: potential application for characterization of small renal masses. Eur Radiol. 2007;17:193–200.
29. Shinmoto H, Yvasa Y, Tanimoto A, et al. Small cell carcinoma: MRI with pathologic correlation. J Magn Reson Imaging. 1998;8:690–4.
30. Yoshimitsu K, Irie H, Tajima T, et al. MR imaging of renal cell carcinoma: its role in determining cell type. Radiat Med. 2004;22: 371–6.
31. Sussmann SK, Glickstein MF, Krzymowski GA. Hypointense renal cell carcinoma: MR imaging with pathologic correlation. Radiology. 1990;177:495–7.
32. Oliva MR, Glickman JN, Zou KH, et al. Renal cell carcinoma: T1 and T2 signal intensity characteristics of papillary and clear cell types correlated with pathology. AJR Am J Roentgenol. 2009;192:1524–30.
33. Sun MR, Ngo L, Genega EM, et al. Renal cell carcinoma: dynamic contrast-enhanced MR imaging for differentiation of tumor subtypes – correlation with pathologic findings. Radiology. 2009;250: 793–802.
34. Cochand-Priollet B, Molinie V, Bougaran J, et al. Renal chromophobe cell carcinoma and oncocytoma: a comparative morphologic, histochemical, and immunohistochemical study of 124 cases. Arch Pathol Lab Med. 1997;121:1081–6.
35. Rosenkrantz AB, Hindman N, Fitzgerald EF, et al. MRI features of renal oncocytoma and chromophobe renal cell carcinoma. AJR Am J Roentgenol. 2010;195:W421–7.
36. Kim JI, Cho JY, Moon KC, et al. Segmental enhancement inversion at biphasic multidetector CT: characteristic finding of small renal oncocytoma. Radiology. 2009;252:441–8.
37. Quinn MJ, Hartman DS, Friedman AC, et al. Renal oncocytoma: new observations. Radiology. 1984;153:49–53.
38. Davidson AJ, Hayes WS, Hartman DS, et al. Renal oncocytoma and carcinoma: failure of differentiation with CT. Radiology. 1993;186:693–6.
39. McGahan JP, Lamba R, Fisher J, et al. Is segmental enhancement inversion on enhanced biphasic MDCT a reliable sign for the noninvasive diagnosis of renal oncocytomas? AJR Am J Roentgenol. 2011;197:W674–9.
40. Harmon WJ, King BF, Lieber MM. Renal oncocytoma: magnetic resonance imaging characteristics. J Urol. 1996;155:863–7.
41. Wagner BJ, Wong-You-Cheong JJ, Davis Jr CJ. Adult renal hamartomas. Radiographics. 1997;17:155–69.
42. Simpfendorfer C, Herts BR, Motta-Ramirez GA, et al. Angiomyolipoma with minimal fat on MDCT: can counts of negative-attenuation pixels aid diagnosis? AJR Am J Roentgenol. 2009; 192:438–43.
43. Kutikov A, Fossett LK, Ramchandani P, et al. Incidence of benign pathologic findings at partial nephrectomy for solitary renal mass presumed to be renal cell carcinoma on preoperative imaging. Urology. 2006;68:737–40.
44. Jinzaki M, Tanimoto A, Narimatsu Y, et al. Angiomyolipoma: imaging findings in lesions with minimal fat. Radiology. 1997; 205:497–502.
45. Israel GM, Bosniak MA, Slywotzky CM, et al. CT differentiation of large exophytic renal angiomyolipomas and perirenal liposarcomas. AJR Am J Roentgenol. 2002;179:769–73.
46. Siegel CL, Middleton WD, Teefey FA, McClennan BL. Angiomyolipoma and renal cell carcinoma: US differentiation. Radiology. 1996;198:789–93.
47. Prasad SR, Humphrey PA, Menias CO, et al. Neoplasms of the renal medulla: radiologic-pathologic correlation. Radiographics. 2005;25:369–80.
48. Chao D, Zisman A, Pantuck AJ, et al. Collecting duct renal cell carcinoma: clinical study of a rare tumor. J Urol. 2002;167:71–4.
49. Pickhardt PJ, Siegel CL, McLarney JK. Collecting duct carcinoma of the kidney: are imaging findings suggestive of the diagnosis? AJR Am J Roentgenol. 2001;176:627–33.
50. Davis Jr CJ, Mostofi FK, Sesterhenn IA. Renal medullary carcinoma: the seventh sickle cell nephropathy. Am J Surg Pathol. 1995;19:1–11.
51. Davidson AJ, Choyke PL, Hartman DS, Davis Jr CJ. Renal medullary carcinoma associated with sickle cell trait: radiologic findings. Radiology. 1995;195:83–5.
52. Hartman DS, David Jr CJ, Goldman SM, et al. Renal lymphoma: radiologic-pathologic correlation of 21 cases. Radiology. 1982; 144:759–66.
53. Urban BA, Fishman EK. Renal lymphoma: CT patterns with emphasis on helical CT. Radiographics. 2000;20:197–212.
54. Zhang J, Lefkowitz RA, Bach A. Imaging of kidney cancer. Radiol Clin North Am. 2007;45:119–47.
55. Cohan RH, Dunnick NR, Leder RA, et al. Computed tomography of renal lymphoma. J Comput Assist Tomogr. 1990;14:933–8.
56. Heiken JP, Gold RP, Schnur MJ, et al. Computed tomography of renal lymphoma with ultrasound correlation. J Comput Assist Tomogr. 1983;7:245–50.
57. Shirkhoda A, Lewis E. Renal sarcoma and sarcomatoid renal cell carcinoma: CT and angiographic features. Radiology. 1987; 162:353–7.
58. Vogelzang NJ, Fremgen AM, Guinan PD, et al. Primary renal sarcoma in adults. A natural history and management study by the American Cancer Society, Illinois Division. Cancer. 1993; 71:804–10.
59. Rha SE, Byun JY, Jung SE, et al. The renal sinus: pathologic spectrum and multimodality imaging approach. Radiographics. 2004;24 Suppl 1:S117–31.
60. Curry NS. Small renal masses (lesions smaller than 3 cm): imaging evaluation and management. AJR Am J Roentgenol. 1995;164: 355–62.
61. Israel GM, Krinsky GA. MR imaging of the kidneys and adrenal glands. Radiol Clin North Am. 2003;41:145–59.
62. Wagle DG, Moore RH, Murphy GP. Secondary carcinomas of the kidney. J Urol. 1975;114:30–2.
63. Zhang J, Israel GM, Krinsky GA, Lee VS. Masses and pseudomasses of the kidney: imaging spectrum on MR. J Comput Assist Tomogr. 2004;28:588–95.
64. Sheth S, Scatarige JC, Horton KM. Current concepts in the diagnosis and management of renal cell carcinoma: role of multidetector CT and three-dimensional CT. Radiographics. 2001;21(spec no):S237–25.
65. Kopka L, Fischer U, Zoeller G, et al. Dual-phase helical CT of the kidney: value of the corticomedullary and nephrographic phase for evaluation of renal lesions and preoperative staging of renal cell carcinoma. AJR Am J Roentgenol. 1997;169:1573–8.
66. Johnson CD, Dunnick NR, Cohan RH, Illescas FF. Renal adenocarcinoma: CT staging of 100 tumors. AJR Am J Roentgenol. 1987;148:59–63.
67. Russo P. Renal cell carcinoma: presentation, staging, and surgical treatment. Semin Oncol. 2000;27:160–76.

68. Kallman DA, King BF, Hattery RR, et al. Renal vein and inferior vena cava tumor thrombus in renal cell carcinoma: CT, US, MRI, and venacavography. J Comput Assist Tomogr. 1992;16:240–7.
69. Staehler G, Brkovic D. The role of radical surgery for renal cell carcinoma with extension into the vena cava. J Urol. 2000; 163:1671–5.
70. Zeman RK, Cronan JJ, Rosenfield AT, et al. Renal cell carcinoma: dynamic thin-section CT assessment of vascular invasion and tumor vascularity. Radiology. 1988;167:393–6.
71. Zagoria RJ, Bechtold RE, Dyer RB. Staging of renal adenocarcinoma: role of various imaging procedures. AJR Am J Roentgenol. 1995;164:363–70.
72. Ng CS, Wood CG, Silverman PM, et al. Renal cell carcinoma: diagnosis, staging, and surveillance. AJR Am J Roentgenol. 2008; 191:1220–32.
73. Dinney CPN, Awad SA, Gajewski JB, et al. Analysis of imaging modalities, staging systems, and prognostic indicators for renal cell carcinoma. Urology. 1992;36:22–9.
74. Thrasher JB, Paulson DF. Prognostic factors in renal cancer. Urol Clin North Am. 1993;20:247–61.
75. Pretorius ES, Siegelman ES, Ramchandani P, et al. Renal neoplasms amenable to partial nephrectomy: MR imaging. Radiology. 1999;212:28–34.
76. Joniau S, Vander Eeckt K, Van Poppel H. The indications for partial nephrectomy in the treatment of renal cell carcinoma. Nat Clin Pract Urol. 2006;3:198–205.
77. Israel GM, Hecht E, Bosniak MA. CT and MR imaging of complications of partial nephrectomy. Radiographics. 2006;26: 1419–29.
78. Gill IS. Minimally invasive nephron-sparing surgery. Urol Clin North Am. 2003;30:551–79.
79. Heye S, Maleux G, Van Poppel H, et al. Hemorrhagic complications after nephron-sparing surgery: angiographic diagnosis and management by transcatheter embolization. AJR Am J Roentgenol. 2005;184:1661–4.
80. Albani JM, Novick AC. Renal artery pseudoaneurysm after partial nephrectomy: three cases and a literature review. Urology. 2003; 62:227–31.
81. Chen KC. Lymphatic abnormalities in patients with chyluria. J Urol. 1971;106:111–4.
82. Miller FH, Keppke AL, Yaghmai V, et al. CT diagnosis of chyluria after partial nephrectomy. AJR Am J Roentgenol. 2007;188:W25–8.
83. Tuck J, Pearce I, Pantelides M. Chyluria after radical nephrectomy treated with N-butyl-2-cyanoacrylate. J Urol. 2000;164:778–9.
84. Ciferri F, Glovsky MM. Chronic chyluria: a clinical study of three patients. J Urol. 1985;133:631–4.
85. Hilton S. Imaging of renal cell carcinoma. Semin Oncol. 2000;27:150–9.
86. Chin AI, Lam JS, Figlin RA, Belldegrun AS. Surveillance strategies for renal cell carcinoma patients following nephrectomy. Rev Urol. 2006;8:1–7.
87. Chae EJ, Kim JK, Kim SH, et al. Renal cell carcinoma: analysis of postoperative recurrence patterns. Radiology. 2005;234:189–96.
88. Kawamoto S, Permpongkosol S, Bluemke DA, et al. Sequential changes after radiofrequency ablation and cryoablation of renal neoplasms: role of CT and MR imaging. Radiographics. 2007;27:343–55.
89. Matsumoto ED, Watumull L, Johnson DB, et al. The radiographic evolution of radiofrequency ablated renal tumors. J Urol. 2004;172:45–8.
90. Gill IS, Remer EM, Hasan WA, et al. Renal cryoablation: outcome at 3 years. J Urol. 2005;173:1903–7.
91. Merkle EM, Nour SG, Lewin JS. MR imaging follow-up after percutaneous radiofrequency ablation of renal cell carcinoma: findings in 18 patients during first 6 months. Radiology. 2005;235: 1065–71.

Upper Tract Oncologic Imaging

2

Vandan Caur, Nathalie Ibrahim, Yulia Lakhman, and Scott Gerst

Urothelial tumors involving the renal pelvis and ureter are relatively uncommon and account for approximately 5 % of all urological malignancies [1]. The vast majority (90 %) are transitional cell carcinoma (TCC) and most arise in the renal pelvis; 9 % are squamous cell carcinoma and 1 % are mucinous adenocarcinoma [2]. Most upper tract urothelial tumors occur in the sixth to seventh decade of life and are seen three times more frequently in men than in women, with a ratio of 3:1 [3].

TCC within the renal pelvis occurs most commonly in the extrarenal part of the pelvis, followed by the infundibulocaliceal region [4]. Within the ureter, the highest incidence is in the distal ureter with decreasing incidence proximally, with a ratio of 70:20:10 for the distal, mid, and proximal ureter, respectively [5].

Several factors contribute to the development of upper urinary tract TCC and are very similar to those for bladder cancer. The most important factor is smoking, which accounts for a two to three times increased likelihood of developing TCC than in nonsmokers [4]. Other factors include environmental exposure to substances, including phenacetin, chemical carcinogens (aniline, benzidine), cyclophosphamide, and Balkan nephropathy [4, 6, 7].

In the case of adenocarcinoma and squamous cell carcinoma, chronic infection, inflammation, obstruction, and stones are associated with increased risk [8, 9].

Presentation

Similar to its presentation in the bladder, upper urothelial tumors most commonly present with hematuria, either frank or microscopic. Other presenting symptoms include dull flank pain or acute renal colic due to obstruction.

Tumor spread occurs by local extension, hematogenous, or lymphatic invasion. Pelvis and upper ureteral TCC initially spread via the paraaortic and pericaval lymph nodes, with distal ureteral TCC spread to pelvic nodes. The most common sites of distant metastases, in decreasing order of frequency, are lung, bone, and liver.

Bilateral upper tract tumor involvement occurs in 2–4 % of upper tract TCC [10]. Furthermore, recurrence at additional ipsilateral sites occurs in approximately 40 % (range, 20–70 %), necessitating cautious urological and radiological follow-up [11].

Staging

Radiological evaluation, in conjunction with ureteroscopy and biopsy, are essential tools for clinical staging. The TNM (tumor, node, metastasis) staging supported by the American Joint Committee on Cancer (AJCC) is most frequently used for pathological staging of upper tract tumors (*see* Table 2.1 and 2.2) [12]. This system only applies to carcinomas and papillomas; nonepithelial or metastatic tumors are excluded.

Many studies have demonstrated strong correlation between survival and tumor stage, grade, and multifocality,

V. Caur, M.D.
Wirral University Teaching Hospitals NHS Foundation Trust, Arrowe park road, Wirral, CH49 5PE, UK
e-mail: v.arora@nhs.net

S. Gerst, M.D. (✉)
Department of Radiology, Memorial Sloan-Kettering Cancer Center, 1275 York Avenue, New York, NY, 10065, USA
e-mail: gersts@mskcc.org

N. Ibrahim, M.D.
Radiology Department, McGill University Health Center, Montreal, QC, Canada
e-mail: natibrahim@yahoo.com

Y. Lakhman, M.D.
Department of Radiology, Memorial Sloan-Kettering Cancer Center, 303 East 66 Street, Room 703, New York, NY, 10065, USA
e-mail: lakhmany@mskcc.org

A.M. Bach, J. Zhang (eds.), *Atlas of Genitourinary Oncological Imaging*, Atlas of Oncology Imaging,
DOI 10.1007/978-1-4614-4872-3_2, © Springer Science+Business Media New York 2013

Table 2.1 TNM staging system for cancer of renal pelvis and ureter [12]

Primary Tumor (T)
Tx: Primary tumor cannot be assessed
T0: No evidence of primary tumor
Ta: Noninvasive papillary carcinoma
Tis: Carcinoma in situ
T1: Tumor invades subepithelial connective tissue
T2 : Tumor invades muscularis
T3 (renal pelvis only): Tumor invades beyond muscularis into peripelvic fat or the renal parenchyma
T3 (ureter only): Tumor invades beyond the muscularis into periureteric fat
T4: Tumor invades adjacent organs or through the kidney into perinephric fat
Regional Lymph Nodes (N)[a]
Nx: Regional lymph nodes cannot be assessed
N0: No Regional lymph node metastasis
N1: Metastasis in a single lymph node, 2 cm or less in greatest dimension
N2: Metastasis in a single lymph node, more than 2 cm but not more than 5 cm in greatest dimension; or multiple lymph nodes, none more than 5 cm in greatest dimension
N3: Metastasis in a lymph node more than 5 cm in greatest dimension
Distant Metastasis (M)
Mx: Distant metastasis cannot be assessed
M0: No distant metastasis
M1: Distant metastasis

Used with the permission of the American Joint Committee on Cancer (AJCC), Chicago, IL. The original source for this material is the *AJCC Cancer Staging Manual*, 7th edn (2010) published by Springer Science and Business Media LLC, www.springer.com

[a]Laterality does not affect the N classification

Table 2.2 Anatomic staging and prognostic groups [12]

	Stage grouping		
Stage 0a	Ta	N0	M0
Stage 0is	Tis	N0	M0
Stage I	T1	N0	M0
Stage II	T2	N0	M0
Stage III	T3	N0	M0
Stage IV	T4	N0	M0
	Any T	N1	M0
	Any T	N2	M0
	Any T	N3	M0
	Any T	Any N	M1

Used with the permission of the American Joint Committee on Cancer (AJCC), Chicago, IL. The original source for this material is the *AJCC Cancer Staging Manual*, 7th edn (2010) published by Springer Science and Business Media LLC, www.springer.com

with staging being the most important factor [13]. The 5-year survival rate for patients with Ta or T1 disease ranges from 60 to 90 %, decreasing to only 5 % in T3 or T4 disease [14].

Table 2.3 Histologic grading [12]

GX	Grade cannot be assessed
G1	Well differentiated
G2	Moderately differentiated
G3-4	Poorly differentiated or undifferentiated

Used with the permission of the American Joint Committee on Cancer (AJCC), Chicago, IL. The original source for this material is the *AJCC Cancer Staging Manual*, 7th edn (2010) published by Springer Science and Business Media LLC, www.springer.com

Furthermore, the histological grade (*see* Table 2.3) has also demonstrated close correlation with staging (*e.g.*, superficial tumors tend to be of lower grade whereas higher grade tumors have higher propensity to be invasive) [15].

Studies suggest that renal pelvis tumors tend to have better prognosis than ureteral tumors; this is thought to be due to the renal parenchyma acting as a barrier [2, 11].

Treatment and prognosis are largely dependent on the depth of tumor infiltration, the degree of lymph node involvement, metastases, and the histology of the tumor, further emphasizing the need for proper staging.

After the detection of hematuria or diagnosis of suspected upper tract TCC, radiological evaluation is important in detecting and determining tumor extent and stage (*see* Table 2.4). Intravenous urography has been largely replaced by computed tomography urography (CTU), capable of detecting lesions larger than 5 mm [18], as this technique can image the entire urinary tract and provide information on locoregional extension, as well as nodal and distant metastases. However, not all filling defects within the collecting system represent urothelial tumors. Although rare, other malignant lesions such as sarcomas (leiomyosarcoma, Ewing's, liposarcoma, rhabdomyosarcoma) and benign conditions (*e.g.*, blood clot, fungus ball, calculi, sloughed papilla, malakoplakia, tuberculosis, ureteritis cystic, and endometriosis) may present in a similar fashion, making differentiation more challenging, sometimes requiring endoscopy and biopsy for differentiation before treatment.

Magnetic resonance imaging (MRI) urography is not currently considered standard due to its inferior spatial resolution to CT, long scanning time and cost [19]. However, it remains an attractive alternative technique that does not involve ionizing radiation. Currently, MR urography is a noninvasive alternative that has found use predominantly in patients allergic to iodinated contrast media.

Management

Traditionally, organ-confined renal pelvis and proximal upper ureteral disease in patients with otherwise normal contralateral kidney has required radical nephroureterectomy with resection of bladder cuff [20]. There are several reasons for this: the synchronous and metachronous nature of TCC,

Table 2.4 Imaging techniques summary

Evaluation of patient with hematuria and staging
Intravenous urography
Largely replaced by CTU
Examination of choice if CTU not available
Does not provide information about surrounding structures
CT urography
Current standard for minimally invasive imaging
Useful for staging and diagnosis
Allows assessment in multiple planes
Evaluates periureteric and renal infiltration
Evaluates for nodal and distant metastasis
Split bolus technique, with two runs may minimize radiation
Prone positioning, intravenous saline bolus and oral water hydration help maximize ureteral opacification and collecting system distension
Currently, there is no single universal standard CTU protocol. However, for the past 5 years there has been an increasing trend toward CTU techniques with improved ureteral opacification and minimal radiation dose. Radiation dose including cumulative dose from repeated examination is a specific point of consideration when utilizing CT urography in imaging work-up, particularly for younger patients who may undergo repeat follow-up examination. The effective dose for CTU is undeniably higher than that of conventional urography. Nawfel et al. [16] calculated an estimated effective dose of 14.8 mSv for CTU utilizing a single bolus three-phase technique compared to 9.7 mSv for conventional urography. However, Martingano et al. [17] demonstrated that CTU estimated effective dose may reach levels up to 17.1 mSv for nephrographic-excretory phase, but with optimization of radiation a value of 6.2 mSv was obtained.
MR urography (MRU)
Less spatial resolution compared to CTU
Alternative for patients with iodinated contrast allergy
Possible alternative in patients with mild renal insufficiency
Exception: patients with severely impaired renal function, due to potential nephrogenic systemic fibrosis (NSF)
Patients must be able to be exposed to the magnetic field without contraindications
Pyelography
Anterograde: Rarely performed when CTU is inconclusive for evaluation of renal pelvis because of theoretical risk of tumor seeding
Retrograde: Indicated if poor renal function, contrast allergy or partial or incomplete visualization of the collecting system, however even then, MRU may prove a superior alternative when not contraindicated.
Representative CTU protocol and technical factors
IV injection:
Saline 2.5 mL/s for 200 mL
Contrast 2.5 mL/s for 150 mL (*e.g.*, iohexol 300), followed by saline 2.5 mL/s 200 mL
Oral contrast:
400 mL H_2O 20 min before scan
Precontrast, parenchymal phase and excretion phase imaging:
Injection to scan delay: parenchymal phase 80 s; excretion phase: 12 min
Scan coverage:
Precontrast: just above kidneys through ischial tuberosity
Parenchymal phase: just above hepatic dome through tuberosity
Excretion phase: same as precontrast
Technical factors:
Exposure:
Precontrast and excretion phases: 0.7 s rotation time; low mA (*e.g.*, 130)
Parenchymal phase: 0.7 s rotation time; auto mA
Pitch/table speed: all phases, 0.984/39.37 mm
Reconstruction thickness: 2.5×2.5 mm standard all phases
Reconstruction 2: 1.25×1 mm standard
Additional delays:
Only scan targeted 12 min supine and/or 18 min prone, if necessary
Additional delays will be determined by the radiologist, if pathology is suspected
(Abdominal compression: none)
Reformats:
Parenchymal phase:
1.6×0.8 mm coronal reformats through kidneys, ureters, and bladder
3D reconstruction: use 1.25×1 mm reconstructions from excretion phases to push to workstation

the high tumor recurrence rate (30–50 %) [21] within the ureteral stump when only a nephrectomy is performed, and the low frequency of contralateral lesions (1–5.8 %) [22].

Regional lymphadenectomy is then performed, especially for patients with high-grade tumors; however, the role and extent of routine lymphadenectomy are still to be determined [23].

Segmental ureteral resection with anastomosis or ureteroneocystostomy for proximal or midureteral tumors and distal ureterectomy for tumors of the distal ureter without evidence of multifocality are feasible options, especially for low-grade, low-stage lesions, and in patients in whom renal function preservation is vital.

There is an increasing trend toward conservative management with recent advances in endoscopic technology and minimally invasive surgery. Such conservative management allowing for renal function preservation is generally accepted for patients with low-grade tumor, solitary kidney, bilateral disease, poor renal function, or comorbidities precluding open surgery [24].

Despite no accepted protocol for radiological follow-up, endoscopic and cytological surveillance for upper urinary tract TCC is essential, irrespective of the surgical procedure employed, to detect local recurrence.

Due to its rarity, recommendation on topical chemotherapy, immunotherapy, and neoadjuvant systemic chemotherapy of upper tract disease extrapolates from the management of lower urothelial tract tumors. Controversy still exists on the role of radiotherapy and chemotherapy in reducing tumor recurrence and lengthening survival, and further confirmation in randomized multicenter trials is needed to ensure efficacy [25].

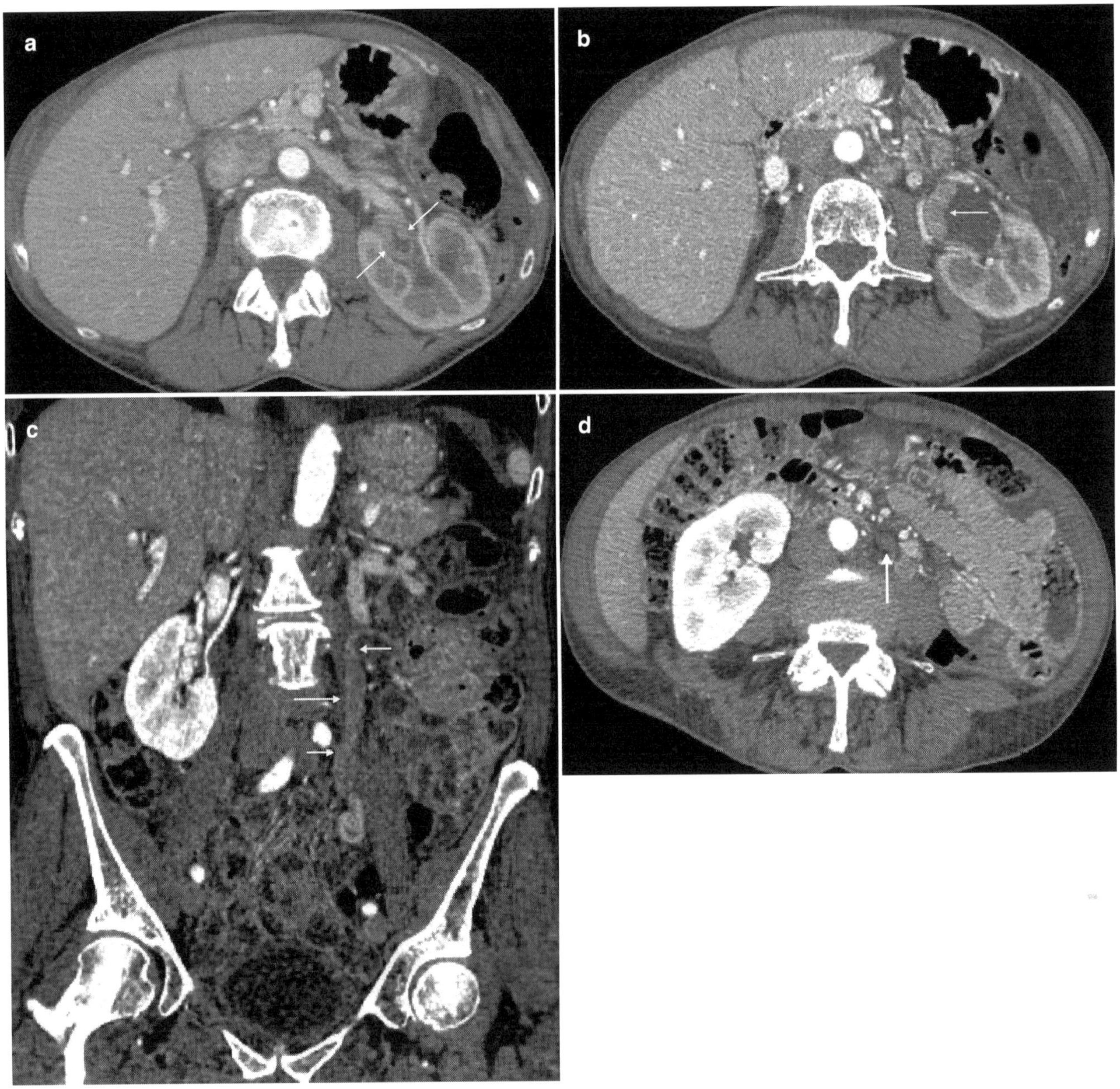

Fig. 2.1 A 68-year-old woman with a history of hematuria with bladder cancer after transurethral resection of bladder tumor (TURBT). CTU demonstrated extensive upper tract tumor and borderline enlarged retroperitoneal lymph nodes. T1 papillary involving the lamina without muscularis invasion was confirmed by histopathologic analysis. (**a**) Axial parenchymal phase images showed multifocal enhancing tumor within the left renal pelvis (*arrows*), as well as involving the upper moiety and upper ureter with moderate hydronephrosis. (**b**) Axial parenchymal phase images at a lower level show eccentric thickening (*arrow*) along the ureteropelvic junction. (**c**) Coronal multiplanar reformatted (MPR) showing the extent of urothelial tumor involving the left ureter (*arrows*) in this patient who also had a delayed nephrogram. (**d**) Axial parenchymal phase images at the level inferior to the left lower pole show prominent, borderline-enlarged para-aortic nodes (*arrow*). Node-positive tumors of the renal pelvis can involve upper retroperitoneal nodes (retrocrural, suprahilar, paracaval, paraaortic, and interaortocaval) and extend caudally to the external iliac lymph nodes. Node-positive tumors of the middle and lower third of the ureter can involve both the retroperitoneal and pelvic lymph nodes. Lymph node metastases have consistently been associated with an adverse prognosis [23]

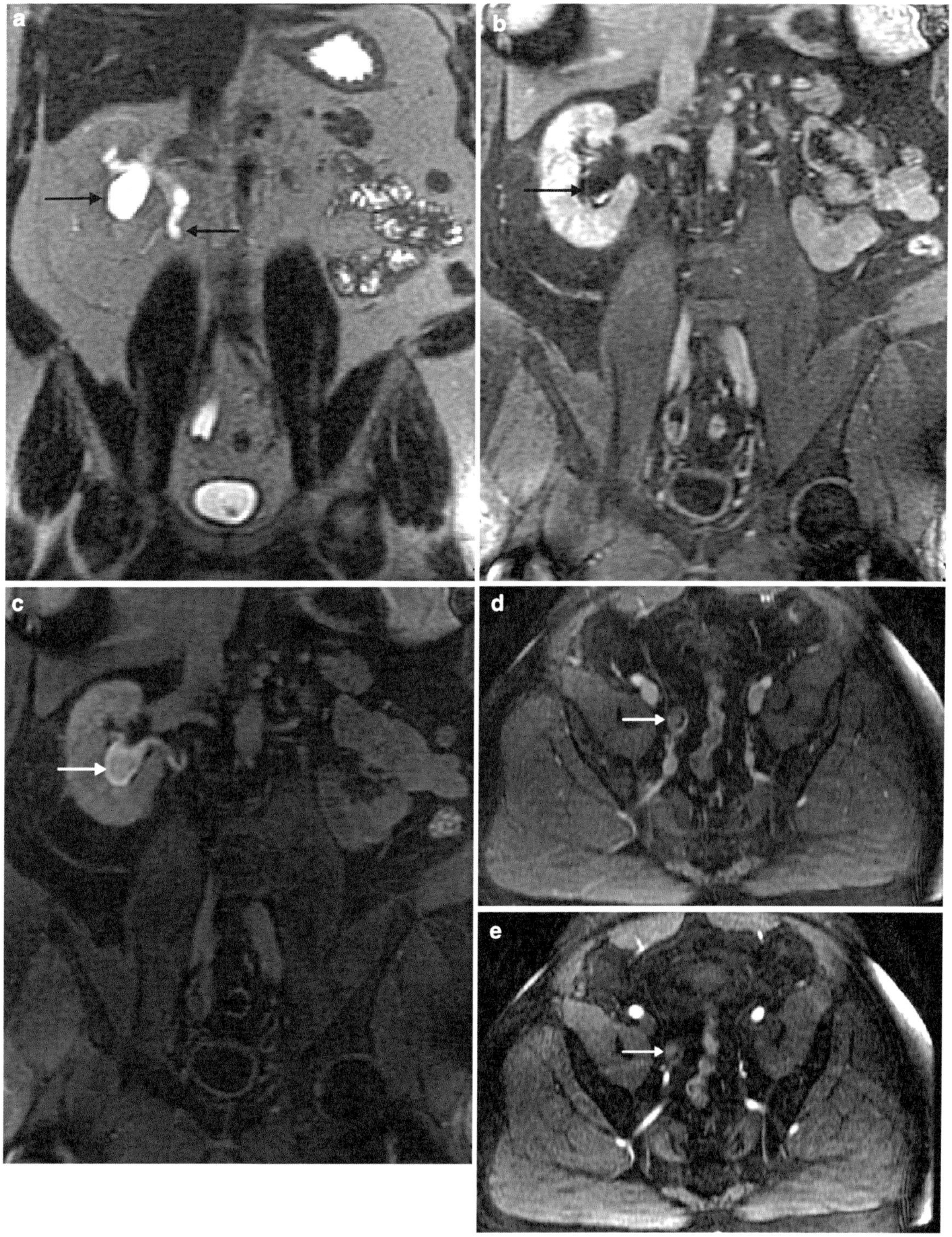

Fig. 2.2 A 55-year-old man with history of low-grade TCC involving the bladder and left upper tract after TURBT and left nephroureterectomy. Routine follow-up MRU revealed new right hydroureteronephrosis and lobulated enhancing lesion obliterating the distal ureteral lumen. Although ureteral washings at time of placement of JJ stent were negative for malignant cells, histopathology from subsequent right distal ureterectomy confirmed noninvasive urothelial carcinoma. (**a**) Coronal T2 image shows dilated renal collecting system and proximal hydroureter (*arrows*) or a variant of "champagne glass sign" related to more distal ureteral disease. Coronal, postintravenous, gadolinium-enhanced early (**b**) and excretory phase (**c**) imaging demonstrates a dilated lower pole moiety with confirmed nonenhancing filling defect consistent with debris (*arrow*). (**d**) Axial T1 fat-saturated postintravenous gadolinium images show distal ureteral enhancing tumor (*arrow*). (**e**) Distal ureteral tumor confirmed on subtraction images (*arrow*). Patients with a history of lower or upper tract urothelial carcinoma are at high risk of developing synchronous or metachronous urothelial carcinoma in the upper tract. MRU is a promising alternative for CTU in the evaluation of upper tract urothelial carcinoma, especially when the patient has a contraindication to iodinated contrast material. When the lesions are obstructive, MRU can detect upper tract urothelial carcinoma with an accuracy of 88 % or higher using gadolinium-enhanced pyelographic phase or T2-weighted single-shot fast spin-echo MRU but has a limited role in accurately staging low-volume tumor (Ta, T1, T2), which may be important in deciding the treatment option (nephroureterectomy versus endoscopic treatment) [26]

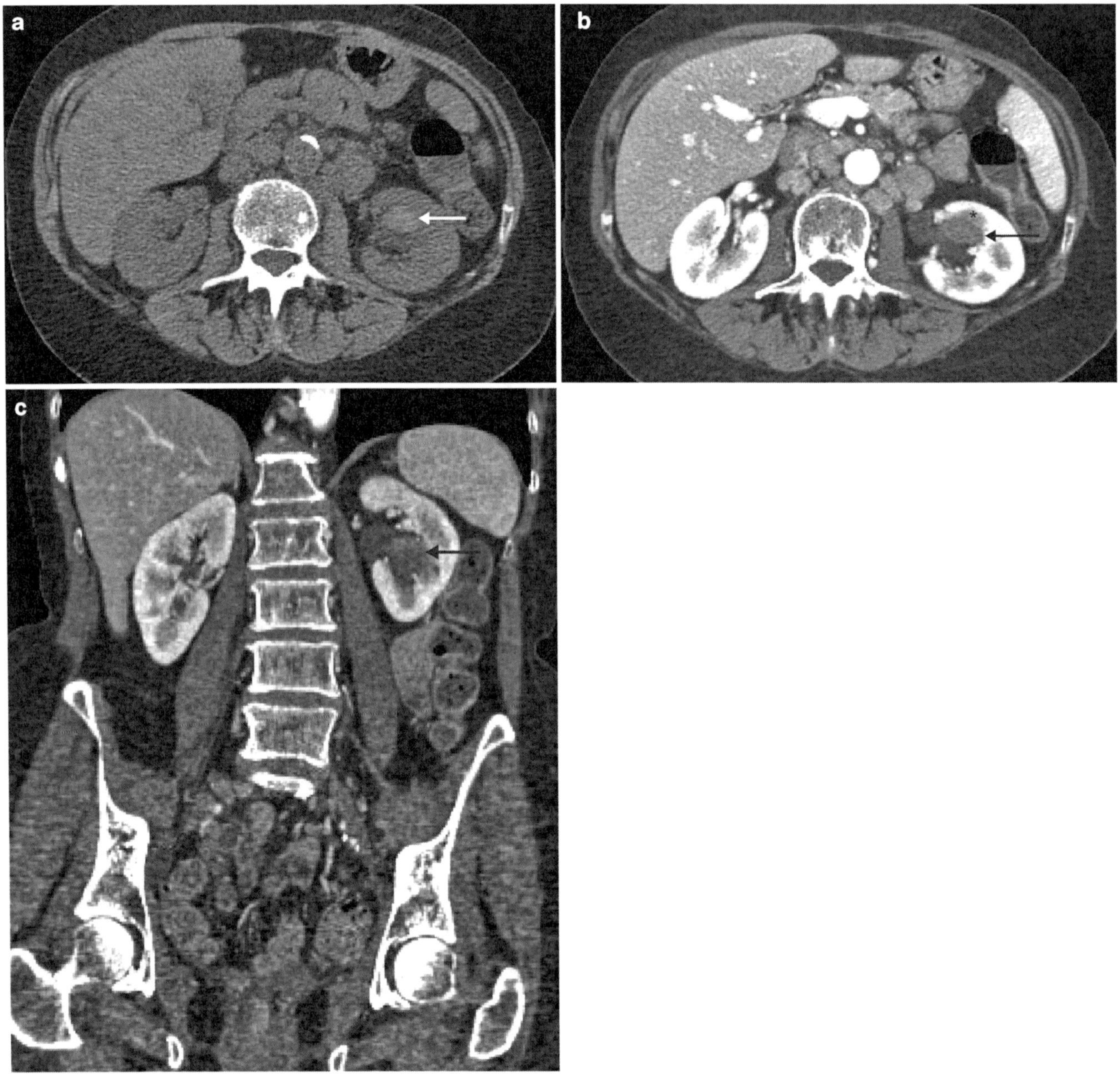

Fig. 2.3 A 69-year-old woman with history of pT3N2 bladder cancer after neoadjuvant chemotherapy and radical cystectomy found to have renal mass and adenopathy on routine follow-up CTU. The patient was managed with adjuvant chemotherapy. (**a**) Axial precontrast images show a hyperattenuating mass (*arrow*) in the anterior lower pole calyx of the left kidney. (**b**) Axial parenchymal phase images show enhancing lower pole mass (*arrow*) with extension into the adjacent renal parenchyma (*asterisk*). (**c**) Coronal maximum intensity projection (MIP) images show tumor filling the lower moiety and mild distortion of the collecting system. (**d**) Axial corticomedullary phase image shows paraaortic adenopathy (*arrows*). (**e**) Axial excretory phase image shows diffuse tumor (*arrows*) with a small amount of excreted contrast centrally. (**f**) Volumetric three-dimensional (3D) excretory phase reconstruction shows truncation, narrowing, and distortion of the left lower and mid-lower moiety (*arrows*) in this diverted patient. Note mild fullness of the right collecting system, which is often seen in diverted patients. The renal contour is preserved. On precontrast images, TCC is typically hyperattenuating (5–30 HU) to urine and renal parenchyma but less attenuating than other pelvic filling defects such as clot (40–80 HU) or calculus (100 HU). Advanced TCC extends into the renal parenchyma in an infiltrating pattern that distorts normal architecture. However, reniform shape is typically preserved, unlike in renal cell carcinoma [26]. With urinary diversion procedures, hydroureter and mild pelvicaliectasis are often seen early and may either resolve or remain stable. However, severe pelvicaliectasis implies obstruction from a stricture, stone, or recurrence [27]. all arrows in all images better delineate margins of tumor / important findings for the target audience / reader

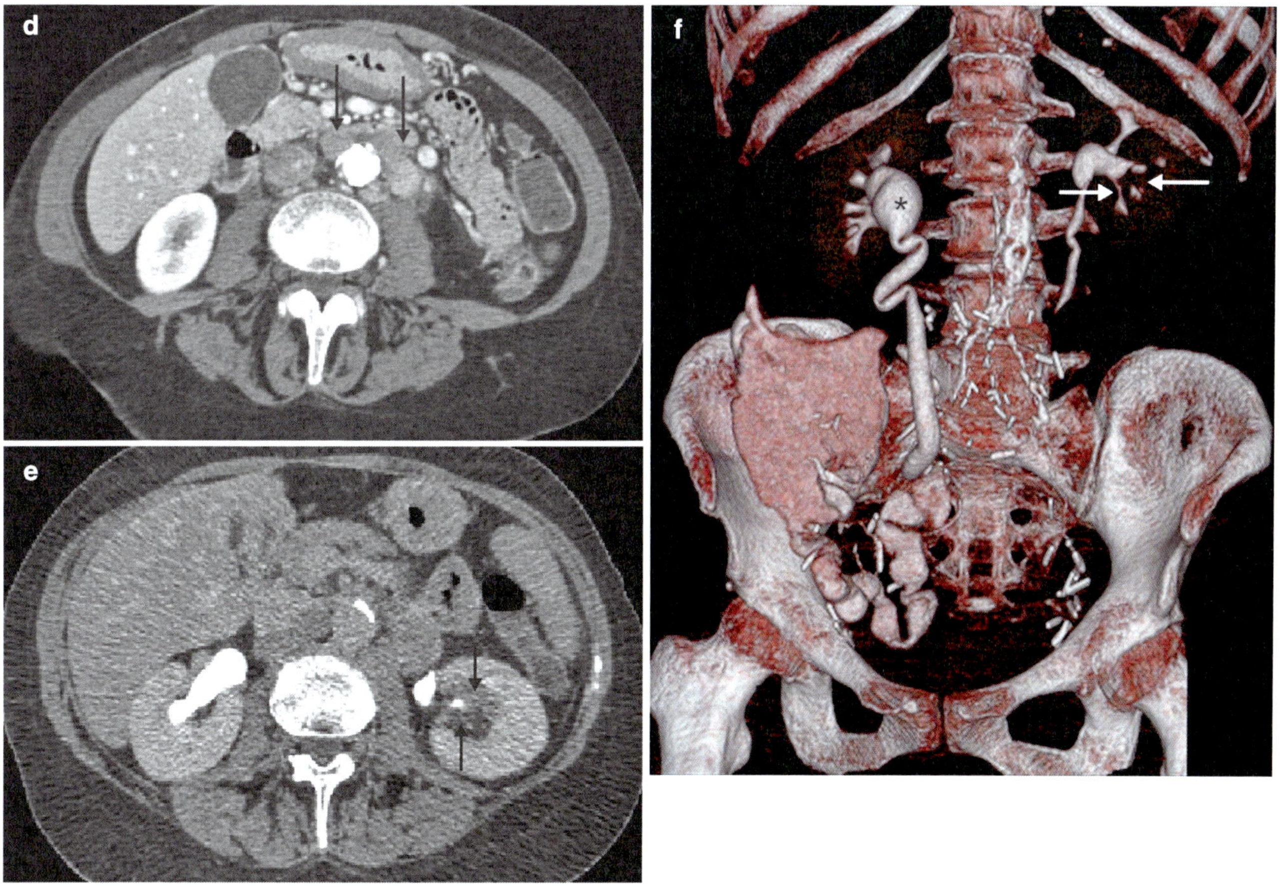

Fig. 2.3 (continued)

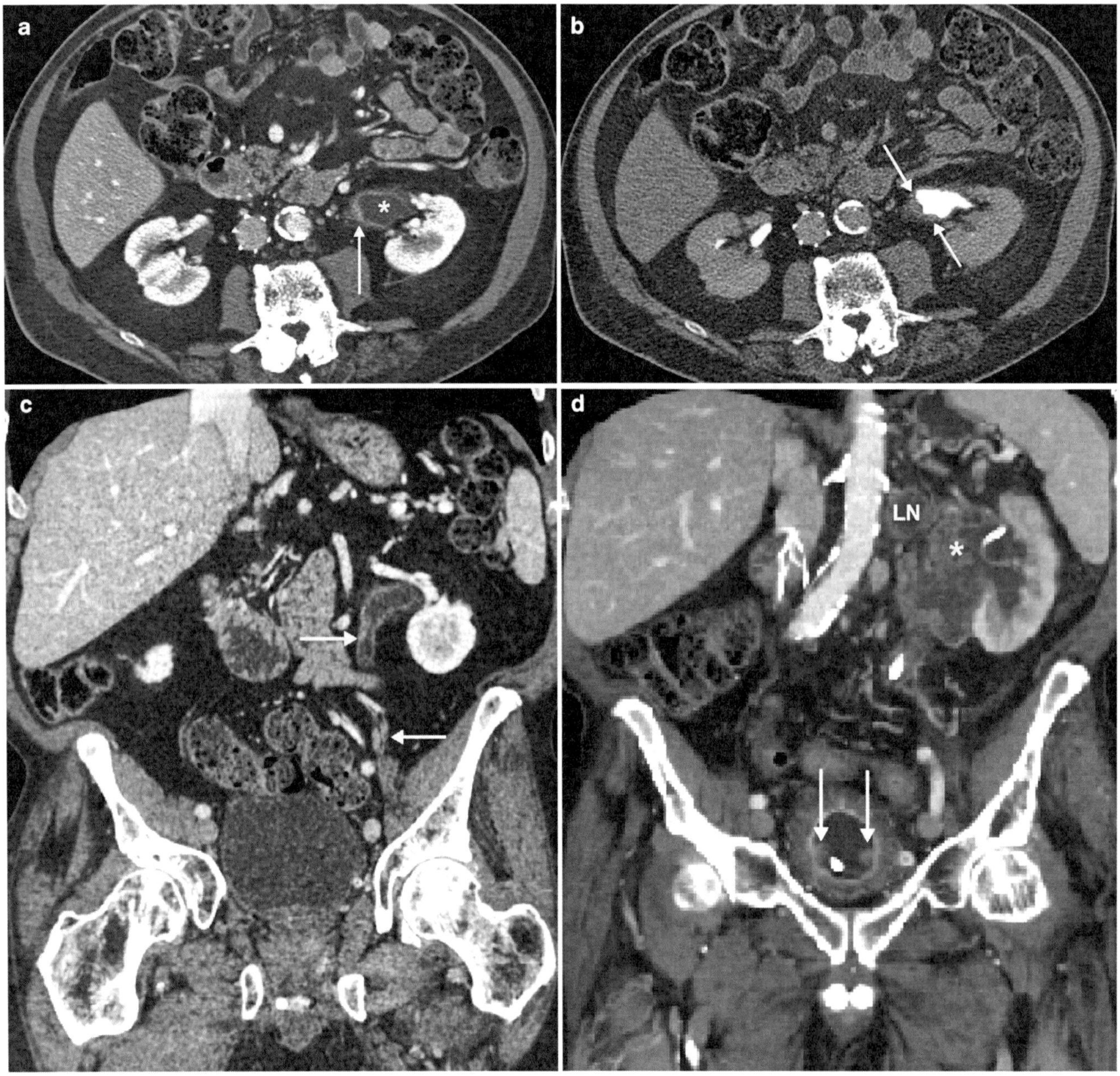

Fig. 2.4 An 83-year-old man with a history of bladder cancer status post-TURBT 20 years prior was found to have incidental hydronephrosis and ureteral thickening on CTU. Ureteroscopic resection and laser fulguration was performed, followed by insertion of a double J stent. Histopathology was positive for invasive pT2 urothelial malignancy; however, there was inability to assess for muscle invasion due to combined superficial biopsy and thermal artifact. Patient subsequently progressed to unresectable disease. (**a**) Axial parenchymal phase images show mild dilation of the left renal pelvis (*asterisk*) with generalized wall-thickening and enhancement most marked at the ureteropelvic junction (*arrow*) and proximal ureter. (**b**) Axial excretory phase images show circumferential wall-thickening most marked at the ureteropelvic junction (*arrows*). (**c**) Coronal MPR parenchymal phase images show the extent of urothelial thickening (*arrows*). Patients with bladder cancer are at lifelong risk for late oncologic recurrence in the upper tract urothelium. Left ureteroscopy and biopsy was positive for high-grade TCC. Tumor progressed to unresectable disease despite laser fulguration. (**d**) Parenchymal phase coronal MIP images show extensive upper tract tumor (*asterisk*), para-aortic adenopathy (*LN*), and circumferential bladder thickening with multifocal polypoid tumor recurrence (*arrows*). Note double J ureteral stent and penile prosthesis in situ. The 3- and 5-year cumulative incidence of upper tract recurrence is 4 and 7 %, respectively [28]. These patients should be monitored with routine upper tract cytology and imaging studies [29]. CTU has been proven to be a sensitive and specific method for the detection of urothelial malignancy, with sensitivity ranging between 88 and 100 %, and specificity between 93 and 100 % [30]

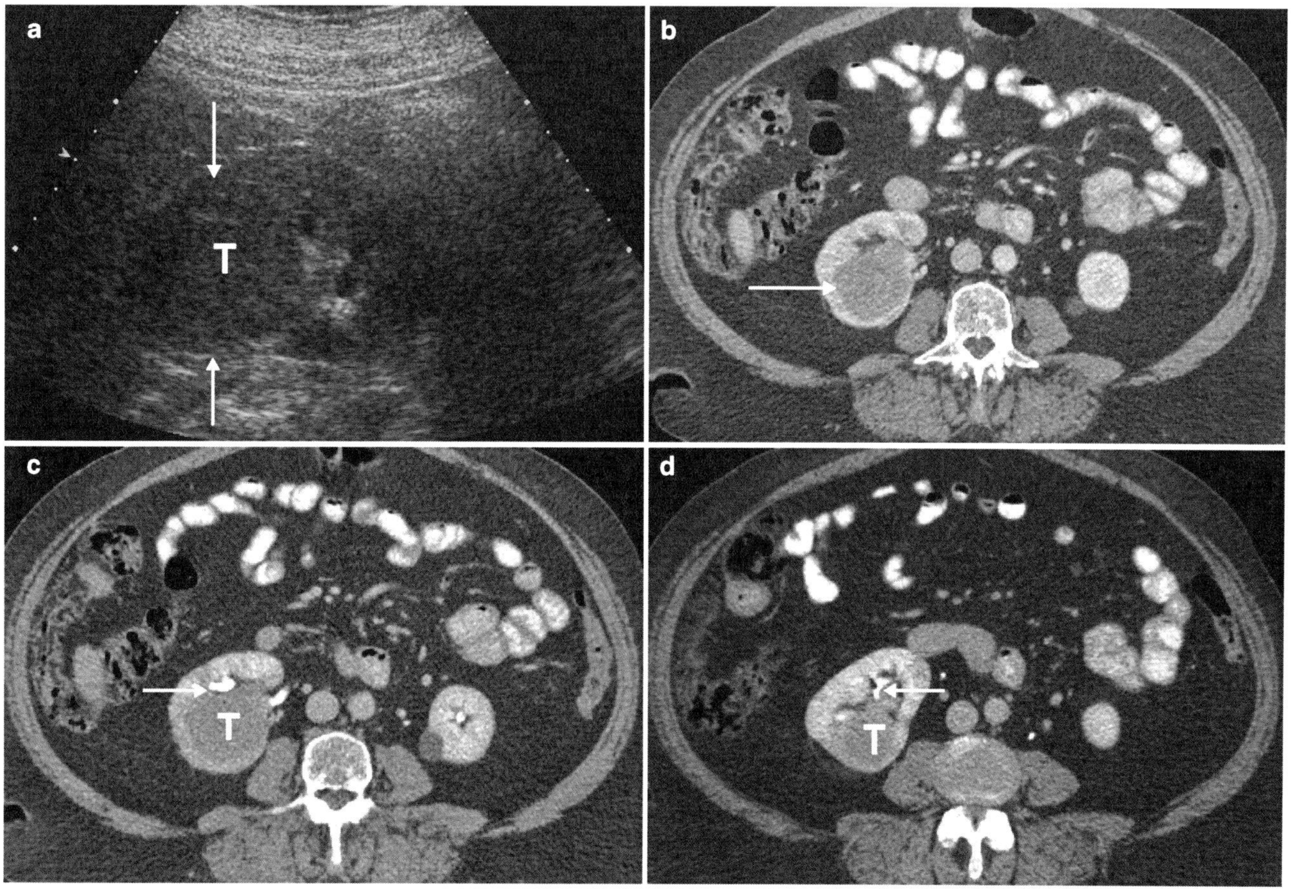

Fig. 2.5 A 56-year-old woman with hematuria underwent cystoscopy with negative findings. Outside CT showed a large upper pole renal mass. Patient underwent radical right nephrectomy and pathology was positive for high-grade urothelial neoplasm (T1N0). Subsequent completion laparoscopic ureterectomy was performed with histopathology showing the specimen to be free of tumor. (**a**) Longitudinal grayscale ultrasound image of the right kidney reveals a solid round isoechoic mass (*T*) measuring just under 5 cm in diameter (*arrows*). The mass displaces central echogenic pelvic fat. (**b**) Axial early parenchymal phase image through the right kidney shows a mass (*arrow*) in the posterior upper pole measuring up to 5 cm and displacing central pelvic fat with associated delayed nephrogram compared to the visualized left kidney, with small left renal cyst. (**c**) and (**d**) Axial excretory phase images confirm distortion of the collecting system (*arrow*) by tumor (*T*). At ultrasound, renal pelvic TCC typically appears as a central soft-tissue mass in the echogenic renal sinus with or without hydronephrosis. Tumor is usually slightly hyperechoic relative to surrounding renal parenchyma and it may be obscured by the surrounding hyperechoic renal sinus fat. Also, small nonobstructing TCCs may be impossible to differentiate from blood clots, sloughed papillae, or a fungus ball [31]. Ultrasound (US) is not as specific as CT in identifying or characterizing renal masses but is frequently requested in the evaluation of patients with hematuria to assess for renal parenchymal masses. A review of more than 1,000 cases in patients with hematuria suggested that US has value for evaluation of upper tract disease, as two patients with upper tract tumors and 21 patients with renal cortical tumors were properly diagnosed using the investigational protocol [32]

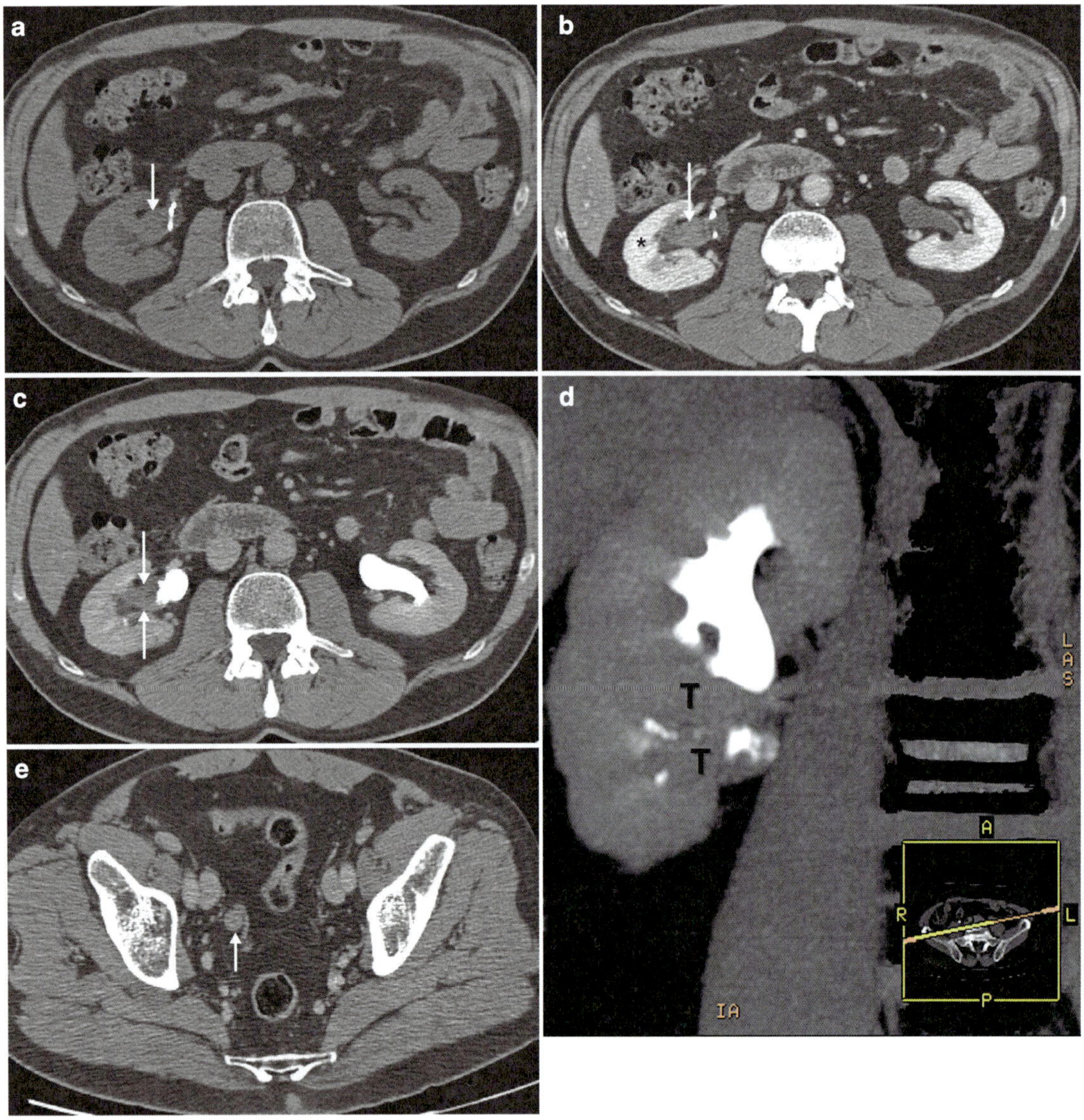

Fig. 2.6 A 63-year-old man with history of high-grade papillary TCC right renal pelvis after nephroureterectomy and TURBT for superficial bladder lesion. One year later, the patient presented with an abnormal CTU, with a tubular soft tissue mass in the region of the anticipated right ureteral stump and vesicle-ureteral junction suspicious for recurrent tumor. TURBT was positive for low-grade papillary (pT1) TCC. (**a**) Axial noncontrast images from baseline CTU reveals a mass (*arrow*) in the right renal pelvis, which is slightly hyperattenuating to urine and renal parenchyma [33]. (**b**) Axial parenchymal phase images show characteristic mild early enhancement (*arrow*) less than that of the renal parenchyma (*asterisk*) [33]. (**c**) Axial images acquired in the excretory phase show the mass (*arrows*) as a filling defect in the renal collecting system [33]. (**d**) Coronal reformatted image showing tumor (*T*) filling the right renal lower moiety and pelvis. (**e**) Ureteral stump recurrence on CTU 1-year after surgical resection. Axial parenchymal phase images show enhancing soft tissue (*arrow*) filling the right distal ureteric stump. (**f**) Coronal MPR image in the nephrographic phase confirms linear enhancing soft tissue (*arrows*). (**g**) Axial excretion phase image demonstrates nodular tumor (*arrow*) within the distal ureteral stump with diminished attenuation consistent with contrast washout when compared with previous parenchymal phase. When nephrectomy alone or incomplete nephroureterectomy is performed, subsequent transitional cell carcinoma can develop in up to 30 % of the ureteral stumps [34]

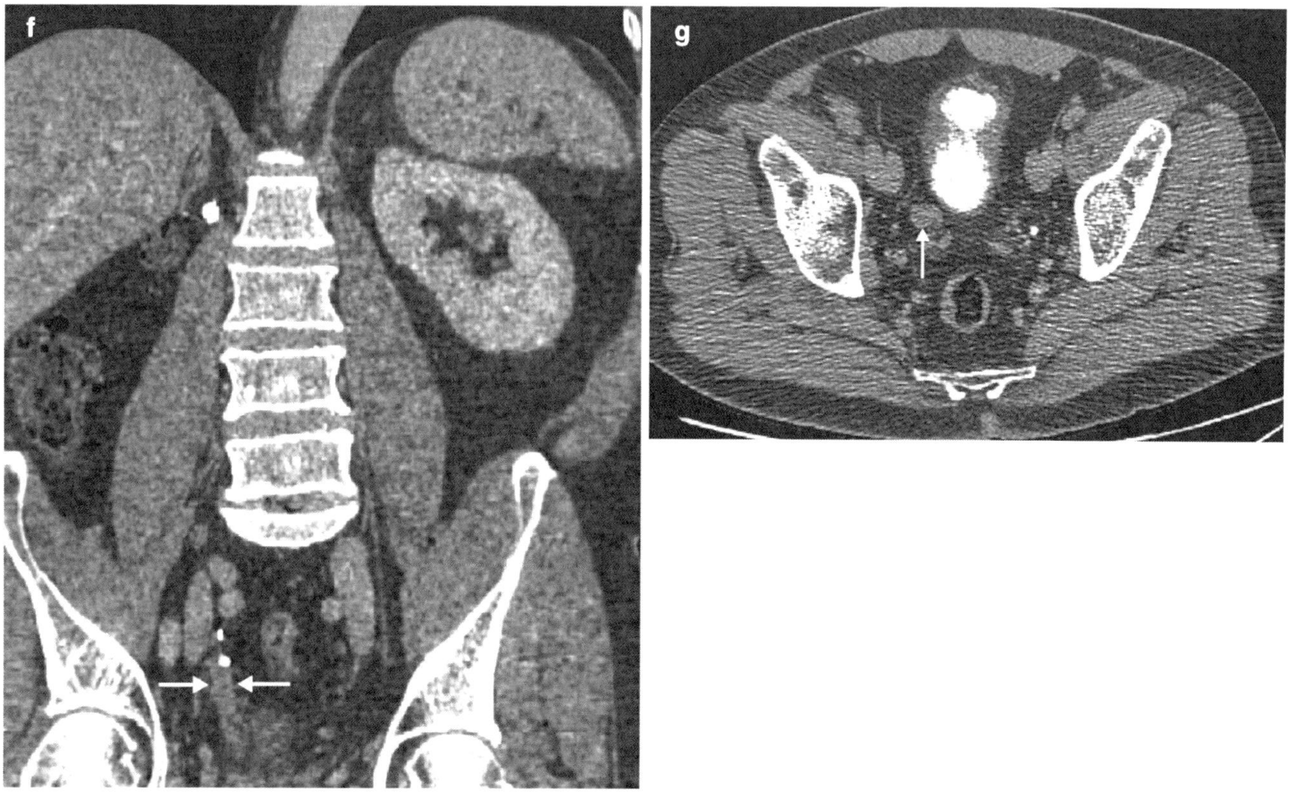

Fig. 2.6 (continued)

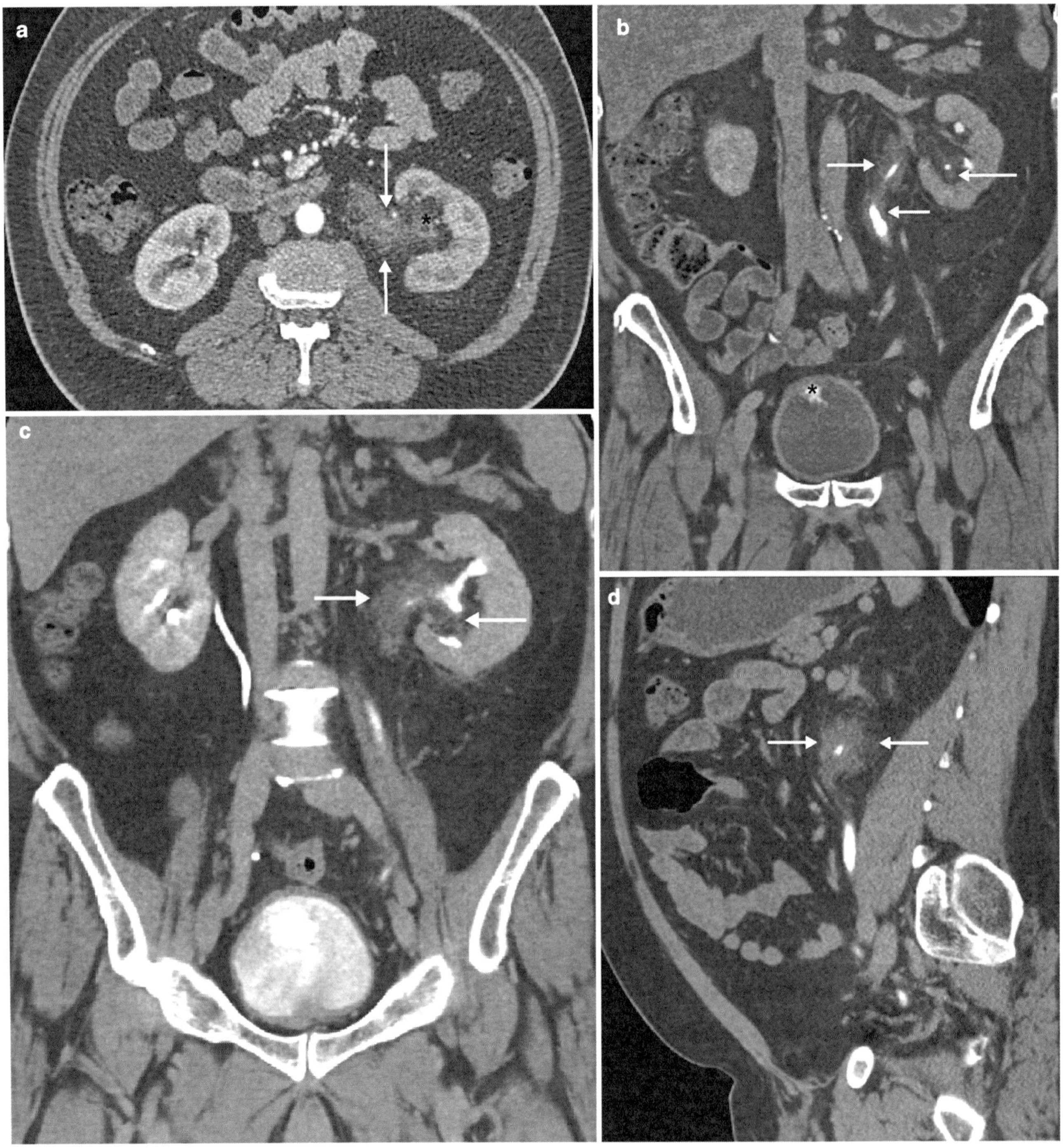

Fig. 2.7 A 59-year-old man with gross hematuria. Cystoscopy at an outside institution revealed carcinoma in situ of the bladder, whereas subsequent CTU imaging revealed marked surrounding fat-stranding and wall-thickening involving the left renal pelvis and lower moiety, as well as proximal ureteral narrowing and nonobstructing renal calculi. No lymphadenopathy was seen. Left nephroureterectomy was performed, with histopathology confirming pT3N0 transitional cell carcinoma within the upper tract. (**a**) Axial CTU parenchymal-phase shows abnormal left ureteropelvic junction thickening and enhancement with indistinct collecting system margins and surrounding fat infiltration (*arrows*). Thickening and circumferential enhancement of the lower moiety is noted en-face (*asterisk*) with delayed left nephrogram. (**b**, **c**) Coronal excretory-phase MPR confirms segmental circumferential tumor involving the proximal left ureter and lower moiety (*arrows*) with marked surrounding fat infiltration and narrowing of the ureteral lumen. Excreted contrast from ureteral jet is noted at bladder dome (*asterisk*). (**d**) Sagittal excretory phase MPR through the left proximal ureteral demonstrates the marked irregular circumferential tumor with ill-defined margins and infiltration involving the periureteral fat (*arrows*). Histopathologic analysis upon subsequent radical nephroureterectomy confirmed invasive high-grade urothelial carcinoma with tumor invasion into renal hilar and peripelvic tissue. Although the majority of focal infiltrative TCCs tend to have a more central location, eccentric or peripheral tumors may occur. In such a situation, the reniform shape can be preserved or distorted. When the reniform shape is distorted or lost, the mass effect of eccentric or peripheral TCC may simulate RCC. In addition, large infiltrative TCCs with both pelvic and parenchymal involvement may simulate other entities such as tuberculosis, lymphoma, metastasis, or xanthogranulomatous pyelonephritis [31]

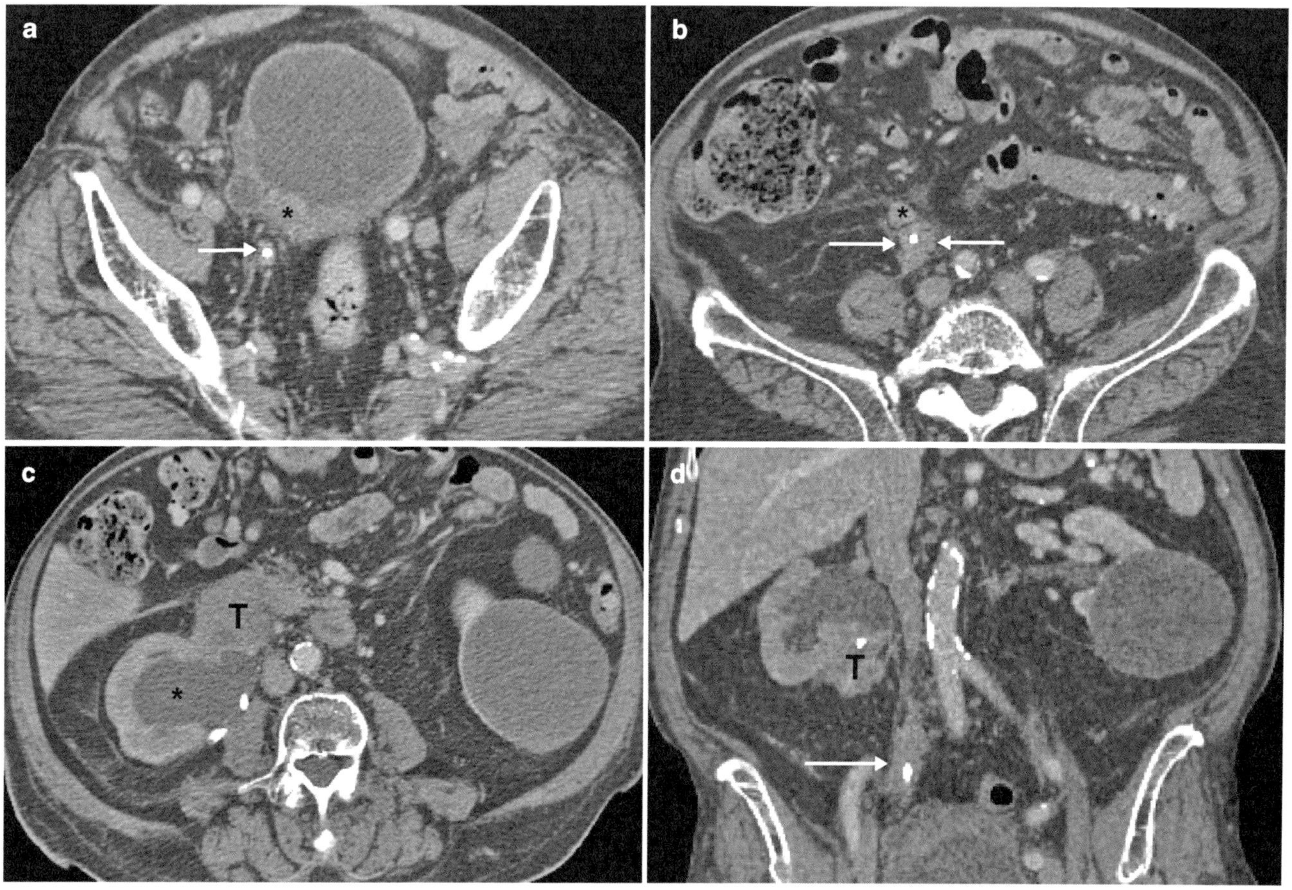

Fig. 2.8 A 92-year-old man with a history of gross hematuria and poorly differentiated muscle invasive pT2 urothelial tumor of the bladder, after TURBT and Bacillus Calmette-Guerin (BCG) over 8 weeks after initial diagnosis, with recurrence and repeat TUR showing poorly differentiated carcinoma with lymphovascular invasion. Urine cytologic fluorescence in situ hybridization (FISH) analysis revealed aneuploidy of chromosomes 3, 7, and 17. FISH analysis, assessing for denatured nuclei counterstain uptake to probe for DNA markers, shows high sensitivity for high-grade tumors and offers good specificity for detecting bladder cancer. It may be utilized in patients recently treated with BCG therapy, in contradistinction to other protein assays. FISH analysis is limited in sensitivity for low-grade tumors, however; it also requires trained personnel and sophisticated instrumentation for accurate performance [35]. (**a**) Axial nephrographic phase image. Despite diffuse trabeculation, focal nodular bladder thickening posteriorly (*asterisk*) was confirmed as focal abnormal bladder thickening on cystoscopy. Thickening and dilation of the distal right ureter is noted, with an indwelling stent (*arrow*). (**b**) Axial nephrographic phase image. Diffuse right periureteric tumor (*arrows*) with adjacent fat infiltration and subjacent lymphadenopathy (*asterisk*) noted just below the pelvic inlet. (**c**) Axial parenchymal phase image at the level of the renal pelvis demonstrates gross tumor mass (*T*) extending anteriorly within the perirenal fat as well as hydronephrosis (*asterisk*). The tumor was inseparable from portions of the inferior vena cava. Stent partially imaged. (**d**) Coronal plane reformatted parenchymal phase image confirms gross perinephric tumor (*T*) extension inferiorly as well, inseparable from the proximal ureteropelvic junction. Midureteral extensive tumor involvement (*arrow*) is also seen. In the bladder, thickened bladder wall with focal nodularity may be seen on CT or MRI after intravesical BCG and is very difficult to differentiate from bladder tumor. It is clinically important for the radiologist to consider the possibility of BCG reaction when local or disseminated masses are visualized on follow-up imaging in bladder cancer patients. If clinical concern for metastatic disease or another primary tumor is high, a biopsy may be needed to provide a definitive diagnosis [36]

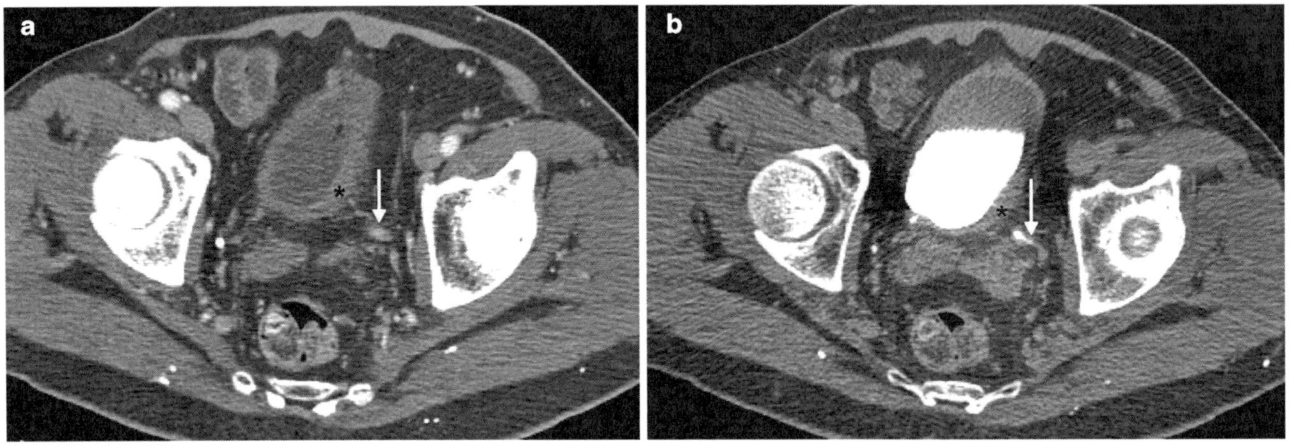

Fig. 2.9 A 74-year-old man with a history of Gleason 6 prostate cancer underwent cystoscopy and biopsy for hematuria; pathology was positive for superficial noninvasive urothelial carcinoma pTa. Surveillance cystoscopy showed tumor of the left distal ureter, and subsequent TURBT and distal ureteral resection confirmed pTa tumor. (**a**) Axial parenchymal phase image shows distal left ureteral thickening (*arrow*) and mild enhancement. Diffuse urinary bladder wall trabeculation and mild left more than right bladder wall thickening is also noted (*asterisk*). (**b**) Axial excretory phase image confirms distal ureter (*arrow*) and bladder wall (*asterisk*) thickening. Although the "gold standard" for urothelial tumors involving the upper urinary tract has been complete excision of the entire kidney and ureter, equivalent oncologic outcomes after conservative endoscopic management of low-grade superficial upper urinary tract TCC have been widely reported, suggesting that the removal of the entire ipsilateral tract is not always necessary. All patients with urothelial tumors require close surveillance of the entire urinary tract [37]

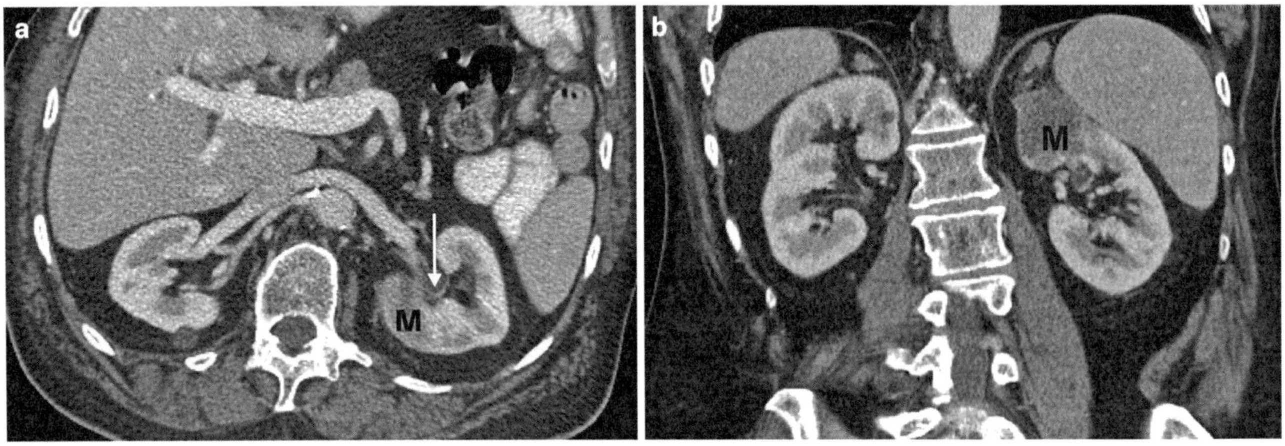

Fig. 2.10 A 69-year-old man with metastatic squamous cell carcinoma of the left lung (with brain, bone, and pleural metastases). An incidentally detected left upper pole renal mass was noted on standard CT, as well as slight urothelial thickening and enhancement of the left renal pelvis and ureter. Prior left video-assisted thoracic surgery procedure for lung lesion was positive for *Mycobacterium xenopi*, hence a differential diagnosis for the renal and upper tract lesion was tuberculosis, metastasis, or primary urothelial or renal cortical tumor. CT-guided biopsy positive for metastatic squamous cell carcinoma. (a) Axial parenchymal phase image shows vague heterogeneity of the medial upper pole posteriorly (*M*) as well as thickening and enhancement of the adjacent collecting system urothelium (*arrow*). (**b**) Coronal nephrographic phase MPR demonstrates a mass (*M*) at the left upper pole

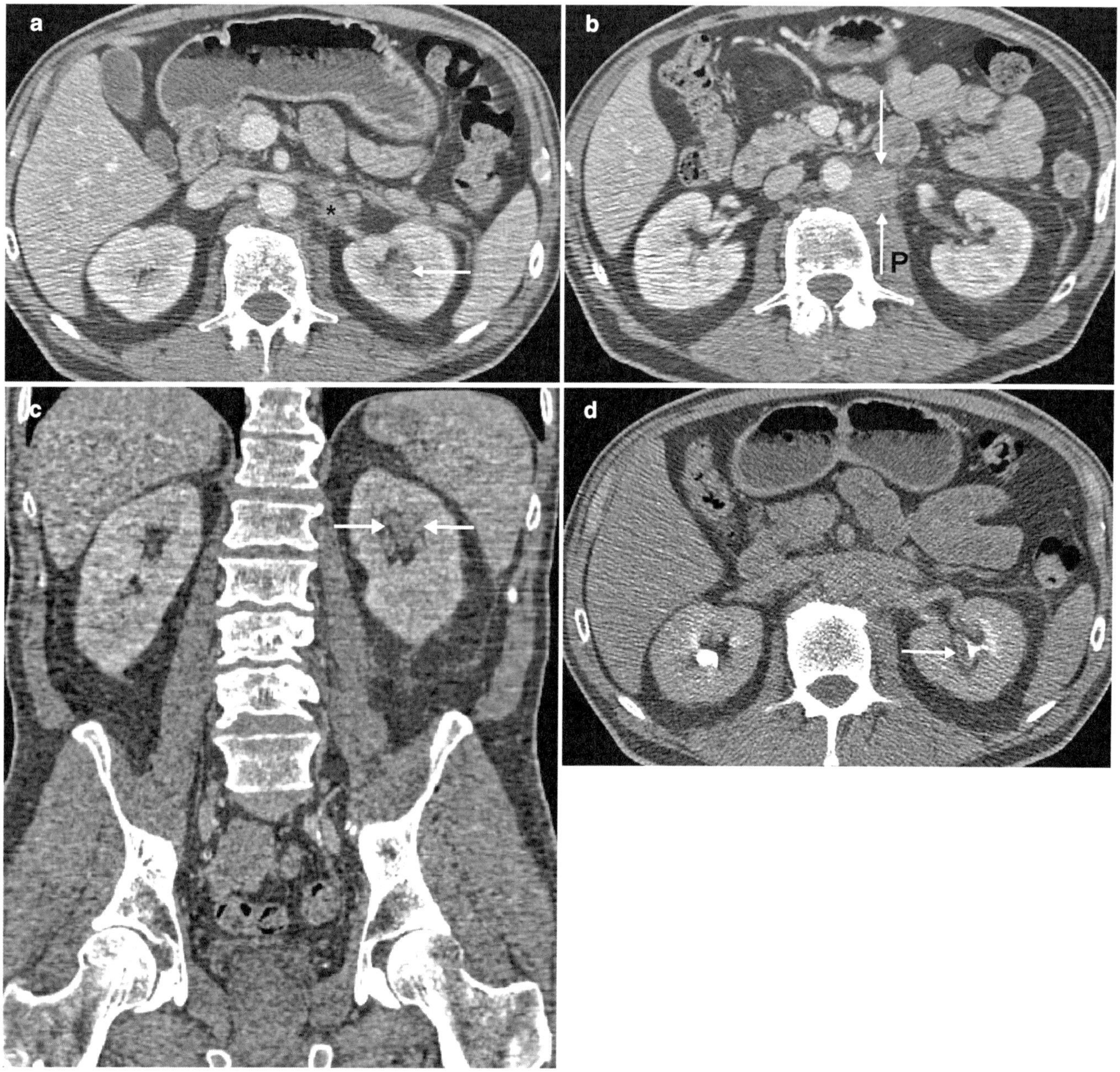

Fig. 2.11 A 62-year-old man with left flank pain (radiating to the left testicle) and unexplained weight loss. Outside institution CT showed a renal mass and retroperitoneal soft tissue masses. CTU performed showed a 1.8 × 1.6 cm soft tissue mass filling the left upper pole renal calyx and a nonobstructing 1.1 cm left renal calculus. Retroperitoneal adenopathy was also noted. Subsequent left retroperitoneal biopsy was positive for metastatic squamous cell carcinoma. Differentials included lung, urothelial, and head and neck primaries. The patient was treated with chemotherapy. (**a**) Axial parenchymal phase image shows abnormal enhancing left calyceal mass (*arrow*) and adjacent paraaortic adenopathy (*asterisk*). (**b**) Axial parenchymal phase image at a lower level shows ill-defined para aortic adenopathy (*arrows*) inseparable from the aorta and psoas muscle (*P*). (**c**) Coronal MPR parenchymal phase image demonstrates expansion and urothelial enhancement involving the left upper moiety (*arrows*). (**d**) Axial delayed phase image shows abnormal urothelial thickening (*arrow*) and distortion of the upper moiety on the left. Upper tract TCCs are more commonly spread by direct invasion and the lymphatic route than hematogenously. Tumors of the right renal collecting system can metastasize to the renal hilar, paracaval, retrocaval, and interaortocaval lymph nodes, as well as the right common iliac lymph nodes. Tumors of the left renal collecting system may involve hilar, paraaortic, inter-aortocaval, and left common iliac lymph nodes [31]

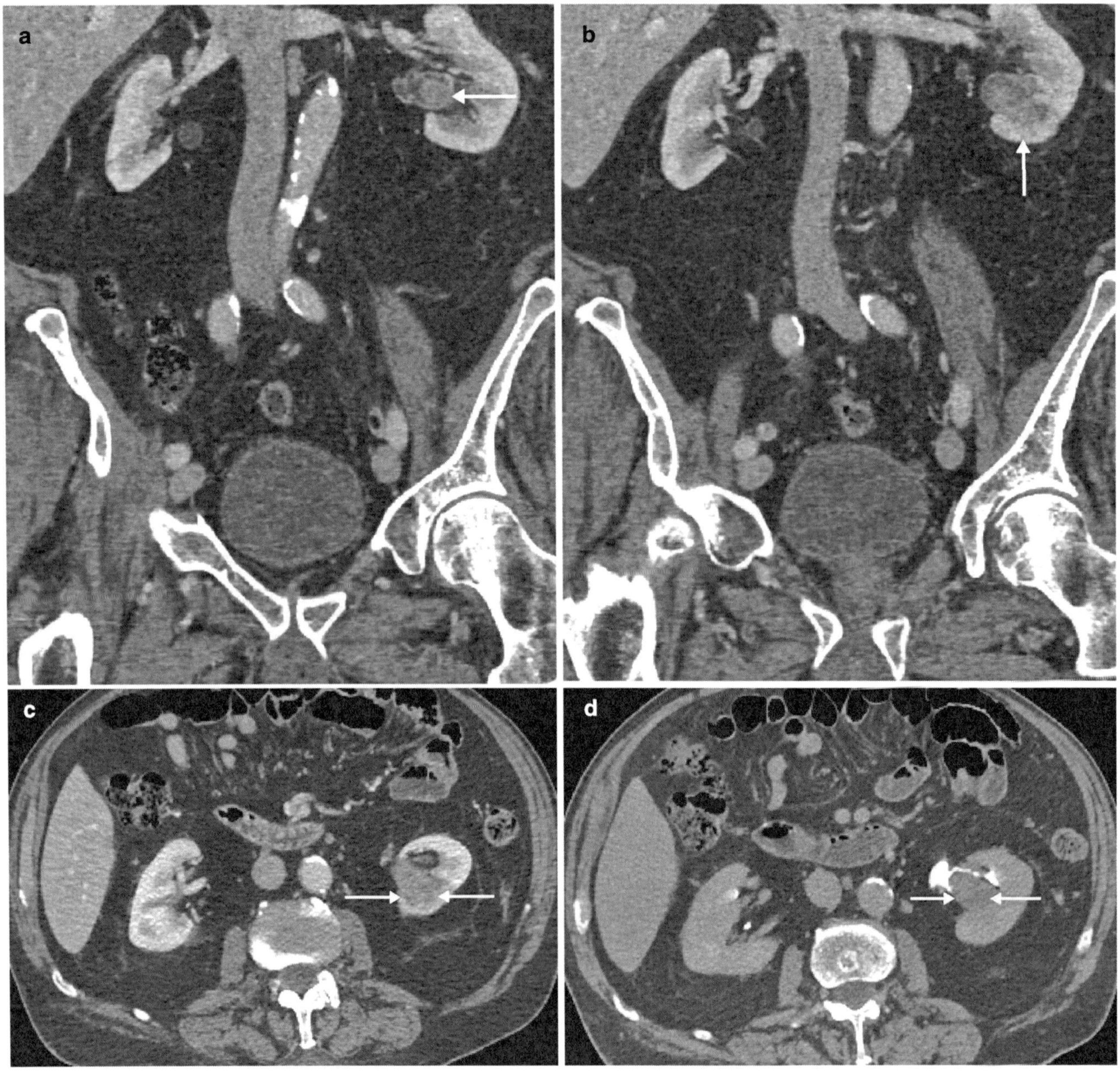

Fig. 2.12 An 87-year-old man with hematuria and left flank pain. CT work-up showed a left renal pelvis mass. Biopsy performed at ureteroscopic stent placement positive for papillary non invasive TCC, initially treated by local resection. Recurrent tumor led to left nephroureterectomy revealing pT3N0 tumor. (**a**) Coronal reformatted parenchymal-phase image shows enhancing tumor (*arrow*) projecting into the proximal left renal pelvis from the lower moiety. (**b**) Coronal reformatted parenchymal phase image in a slightly different plane suggests tumor involvement of adjacent renal parenchyma (*arrow*) with vague, irregular margins extending into the parenchyma. (**c**) Axial parenchymal phase image confirms involvement of the surrounding renal parenchyma (*arrows*) in the left lower pole. (**d**) Axial delayed phase image showing collecting system distortion due to the mass, as evidenced as a filling defect (*arrows*). Loss of renal sinus fat and abnormal enhancement of the adjacent parenchyma are signs of a T3 tumor. Advanced TCC extends into the renal parenchyma in an infiltrating pattern that distorts normal architecture. However, reniform shape is typically preserved unlike in renal cell carcinoma [2]

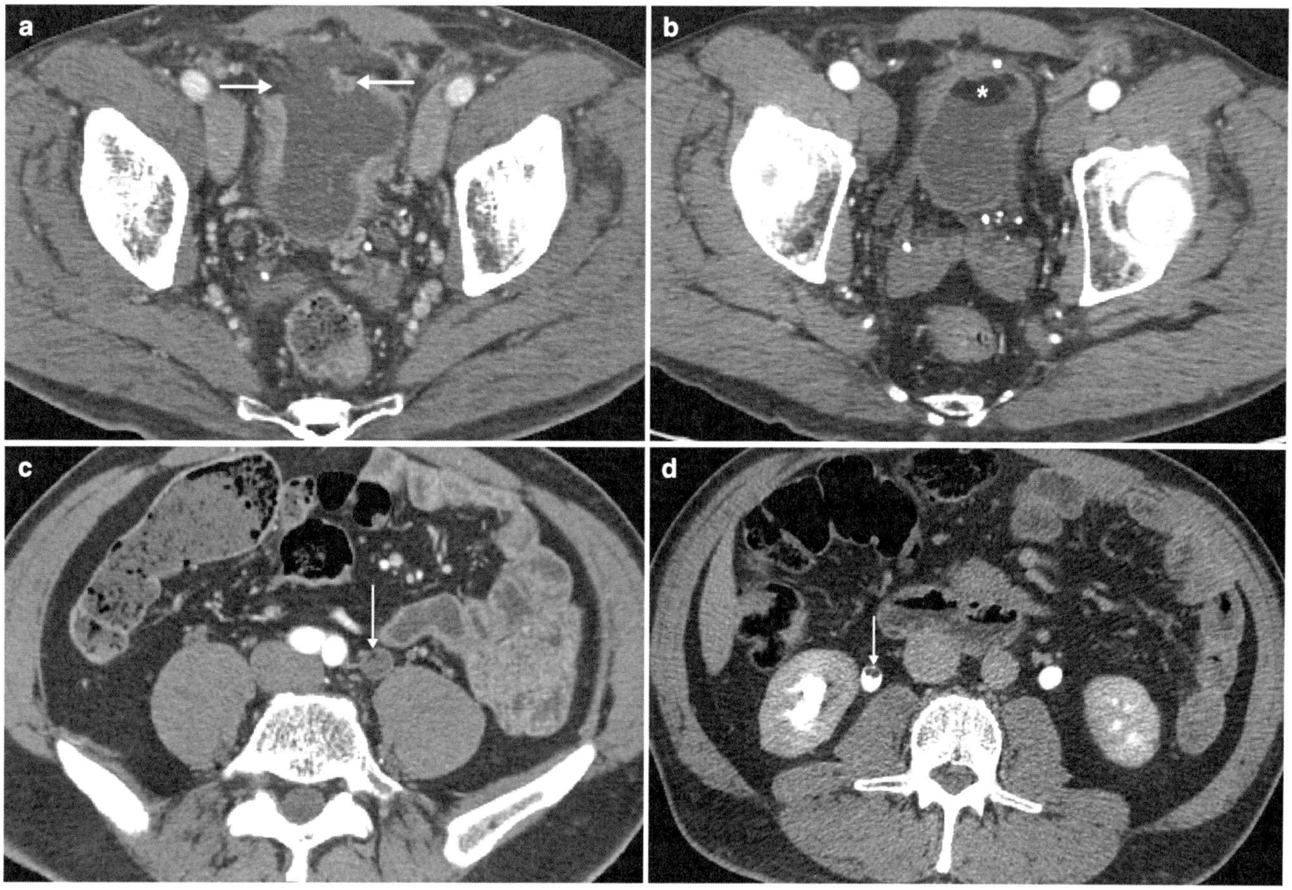

Fig. 2.13 A 58-year-old man with history of multifocal recurrent bladder cancer. TURBT at an outside institution was complicated by perforation. CTU showed walled off perforation of the bladder and bilateral hydroureteronephrosis. Mobile nondependent fat in the right collecting system and intraluminal fat in the urinary bladder near the dome. (**a**) Axial parenchymal phase image shows anterior bladder wall defect (*arrows*). (a) Axial late arterial phase shows intraluminal pelvic fat (*asterisk*) within the bladder. (**c**) Axial parenchymal phase image shows a punctate focus of fat within the left ureter anteriorly (*arrow*). (**d**) Axial excretory phase image at the level of the proximal right ureter shows nondependent intraluminal fat (*arrow*) confirmed by density measurements on earlier phases anterior to opacified urine. Follow-up CT scan 6 months later showed near complete closure of the bladder defect. Although small and clinically innocuous bladder perforations may be encountered in up to 58 % of patients undergoing transurethral resection [38], large perforations requiring open surgical repair are rare. Despite its potential for associated morbidity, bladder perforation does not seem to substantially increase the risk of extravesical tumor seeding [39]

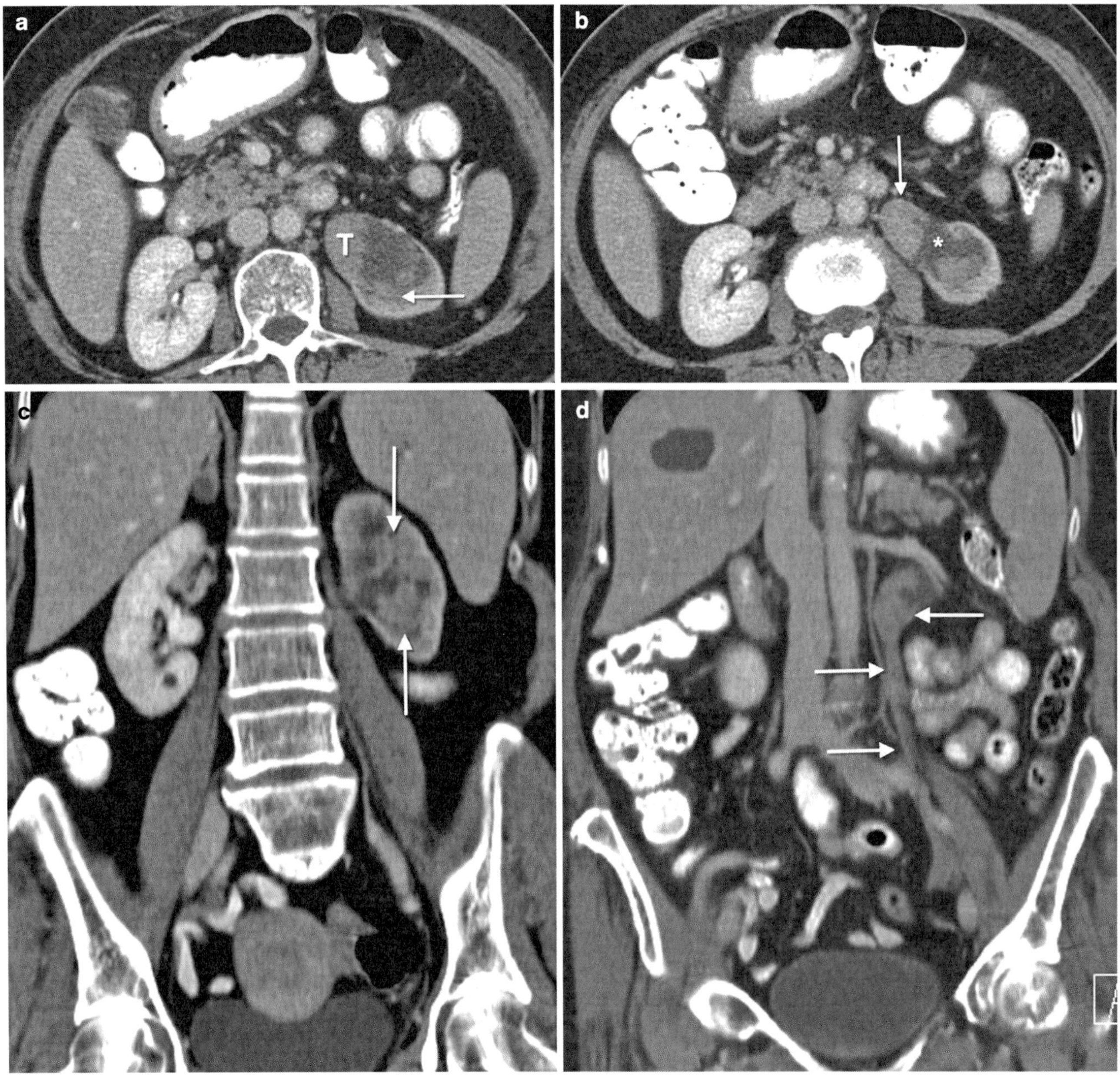

Fig. 2.14 A 70-year-old woman with history of hematuria. CT revealed a lobulated infiltrative appearing mass within the left renal pelvis, calyces, and proximal ureter. By CT imaging, invasion of the parenchyma was suspected. Patient underwent radical nephroureterectomy with histopathology revealing high-grade flat and papillary multifocal urothelial cancer in the renal pelvis and calyces with invasion of the lamina propria, stage pT1N0M0. (**a**) Axial parenchymal phase image shows irregular enhancing left collecting system tumor (*T*) with poorly defined margins posteriorly (*arrow*) suspicious for renal parenchymal involvement. (**b**) Axial parenchymal phase image at the level of the left renal pelvis shows tumor extension (*arrow*) into renal pelvis. Left hydronephrosis (*asterisk*) is present. (**c**) Coronal MPR parenchymal phase image showing extensive tumor (*arrows*) filling the dilated left collecting system at the level of the left kidney. (**d**) Coronal MPR parenchymal phase image of the left ureter demonstrates extensive ureteral tumor (*arrows*) to the pelvic inlet

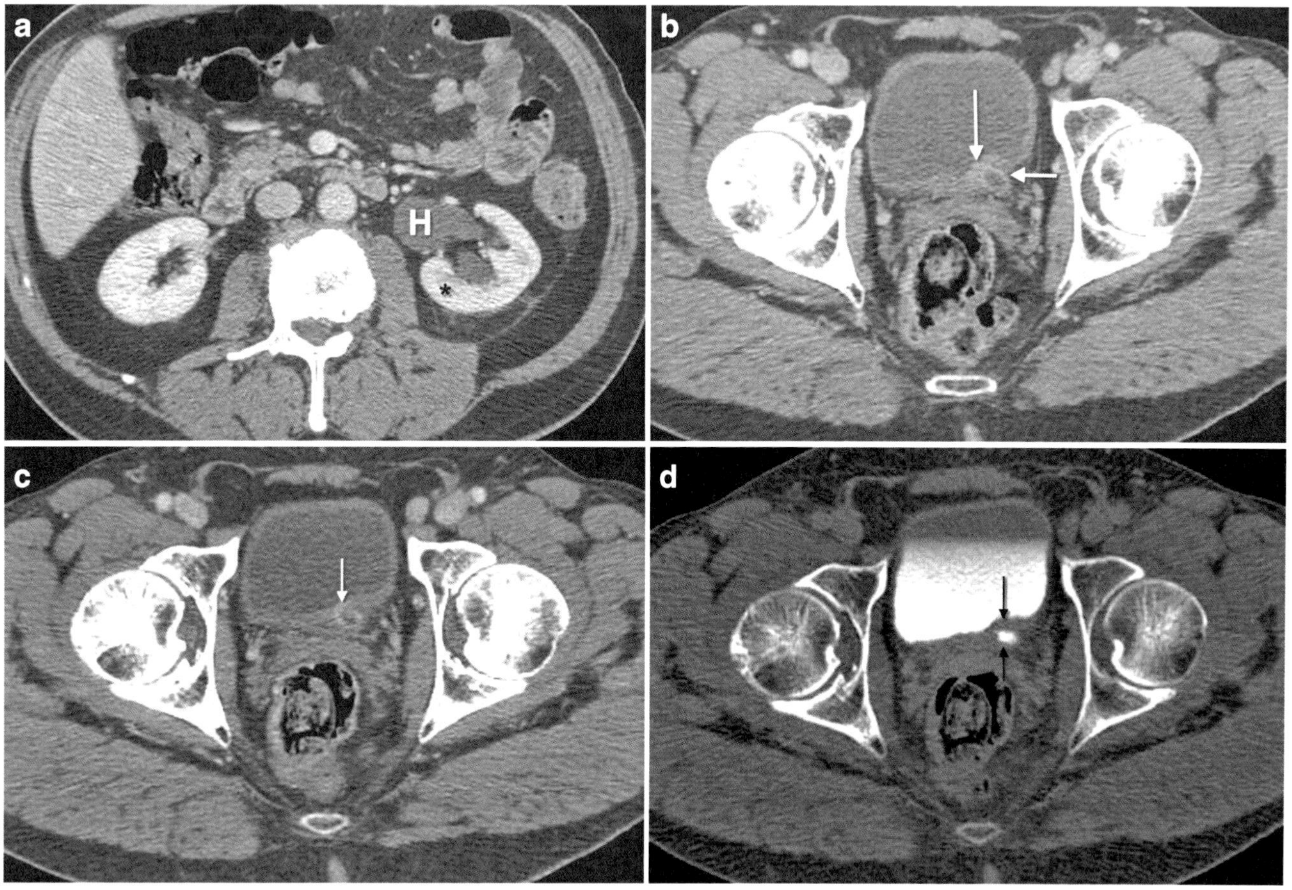

Fig. 2.15 A 64-year-old man with recurrent high-grade Ta and Tis of the bladder refractory to induction treatments with BCG, presenting with left hydronephrosis. (**a**) Axial parenchymal phase image at the level of the kidney shows moderate left hydronephrosis (*H*) and subtly delayed nephrogram (*asterisk*). (**b**) Axial parenchymal phase image at the level of the left ureteral vesicle junction (UVJ) shows thickening and enhancement of the urothelium (*arrows*). (**c**) Axial parenchymal phase image at slightly more inferior level shows avidly enhancing abnormal thickened urothelium at the left UVJ (*arrow*). (**d**) Axial excretory phase image at the level of the VUJ confirms circumferential wall thickening (*arrows*). Patient underwent radical cystoprostatectomy with resection of the distal ureter and nodal dissection confirmed noninvasive high-grade urothelial carcinoma pathologic stage Tis. Patients with CIS that involves the ureteral margin are at increased risk for upper tract recurrence and progression with an ipsilateral recurrence rate of up to 42 %. Aggressive follow-up with scheduled ureteroscopy may identify recurrences at an earlier stage [40]

References

1. Munoz JJ, Ellison LM. Upper tract urothelial neoplasms: incidence and survival during the last 2 decades. J Urol. 2000;164:1523–5.
2. Guinan P, Vogelzang NJ, Randazzo R, et al. Renal pelvic cancer: a review of 611 patients treated in Illinois 1975–1985. Cancer incidence and End results committee. Urology. 1992;40:393–9.
3. Gittes RF. Management of transitional cell carcinoma of the upper tract: case for conservative local excision. Urol Clin North Am. 1980;7:559–68.
4. Wong-You-Cheong JJ, Wagner BJ, Davis Jr CJ. Transitional cell carcinoma of the urinary tract: radiologic-pathologic correlation. Radiographics. 1998;18:123–42. quiz 148.
5. Vogelzang N. Comprehensive textbook of genitourinary oncology. 2nd ed. Philadelphia: Lippincott Williams & Wilkins; 2000. p. 1177. xxxiii.
6. Radovanovic Z, Jankovic S, Jevremovic I. Incidence of tumors of urinary organs in a focus of Balkan endemic nephropathy. Kidney Int Suppl. 1991;34:S75–6.
7. Ross RK, Paganini-Hill A, Landolph J, et al. Analgesics, cigarette smoking, and other risk factors for cancer of the renal pelvis and ureter. Cancer Res. 1989;49:1045–8.
8. Kobayashi S, Ohmori M, Akaeda T, et al. Primary adenocarcinoma of the renal pelvis. Report of two cases and brief review of literature. Acta Pathol Jpn. 1983;33:589–97.
9. Talwar N, Dargan P, Arora MP, et al. Primary squamous cell carcinoma of the renal pelvis masquerading as pyonephrosis: a case report. Indian J Pathol Microbiol. 2006;49:418–20.
10. Kirkali Z, Tuzel E. Transitional cell carcinoma of the ureter and renal pelvis. Crit Rev Oncol Hematol. 2003;47:155–69.
11. Vikram R, Sandler CM, Ng CS. Imaging and staging of transitional cell carcinoma: part 2, upper urinary tract. AJR Am J Roentgenol. 2009;192:1488–93.
12. American Joint Committee on Cancer. Purposes and principles of staging. In: Edge SB, Byrd DR, Compton CC, editors. AJCC Cancer Staging Manual. 7th ed. New York, NY: Springer; 2010.
13. Arocena García-Tapia J, Zudaire Bergera JJ, Sanz-Prez G, et al. Upper tract urothelial tumor. Factors that influence survival. Actas Urol Esp. 1999;23:751–6.
14. Argyropoulos AN, Tolley DA. Upper urinary tract transitional cell carcinoma: current treatment overview of minimally invasive approaches. BJU Int. 2007;99:982–7.
15. Brown GA, Matin SF, Busby JE, et al. Ability of clinical grade to predict final pathologic stage in upper urinary tract transitional cell carcinoma: implications for therapy. Urology. 2007;70:252–6.
16. Nawfel RD, Judy PF, Schleipman AR, Silverman SG. Patient radiation dose at CT urography and conventional urography. Radiology. 2004;232:126–32.
17. Martingano P, Stacul F, Cavallaro MF, et al. 64-Slice CT urography: optimisation of radiation dose. Radiol Med. 2011;116:417–31.
18. Sadow CA, Silverman SG, O'Leary MP, Signorovitch JE. Bladder cancer detection with CT urography in an academic medical center. Radiology. 2008;249:195–202.
19. Silverman S, Leyendecker J, Amis EJ. What is the current role of CT urography and MR urography in the evaluation of the urinary tract? Radiology. 2009;250:309–23.
20. Tawfiek ER, Bagley DH. Upper-tract transitional cell carcinoma. Urology. 1997;50:321–9.
21. Oldbring J, Glifberg I, Mikulowski P, Hellsten S. Carcinoma of the renal pelvis and ureter following bladder carcinoma: frequency, risk factors and clinicopathological findings. J Urol. 1989;141:1311–3.
22. Charbit L, Gendreau MC, Mee S, Cukier J. Tumors of the upper urinary tract: 10 years of experience. J Urol. 1991;146:1243–6.
23. Kundu SD, Eggener SE. Retroperitoneal lymph nodes in transitional cell carcinoma of the kidney and ureter. Adv Urol. 2009;1819–27.
24. Viprakasit DP, Macejko AM, Nadler RB. Laparoscopic nephroureterectomy and management of the distal ureter: a review of current techniques and outcomes. Adv Urol. 2009;721371.
25. O'Donnell PH, Stadler WM. The role of chemotherapy in upper tract urothelial carcinoma. Adv Urol. 2009;419028.
26. Takahashi N, Kawashima A, Glockner J, et al. MR urography for suspected upper tract urothelial carcinoma. Eur Radiol. 2009; 19:912–23.
27. Kundra V, Silverman PM. Imaging in the diagnosis, staging, and follow-up of cancer of the urinary bladder. Am J Roentgenol. 2003;180:1045–54.
28. Tran W, Serio AM, Raj GV, et al. Longitudinal risk of upper tract recurrence following radical cystectomy for urothelial cancer and the potential implications for long-term surveillance. J Urol. 2008; 179:96–100.
29. Sanderson KM, Cai J, Miranda G, et al. Upper tract urothelial recurrence following radical cystectomy for transitional cell carcinoma of the bladder: an analysis of 1069 patients with 10-year followup. J Urol. 2007;177:2088–94.
30. Chlapoutakis K, Theocharopoulos N, Yarmenitis S, Damilakis J. Performance of computed tomographic urography in diagnosis of upper urinary tract urothelial carcinoma, in patients presenting with hematuria: systematic review and meta-analysis. Eur J Radiol. 2010;73:334–8.
31. Prando A, Prando P, Prando D. Urothelial cancer of the renal pelvicaliceal system: unusual imaging manifestations. Radiographics. 2010;30:1553–66.
32. Datta SN, Allen GM, Evans R, et al. Urinary tract ultrasonography in the evaluation of haematuria—a report of over 1000 cases. Ann R Coll Surg Engl. 2002;84:203–5.
33. Browne RFJ, Meehan CP, Colville J, et al. Transitional cell carcinoma of the upper urinary tract: spectrum of imaging findings. Radiographics. 2005;25:1609–27.
34. Strong DW, Pearse HD. Recurrent urothelial tumors following surgery for transitional cell carcinoma of the upper urinary tract. Cancer. 1976;38:2173–83.
35. Lokeshwar VB, Selzer MG. Urinary bladder tumor markers. Urol Oncol. 2006;24:528–37.
36. Ma W, Kang SK, Hricak H, et al. Imaging appearance of granulomatous disease after intravesical bacille calmette-guerin (BCG) treatment of bladder carcinoma. Am J Roentgenol. 2009;192: 1494–500.
37. Rouprêt M, Harmon JD, Sanderson KM, et al. Laparoscopic distal ureterectomy and anastomosis for management of low-risk upper urinary tract transitional cell carcinoma: preliminary results. BJU Int. 2007;99:623–7.
38. Balbay MD, ÇImentepe E, ÜNsal ALI, et al. The actual incidence of bladder perforation following transurethral bladder surgery. J Urol. 2005;174:2260–3.
39. Golan S, Baniel J, Lask D, et al. Transurethral resection of bladder tumour complicated by perforation requiring open surgical repair—clinical characteristics and oncological outcomes. BJU Int. 2011;107:1065–8.
40. Palou J, Salvador J, MillÁN F, et al. Management of superficial transitional cell carcinoma in the intramural ureter: what to do? J Urol. 2000;163:744–7.

Bladder Cancer Imaging

3

Yulia Lakhman, Joshua Chaim, and Michael J. Sohn

Bladder cancer is the second-most common genitourinary malignant disease in the United States, with an estimated 70,530 newly diagnosed cases and 14,680 cancer-related deaths in 2010. The incidence of bladder cancer increases with age, peaking between 50 and 70 years old. It is three times more common in men than in women, and twice more frequent in Caucasians than in African Americans [1].

Bladder cancer has several risk factors, though many cases occur with no apparent inciting exposures (see Table 3.1) [2]. Cigarette smoking is the most important environmental risk factor for the development of urothelial carcinoma. Heavy smokers (>40 pack years) are five times more likely to develop urothelial carcinoma than nonsmokers [3]. Occupational and environmental exposure to chemicals such as aromatic amines, aniline dyes, coal, and arsenic in drinking water is the second most important risk factor accounting for increased incidence of urothelial carcinoma among workers in the painting, leather, rubber, metal, and automotive industries [4].

Chronic bladder irritation from recurrent urinary tract infections (including bladder infestation by the *Schistosoma haematobium* parasite in endemic areas), indwelling catheters or bladder stones, and neurogenic bladder with superimposed chronic cystitis are associated with increased risk of squamous cell carcinoma (SCC). Persistent urachal remnant and cystitis glandularis in the setting of the bladder extrophy are risk factors for adenocarcinoma [5].

Prior pelvic irradiation also increases subsequent risk of bladder cancer [6]. No strong epidemiologic evidence exists to support a hereditary cause of most bladder cancers [2].

Y. Lakhman, M.D. • J. Chaim, DO
Department of Radiology, Memorial Sloan-Kettering Cancer Center, 303 East 66 Street, Room 703, New York, NY, 10065, USA
e-mail: lakhmany@mskcc.org; chaimj@mskcc.org

M.J. Sohn (✉)
Department of Radiology, Breast and Imaging Center, Memorial Sloan-Kettering Cancer Center, 1275 York Avenue, New York, NY, 10065, USA
e-mail: sohnmj@mskcc.org

Table 3.1 Risk factors associated with bladder cancer

Risk factors
Tobacco use
Exposure to aromatic amines and aniline dyes
Arsenic ingestion
Cyclophosphamide treatment
Recurrent severe urinary tract infections, indwelling catheters, or stones (squamous cell carcinoma)
Schistosomiasis (squamous cell carcinoma)
Urachal remnant and cystitis glandularis/bladder extrophy (adenocarcinoma)
Pelvic Radiation

Diagnosis

Anatomy

The urinary bladder wall consists of four layers: (1) urothelium lining the bladder lumen; (2) the vascular lamina propria; (3) the muscularis propria consisting of bundles of smooth detrusor muscle; and (4) the outermost adventitia formed by the connective tissue. The bladder is surrounded by pelvic fat and its dome is covered by the peritoneum.

More than 95 % of bladder tumors arise from the urothelium. They include urothelial carcinomas (>90 %), squamous cell carcinomas (5 %), and adenocarcinomas (<2 %). Other rare epithelial tumors are metastases, small cell or neuroendocrine carcinoma, carcinoid tumors, and melanoma.

Less than 5 % of bladder tumors are mesenchymal in origin. Benign mesenchymal bladder tumors include leiomyoma (most common), paraganglioma, fibroma, plasmocytoma, hemangioma, solitary fibrous tumor, neurofibroma, and lipoma. Malignant mesenchymal bladder tumors are rhabdomyosarcoma, leiomyosarcoma, lymphoma, and osteosarcoma.

Presentation

Bladder cancer may be detected incidentally or because of symptoms. Found in about 85 % of patients, intermittent

A.M. Bach, J. Zhang (eds.), *Atlas of Genitourinary Oncological Imaging*, Atlas of Oncology Imaging, DOI 10.1007/978-1-4614-4872-3_3, © Springer Science+Business Media New York 2013

gross painless hematuria is the most common presenting symptom. Unexplained irritative voiding symptoms such as increased urinary frequency, urgency, or dysuria may also be a sign of bladder cancer, particularly carcinoma in situ (Tis). Flank pain and other symptoms related to hydronephrosis can be present with tumors involving the ureterovesical junction.

Staging

Clinical Staging

Clinical staging of bladder cancer is an important but imperfect evaluation with a 30–50 % rate of understaging at the time of cystectomy [7]. When bladder cancer is suspected, the initial work-up consists of voided urine cytology, cystoscopy, and radiological evaluation of the upper tracts with computed tomography urography (CTU) or magnetic resonance urography (MRU). Voided urine cytology is the noninvasive diagnostic test of choice but suffers from low sensitivity, particularly for low-grade tumors [8]. Conventional or white-light cystoscopy—with endoscopic evaluation of the bladder and urethra—is the "gold standard" for the detection of bladder cancer. Tissue from any suspicious area is removed with either bladder biopsy or transurethral resection of bladder tumor (TURBT).

TURBT should include muscularis propria, especially if the tumor is high grade or lamina propria is involved. If TURBT demonstrates lamina propria invasion but the specimen does not have sufficient muscularis propria, a repeat resection is required to exclude muscle-invasive disease. A second TURBT should be considered in all patients with high-grade or lamina propria invasive tumors to prevent understaging and possible progression to metastatic disease [9].

During TURBT, a bimanual examination is done to assess the degree of mobility of the bladder and other pelvic organs. In the setting of muscle-invasive disease, a metastatic work-up should be performed including chest, abdomen, and pelvic CT, liver function tests, and assessment of serum creatine and electrolytes.

Table 3.2 TNM staging of bladder cancer

Primary Tumor (T)
Tx Primary tumor cannot be assessed
T0 No evidence of primary tumor
Ta Noninvasive papillary carcinoma
Tis Carcinoma in situ: "flat tumor"
T1 Tumor invades subepithelial connective tissue
T2 Tumor invades muscularis propria
pT2a Tumor invades superficial muscularis propria (inner half)
pT2b Tumor invades deep muscularis propria (outer half)
T3 Tumor invades perivesicular fat
pT3a Microscopically
pT3b Macroscopically (extravesical mass)
T4 Tumor invades any of the following: prostatic stroma, seminal vesicles, uterus, vagina, pelvic wall, or abdominal wall
T4a Tumor invades prostatic stroma, uterus, or vagina
T4b Tumor invades pelvic wall or abdominal wall
Regional Lymph Nodes (N)
Nx Lymph nodes cannot be accessed
N0 No lymph node metastasis
N1 Single regional lymph node metastasis in the true pelvis (internal iliac, obturator, external iliac, or presacral lymph node metastasis)
N2 Multiple regional lymph node metastasis in the true pelvis
N3 Lymph node metastasis to the common iliac lymph nodes
Distant Metastasis (M)
M0 No distant metastasis
M1 Distant metastasis

Table 3.3 Anatomic stage/prognostic groups

Stage 0a
Ta, N0, M0
Stage 0is
Tis, N0, M0
Stage I
T1, N0, M0
Stage II
T2a, N0, M0
T2b, N0, M0
Stage III
T3a, N0, M0
T3b, N0, M0
T4a, N0, M0
Stage IV
T4b, N0, M0
Any T, N1-3, M0
Any T, Any N, M1

Pathologic Staging

Histologic staging of bladder cancer is determined by the tumor-node-metastasis (TNM) staging system (see Tables 3.2 and 3.3). Tumor (T) stage is based on the extent of primary tumor penetration into the bladder wall [10].

Urothelial carcinomas comprise the vast majority of bladder tumors (90 %) and are classified into four categories by the World Health Organization (WHO) and the International Society of Urologic Pathology consensus: (1) papilloma; (2) papillary urothelial neoplasm of low malignant potential; (3) low-grade carcinoma; and (4) high-grade carcinoma [11].

Of all newly diagnosed urothelial carcinomas, 70 % present as non–muscle-invasive (superficial) tumors (stages Ta, Tis, or T1) and 30 % as muscularis propria invasive disease (stages T2–T4), which is associated with a high risk of distant metastases. Around 50–70 % of non-muscle-invasive tumors recur and 10–20 % progress to muscularis propria invasive disease [7]. It remains a challenge to predict which patients will progress from non–muscle-invasive to muscle-invasive disease.

The TNM staging system provides important prognostic information that helps to predict outcome and guide clinical management. Several additional predictive factors (not included in the TNM staging system) such as tumor grade, multifocality, recurrence at 3 months, presence of Tis, and size of the initial tumor (>3 cm) should also be considered in the clinical decision making [12, 13].

Management

Non–muscle-Invasive Bladder Cancer

Current data suggest that patients with all types of non–muscle-invasive bladder cancer benefit from one-time intravesical instillation of a chemotherapeutic agent immediately after TURBT because of the decrease in the rate of recurrence [14].

Patients with high-risk disease (high-grade Ta, multifocal Tis, T1 tumors with associated Tis, and tumors that rapidly recur after TURBT) are candidates for further adjuvant intravesical drug therapy. Compared to other chemotherapeutic agents, intravesical Bacillus Calmette-Guerin (BCG) therapy is the most effective in the prevention of recurrence, but its role in slowing down disease progression is controversial [15, 16].

Close clinical follow-up is required for patients with non–muscle-invasive bladder cancer because of a high rate of recurrence and a risk of disease progression. After initial TURBT, patients should have follow-up cystoscopy and voided urine cytology every 3 months for 2 years, then every 6 months for 2 years, and then annually indefinitely. Upper tract imaging should be done every 12–24 months because of the 5 % lifetime risk for development of upper tract urothelial carcinoma after a diagnosis of bladder cancer [17].

Muscle-Invasive Bladder Cancer

The standard treatment for muscularis propria invasive bladder cancer is radical cystoprostatectomy in men and anterior exenteration (including the bladder, urethra, uterus, and anterior vaginal wall) in women. Additionally, in men, urethrectomy is performed if the prostatic stroma is invaded or Tis is present. In women, the uterus, vagina, and urethra are occasionally spared if they are uninvolved by the tumor and an orthotopic continent urinary diversion is planned.

Pelvic lymphadenectomy is done in all cases of radical cystectomy. Many investigators also advocate an extended lymphadenectomy that includes aortic bifurcation cranially and presacral lymph nodes caudally because it improves tumor staging and survival [18, 19].

After radical cystectomy, a segment of bowel is used for either noncontinent (ileal conduit) or continent (orthotopic neobladder or an abdominal pouch) urinary diversion. The ileal conduit is usually done in elderly patients with multiple comorbidities and increased operative risk; the continent diversion is preferred in young and healthy patients. At present, the role of neoadjuvant and adjuvant chemotherapy for improving survival is still uncertain [20–23].

Alternative treatment strategies for well-selected patients with muscle-invasive disease who strongly desire bladder preservation include TURBT alone, combined chemotherapy and radiation therapy, or trimodality approach consisting of TURBT, chemotherapy, and radiation. Further studies are needed to determine whether bladder preservation can occur while obtaining survival rates similar to those achieved after radical cystectomy.

Patients with muscle-invasive bladder cancer must be closely followed because up to 50 % of patients undergoing radial cystectomy for urothelial carcinoma will develop local or metastatic recurrence, typically within the first 2–3 years after surgery [24]. According to the National Comprehensive Cancer Network (NCCN) bladder cancer guidelines, after cystectomy patients should have urine cytology, electrolytes, and creatine every 3–6 months as well as upper tract and chest, abdomen, and pelvis imaging every 3–12 months for 2 years based on the risk of recurrence and then as clinically indicated [25].

Imaging Techniques

Table 3.4 Role of imaging

Evaluation of patient with hematuria and detection of urothelial lesions
Intravenous Urography (IVU) has largely been replaced by CT Urography (CTU)
MR Urography is preferred in patients with renal insufficiency
Exception: patients with severely impaired renal function due to concern for nephrogenic systemic fibrosis (NSF)
Pretreatment staging of muscle-invasive bladder cancer
Imaging is indicated only if it will affect clinical management
Purpose of imaging
Assess the extent of local tumor invasion
MRI is superior to contrast-enhanced CT (CE-CT)
Better soft tissue resolution leading to higher accuracy in assessing depth of bladder wall and adjacent organ invasion
Multiplanar capabilities resulting in improved visualization of bladder base and dome tumors
Detection of nodal and distant metastases
At present, CE-CT is the preferred imaging modality
In the future, MRI with ultrasmall superparamagnetic iron oxide (USPIO) contrast agents may improve detection of metastatic lymph nodes
CTU or MRU serves as a one-stop-shop examination
Evaluates upper urinary tract to exclude synchronous urothelial lesions and assesses abdomen and pelvis for nodes and distant metastases
Bone scintigraphy or focused MRI
If bone pain or abnormal biochemical markers (serum calcium and alkaline phosphatase)
Role of ^{18}F-FDG-PET
Refer to Chap. 9
Post-treatment follow-up of patients with non-invasive and muscle-invasive bladder cancer
Detection of post-surgical or post-treatment complications
Evaluation for tumor recurrence or tumor progression
Exclusion of metachronous upper tract and bladder urothelial carcinoma

Table 3.5 CT: imaging techniques

Routine CE-CT is useful for detecting nodal or distant metastases but may be inadequate for detection and staging of urothelial lesions
CTU is a one-stop-shop evaluation
Examines entire urinary tract and diagnoses possible causes of hematuria
Detects and stages upper tract and bladder urothelial lesions
Evaluates the rest of the abdomen and pelvis
Refer to the imaging technique section in chapter 2 for more information on CTU techniques
Virtual cystoscopy
Obtained by manipulating CTU data acquired during the excretory phase through the contrast-filled bladder
Allows navigation within a three-dimensional model
Further investigations are needed to study its added value

Table 3.6 MRI: imaging techniques

Patients should void 1–2 h prior to the scan
Prevents under or overdistention of the urinary bladder which compromise image quality
Phase-array pelvic coil
Improves signal-to-noise ratio
Enables to obtain smaller field-of-view, high resolution images
T1-WI
Helps to demonstrate bladder cancer extension into perivesicular fat and to evaluate for pelvic adenopathy and osseous metastases
T2-WI in three orthogonal planes
Optimizes tumor detection and staging
Plane(s) orthogonal to the tumor-bladder interface most accurately demonstrates the presence and extent of the bladder wall invasion
DWI (b values: 0 and 1,000 s/mm^2)
Potential to improve tumor detection and staging accuracy
Multiphasic contrast-enhanced MRI
Improves tumor detecting and local staging such as assessment of depth of bladder wall invasion and adjacent organ involvement

Normal Anatomy

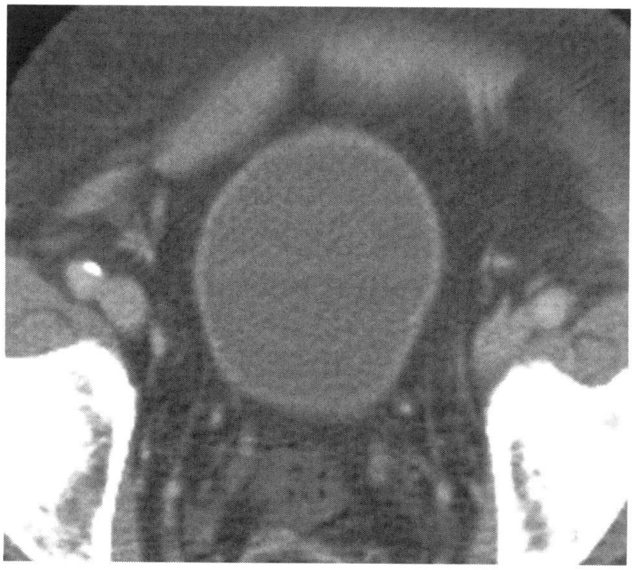

Fig. 3.1 CT appearance of normal urinary bladder. Four layers of the urinary bladder wall (mucosa, submucosa, detrusor muscle, and serosa) are not resolved on CT. As demonstrated on this axial CE-CT image, normal urinary bladder should have smooth wall with thickness varying with distention. Perivesicular fat should be pristine

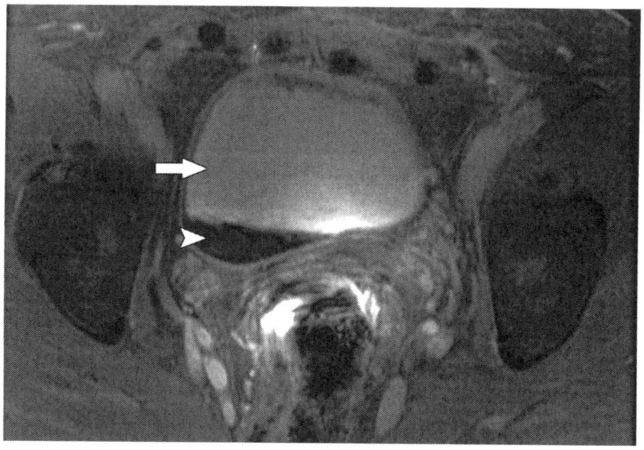

Fig. 3.3 MR illustration of T2-shortening and susceptibility effect of concentrated gadolinium. Gadolinium is a paramagnetic substance and produces both T1 and T2 shortening. As demonstrated on this contrast-enhanced T1-WI image, dilute gadolinium is hyperintense on T1-WI (*arrow*), whereas concentrated gadolinium may have lower SI on T1-WI (*arrowhead*) due to T2-shortening and susceptibility effect

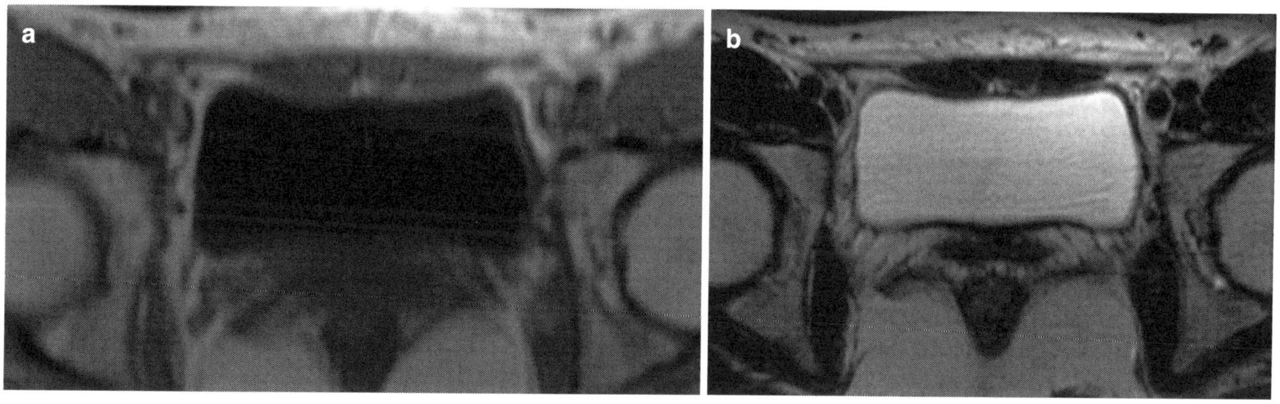

Fig. 3.2 MR appearance of normal bladder. Axial T1 weighted image (**a**) and axial T2-weighted image (**b**). Like other stagnant fluids, urine has low signal intensity (SI) on T1-WI and high SI on T2-WI sequences. Urinary bladder wall has homogenous low-to-intermediate T1 SI and low T2 SI due to dominant detrusor muscle component. Mucosa, submucosa, and serosa are not normally seen as distinct layers. Submucosal edema is hyperintense to detrusor muscle and mildly hypointense to urine on T2-WI. In the presence of submucosal edema, mucosa is seen as thin low SI layer surrounding the bladder lumen. Bladder mucosa, submucosa, and urothelial carcinoma enhance on early dynamic post-contrast images, whereas the detrusor muscle enhances on delayed images

Diagnosis

Table 3.7 Tumor detection [26, 27]

Cystoscopy is the "reference standard"
Detection of bladder cancer with multidetector CTU
Sensitivity 79–93 %
Specificity 91–99 %
High specificity (96 %) and negative predictive value (98 %) of CTU in patients with hematuria and no history of bladder cancer
Normal urinary bladder evaluation on CTU may eliminate the need for further evaluation with cystoscopy
Patients with CTU findings suspicious for bladder cancer may go directly to rigid cystoscopy, biopsy, and/or resection omitting preliminary evaluation with flexible cystoscopy
Accuracy of CTU for bladder cancer detection is substantially lower in patients with a prior bladder cancer (78 %) because of post treatment changes from TURBT or intravesical therapy
In this patient population cystoscopy is the test of choice
Factors limiting detection of bladder cancer on CTU
Bladder underdistention
Pseudo-thickening of the bladder wall
Bladder overdistention
Flattening of some tumors
Tumor characteristics
Size < 1 cm
Carcinoma in situ which is typically plaque-like in appearance
Tumor location
Bladder neck, especially if benign prostatic hypertrophy
DW- MRI is a new useful technique for bladder cancer detection in patients with hematuria and no history of bladder cancer
Tumor appears as high signal intensity mass on high b-value DW-MR images
Sensitivity, 98.1 %; specificity, 92.3 %; PPV, 100 %; NPV, 92.3 %; accuracy, 97 % [28]
Excellent correlation between DW-MRI and cystoscopic findings (k = 0.94) [28]

Imaging Appearance of Urothelial Carcinomas

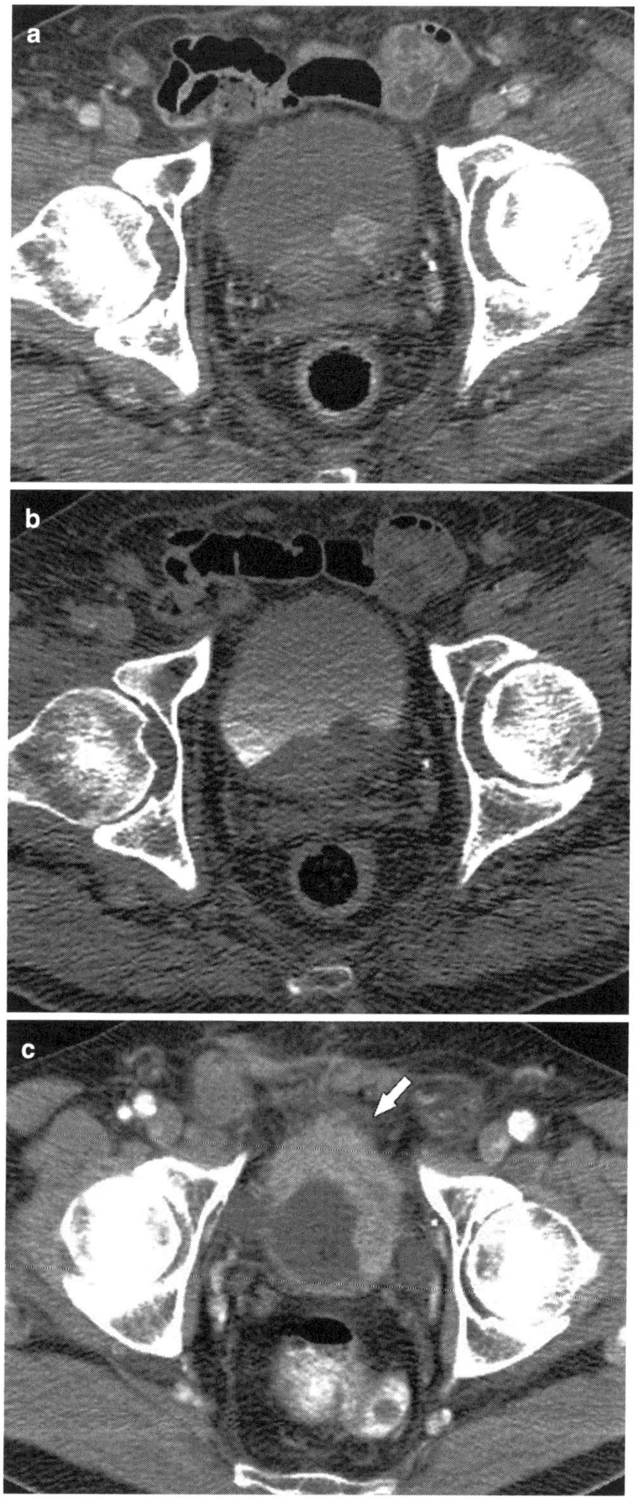

Fig. 3.4 CT illustrations of urothelial carcinoma. Primary tumor may manifest as intraluminal papillary or nodular mass, or plaque-like wall thickening. Images should be acquired 60–80 s after intravenous contrast administration to optimally show tumor enhancement [29]. Axial CTU shows enhancing intraluminal mass on parenchymal phase image (**a**) and nodular filling defect on excretory phase image (**b**). (**c**) Axial parenchymal phase CTU in a different patient demonstrates enhancing thickening of the anterior and left lateral bladder wall. Associated perivesicular fat infiltration (*arrow*) is compatible with pathologically proven tumor invasion into adjacent fat

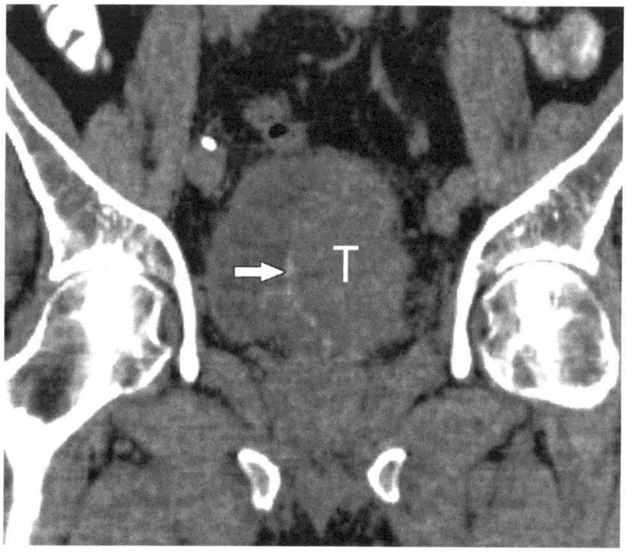

Fig. 3.5 Tumoral calcifications in urothelial carcinoma. Tumoral calcifications may be seen on CT in approximately 5 % of urothelial carcinoma [30]. Calcifications typically encrust the surface of the tumor. Coronal noncontrast CT shows large left intraluminal bladder mass (*T*) with thin peripheral calcifications (*arrow*)

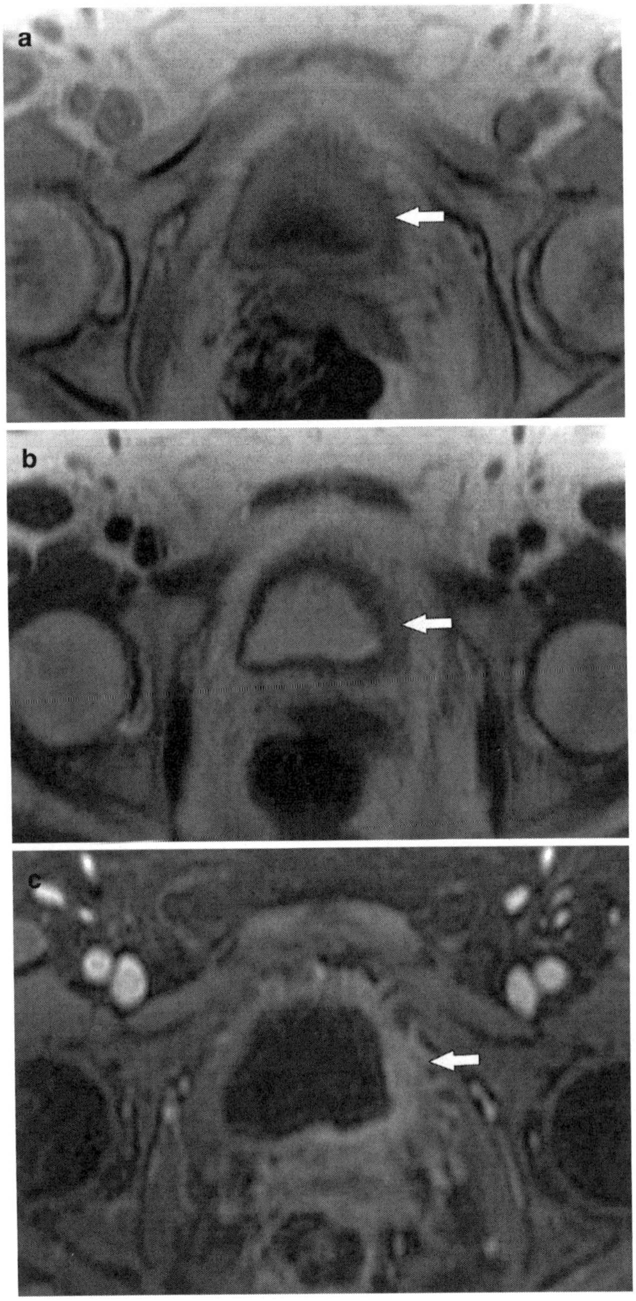

Fig. 3.6 MR illustration of urothelial carcinoma. Urothelial carcinoma is usually isointense to muscle on T1-WI, isointense to slightly hyperintense to muscle on T2-WI, and enhances earlier and more avidly than normal bladder wall or post-biopsy changes such as edema or fibrosis [31]. (**a**) Axial T1-WI shows a small mass with SI similar to that of detrusor muscle (*arrow*). Therefore, it is poorly delineated on this sequence. (**b**) Axial T2-WI demonstrates focal wall thickening that is mildly hyperintense to detrusor muscle (*arrow*). (**c**) Axial CE T1-WI image illustrates left lateral and posterior bladder wall thickening (*arrow*) that enhances greater than normal right lateral bladder wall

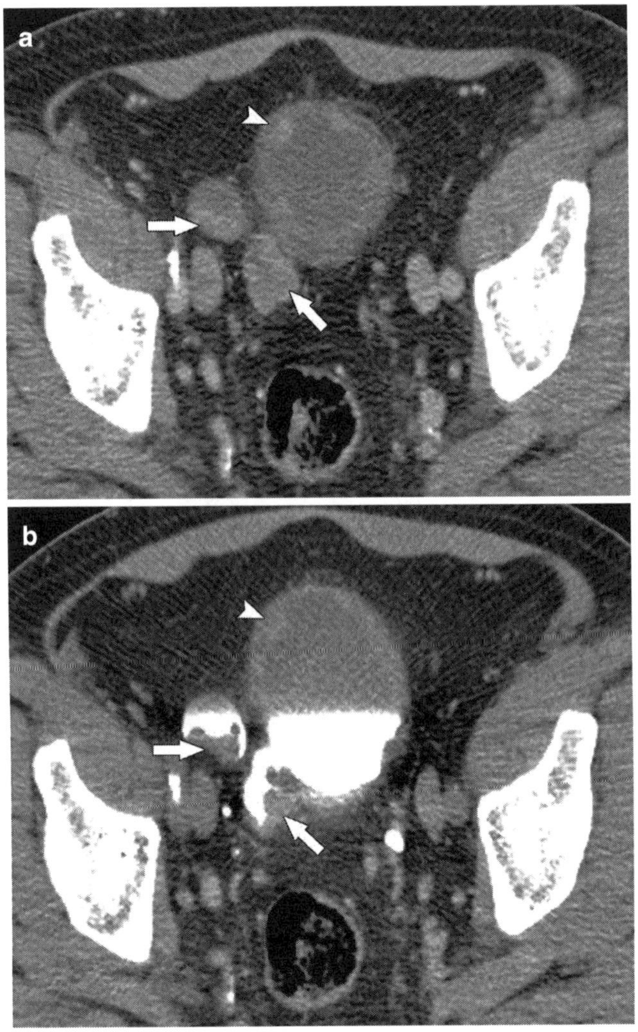

Fig. 3.7 Diverticular urothelial carcinoma. Cross-sectional imaging is useful in detecting neoplasms arising in bladder diverticula, especially when they cannot be accessed at cystoscopy. Bladder diverticula are associated with increased risk of developing bladder cancer (2–10 %), especially urothelial carcinoma, because of urine stasis [32]. Diverticular urothelial carcinoma has worse overall prognosis because of absent muscle layer in the diverticular wall and early tumor invasion into perivesicular fat. (**a**, **b**) Axial parenchymal and excretory phase CTU images show urothelial carcinomas (*arrows*) within bladder diverticula. Additional small intraluminal mass is seen in the anterior bladder wall (*arrowhead*) (Image courtesy of Dr. Robert Lefkowitz, M.D.)

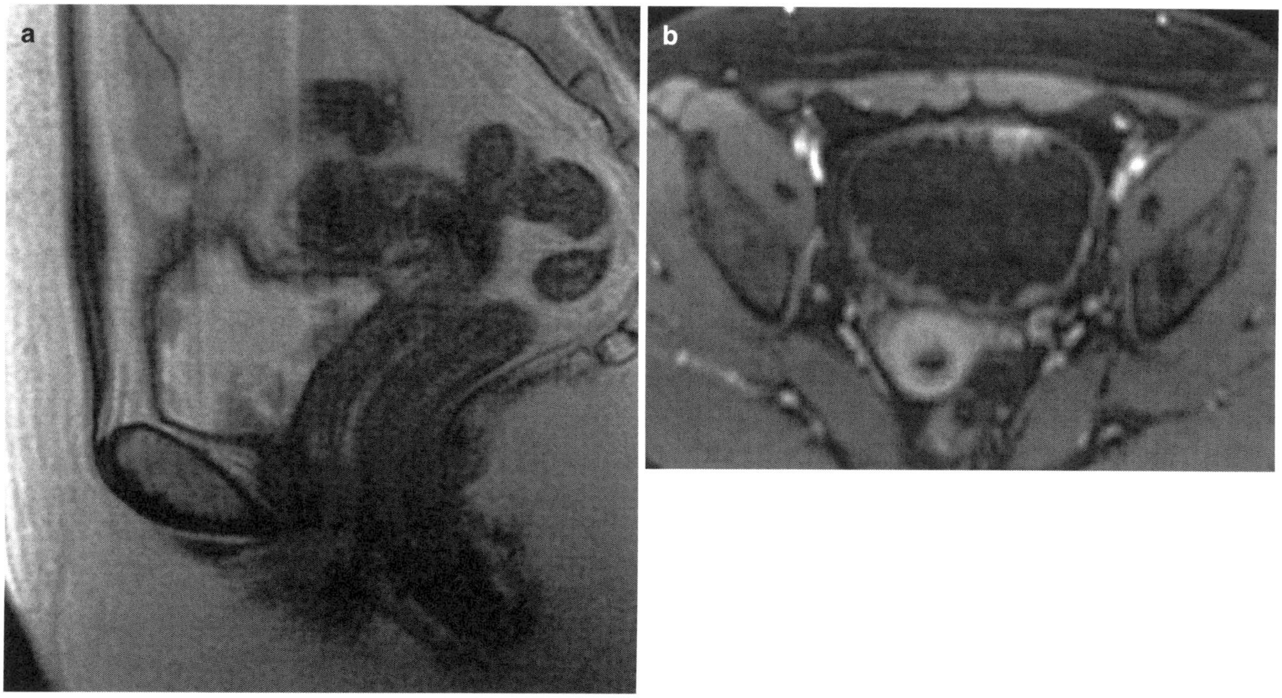

Fig. 3.8 Multicentric urothelial carcinoma. Urothelial carcinoma has a tendency to be multicentric with synchronous and metachronous bladder and upper tract lesions. Multiple bladder tumors are seen in up to 30–40 % of cases [33]. Upper tract tumors occur in 3–5 % of bladder tumor cases and are more common in the setting of multiple bladder lesions [34, 35]. (**a**, **b**) Sagittal T2-WI and axial CE T1-WI demonstrate multiple enhancing intraluminal papillary lesions consistent with synchronous low grade non–muscle-invasive papillary carcinomas

Teaching Points
Urothelial carcinoma is by far the most common bladder tumor.
Urothelial carcinoma has a tendency to be multicentric with synchronous and metachronous bladder and upper tract lesions. It is critical to evaluate the entire urothelium.

Imaging Appearance of Other Select Epithelial Bladder Neoplasms

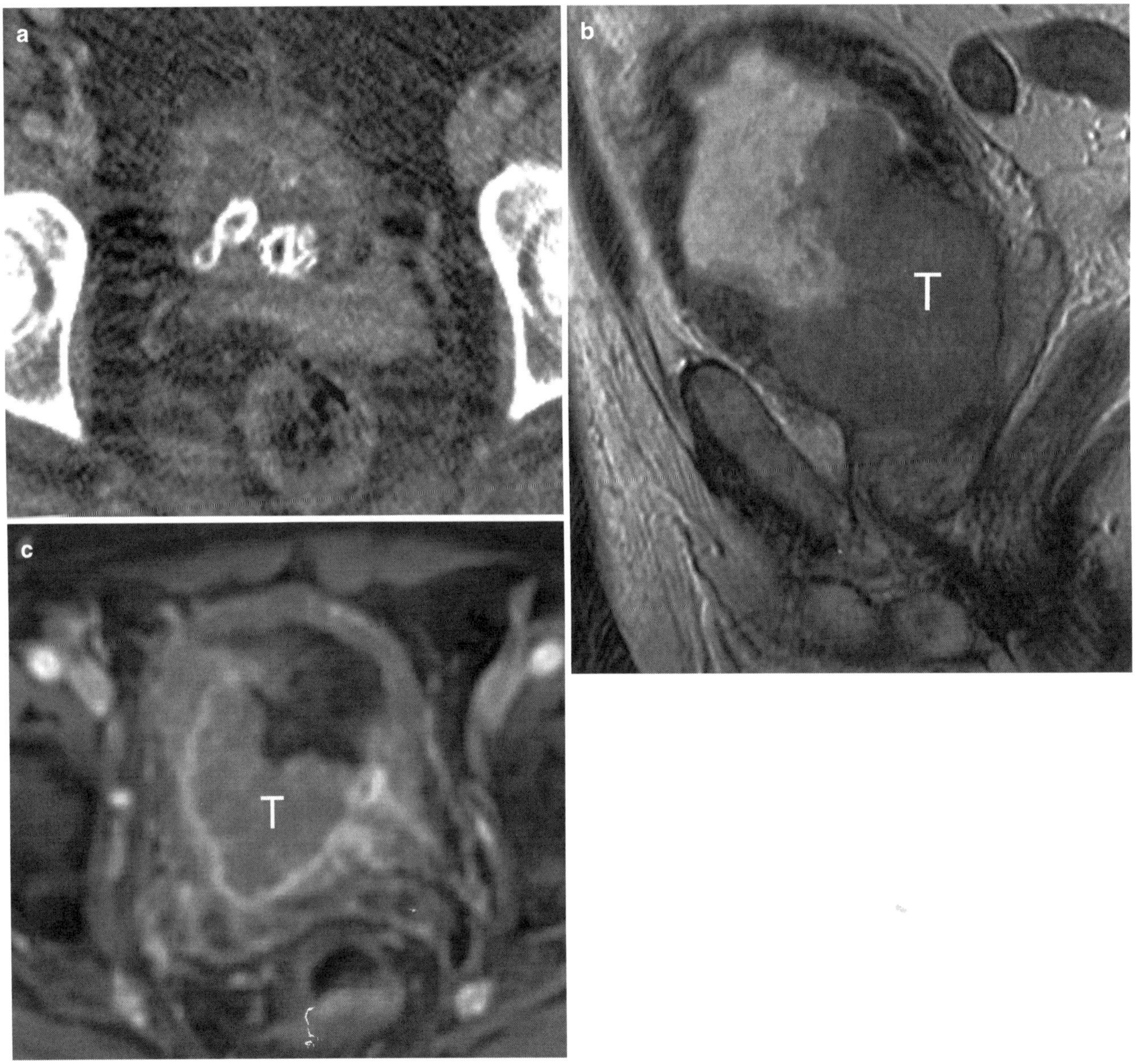

Fig. 3.9 Squamous cell carcinoma. SCC accounts for 5 % of bladder cancers in the United States but is responsible for more than 50 % of bladder tumors in parts of the world where schistosomiasis is endemic [32, 36]. The imaging appearance of SCC is nonspecific. Bladder wall thickening and calcifications from chronic inflammation and/or infection (especially in the setting of schistosomiasis) frequently coexist and make diagnosis more difficult. Muscle invasion is common (about 80 % of cases) and extensive extravesical spread into adjacent organs may be present [37]. (**a**) Axial CE-CT shows partially decompressed urinary bladder with multiple intraluminal calculi, thickened bladder wall due to biopsy-proven SCC, and mild perivesicular fat infiltration from chronic inflammation. (**b**, **c**) Sagittal T2–WI and axial CE T1–WI demonstrate large tumor (*T*) with invasion into perivesicular fat, prostate gland, and right seminal vesicle

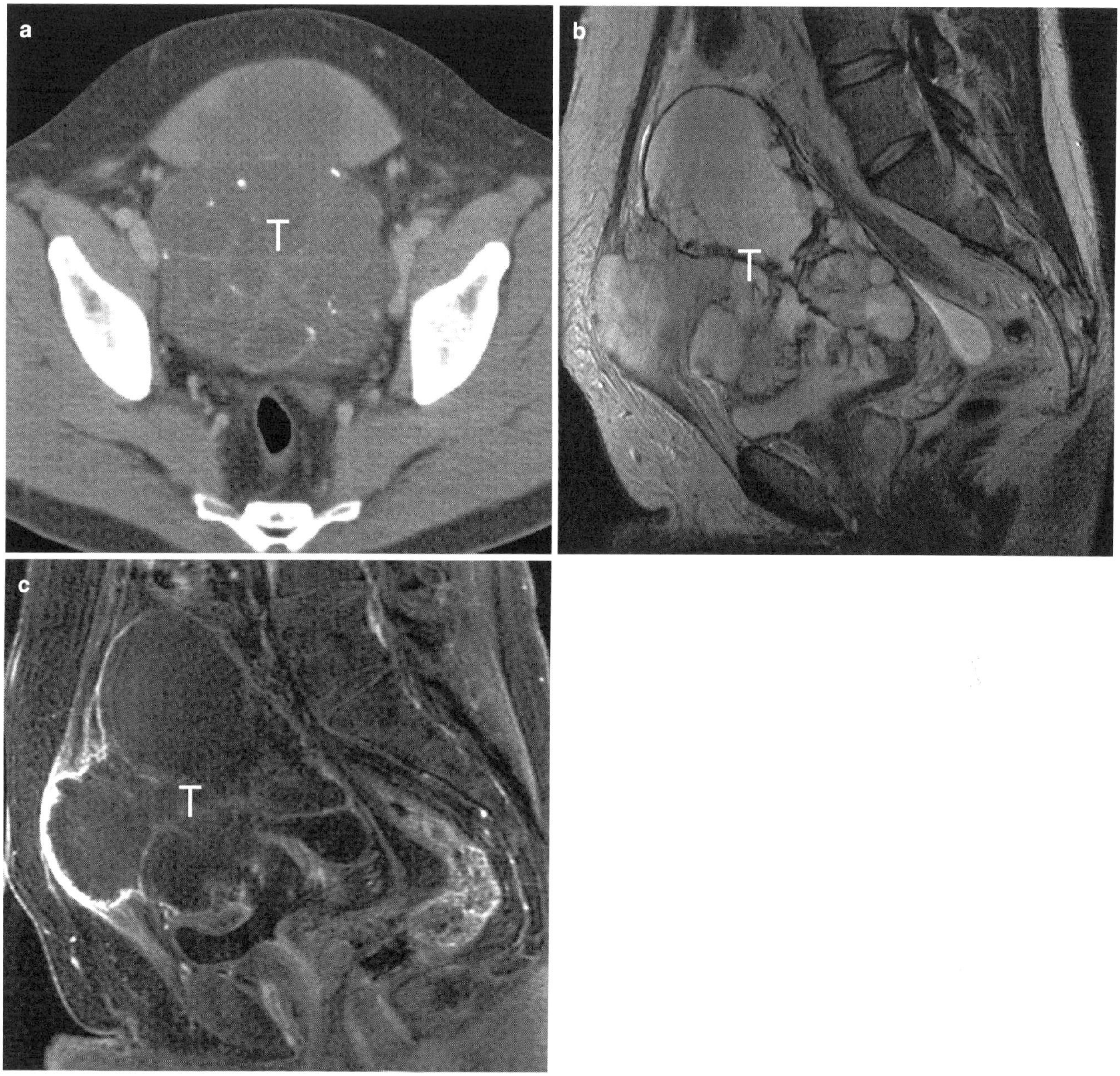

Fig. 3.10 Urachal adenocarcinoma. Adenocarcinomas are rare tumors and represent less than 2 % of bladder cancers. They are subdivided into metastases, as well as primary bladder, and urachal neoplasms. Metastatic adenocarcinoma to the bladder is more common than primary bladder adenocarcinoma. Metastases can invade the bladder by direct extension from other pelvic organs such as the colon, rectum, or prostate gland. Alternatively, metastases may involve the bladder via hematogenous or lymphatic spread from breast, lung, or stomach [38]. Primary adenocarcinomas may be histologically identical to adenocarcinoma of the colon. On CT, diffuse bladder wall thickening and perivesicular fat stranding are common imaging features. Unlike urothelial carcinoma, adenocarcinomas have propensity for peritoneal metastases [39]. Urachal adenocarcinomas are classically large midline, infraumbilical cystic and solid, or solid masses with calcifications. Ninety percent (90 %) of tumors occur near the bladder dome and the rest occur along the course of the urachus or near the umbilicus. (**a**) Axial CE-CT shows a large cystic midline urachal adenocarcinoma with scattered calcifications and cystic areas representing mucin. (**b, c**) Sagittal T2-WI and sagittal CE T1-WI demonstrate the same cystic multiseptate peripherally enhancing tumor (*T*)

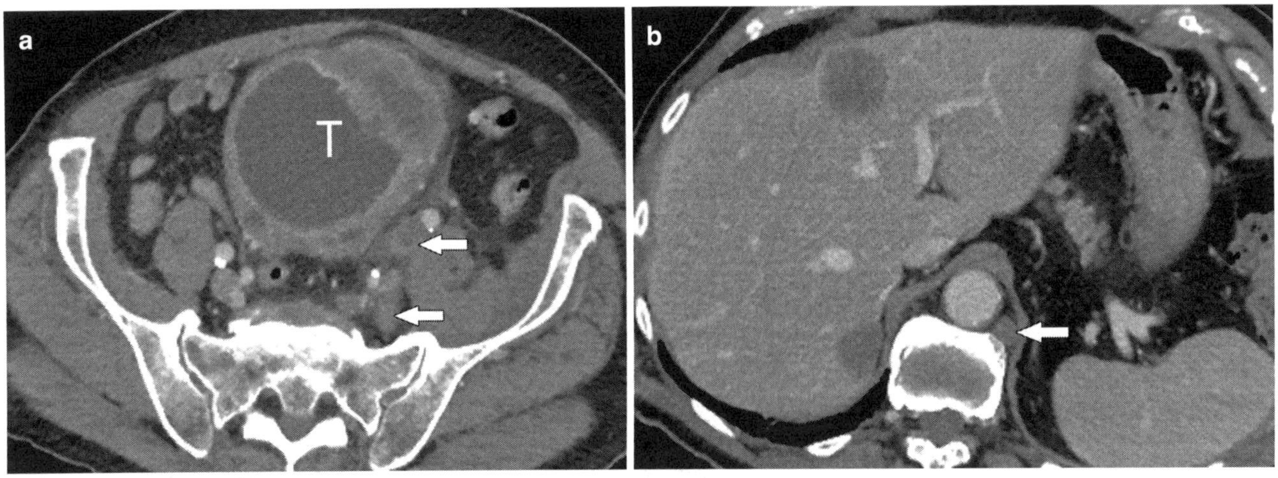

Fig. 3.11 Small cell/neuroendocrine carcinoma. These rare neoplasms are responsible for less than 0.5 % of bladder tumors. At presentation, they are usually large polypoid or nodular masses that may demonstrate central necrosis. Rapid growth with bladder wall and extensive local invasion, as well as peritoneal, lymph node, and distant metastases are common [40]. (**a**) Axial CE-CT illustrates large centrally necrotic bladder tumor (*T*) and metastatic left external and internal iliac lymph nodes (*arrows*). (**b**) Axial CE-CT in the same patient shows enlarged left retrocrural node (*arrow*) and hepatic metastases

Imaging Appearance of Select Nonepithelial (Mesenchymal) Bladder Neoplasms

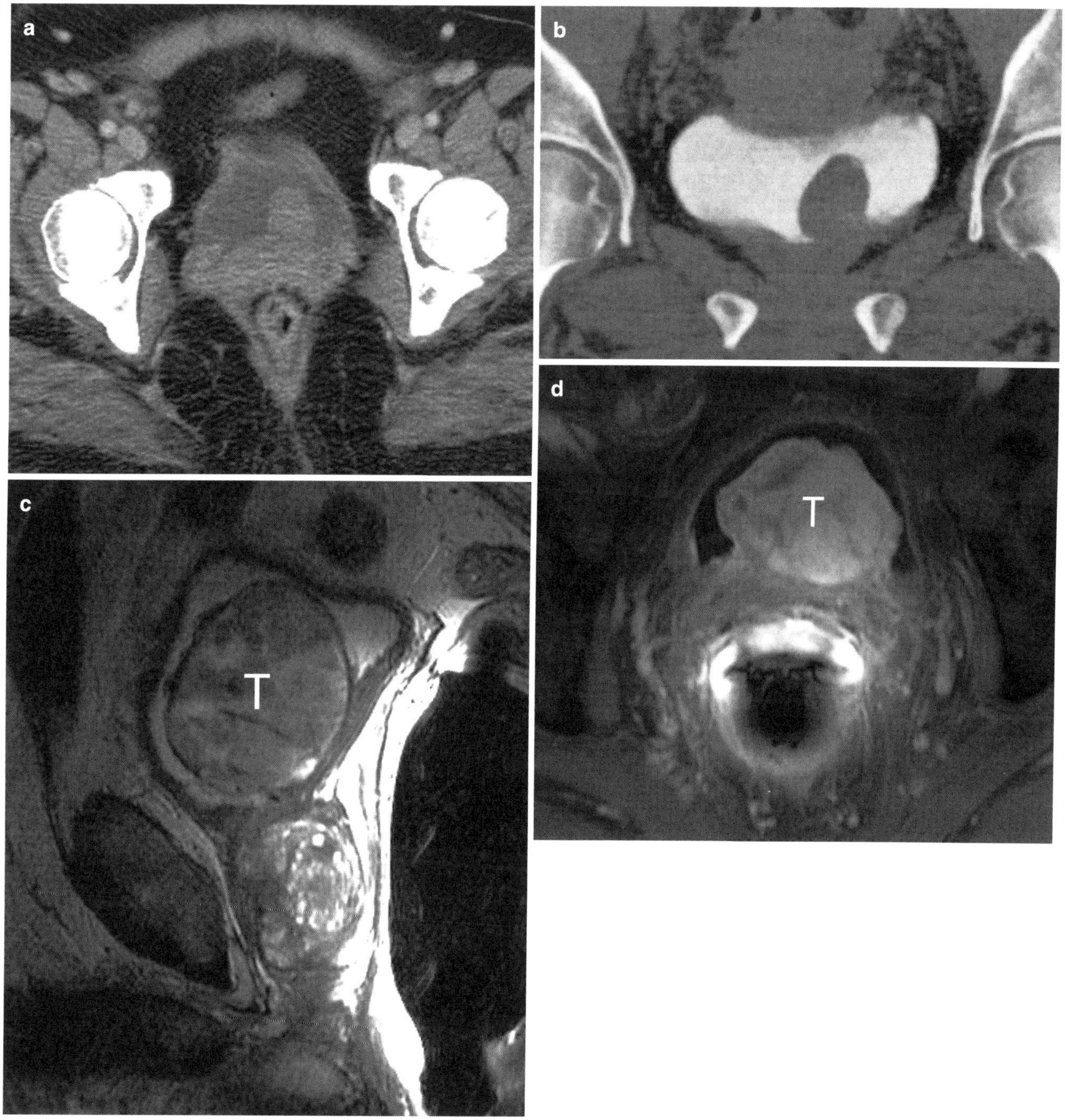

Fig. 3.12 Leiomyoma. Leiomyoma is the common mesenchymal neoplasm of the bladder, but it accounts for less than 0.5 % of all bladder tumors. Leiomyomas are of equal prevalence among both sexes. They are usually asymptomatic except for the large masses that may produce symptoms from mass effect and urinary obstruction. Bladder leiomyomas are submucosal in origin. On CT and MRI they have similar imaging features to uterine fibroids. They are well-circumscribed solid lesions with occasional cystic degeneration producing either smooth indentation of the bladder wall or intraluminal mass. MRI is most specific for characterization of these neoplasms showing their submucosal origin, preserved muscle layer, and low SI on T2-WI images [41]. (**a**, **b**) Axial CTU demonstrates well-circumscribed solid intraluminal mass on axial parenchymal phase image (**a**) and intraluminal filling defect on coronal excretory phase image (**b**). (Images courtesy of Dr. Robert Lefkowitz, M.D.) (**c**, **d**) Sagittal T2-WI and axial CE T1-WI demonstrate well-circumscribed heterogenous T2 SI avidly enhancing submucosal tumor (*T*) extending into the bladder lumen. Areas of increased T2 SI are likely related to cystic degeneration within the tumor

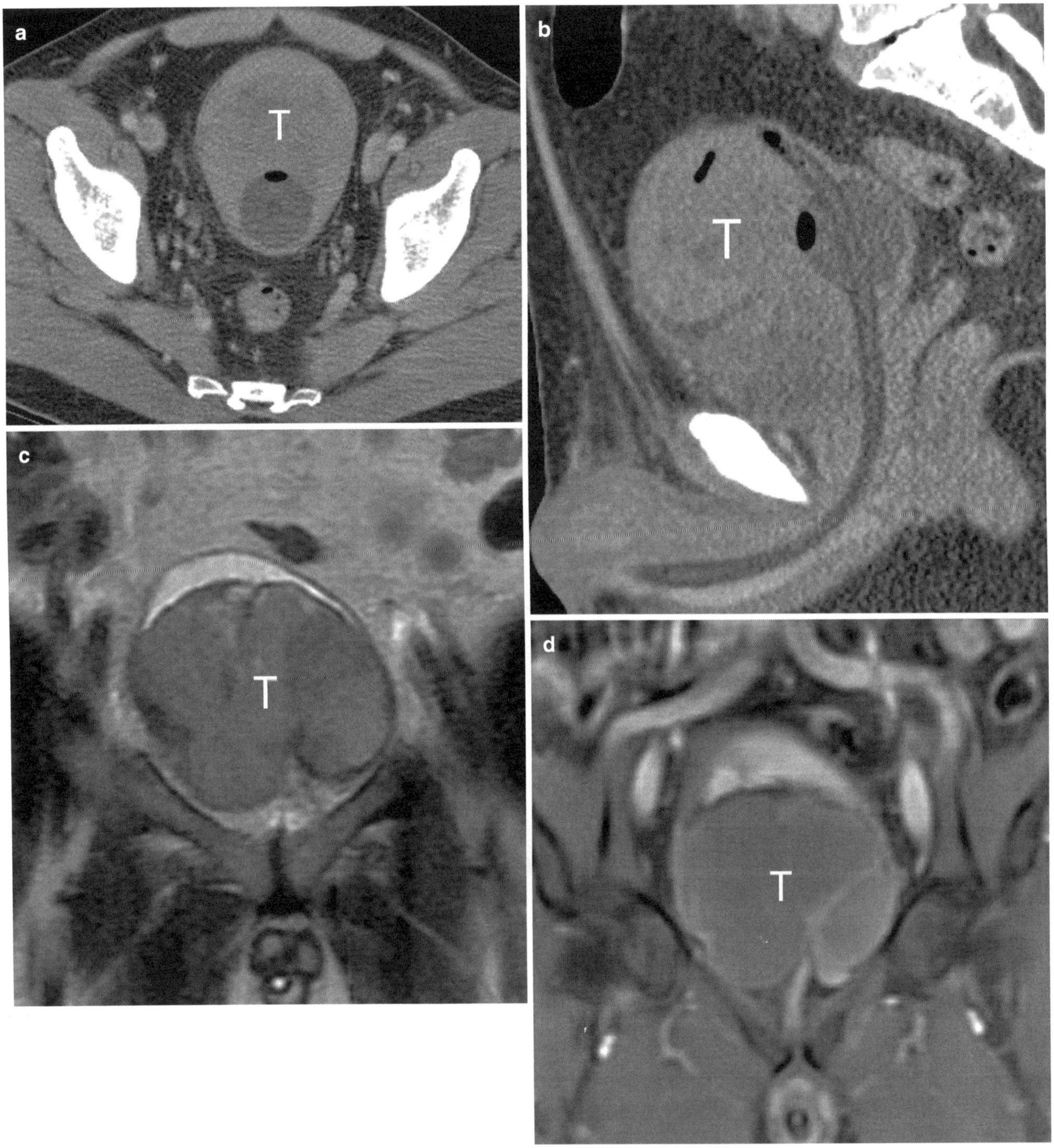

Fig. 3.13 Leiomyosarcoma. Leiomyosarcoma is the most common malignant mesenchymal bladder neoplasm in adults. Risk factors are prior radiation therapy or systemic chemotherapy with cyclophosphamide. Patients present relatively early due to hematuria and urinary obstruction. These are aggressive tumors with frequent local recurrence and distant metastases. They are difficult to distinguish from leiomyomas because of similar imaging features. Several clues are large size (mean diameter, 7 cm), poorly circumscribed borders, and central necrosis [42, 43]. (**a**, **b**) Axial and sagittal CE-CT show a large slightly heterogenous mass (T) filling urinary bladder lumen and producing bladder outlet obstruction. (**c**, **d**) Coronal T2-WI and coronal CE T1-WI demonstrate the same large bladder tumor (*T*) (Image courtesy of Dr. Robert Lefkowitz, M.D.)

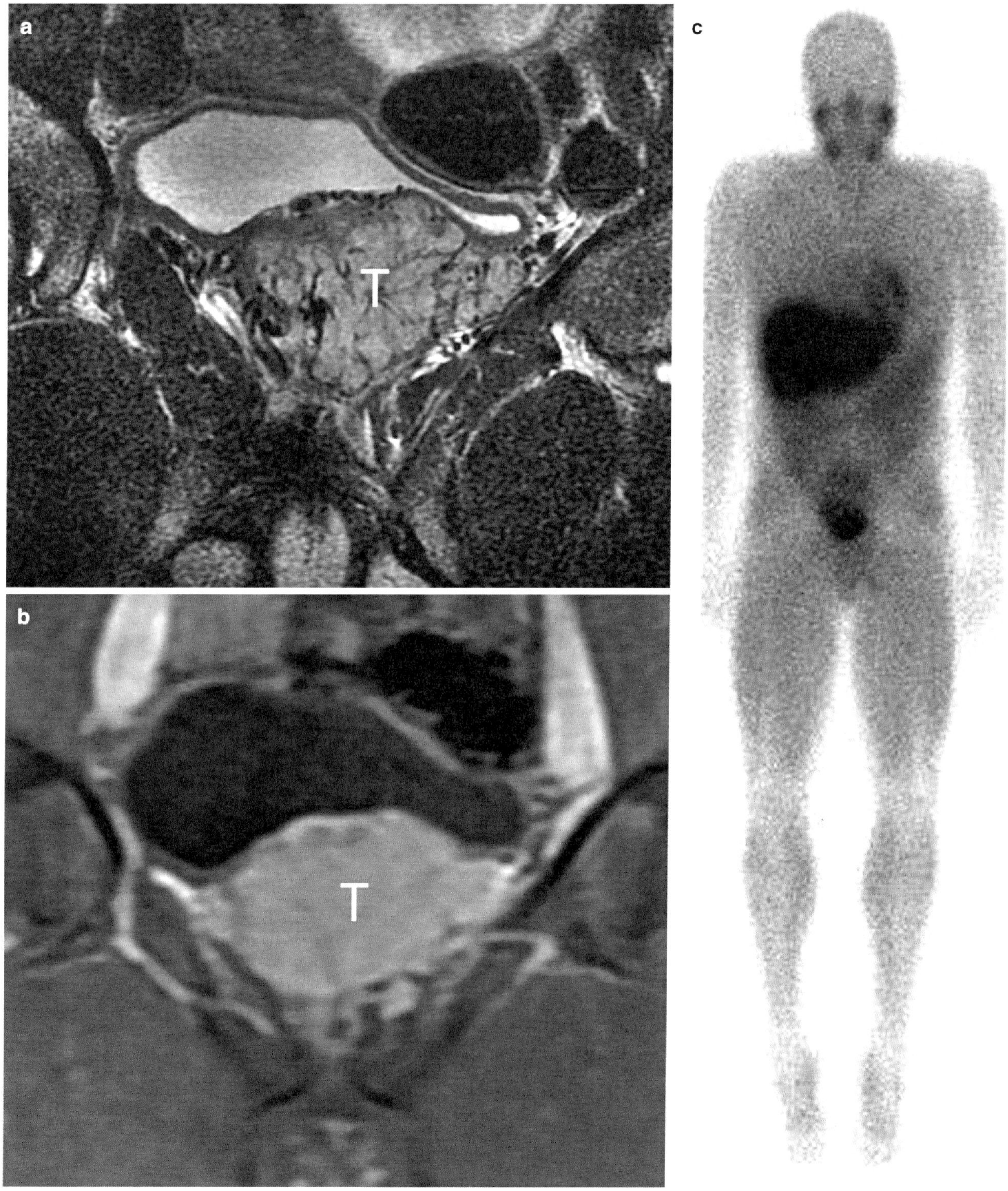

Fig. 3.14 Paraganglioma. Paragangliomas (i.e., extra-adrenal pheochromocytomas) compose only 0.1 % of all bladder neoplasms and 1 % of all pheochromocytomas. Most cases are sporadic. Paragangliomas originate from the chromaffin cells in the detrusor muscle. Most are benign, but 5–18 % are malignant [32]. Fifty percent (50 %) of patients present with characteristic clinical symptoms due to catecholamine release during micturition such as severe headache, anxiety, sweating, tremor, hypertension, syncope, and increased urine catecholamines. At cross-sectional imaging, key features that suggest a paraganglioma are a well-circumscribed homogenous solid submucosal mass (with occasional cystic change due to necrosis or hemorrhage) and marked contrast enhancement [44]. On CT, dense peripheral rim calcifications are also suggestive of a bladder paraganglioma [45]. On MRI, these neoplasms are T1 hypointense and moderately T2 hyperintense submucosal lesions with avid contrast enhancement [45]. I^{131} metaiodobenzylguanidine (MIBG) scan is highly specific (>96 %) but not very sensitive (64 %) for the detection of paraganglioma [46]. (**a**, **b**) Coronal T2-WI and coronal CE T1-WI images show solid well-circumscribed T2 hyperintense submucosal tumor (*T*) with prominent homogenous contrast enhancement. (**c**) Frontal I^{131} MIBG image demonstrates trace uptake in the same tumor

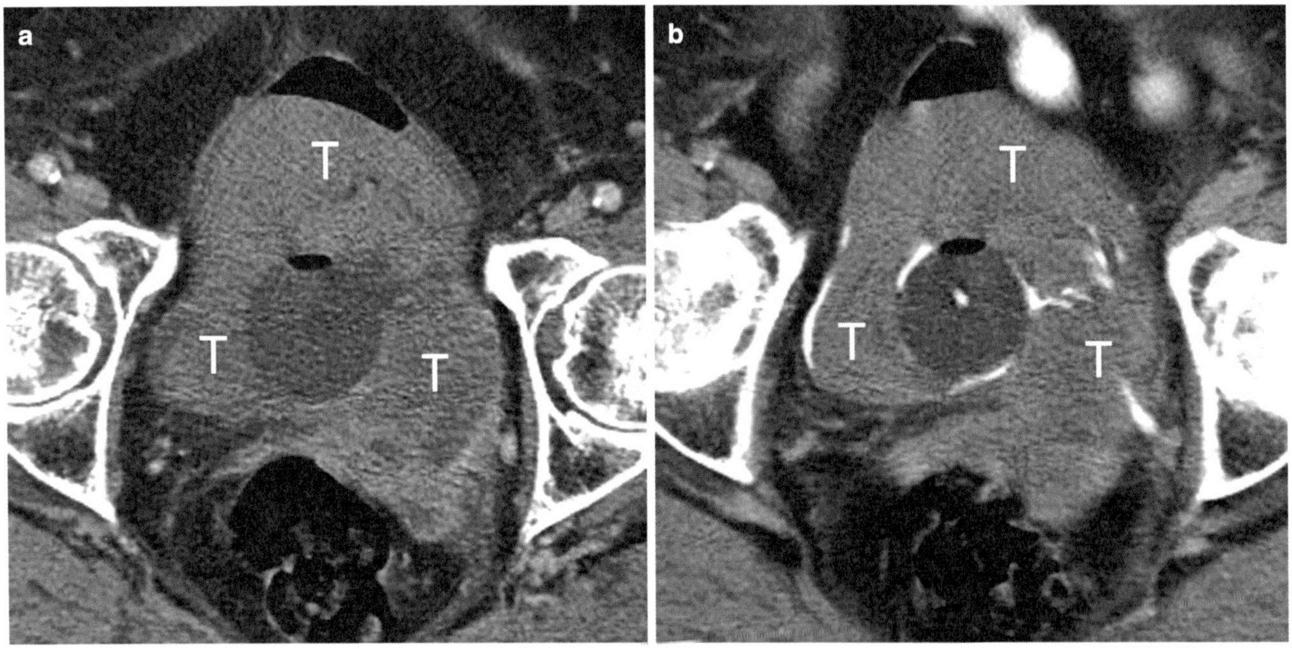

Fig. 3.15 Primary lymphoma of the urinary bladder. Secondary lymphomatous involvement of the urinary bladder is more common than primary bladder lymphoma. Primary bladder lymphomas are rare and are usually of non-Hodgkin subtype. At imaging, they more commonly manifest as well-defined masses rather than diffuse wall thickening or infiltration [47]. (**a**, **b**) Axial parenchymal and excretory phase CTU images show multiple urinary bladder masses (*T*) in keeping with biopsy proven malignant lymphoma of large B-cell type

Teaching Points

- Epithelial bladder tumors other than urothelial carcinoma and mesenchymal bladder neoplasms are relatively rare. Awareness of these tumors is important.
- Ultimate diagnosis requires biopsy due to significant overlap in clinical history and imaging findings.
- Some tumors including urachal adenocarcinoma, leiomyomas and paragangliomas have imaging features that may alert the radiologist as to the correct diagnosis.

Staging

Table 3.8 Local or T staging

- T staging accuracy is limited as current imaging techniques may not accurately resolve various bladder wall layers
  - CT is unable to determine the depth of bladder wall invasion
    - It is best at distinguishing between organ-confined ($\leq$ T2) versus non–organ-confined disease * ($\geq$T3b)
  - MRI is preferred for evaluating depth of bladder wall invasion and detecting organ invasion due to its superior soft tissue contrast or multiplanar capabilities
- Overall accuracy
  - Local bladder cancer staging
    - CT: 40–85 % [48, 49]
    - MRI: 73–96 % [48, 50]
    - DW-MRI may have incremental value in improving T-staging
      - Diagnostic accuracy: T2WI + high b-value DW-MRI (88 %), T2 WI alone (67 %), T2WI + DCE (79 %), T2WI + DW-MRI + DCE (92 %) [51].
  - Organ-confined versus non–organ-confined disease
    - CT: 55–92 % [52]
    - MRI: 82 % [50]
    - DW-MRI may have incremental value in distinguishing organ-confined versus non-organ-confined disease
      - Diagnostic accuracy: T2WI + high b-value DW-MRI (69.6 %) versus T2 WI alone (15.1 %) [53]
- Both CT and MRI tend to overstage (in about 30 % of cases)
  - Because bladder wall and perivesicular fat edema or inflammation after recent biopsy or resection may mimic tumor
- Strategies to improve local staging accuracy
  - Image prior to or at least 7 days after intervention such as TURBT [30]

* Both CT and MRI are unable to detect microscopic invasion of perivesicular fat or T3a disease

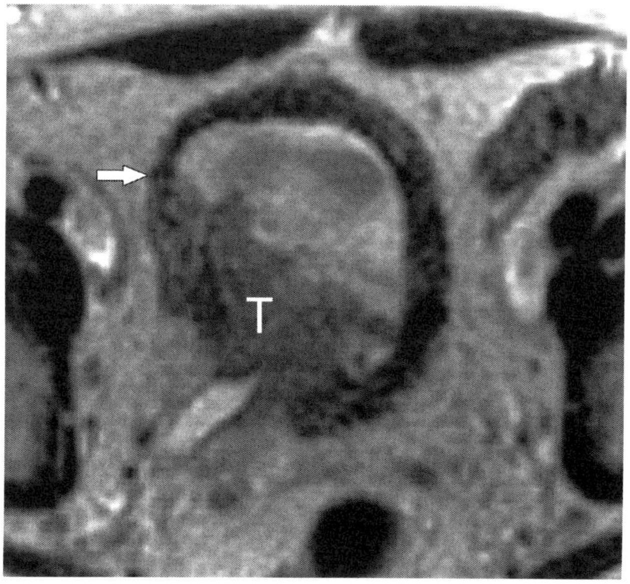

Fig. 3.17 MR demonstration of muscle-invasive urothelial carcinoma. Muscle-invasive disease is suggested when intermediate SI tumor interrupts low SI detrusor muscle layer ("the black line") on T2-WI. Ureteral obstruction is also consistent with muscle-invasive tumor. Axial T2-WI shows intermediate SI tumor (*T*) interrupting low SI muscle layer (*arrow*) and obstructing right distal ureter

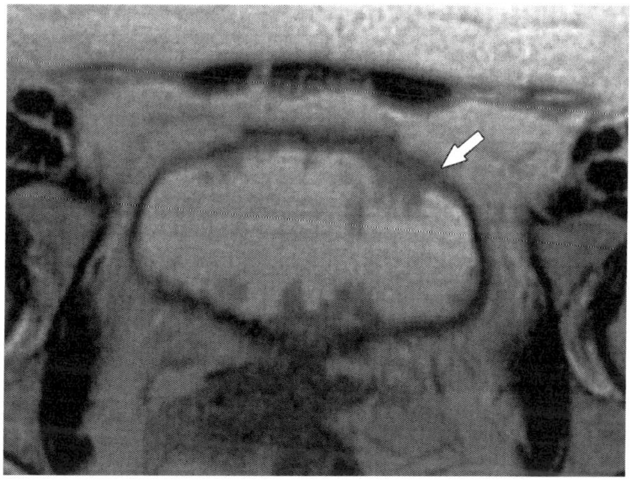

Fig. 3.16 MR illustration of non muscle-invasive urothelial carcinoma. MRI is the preferred imaging modality for assessing depth of tumor invasion. Presence of intact low SI muscle layer at the base of the intermediate SI tumor on T2-WI suggests non–muscle-invasive disease (i.e., stage Ta or T1). Axial T2-WI demonstrates multifocal papillary lesions projecting into the bladder lumen. Intact, low SI muscle layer is present at the bases of the tumors (*arrow*)

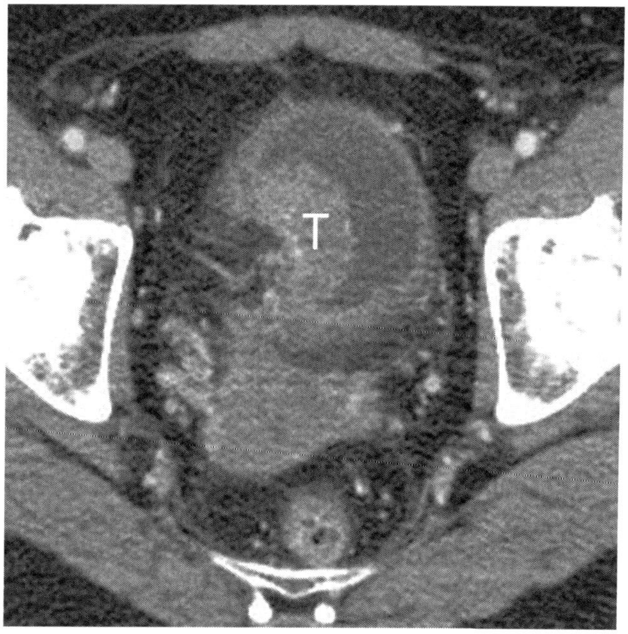

Fig. 3.18 CT findings of muscle-invasive urothelial carcinoma. CT cannot reliably determine the depth of bladder wall invasion. However, when present, such imaging features as retraction of the outer bladder wall and/or ureteral obstruction are suggestive of muscle-invasive disease. Axial parenchymal phase CTU demonstrates right posterolateral tumor (*T*) with prominent associated outer wall retraction consistent with pathologically proven bladder cancer invading deep half of muscularis propria (i.e., stage T2b)

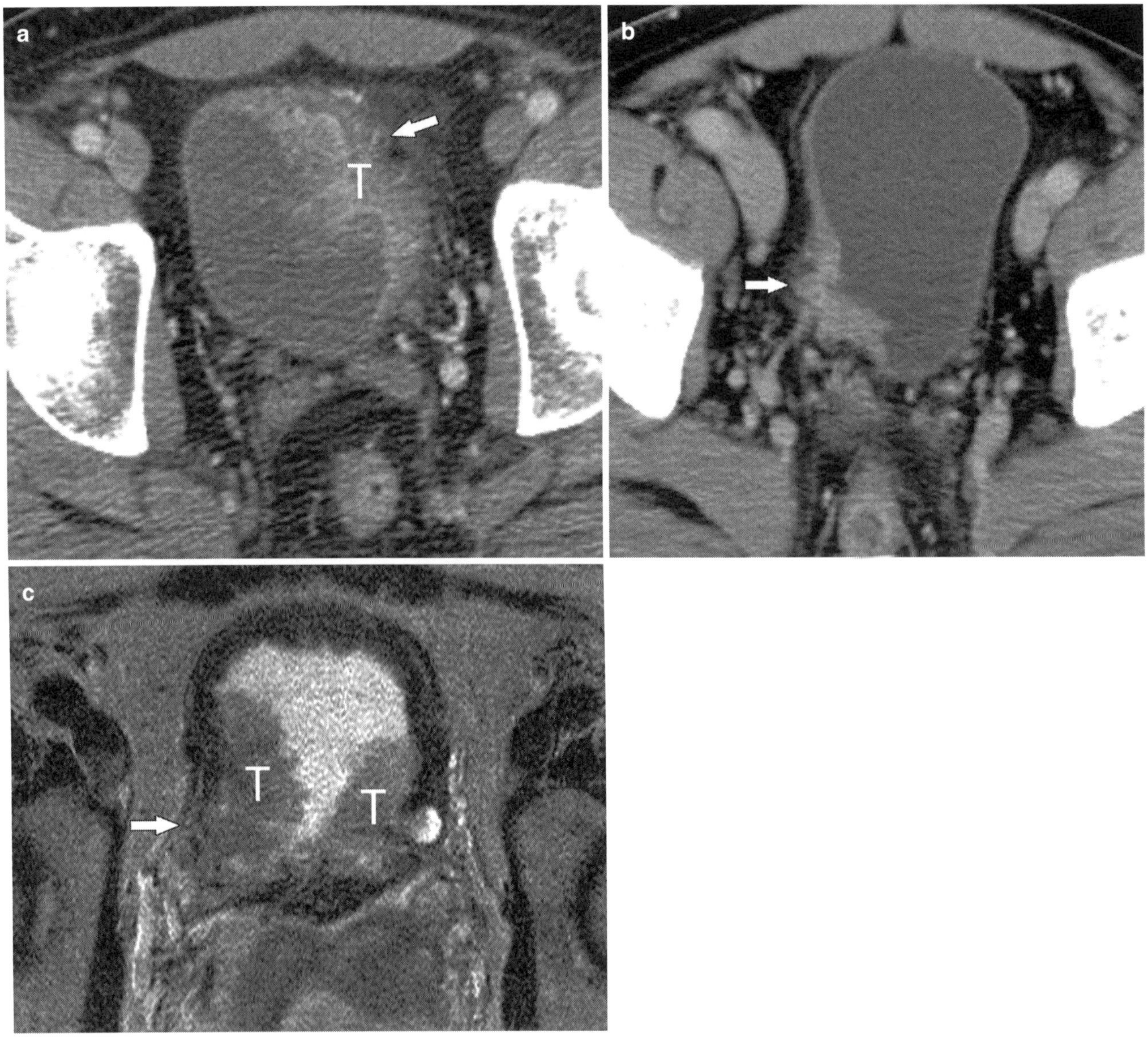

Fig. 3.19 CT and MR illustrations of muscle-invasive urothelial carcinomas with perivesicular fat invasion. On CT and MR, irregular, ill-defined outer bladder wall and adjacent perivesicular fat soft-tissue nodules or stranding are suggestive of macroscopic extravesical tumor extension (i.e., stage T3b). Microscopic fat invasion (i.e., stage T3a) cannot be detected at imaging. (**a**) Axial parenchymal phase CTU shows bladder tumor (*T*) producing nodular ill-defined outer bladder wall thickening, perivesicular fat nodularity and stranding (*arrow*). (**b**) Axial CE-CT in another patient demonstrates right posterolateral tumor involving right UVJ and invading adjacent perivesicular fat (*arrow*). (**c**) Axial T2-WI in a different patient shows bilateral muscle-invasive bladder tumors (*T*) with tumor involvement of entire thickness of low SI detrusor muscle and tumor extension into perivesicular fat (*arrow*)

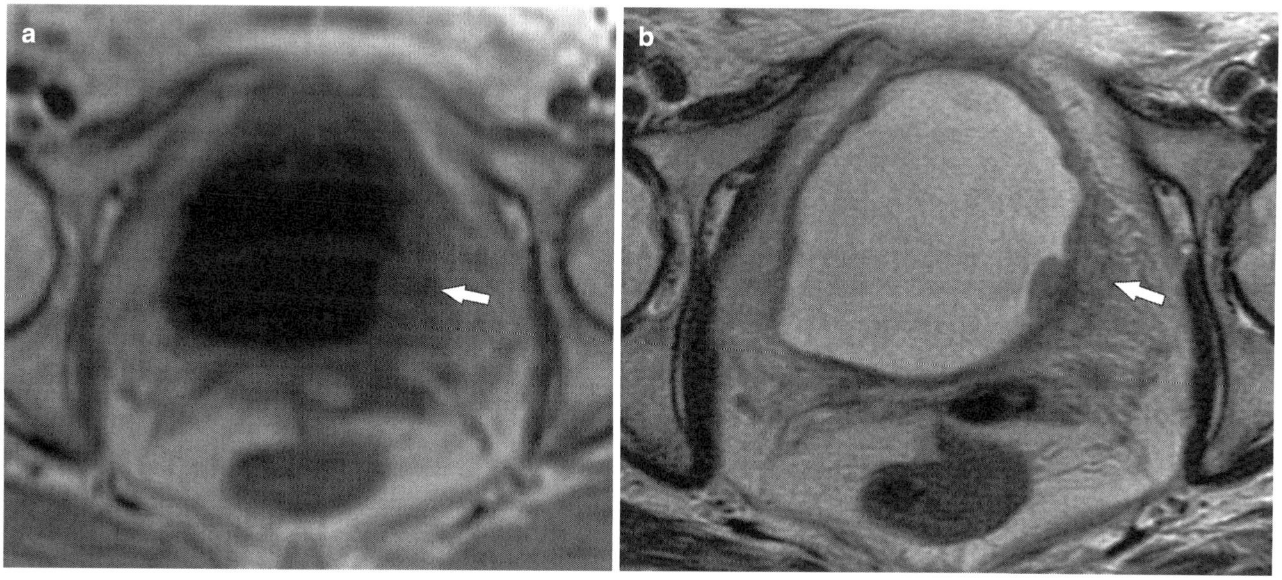

Fig. 3.20 MR demonstration of perivesicular fat edema and inflammation mimicking tumor infiltration. Recent procedures such as biopsy or TURBT may produce focal bladder wall thickening and perivesicular fat stranding that can mimic extravesical tumor extension resulting in overstaging. Therefore, in order to improve specificity it is best to perform staging examinations (e.g., CT or MRI) either before or at least 7 days after any procedure. (**a**, **b**) Axial T1-WI and T2-WI images show pathologically proven superficially invasive (i.e., T2a) urothelial carcinoma. Adjacent extensive perivesicular fat stranding (*arrow*) is from edema and inflammation secondarily to TURBT performed 4 days prior to the imaging

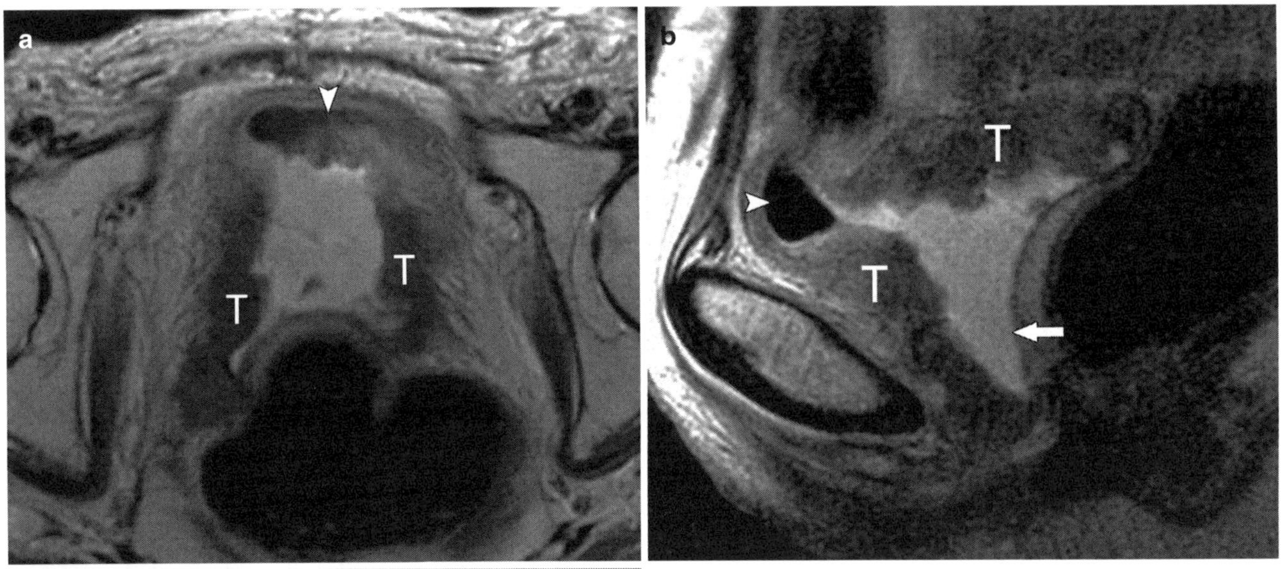

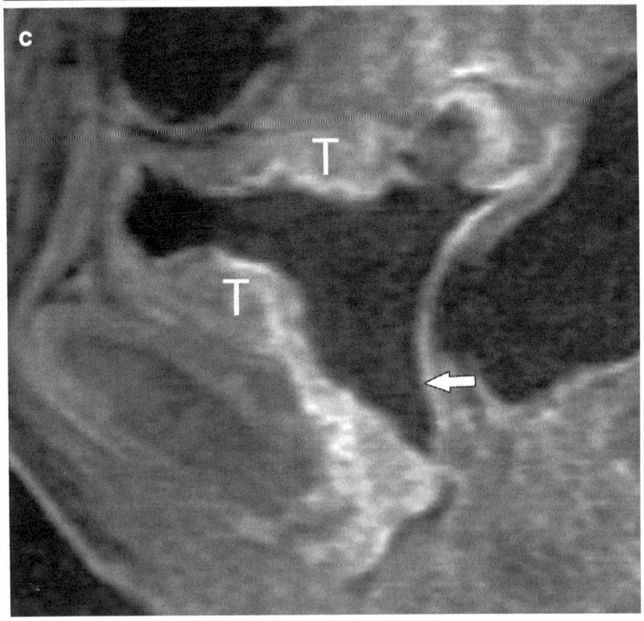

Fig. 3.21 MR illustration of muscle-invasive urothelial carcinoma. CT and MRI can be helpful in identifying T4 bladder cancers invading adjacent organs (i.e., stage T4a) and abdominal or pelvic walls (i.e., stage T4b). Involvement of adjacent organs or abdominopelvic wall is suggested by loss of clear separating fat plane. MRI is superior to CT in identifying adjacent organ involvement, especially in the pelvis, because of its better soft tissue contrast and multiplanar capabilities. (**a–c**) Axial T2-WI, sagittal T2-WI, and sagittal CE T1-WI demonstrate large urothelial carcinoma (*T*) invading upper to mid vagina with secondary large vesicovaginal fistula (*arrow*) and intraluminal bladder air (*arrowhead*) (see Fig. 3.9)

Table 3.9 Nodal staging

Most frequently involved regional lymph nodes
Prevesical, presacral, obturator, internal and external iliac lymph nodes
Diagnosis of nodal metastases on CT and MRI is primarily based on size criteria (i.e., short axis ≥0.8 cm for pelvic nodes and ≥1 cm for abdominal nodes) [54, 55]
Rounded nodes are more likely to be metastatic than oval nodes
CT and MRI have similar N staging accuracy
73–92 % on CT and 73–90 % on MRI
Both modalities have a tendency to understage
Diagnostic limitations
Normal-sized lymph nodes with low-volume metastases
Nodal enlargement due to a benign process
Promising MRI techniques with potential to improve N staging accuracy
Lymphographic MR contrast agents with ultrasmall iron oxide particles (USPIO) [56]

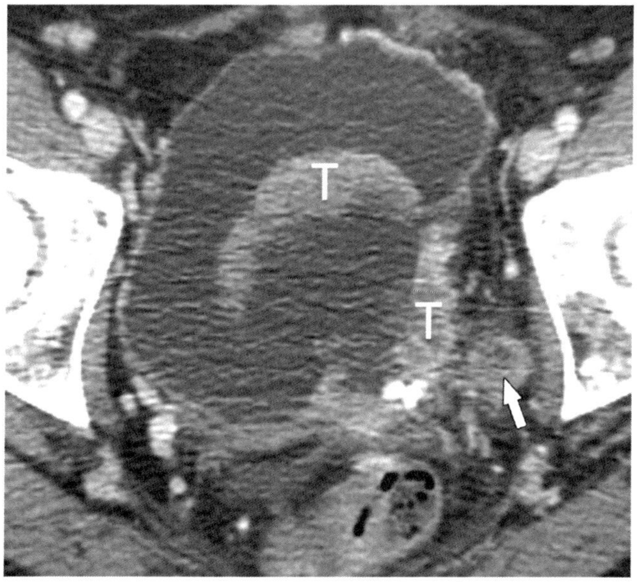

Fig. 3.22 Urothelial carcinoma with nodal metastases. Incidence of lymph node metastasis is about 30 % with deep muscle invasive tumors and 60 % with tumors involving extravesical soft tissues [57]. Lymphatic spread is initially to perivesicular and presacral nodes, followed by internal iliac, obturator, and external iliac nodes. Subsequent spread is to common iliac and retroperitoneal lymph nodes [58]. Axial CE-CT shows enlarged heterogeneously enhancing metastatic left internal iliac lymph node (*arrow*). Large biopsy-proven muscle-invasive primary bladder tumor (*T*) is only partially imaged

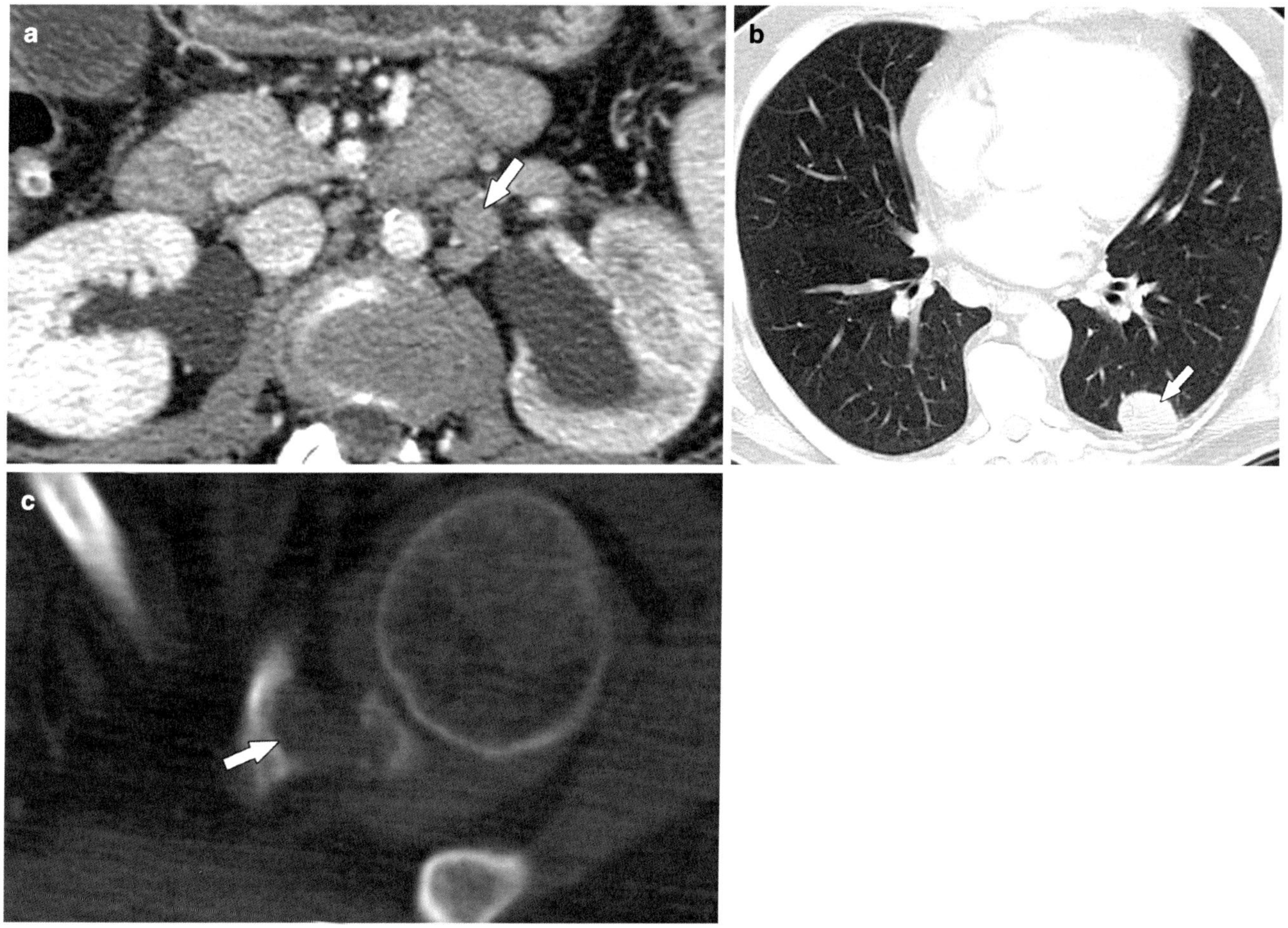

Fig. 3.23 Urothelial carcinoma with distant metastases. Retroperitoneal and inguinal lymph node involvement is considered distant metastasis. Other most common sites of metastases are liver, bone, and lungs in decreasing order of frequency [59]. (**a**) Axial CE-CT demonstrates enlarged left paraaortic lymph node (*arrow*). Primary tumor is not shown. (**b**) Axial CE-CT in a different patient shows biopsy proven left lower lobe metastasis (*arrow*). (**c**) Axial CT in another patient demonstrates lytic osseous metastasis involving left scapula (*arrow*)

Postoperative/Post-treatment Findings and Tumor Recurrence

Table 3.10 Post-treatment follow-up of patients with noninvasive and muscle-Invasive bladder cancer

Detection of post-surgical or post-treatment complications
Evaluation for tumor recurrence or tumor progression
Exclusion of metachronous upper tract and bladder urothelial carcinoma

See Figs. 3.20 and 3.26. Recent procedures or treatments such as biopsy or intravesical medications may cause inflammation with secondary bladder wall thickening, mucosal and submucosal hyperenhancement after intravenous contrast, and adjacent perivesicular fat stranding [50]. Clinical history and imaging follow-up may be helpful in distinguishing these inflammatory changes from the neoplastic process.

Perforation of the urinary bladder is the most common complication after TURBT occurring in about 5 % of cases [60].

Table 3.11 Postsurgical complications [61, 62]

Early (<30 days)
Bowel complications
Ileus, obstruction, anastomotic leak, and ischemia
Infectious complications
Acute pyelonephritis, pelvic, or retroperitoneal abscess
Postsurgical fluid collections
Urinomas, hematomas, and lymphoceles
Ureterointestinal complications
Anastomotic leak, obstruction, or ischemia
Late complications
Tumor recurrence
Deterioration of renal function, ureteral stricture or reflux with secondary hydronephrosis, stone formation (especially patients with ileal conduits), fistulas, metabolic disorders (metabolic acidosis, vitamin B12 deficiency), pouch necrosis, and retroperitoneal fibrosis

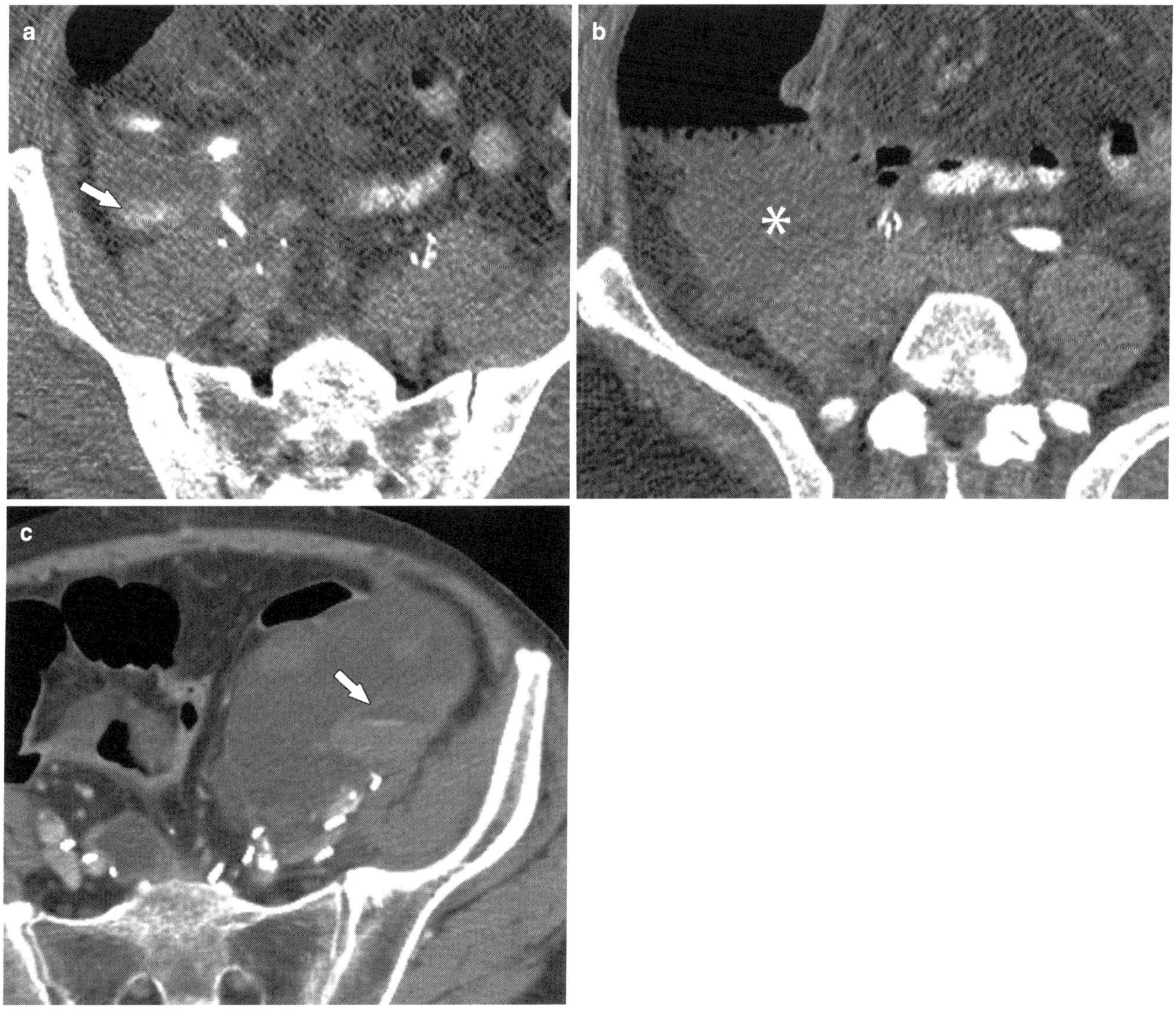

Fig. 3.24 Early postsurgical complications after urinary diversion. In most cases, acute complications manifest clinically and may require urgent radiographic evaluation, typically with contrast-enhanced CT. (**a**, **b**) Axial excretory phase CTU show extravasation of the excreted intravenous contrast (*arrow* in **a**) into right lower quadrant air-fluid collection consistent with ureterointestinal anastomotic leak and secondary right lower quadrant abscess (*asterisk* in **b**) in a 55-year-old man with invasive urothelial carcinoma 12 days after radical cystoprostatectomy, bilateral pelvic lymph node dissection, and ileal conduit urinary diversion. (**c**) Axial CE-CT in a different postsurgical patient demonstrates large acute hematoma in the left pelvis with a hematocrit level (*arrow*). Diagnostic angiography (*not shown*) was consistent with a left external iliac artery pseudoaneurysm

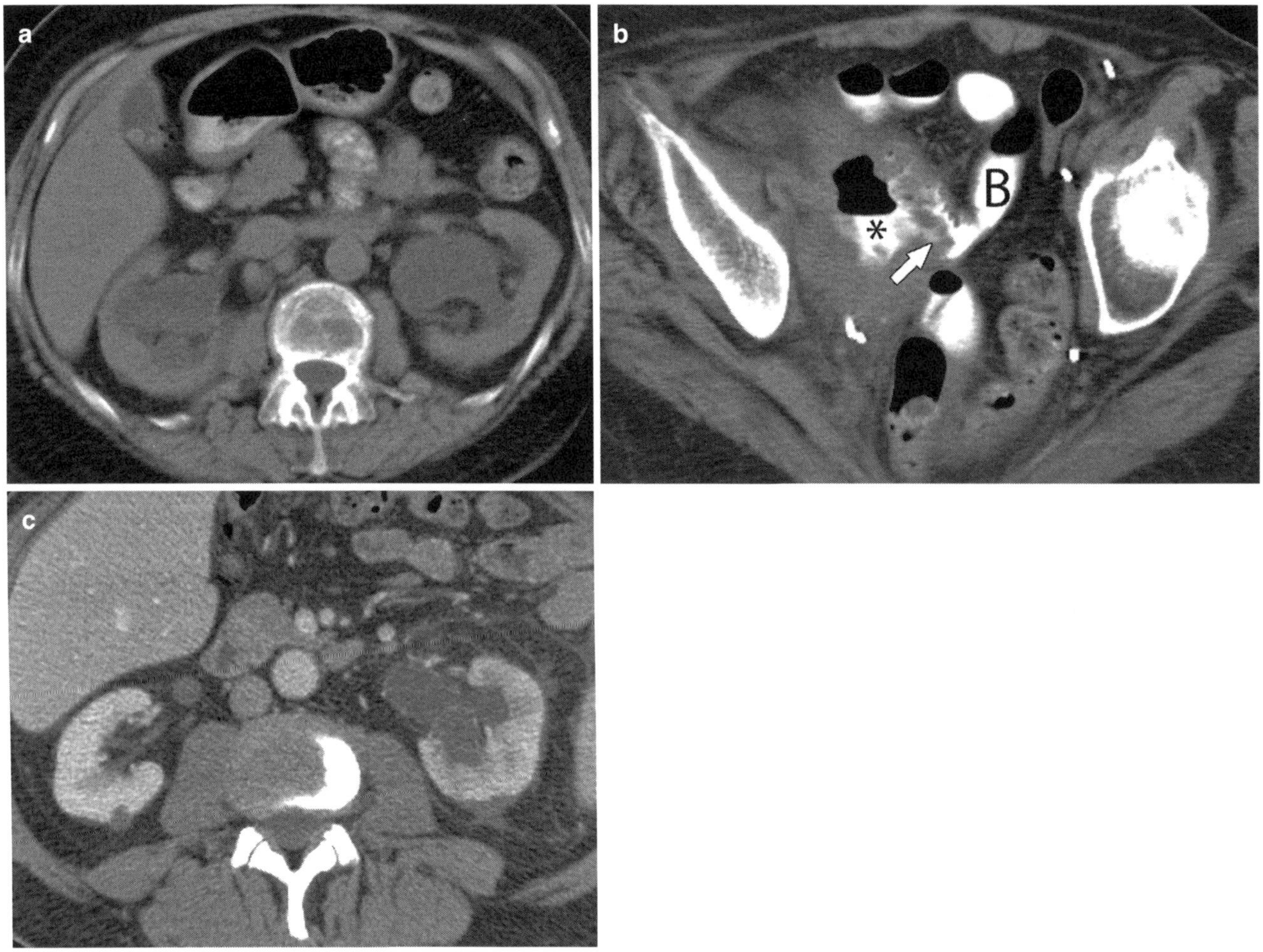

Fig. 3.25 Late postsurgical complications. (**a, b**) Axial noncontrast CT and axial CE-CT in a patient with squamous carcinoma of the bladder after radical cystectomy and ileal conduit reconstruction 6 years earlier demonstrate bilateral hydronephrosis due to presumed bilateral ureteral strictures and a fistula (*arrow*) between ileal conduit (*asterisk*) and small bowel (*B*). (**c**) Axial CE-CT in a different patient with radical cystectomy and neobladder formation for bladder cancer shows left hydronephrosis, delayed left nephrogram and perinephric stranding secondary to the surgically proven left ureterointestinal anastomotic stricture (*not shown*)

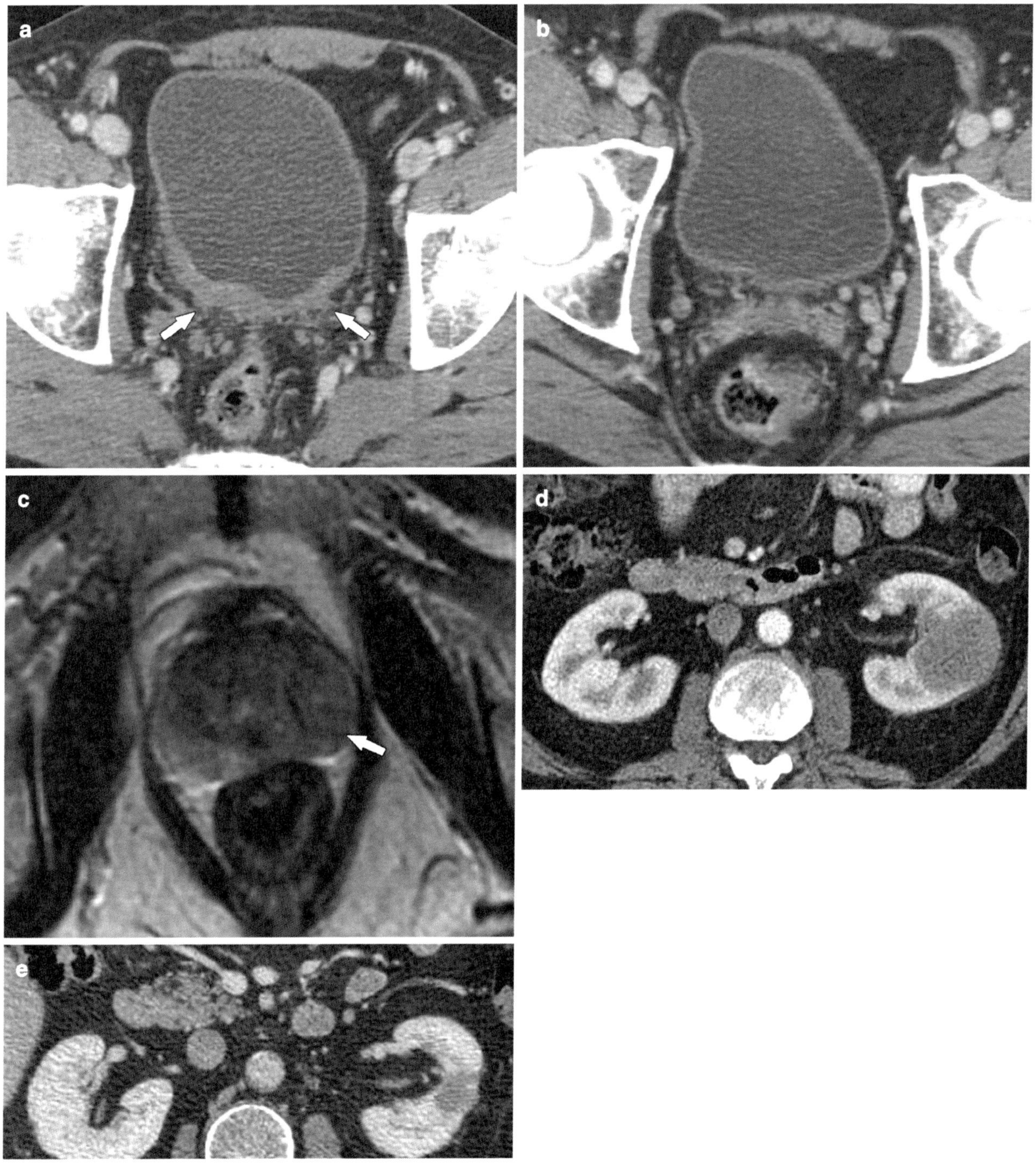

Fig. 3.26 BCG granulomatosis. After intravesical BCG instillation for treatment of superficial bladder cancer, some patients may develop BCG granulomatosis. Awareness of this entity is important as it may present with focal imaging abnormalities, primarily in the genitourinary system, mimicking primary or metastatic tumors. The most common BCG-related complication is granulomatous cystitis, which may manifest as bladder wall thickening and nodularity indistinguishable from bladder cancer. Less common complications are granulomatous prostatitis, epididymo-orchitis, and renal granulomas or abscesses. Granulomatous prostatitis is frequently accompanied by elevated PSA and focal or diffuse T2 hypointensity in the prostate gland on MRI. Therefore, it cannot be reliably distinguished from prostate cancer by either digital rectal examination or imaging and definite diagnosis may require biopsy. Renal granulomas and abscesses are extremely rare, occurring in less than 0.1 % of BCG-treated patients. The mechanism of their formation is controversial, but they may be related to vesicoureteral reflux or systemic spread. On CE-CT, they present as homogenous or heterogenous hypoattenuating lesions, and can be either segmental in appearance similar to pyelonephritis or expansile and mass-like mimicking a tumor. It is critical to consider the possibility of BCG-induced granulomatous renal mass in bladder cancer patients treated with BCG to institute appropriate medical treatment and to avoid unnecessary invasive procedures [63]. (**a**, **b**) Axial CE-CT demonstrates nodular bladder wall thickening, mucosal hyperenhancement, and perivesicular fat stranding (*arrow*) due to presumed granulomatous cystitis after intravesical BCG for bladder cancer (**a**). These findings resolve after empiric anti-mycobacterial treatment (**b**). (**c**) Axial T2-WI from a different patient with prior intravesical BCG therapy shows decreased T2 SI in the peripheral zone of the prostate gland on the left side (*arrow*) consistent with biopsy-proven granulomatous prostatitis. (**d**, **e**) Axial CE-CT images in another patient with prior intravesical BCG treatment demonstrate homogenous mass-like left renal lesion (**d**) which substantially improves after empiric antimycobacterial treatment (**e**)

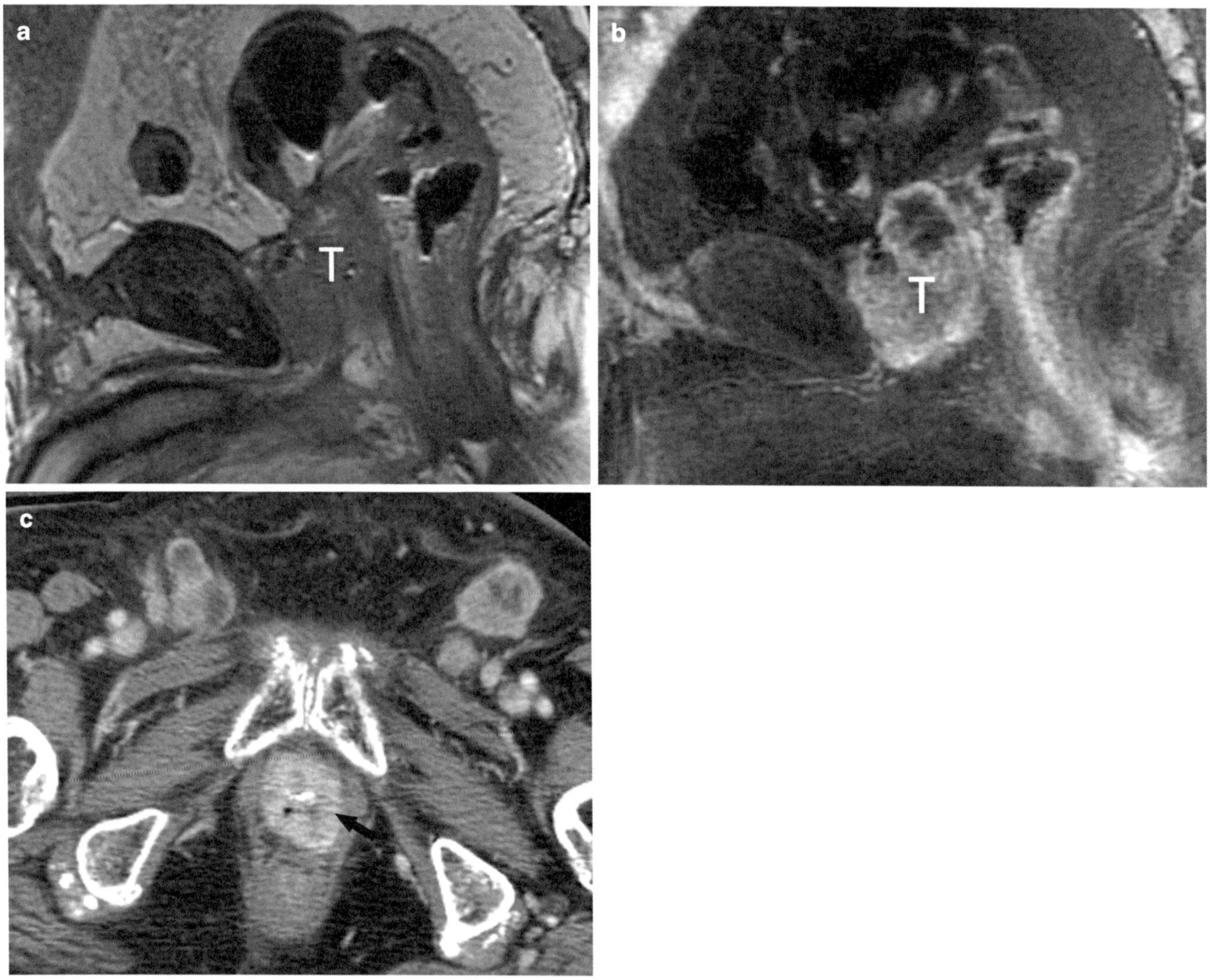

Fig. 3.27 Recurrent urothelial carcinoma after cystectomy. Recurrent disease may present as metachronous upper tract tumors, pelvic mass at or adjacent to the urethral-reservoir anastomosis, and metastases to abdominal and pelvic lymph nodes or other organs [62]. Patients with high-grade and high-stage tumors are at a higher risk for both local and distal recurrence. Involvement of the prostate gland by urothelial carcinoma increases the risk of recurrence at the urethral-reservoir anastomosis. (**a**, **b**) Sagittal T2WI and sagittal CE T1WI show large centrally necrotic locally recurrent tumor (*T*) in a 69-year-old man with muscle-invasive urothelial carcinoma treated 6 months earlier with radical cystoprostatectomy and ileal conduit urinary diversion. (**c**) Axial CE-CT demonstrates recurrent tumor in the cystectomy bed (*arrow*) and bilateral metastatic superficial inguinal adenopathy in a 90-year-old woman with muscle-invasive urothelial carcinoma status post anterior exenteration and ileal conduit urinary diversion 4 years prior

Radiology Report

Table 3.12 Key radiology report elements: initial staging [64]

- **T:** Primary Tumor
  - Location and size
    - Specify if multiple synchronous tumors
  - Tumor appearance
    - Papillary or plaque-like
  - Local extent
    - Presence of bladder wall retraction
      - Suggests muscle-invasive tumor
    - Perivesicular fat infiltration
      - Indicates perivesicular tumor extension versus post-procedural or post-treatment inflammation
    - Invasion of adjacent organs
      - Seminal vesicles, prostate gland, rectum, uterus, vaginal, and pelvic floor
- **N:** Lymph nodes
  - Location and dimensions of any regional lymph nodes
    - Most frequently involved regional nodes
      - Perivesicular, presacral, internal iliac, obturator, and external iliac nodes
- **M:** Metastases
  - Retroperitoneal and inguinal nodes indicate distant metastasis
  - Liver
    - Usually in the setting of pelvic or abdominal nodal disease
  - Bone
    - Especially with a squamous histology
  - Lung

Table 3.13 Key radiology report elements: follow-up examinations [62, 64]

- Date of each comparison study used
- If no prior cystectomy
  - See Table 3.12
- If prior cystectomy and urinary diversion
  - Acute or late complications
  - Local tumor recurrence
    - Ureteral stricture (without or with associated soft tissue mass), pelvic mass, pelvic lymphadenopathy, stricture (without or with associated mass) at the urethro-intestinal anastomosis if orthotopic neobladder
  - Metastatic tumor recurrence
    - If prior pelvic lymphadenectomy, carefully evaluate retroperitoneal and inguinal regions for nodal metastases
- Indicate change in previous and list new sites of disease since prior study
- If measurable disease is present
  - Measure same lesions as on prior scans
  - Give overall assessment of response
    - Increase, decrease, or no change in size and number of lesions
    - Incorporate Response Evaluation Criteria in Solid Tumors (RECIST) or World Health Organization (WHO) guidelines, if institution or clinical trial uses them.

Acknowledgment The authors thank Ada Muellner, MS, for editing the manuscript.

References

1. Jemal A, Siegel R, Xu J, Ward E. Cancer statistics. CA Cancer J Clin. 2010;60(5):277–300.
2. Golijanin DJ, Kakishvili D, Madeb RR, et al. Chemoprevention of bladder cancer. World J Urol. 2006;24:445–72.
3. Fleshner N, Kondylis F. Demographics and epidemiology of urothelial cancer of urinary bladder. In: Droller MJ, editor. Urothelial tumors. Hamilton, Ontario, Canada: Decker; 2004. p. 1–16.
4. Vineis P, Simonato L. Proportion of lung and bladder cancers in males resulting from occupation: a systematic approach. Arch Environ Health. 1991;46(1):6–17.
5. Mostofi F, Davis CJ, Sesterhenn I. Histological typing of urinary bladder tumors. 2nd ed. Berlin: Springer; 1999.
6. Sandhu JS, Vickers AJ, Bochner B, et al. Clinical characteristics of bladder cancer patients previously treated with radiation for prostate cancer. BJU Int. 2006;98:59–62.
7. Ficarra V, Dalpiaz O, Alrabi N, et al. Correlation between clinical and pathologic staging in a series of radical cystectomics for bladder carcinoma. BJU Int. 2005;95.786–90.
8. McDougal WS, Shipley WU, Kaufman DS, et al. Cancer of the bladder, ureter, and renal pelvis. In: DeVita VT, Hellman S, Rosenberg SA, editors. Cancer: principles and practice of oncology. 8th ed. Philadelphia: Lippincott Williams and Wilkins; 2008. p. 1358–84.
9. Nieder AM, Brausi M, Lamm D, et al. Management of stage T1 tumors of the bladder. Int Consens Panel Urol. 2005;66:108–25.
10. American Joint Committee on Cancer (AJCC). Cancer staging manual. 6th ed. Philadelphia: Lippincott-Raven Publishers; 2002.
11. Epstein JI, Amin MB, Reuter VE, et al. The world health organization/international society of urologic pathology consensus on classification of urothelial (transitional cell) neoplasms of the urinary bladder. Am J Surg Pathol. 1998;22:1435–8.
12. Milan-Rodriguez F, Chechile-Toniolo G, Salvador-Bayarri J, et al. Primary superficial bladder cancer risk groups according to progression, mortality and recurrence. J Urol. 2000;164:680–4.
13. Milan-Rodriguez F, Chechile-Toniolo G, Salvador-Bayarri J, et al. Multivariate analysis of the prognostic factors of primary superficial bladder cancer. J Urol. 2000;163:73–8.
14. Sylvester RJ, Oosterlinck W, van der Meijden AP. A single immediate postoperative instillation of chemotherapy decreases the risk of recurrence in patients with stage Ta T1 bladder cancer: a meta-analysis of published results of randomized clinical trials. J Urol. 2004;171:2186–90.
15. Bohle A, Jocham D, Bock PR. Intravesical bacillus Calmette-Guerin versus mitomycin C for superficial bladder cancer: a formal meta analysis of comparative studies on recurrence and toxicity. J Urol. 2003;169:90–5.
16. Lamm DL, Blumenstein BA, Crawford ED, et al. A randomized trial of intravesical doxorubicin and immunotherapy with bacillus Calmette-Guerin for transitional cell carcinoma of the bladder. J Urol. 2000;163(4):1124–9.
17. Smith H, Weaver D, Barjenbruch O, et al. Routine excretory urography in follow-up of superficial transitional cell carcinoma of bladder. Urology. 1989;34:193–6.
18. Wright JL, Lin DW, Porter MP. The association between extent of lymphadenectomy and survival among patients with lymph node metastases undergoing radical cystectomy. Cancer. 2008;112:2332–3.
19. Dhar NB, Klein EA, Reuther AM, et al. Outcome after radical cystectomy with limited or extended pelvic lymph node dissection. J Urol. 2008;179:873–8.
20. Black PC, Brown GA, Grossman HB, et al. Neoadjuvant chemotherapy for bladder cancer. World J Urol. 2006;24:531–42.
21. Grossman HB, Natale RB, Tangen CM, et al. Neoadjuvant chemotherapy plus cystectomy compared to cystectomy alone for locally advanced bladder cancer. N Engl J Med. 2003;34:859–66.
22. Winquist E, Waldron T, Segal R, et al. Neoadjuvant chemotherapy in transitional cell carcinoma of the bladder: a systemic review and meta-analysis. J Urol. 2004;171:561–9.
23. Vale CL, Adjuvant chemotherapy in invasive bladder cancer: a systematic review and meta-analysis of individual patient data: Advance Bladder Cancer (ABC) Meta-analysis Collaboration. Eur Urol. 2005;48(2):189–199.
24. Hassan JM, Cookson MS, Smith Jr JA, et al. Patterns of initial transitional cell recurrence in patients after cystectomy. J Urol. 2006;175:2054–7.
25. Montie JE, Clark PE, Eisenberger MA, et al. Bladder cancer. J Natl Compr Canc Netw. 2009;7:8–39.
26. Sadow CA, Silverman SG, O'Leary MP, et al. Bladder cancer detection with CT urography in an academic medical center. Radiology. 2008;249:195–202.
27. Turney BW, Willatt JMG, Nixon D, et al. Computed tomography urography for diagnosing bladder cancer. BJU Int. 2006;98:345–8.
28. Abou-El-Ghar ME, El-Assmy A, Refaie HF, et al. Bladder cancer: diagnosis with diffusion-weighted MR imaging in patients with gross hematuria. Radiology. 2009;251:415–21.
29. Kim JK, Park SY, Ahn HJ, et al. Bladder cancer: analysis of multidetector row helical CT enhancement pattern and accuracy in tumor detection and perivesical staging. Radiology. 2004;231:725–31.
30. Moon WK, Kim SH, Cho JM, et al. Calcified bladder tumors: CT features. Acta Radiol. 1992;33:440–3.
31. Barentsz JO, Engelbrecht M, Jager GJ, et al. Fast dynamic gadolinium-enhanced MR imaging of urinary bladder and prostate cancer. J Magn Reson Imaging. 1999;10:295–304.
32. Murphy WM, Grignon DJ, Perlman EJ. Tumors of the kidney, bladder, and related urinary structures. Washington, DC: American Registry of Pathology; 2004.
33. Huguet-Perez J, Palou J, Millan-Rodriguez F, et al. Upper tract transitional cell carcinoma following cystectomy for bladder cancer. Eur Urol. 2001;40:318–23.
34. Millan-Rodriguez F, Chechile-Toniolo G, Salvador-Bayarri J, et al. Upper urinary tract tumors after primary superficial bladder tumors: prognostic factors and risk groups. J Urol. 2000;164:1183–7.
35. Shokeir AA. Squamous cell carcinoma of the bladder: pathology, diagnosis and treatment. BJU Int. 2004;93:216–20.
36. Wong JT, Wasserman NF, Padurean AM. Bladder squamous cell carcinoma. Radiographics. 2004;24:855–60.
37. Bates AW, Baithun SI. Secondary neoplasms of the bladder are histologic mimics of nontransitional cell primary tumours: clinicopathological and histological features of 282 cases. Histopathology. 2000;36:32–40.
38. Hughes MJ, Fischer C, Sohaib SA. Imaging features of primary nonurachal adenocarcinoma of the bladder. AJR Am J Roentgenol. 2004;183:1397–401.
39. Wong-You-Cheong JJ, Woodard PJ, Manning MA, et al. From the archives of the AFIP. Neoplasms of the urinary bladder: radiologic-pathologic correlation. Radiographics. 2006;26:553–80.
40. Sundaram CP, Rawal A, Saltzman B. Characteristics of bladder leiomyoma as noted on magnetic resonance imaging. Urology. 1998;52:1142–3.
41. Martin SA, Sears DL, Sebo TJ, et al. Smooth muscle neoplasms of the urinary bladder: a clinicopathologic comparison of leiomyoma and leiomyosarcoma. Am J Surg Pathol. 2002;26:292–300.

42. Mallampati GK, Siegelman ES. MR imaging of the bladder. Magn Reson Imaging Clin N Am. 2004;12:545–55.
43. Chen M, Lipson SA, Hricak H. MR imaging evaluation of benign mesenchymal tumors of the urinary bladder. AJR Am J Roentgenol. 1997;168:399–403.
44. Asbury Jr WI, Hatcher PA, Gould HR, et al. Bladder pheochromocytoma with ring calcification. Abdom Imaging. 1996;21:275–7.
45. Crecelius SA, Bellah R. Pheochromocytoma of the bladder in an adolescent: sonographic and MR imaging features. AJR Am J Roentgenol. 1995;165:101–3.
46. Jalil ND, Pattou FN, Combemale F, et al. Effectiveness and limits of preoperative imaging studies for the localization of pheochromocytomas and paragangliomas: a review of 282 cases. French Association Of Surgery (AFC), and French Association of Endocrine Surgeons (AFCE). Eur J Surg. 1998;164:23–8.
47. Bates AW, Norton AJ, Baithun SI. Malignant lymphoma of the urinary bladder: a clinicopathologic study of 11 cases. J Clin Pathol. 2000;53:458–61.
48. Barentsz JO, Witjes JA, Ruijs JH. What is new in bladder cancer imaging. Urol Clin North Am. 1997;24:583–602.
49. Kim B, Semelka RC, Ascher SM, et al. Bladder tumor staging: comparison of contrast enhanced CT, T1 and T2 weighted MR imaging, dynamic gadolinium-enhanced imaging, and late gadolinium-enhanced imaging. Radiology. 1994;193:239–45.
50. Tekes A, Kamel I, Imam K, et al. Dynamic MRI of bladder cancer: evaluation of staging accuracy. AJR Am J Roentgenol. 2005; 184:121–7.
51. Takeuchi M, Sasaki S, Ito M, et al. Urinary bladder cancer: diffusion-weighted MR imaging: accuracy for diagnosing T stage and estimating histologic grade. Radiology. 2009;251(1):112–21.
52. Kundra V, Silverman PM. Imaging in oncology from the University of Texas M.D. Anderson Cancer Center. Imaging in the diagnosis, staging, and follow-up of cancer of the urinary bladder. AJR Am J Roentgenol. 2003;180:1045–54.
53. El-Assmy A, Abou-El-Ghar ME, Mosbah A, et al. Bladder tumour staging: comparison of diffusion- and T2-weighted MR imaging. Eur Radiol. 2009;19:1575–81.
54. Hall TB, MacVicar AD. Imaging of bladder cancer. Imaging. 2001;13:1–10.
55. Barentsz JO, Jager GJ, van Vierzen PB, et al. Staging urinary bladder cancer after transurethral biopsy: value of fast dynamic contrast-enhanced MR imaging. Radiology. 1996;201:185–93.
56. Deserno WM, Harisinghani MG, Taupitz M, et al. Urinary bladder cancer: preoperative nodal staging with ferumoxtran-10-enhanced MR imaging. Radiology. 2004;233:449–56.
57. MacVicar AD. Bladder cancer staging. BJU Int. 2000;86 suppl 1:111–22.
58. Husband JES, Reznek RH. Imaging in oncology. 2nd ed. London: Taylor & Francis; 2004.
59. Knap MM, Lundbeck F, Overgaard J. Prognostic factors, pattern of recurrence and survival in a Danish bladder cancer cohort treated with radical cystectomy. Acta Oncol. 2003;42:160–8.
60. Dick A, Barnes R, Hadley H, et al. Complications of transurethral resection of bladder tumors: prevention, recognition and treatment. J Urol. 1980;124:810–1.
61. Sudakoff GS, Guralnick M, Langenstroer P, et al. CT urography of urinary diversions with enhanced CT digital radiography: preliminary experience. AJR Am J Roentgenol. 2005;184: 131–8.
62. Catala V, Sola M, Samaniego J, et al. CT findings in urinary diversion after radical cystectomy: postsurgical anatomy and complications. Radiographics. 2009;29:461–76.
63. Ma W, Kang SK, Hricak H, et al. Imaging appearance of granulomatous disease after BCG treatment of bladder carcinoma. AJR Am J Roentgenol. 2009;192:1494–500.
64. Hricak H, Husband JES, Panicek DM, et al. Oncologic imaging: essentials of reporting common cancers. Philadelphia: Saunders Elsevier; 2007.

Prostate Cancer Imaging

4

Hebert Alberto Vargas, Joshua Chaim, and Oguz Akin

The prostate is an exocrine gland that is part of the male reproductive system. It is located in the pelvis, just below the urinary bladder and anterior to the rectum surrounding the prostatic segment of the urethra. Its shape is described as an "inverted pyramid," with the widest portion situated cranially (prostatic base) and its narrowest portion caudally (prostatic apex). Between the prostatic base and apex lies the "midgland." Its function is to contribute to semen production, together with the seminal vesicles and testes, and it also plays a role in male ejaculation.

The prostate is also the most common site of noncutaneous cancer in men [1]. Since the introduction of the prostate-specific antigen (PSA) test in the late 1980s, there has been a dramatic increase in the incidence of prostate cancer, but also a shift toward earlier detection and improved survival. In fact, although about 17 % of men will be diagnosed with prostate cancer during their lifetime, only 3 % of men will die from the disease [1]. In some patients the disease follows a relatively indolent course, whereas in others it can be extremely aggressive and sometimes lethal. Due to this extreme variability in outcomes, risk-stratification is important to identify patients who are more likely to benefit from aggressive intervention and those in whom other management approaches, such as active surveillance, would suffice. This requires adequate interpretation of multiple variables such as the presence of known risk factors (e.g., increasing age, African-American race, and family history of prostate cancer) and findings from clinical examination, laboratory tests, and imaging studies. Several prediction tools have been developed to aid the decision-making process in patients with suspected or confirmed prostate cancer. Nomograms, which are graphical representations of a logistic regression analysis, are one such tool widely used to predict outcomes in various scenarios before and after treatment for prostate cancer. The main role of imaging in patients with biopsy-proven prostate cancer is to detect and localize the tumor(s) and to define the extent of the disease (mainly extracapsular extension, seminal vesicle invasion, lymph node involvement, and distant metastases), and thereby aid in treatment planning. Imaging also plays a role in post-treatment follow-up.

In this chapter, we present an overview of the imaging techniques used to assess the normal and the treated prostate, together with the typical and atypical imaging features of primary and recurrent prostate cancer and its mimics.

H.A. Vargas, M.D. • J. Chaim, DO • O. Akin, M.D. (✉)
Department of Radiology, Memorial Sloan-Kettering Cancer Center, 1275 York Avenue, New York, NY, 10065, USA
e-mail: vargasah@mskcc.org; chaimj@mskcc.org; akino@mskcc.org

A.M. Bach, J. Zhang (eds.), *Atlas of Genitourinary Oncological Imaging*, Atlas of Oncology Imaging, DOI 10.1007/978-1-4614-4872-3_4, © Springer Science+Business Media New York 2013

Normal Anatomy

Table 4.1 Zonal anatomy and seminal vesicles

Structure	Location	Normal T2-weighted MRI appearance	Other
Peripheral zone	Surrounds the central zone and the distal prostatic urethra	Homogeneous high signal intensity	Most common site of prostate cancer
Transition zone	Forms two bulges on either side of the urethra that extend superiorly, anteriorly, and laterally from the verumontanum	Heterogeneous appearance owing to variable mix of stromal and glandular components	Most common site of benign prostatic hyperplasia (BPH)
Central zone	Surrounds the ejaculatory ducts, enclosing both the transition zone and the urethra proximal to the verumontanum	Most commonly of homogeneous low signal intensity	Embryologically more akin to seminal vesicles than to the rest of the prostate
Seminal vesicles	Postero-superior to the prostate	High signal intensity; convoluted "tubular" appearance	Drain into the midprostatic urethra via ejaculatory ducts at the verumontanum

The prostate is divided into distinct anatomical "zones," based on their location with respect to the prostatic urethra and their histological and embryological features [2]. The anatomy of the prostatic region including prostate zonal anatomy is best depicted on endorectal T2-weighted magnetic resonance imaging (MRI) [3]

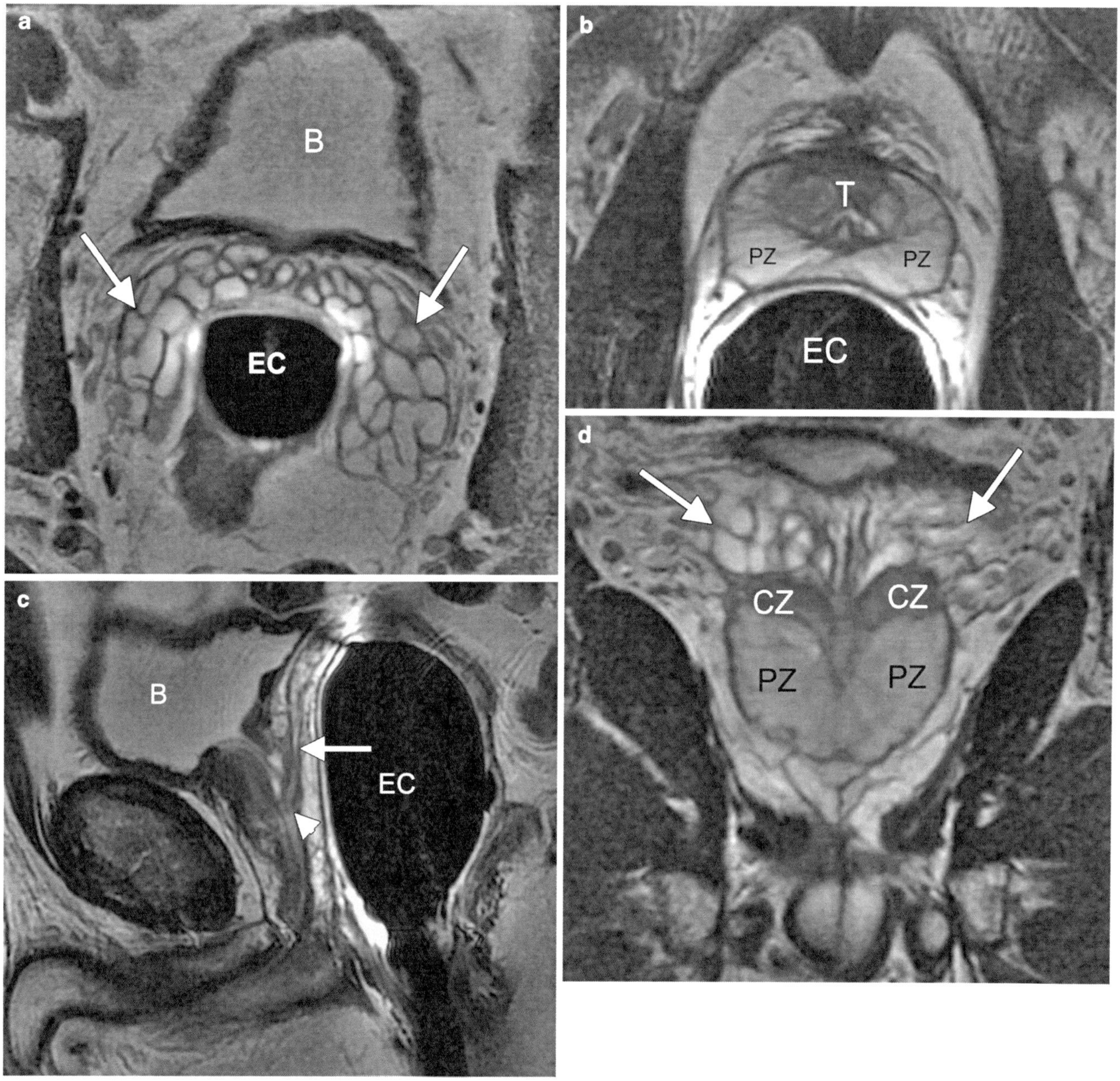

Fig. 4.1 Normal prostate anatomy on MRI. Axial (**a**, **b**), sagittal (**c**), and coronal (**d**) T2-weighted MR images of the male pelvis. The seminal vesicles (*arrows* in **a** and **d**) drain into the midprostatic urethra via the ejaculatory ducts (*arrow* in **c**) at the level of the verumontanum (*arrowhead* in **c**). The transition zone (*T*) extends superiorly, anteriorly, and laterally from the verumontanum. The central zone (*CZ*) surrounds the ejaculatory ducts and the peripheral zone (*PZ*) surrounds both the central zone and the distal prostatic urethra. *B* bladder; *EC* endorectal coil

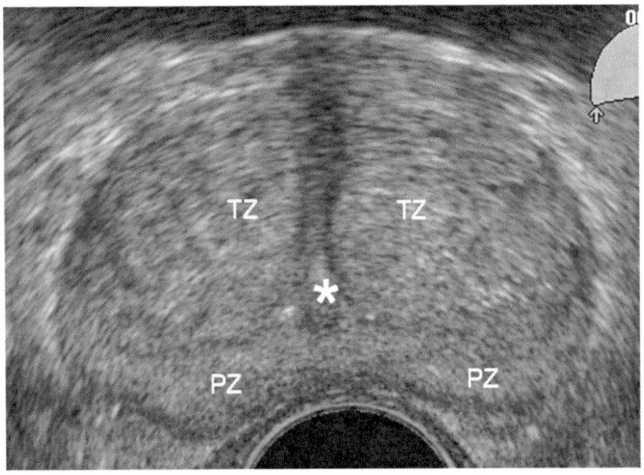

Fig. 4.2 Normal prostate anatomy on transrectal ultrasound (TRUS). TRUS image at the level of the midgland showing the peripheral zone (*PZ*), transition zone (*TZ*) and urethra (*asterisk*). TRUS has a limited accuracy for the detection of prostate cancer, but is typically used to guide prostate biopsies when cancer is suspected based on abnormal digital rectal examination or raised serum PSA

Prostate Cancer Diagnosis

Table 4.2 Typical appearance of prostate cancer according to imaging modality

Technique	Imaging appearance
Ultrasound	Hypoechoic compared to adjacent prostate tissue. Ultrasound is primarily used for guidance of transrectal prostate biopsies and focal therapies
CT	Hypoattenuating compared to adjacent prostate tissue, with enhancement following intravenous contrast. Not routinely used for primary diagnosis due to lack of sensitivity and specificity, however is useful for assessment of lymphadenopathy and in the post-treatment setting
PET	Increased uptake of FDG; however, this finding is not always present and artifact from FDG accumulation in the adjacent bladder limit the use of FDG PET-CT in diagnosis
T2-weighted MRI	Hypointense compared to adjacent prostate tissue
Diffusion-weighted MRI	High signal intensity on diffusion-weighted images and low signal intensity on apparent diffusion coefficient (ADC) map (restricted diffusion)
Dynamic contrast-enhanced MRI	Early enhancement, early washout
MR spectroscopy	Alteration in the ratio of prostate metabolites: citrate, choline, creatine, polyamines

Computed tomography (CT) and fluorodeoxyglucose (FDG) positron emission tomography (PET) are not routinely used for primary diagnosis due to lack of sensitivity and specificity; however, they are more often used for the assessment of lymphadenopathy and in the post-treatment setting [3]

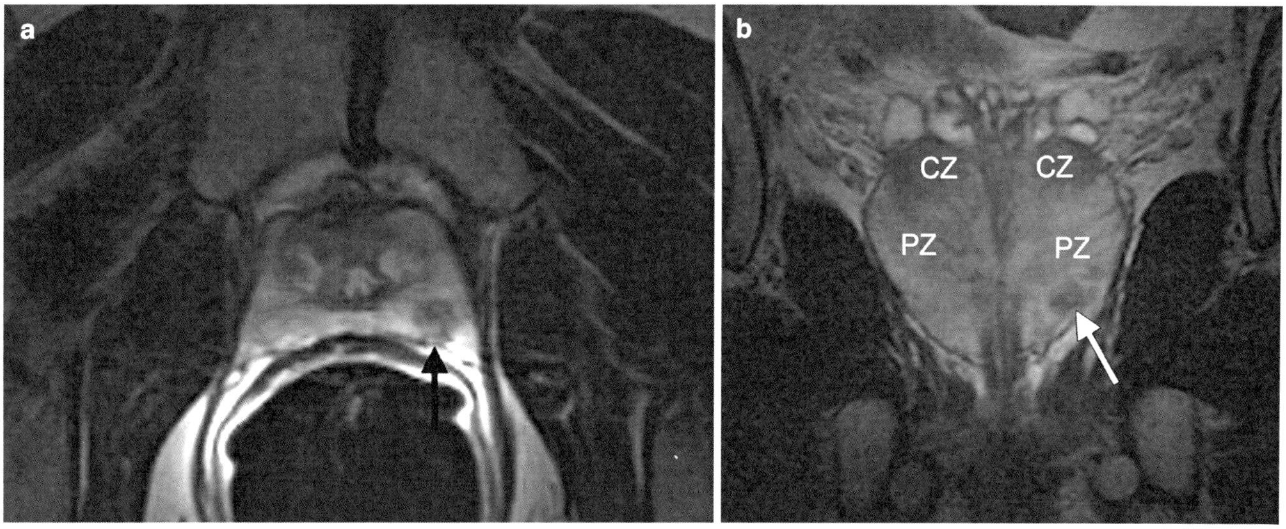

Fig. 4.3 MRI appearance of peripheral zone prostate cancer [4]. Axial (**a**) and coronal (**b**) T2-weighted images show the typical appearance of prostate cancer in the peripheral zone (*arrow*): low signal intensity compared to homogeneous high signal intensity of the normal peripheral zone (*PZ*). *CZ* central zone

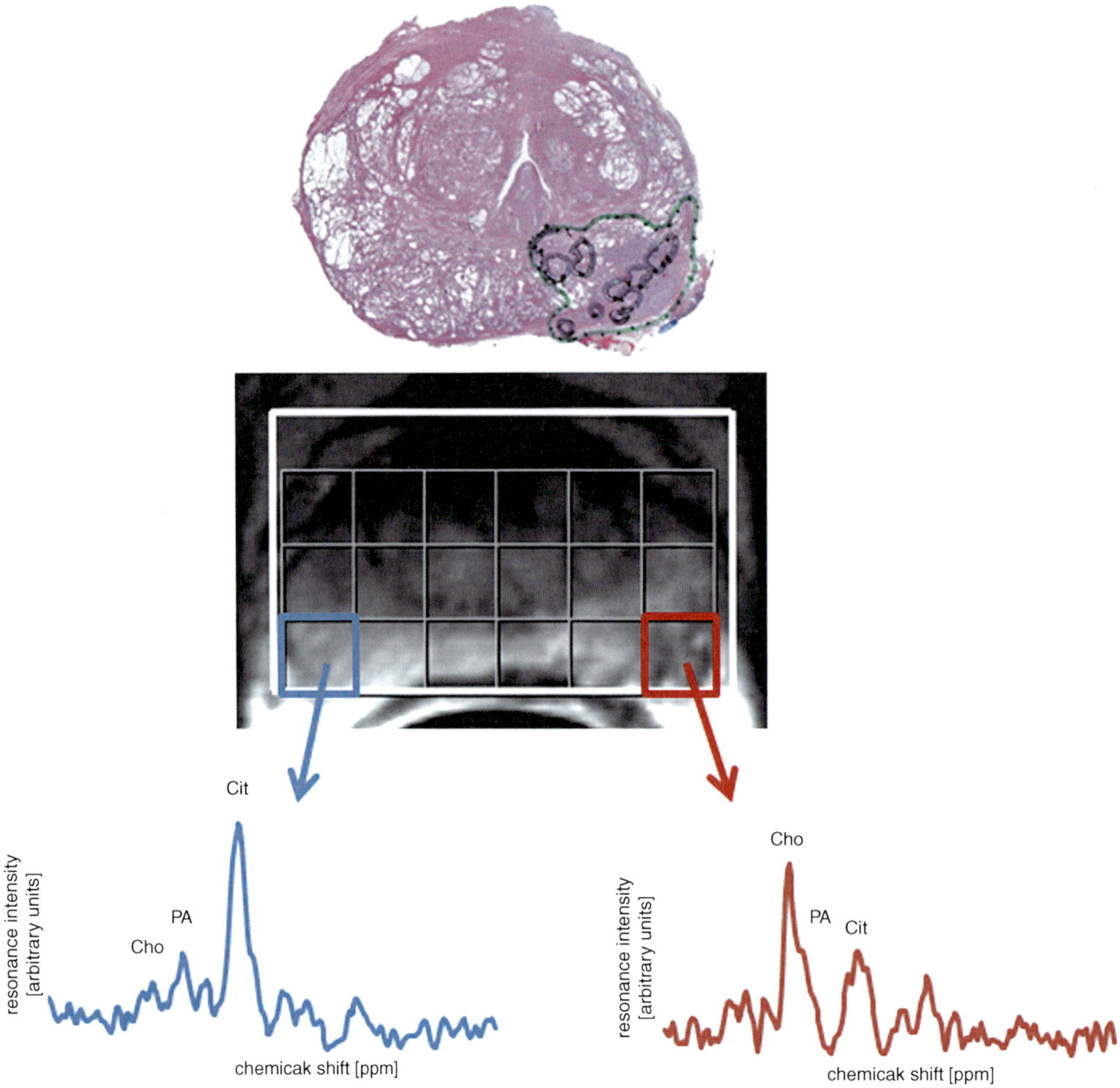

Fig. 4.4 MR spectroscopy (MRSI) appearance of prostate cancer [5]. MRSI spectral grid overlaid on T2-weighted MR image (*bottom row*) showing metabolite peaks from healthy (*blue*) and cancerous (*red*) voxels and corresponding whole-mount pathology map (*top row*) outlining a cancer focus in the left peripheral zone (*green and black lines*). Typically, the citrate level is high in normal prostatic tissue owing to the fact that the presence of zinc inhibits the first enzyme in the Krebs cycle. Citrate levels are reduced in prostate cancer but they can also be decreased as a result of prostatitis or hemorrhage. Choline is a constituent of the cell membrane, and as such its levels increase with the increased membrane turnover and phospholipids metabolism seen in prostate cancer. The polyamine level peak occurs between the creatine and choline level peaks and is typically decreased in prostate cancer

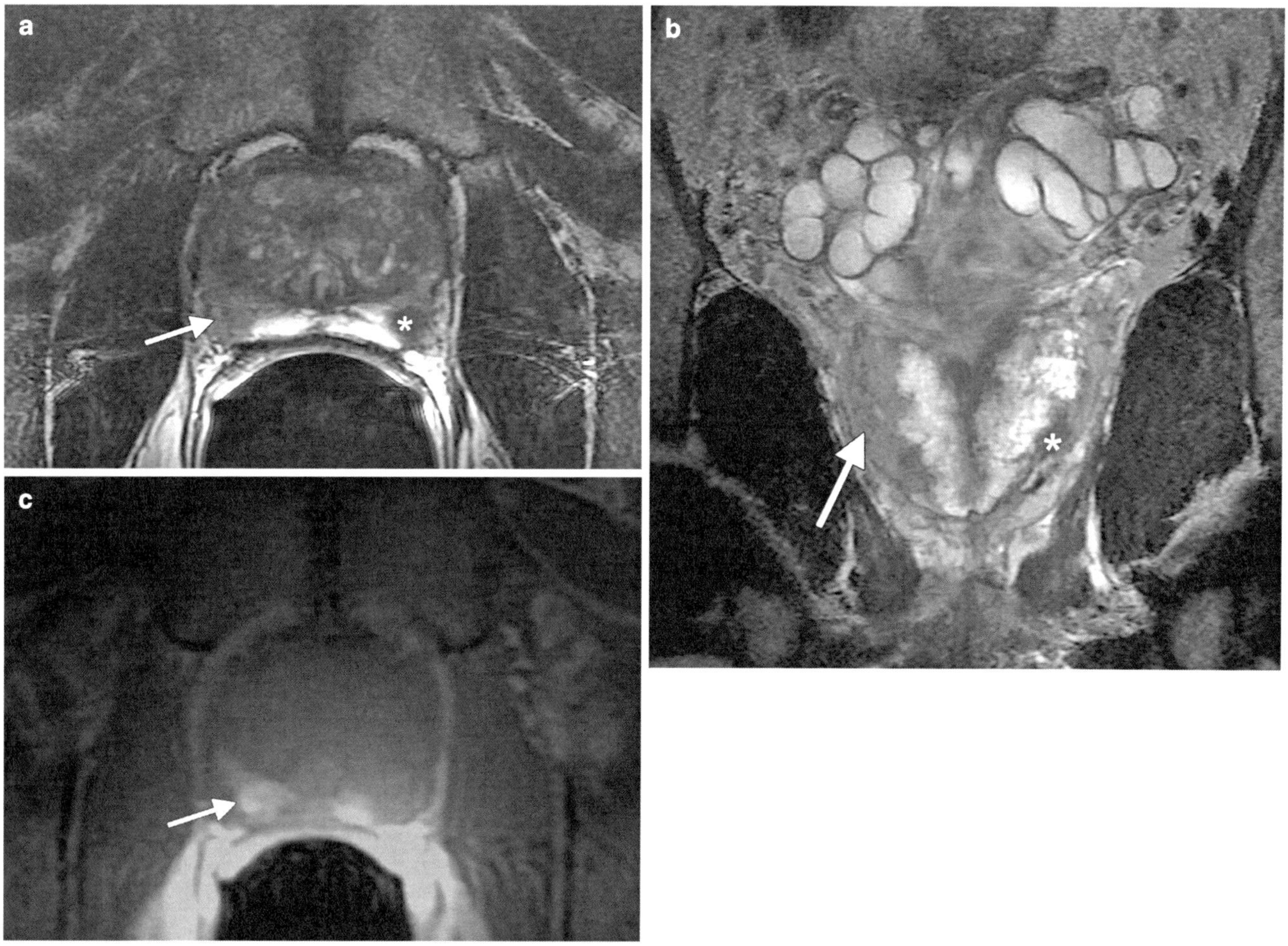

Fig. 4.5 Potential pitfall in prostate cancer detection on MRI: in the first few weeks after prostate biopsy, postbiopsy changes may be observed as areas of low, intermediate, or high signal intensity depending on the interval between biopsy and imaging, and in some cases may hinder identification of prostate cancer [6]. In this case, a clear low signal intensity tumor focus could be identified in the left peripheral zone (*asterisk*) despite the extensive low signal intensity regions on axial (**a**) and coronal (**b**) T2-weighted images, and high signal intensity regions on axial T1-weighted images (**c**) representing postbiopsy changes (*arrows*)

Table 4.3 Transition zone cancer

Prostate cancer most commonly occurs in the peripheral zone; however, about 25 % of cancers occur in the transition zone (TZ) [7]. On T2-weighted images (T2WI), the normal TZ is of heterogeneous signal intensity owing to variable amounts of glandular and stromal components. Features that aid the MRI detection of cancer in the TZ include:
1. Homogeneous low signal intensity
2. Ill-defined margins
3. Lack of a capsule (a feature associated with BPH nodules)
4. Lenticular shape
5. Invasion of the anterior fibromuscular stroma
6. Homogeneous enhancement following intravenous contrast

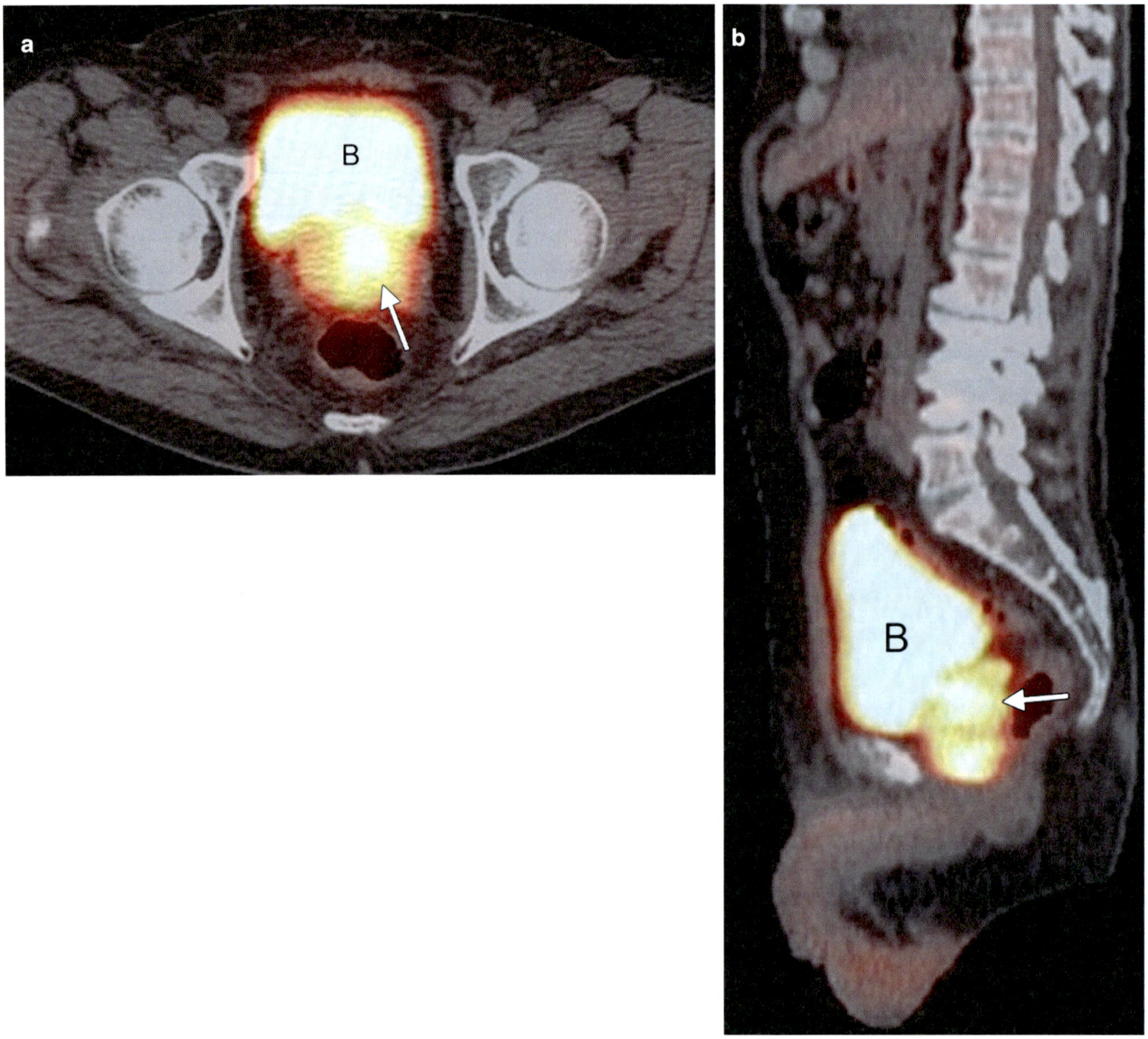

Fig. 4.6 FDG PET-CT in prostate cancer. Fused axial (**a**) and sagittal (**b**) PET-CT images demonstrate increased FDG uptake corresponding to prostate cancer with seminal vesicle invasion (*arrows*). Uptake in the bladder (*B*) due to renal excretion of FDG and the lack of FDG avidity in some prostate cancers limit the routine use of FDG PET-CT in the diagnosis of prostate cancer; however FDG PET-CT is useful in the detection of metastatic or recurrent disease in lymph nodes and bones, the two most common sites of spread of prostate cancer. Novel radiotracers (e.g., acetate, FLT [fluorothymidine], FACBC [fluorocyclobutane-1-carboxylic acid]) are currently being investigated and may play a role in imaging of prostate cancer in the future

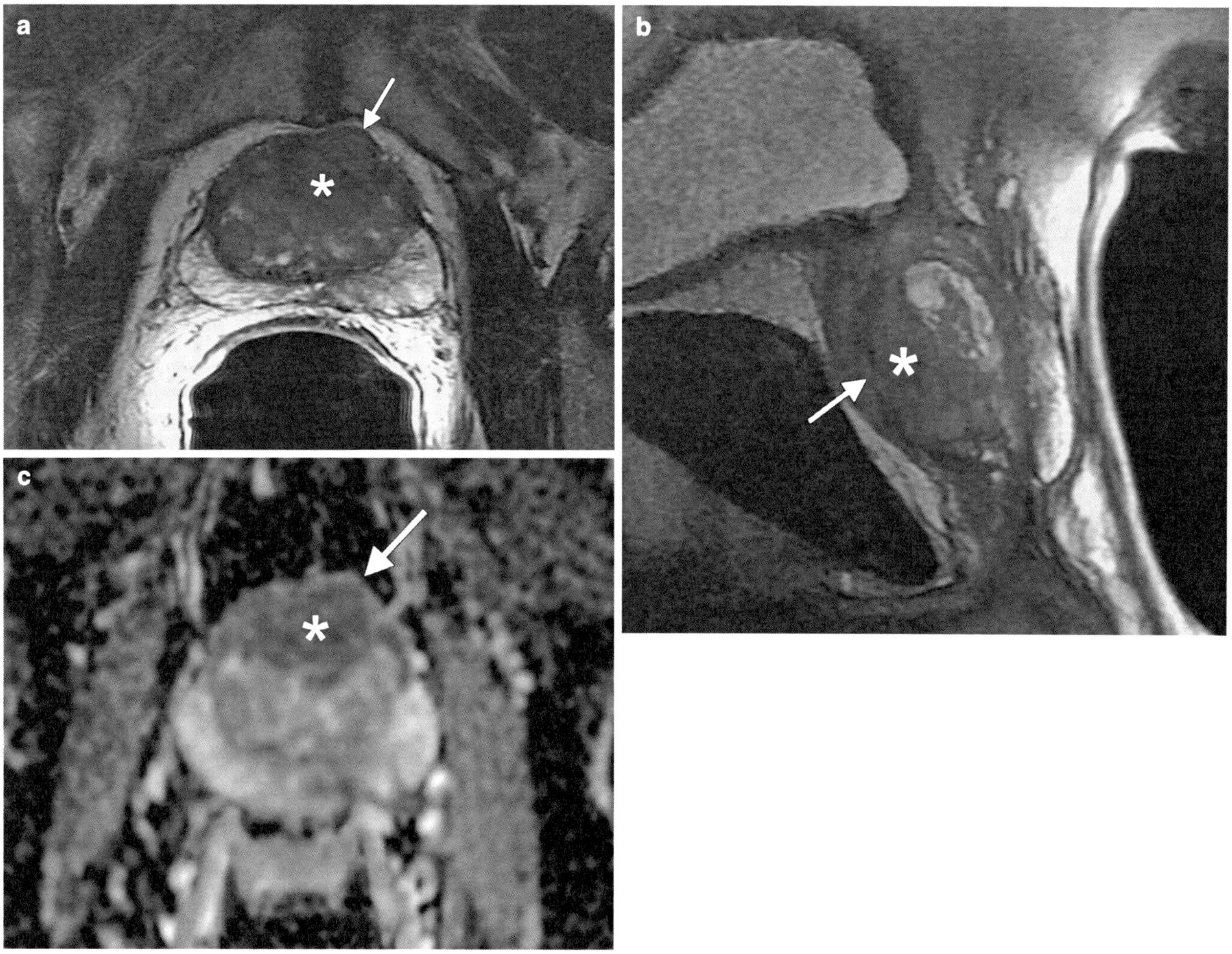

Fig. 4.7 Transition zone cancer. Axial (**a**) and sagittal (**b**) T2-weighted MRI and ADC map (**c**) derived from DW-MRI demonstrate an ill-defined area of homogeneous low signal intensity corresponding to a transition zone tumor (*asterisk*) with extension to the anterior fibromuscular stroma (*arrows*)

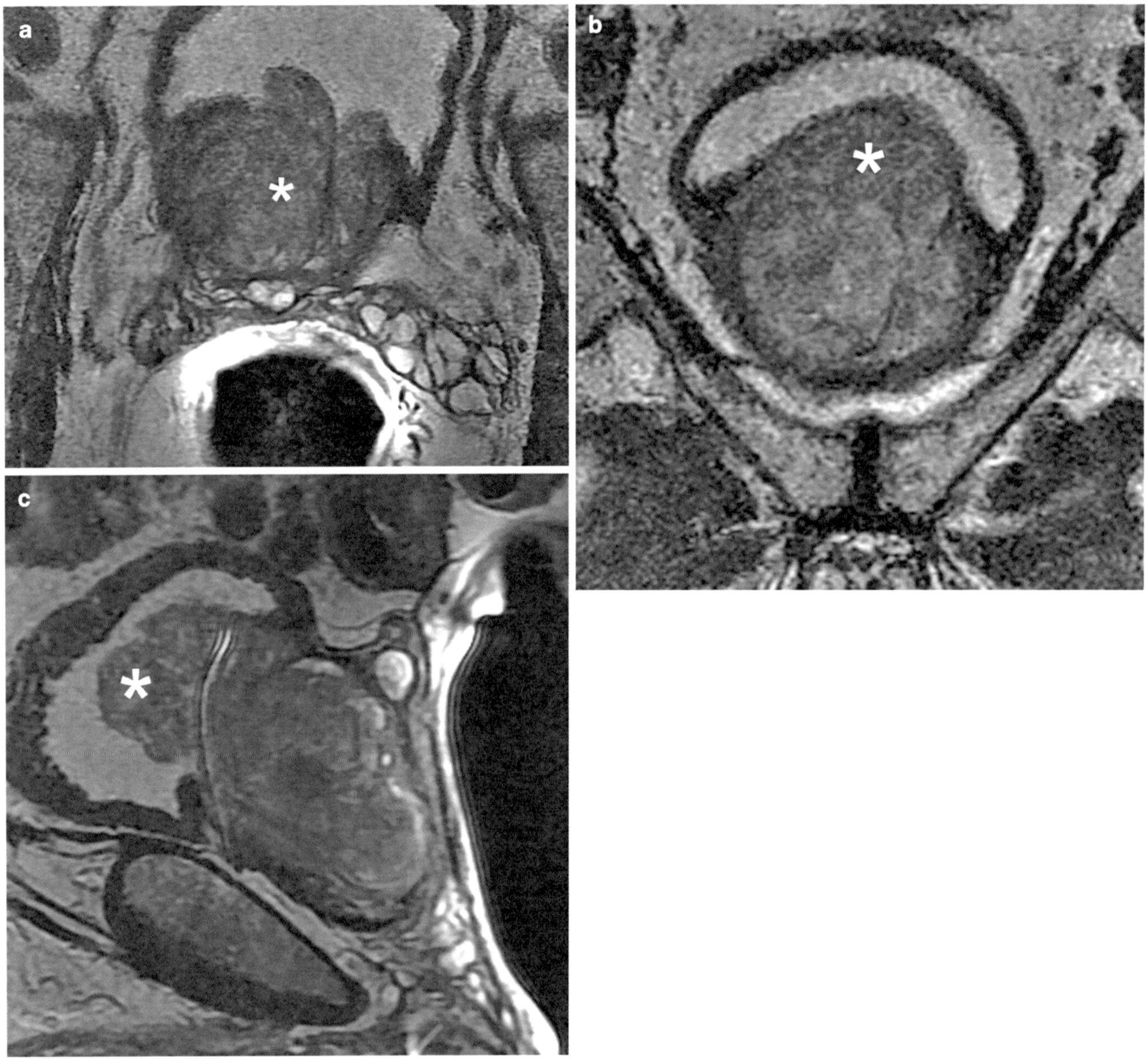

Fig. 4.8 Differential diagnosis of cancer. Axial (**a**), coronal (**b**), and sagittal (**c**) T2-weighted images demonstrate the typical heterogeneous appearance of BPH, in this case compressing the bladder wall (*asterisk*). BPH is more common with increasing age and can cause symptoms (e.g., urinary hesitancy, frequency, dysuria, and urinary retention). PSA levels may be elevated. BPH is not considered a premalignant condition. Prostatitis may also have MRI features that mimic those of prostate cancer

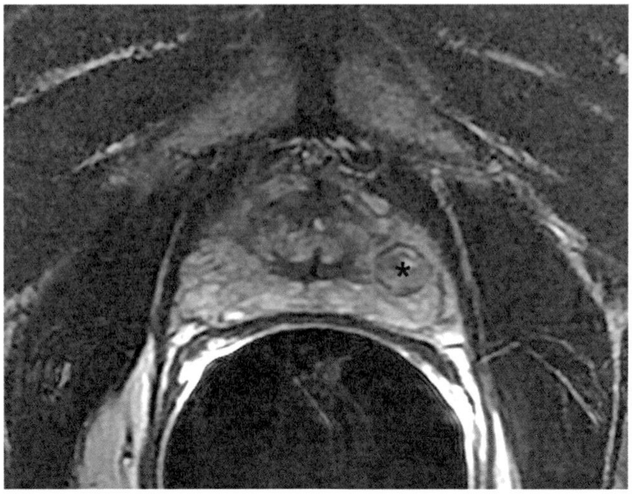

Fig. 4.9 Benign prostatic hyperplasia. Axial T2-weighted image demonstrates BPH in the peripheral zone (*asterisk*). Although BPH most commonly occurs in the transition zone, the peripheral zone is occasionally affected. Typical features such as the presence of a hypointense capsule and heterogeneous signal intensity aid its diagnosis

Prostate Cancer Staging

Table 4.4 American Joint Committee on Cancer (AJCC) TNM staging system (edn 7) [3]

T- stage	Notes
T1: Organ-confined tumor that is clinically and radiologically inapparent	
T2: Organ-confined tumor that is clinically or radiologically apparent	T2a: Tumor localized to a quadrant
	T2b: Tumor localized to one side
	T2c: Bilateral tumor
T3: Locally advanced tumor, with extraprostatic extension	T3a: Unilateral extracapsular extension
	T3b: Bilateral extracapsular extension
	T3c: Seminal vesicle invasion
T4: Invasion of the bladder, external sphincter, or rectum	**Microscopic bladder neck invasion is included in stage T3a**
N: Nodal evaluation	N0: No nodal metastases
	N1: Microscopic regional nodal metastases
	N2: Macroscopic regional nodal metastases
	N3: Extraregional nodal metastases
M: Metastasis evaluation	M1a: Nonregional lymph nodes
	M1b: Bones
	M1c: Others

Used with the permission of the American Joint Committee on Cancer (AJCC), Chicago, IL. The original source for this material is the *AJCC Cancer Staging Manual*, Seventh Edition (2010) published by Springer Science and Business Media LLC, www.springer.com

Table 4.5 AJCC stage groupings [3]

Stage I	T1a, N0, M0
Stage II	T1b, N0, M0
	T1c, N0, M0
	T2, N0, M0
Stage III	T3, N0, M0
Stage IV	T4, N0, M0
	Any T, N1, M0
	Any T, any N, M1

Used with the permission of the American Joint Committee on Cancer (AJCC), Chicago, IL. The original source for this material is the *AJCC Cancer Staging Manual*, Seventh Edition (2010) published by Springer Science and Business Media LLC, www.springer.com

Table 4.6 Information to include in the prostate MRI report

Clinical statement	Including PSA, biopsy positive locations, and Gleason grades
MRI technique	1. Magnetic field strength
	2. Imaging sequences: axial T1-weighted, axial, coronal, and sagittal T2-weighted
	3. Additional sequences: MR spectroscopy, diffusion-weighted MRI (DW-MRI), dynamic contrast-enhanced MRI (DCE-MRI)
	4. Coils used (e.g., endorectal and pelvic coils)
Prostate measurements	1. Anteroposterior (AP) × transverse (TR) × cranio-caudal (CC) in cm
	2. Volume: (AP × TR × CC)/2
	3. PSA density: PSA/volume
Postbiopsy changes	Indicate whether mild, moderate, or extensive
Suspicious lesion location	1. Right–left
	2. Base, mid-gland, or apex
	3. Prostate zone(s) involved
	4. Anterior, anterolateral, posterior, posterolateral
Local extent	1. Extracapsular extension
	2. Seminal vesicle invasion
	3. Adjacent organ invasion
Lymph nodes	Size and location
Bone lesions	Indicate presence of suspicious bone lesions

Table 4.7 MRI evaluation of extracapsular extension

Prostate tumors demonstrating the following MRI features indicate the presence of extracapsular extension [8]:
1. Broad capsular contact
2. Capsular bulging
3. Irregular, spiculated, or angulated margin
4. Gross extension
5. Obliteration of rectoprostatic angle
6. Asymmetry, traction, and/or thickening of the neurovascular bundles

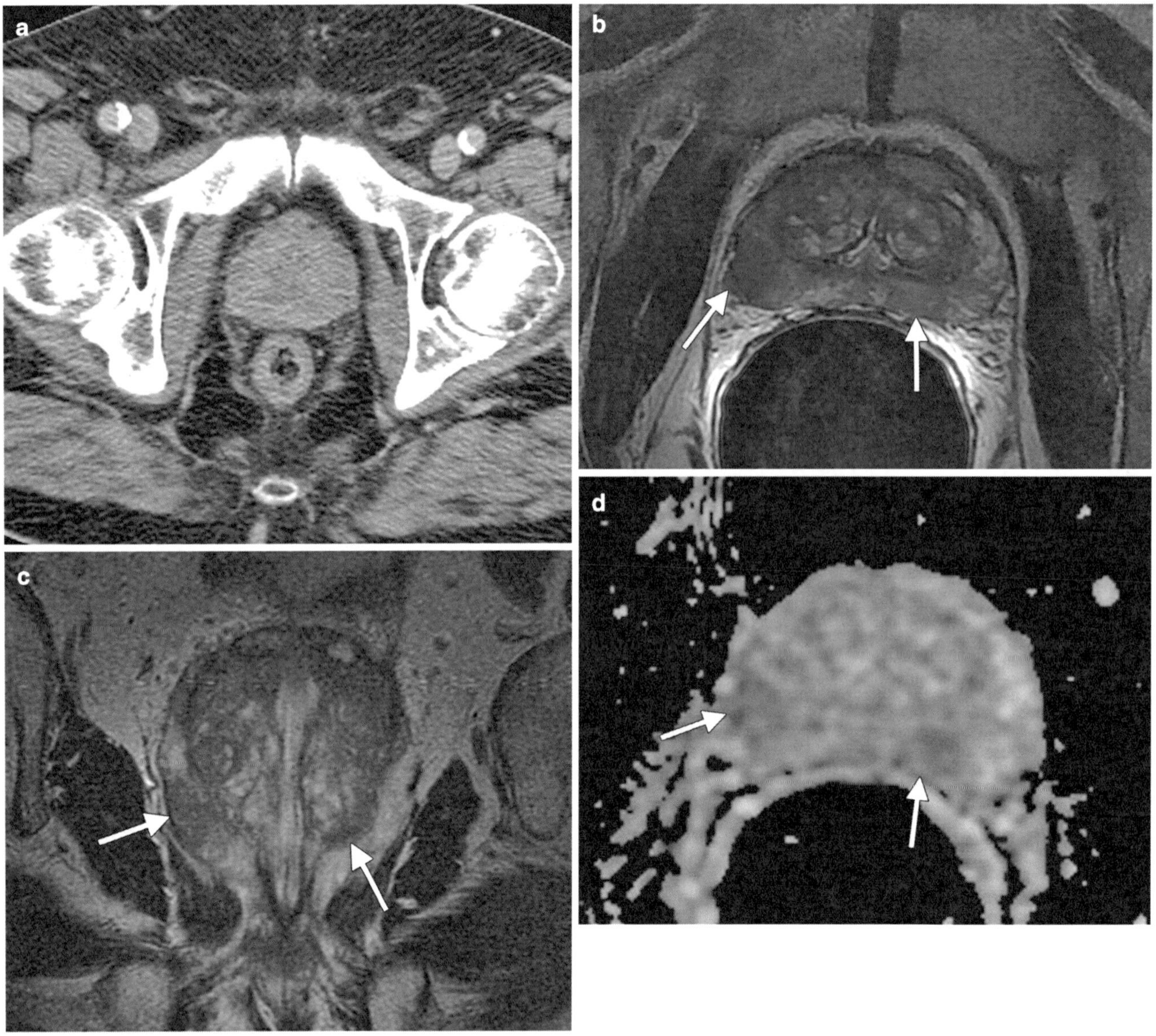

Fig. 4.10 Extracapsular extension (T3a disease). Axial CT (**a**) findings in the prostate are noncontributory. Axial (**b**) and coronal (**c**) T2-weighted images and ADC map (**d**) demonstrate suspicious tumors in the right and left peripheral zone (*arrows*), with gross extracapsular extension from the right peripheral zone tumor

Table 4.8 MRI criteria for detecting seminal vesicle invasion [9]

1. Focal or diffuse low T2 signal intensity
2. Expansion with low T2 signal intensity
3. Loss of seminal vesicle architecture and wall thickening
4. Direct tumor extension from base or through ejaculatory ducts
5. Obliteration of angle between seminal vesicle, bladder, and prostate

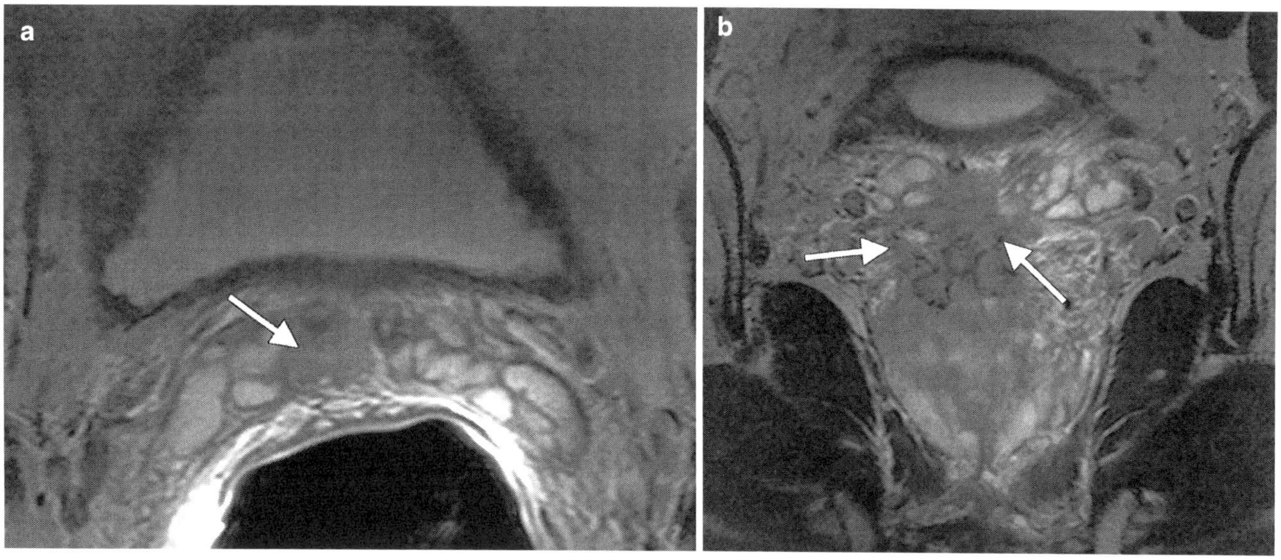

Fig. 4.11 Seminal vesicle invasion (T3c disease). Axial (**a**) and coronal (**b**) T2-weighted MRI demonstrates gross prostate tumor with direct extension into the seminal vesicles bilaterally (*arrows*)

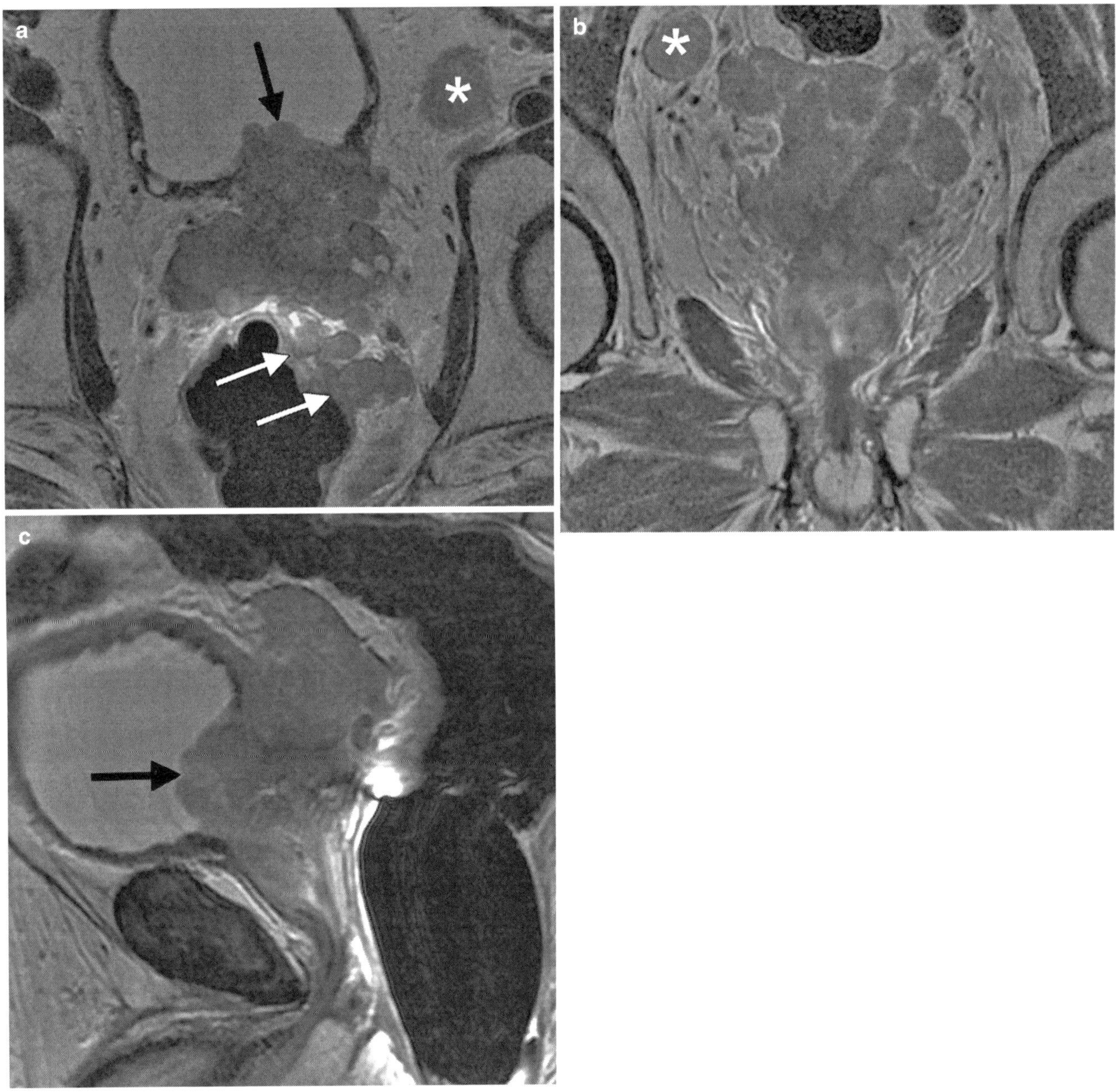

Fig. 4.12 Invasion of adjacent organs (T4 disease) and lymphadenopathy. Axial (**a**), coronal (**b**), and sagittal (**c**) T2-weighted images demonstrate invasion of the bladder (*black arrows*), rectum (*white arrows*), and metastatic lymph nodes (*asterisk*)

Table 4.9 Lymph node involvement in prostate cancer

1. Size: No absolute size cutoff exists for differentiating benign and malignant nodes. However, a size larger than 5 mm or asymmetry of lymph nodes on the same side as extracapsular extension are features suspicious for metastasis.
2. Location:
Regional lymph nodes (N1-N2): pelvic, obturator, external iliac, internal iliac, sacral
Distant lymph nodes (M): paraortic nodes, common iliac, superficial, and deep inguinal

Table 4.10 Prostate cancer metastases

1. Lymph nodes
2. Bone
3. Liver
4. Lungs
Lymph nodes and bones account for the majority of prostate cancer metastases, with other organs much less commonly affected

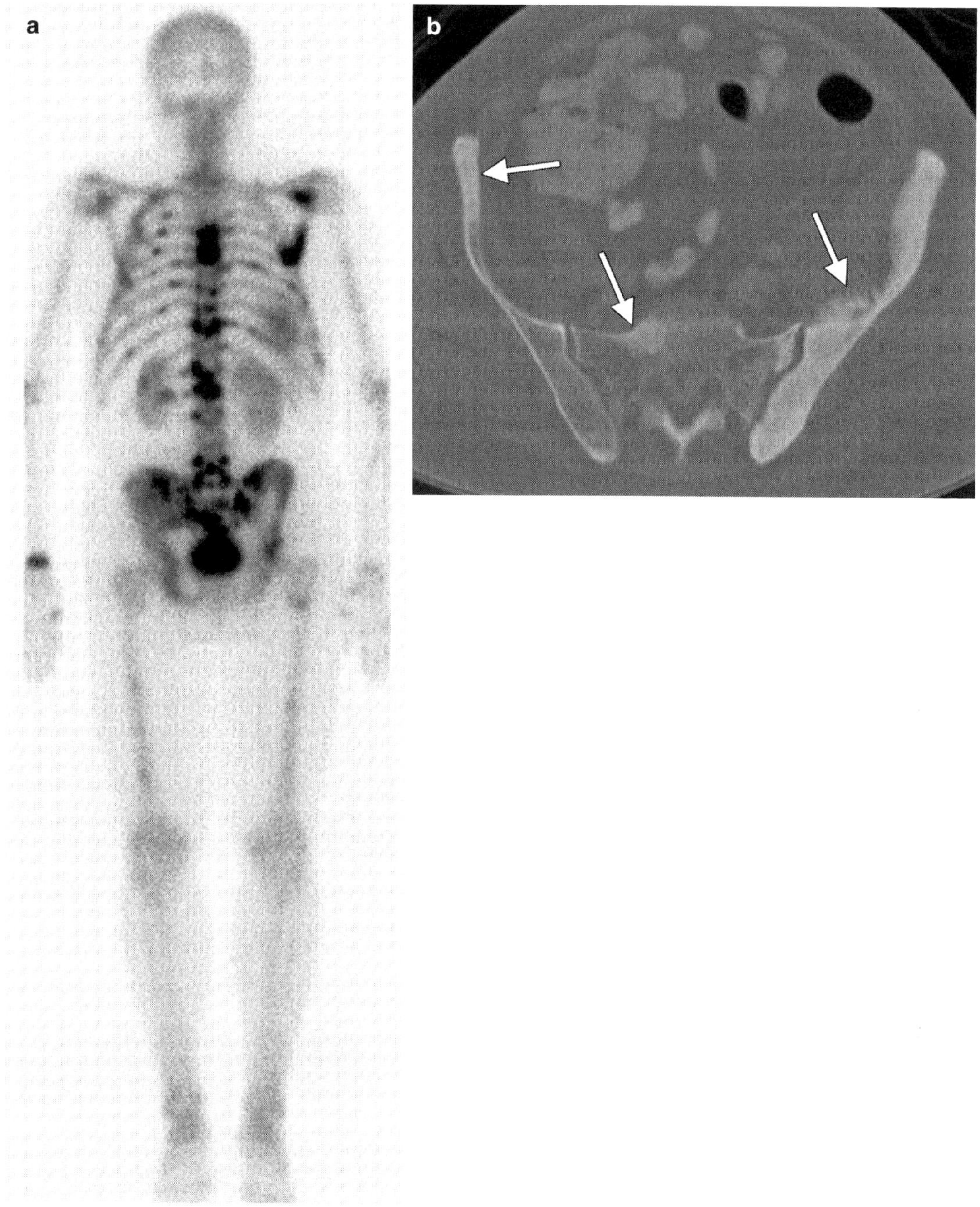

Fig. 4.13 Distant metastases: bone. 99 m technetium-methylene diphosphonate (Tc-99 m-MDP) bone scintigram (**a**) demonstrating multiple areas of increased uptake corresponding to prostate cancer bone metastases. Axial CT (**b**) demonstrates metastasis in the iliac bones bilaterally and the sacrum (*arrows*)

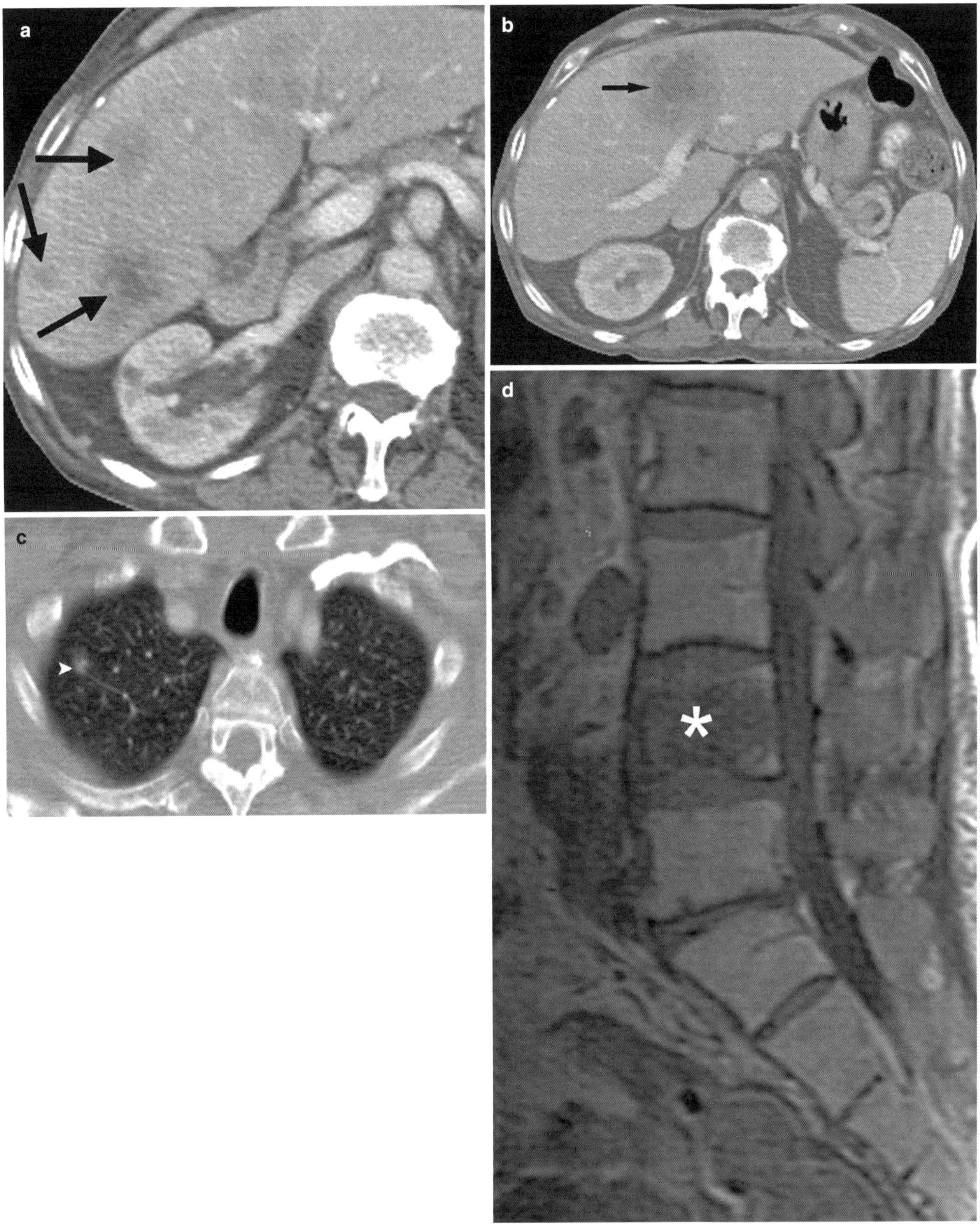

Fig. 4.14 Distant metastases: liver, lung, and bone. Axial CT images (**a–c**) demonstrating hypoattenuating liver lesions (*arrows*) and a right pulmonary nodule (*arrowhead*), all representing metastases. Sagittal T1-weighted MRI of the spine (**d**) demonstrates the typical T1-hypointense appearance of bone metastases, in this case affecting the L4 vertebral body (*asterisk*)

Prostate Cancer Treatment and Recurrence Assessment

Table 4.11 Prostate cancer management options

1. Active surveillance
2. Surgery (radical prostatectomy)
3. Radiation therapy (external-beam or brachytherapy)
4. Androgen deprivation therapy
5. Focal treatments
Cryotherapy
High-intensity focused ultrasound (HIFU)
Photodynamic therapy
Laser ablation

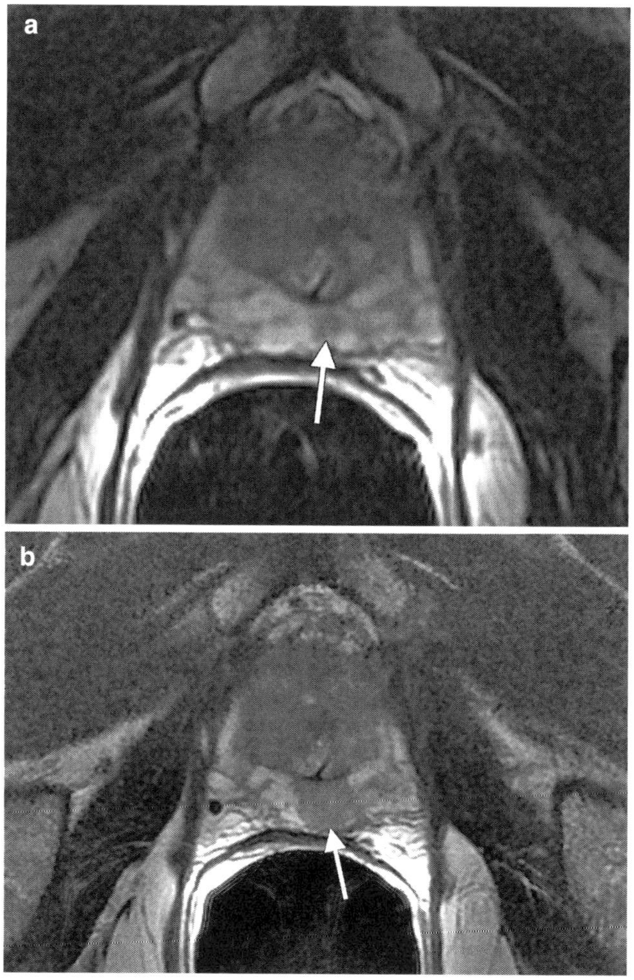

Fig. 4.15 Active surveillance is an option for patients with low-risk prostate cancer (e.g., Gleason score 6, clinical stage<T2a, and PSA<10 ng/mL) [10]. Definitive treatment may be delayed until there is evidence of disease progression. Axial T2-weighted images performed at diagnosis (**a**) and repeated 3 years later (**b**) show an increase in the size of a peripheral zone tumor (*arrows*) in a patient on active surveillance

Table 4.12 Imaging after radical prostatectomy [11]

Normal post-treatment appearance:
The bladder descends to occupy the space created by the absent prostate
Low signal intensity compared to muscle on all sequences may be present at the site of vesicourethral anastomosis, indicating normal postoperative scarring
Increased signal intensity compared to muscle may be present in the pelvic sidewall on T2-weighted MRI secondary to edema, particularly during the early stages of postoperative follow-up
Typical appearance of recurrence:
Soft tissue nodule in the prostatectomy bed (isointense to muscle on T1WI and hyperintense to muscle on T2-weighted MRI)
Early and avid enhancement following IV contrast
Typical sites of recurrence are the vesicourethral anastomosis, posterior bladder wall, and residual seminal vesicles
Differential diagnosis and potential pitfalls:
Postoperative fibrosis (low signal intensity on all sequences)
Granulation tissue (may mimic signal intensity of tumor recurrence)
Retained seminal vesicles may mimic soft tissue recurrence
Metallic clips (low signal intensity on T1 and T2-weighted MRI) may interfere with evaluation
“Residual prostate” after prostatectomy
Prominent periprostatic venous plexus should not be confused with “enhancing” recurrent tumor

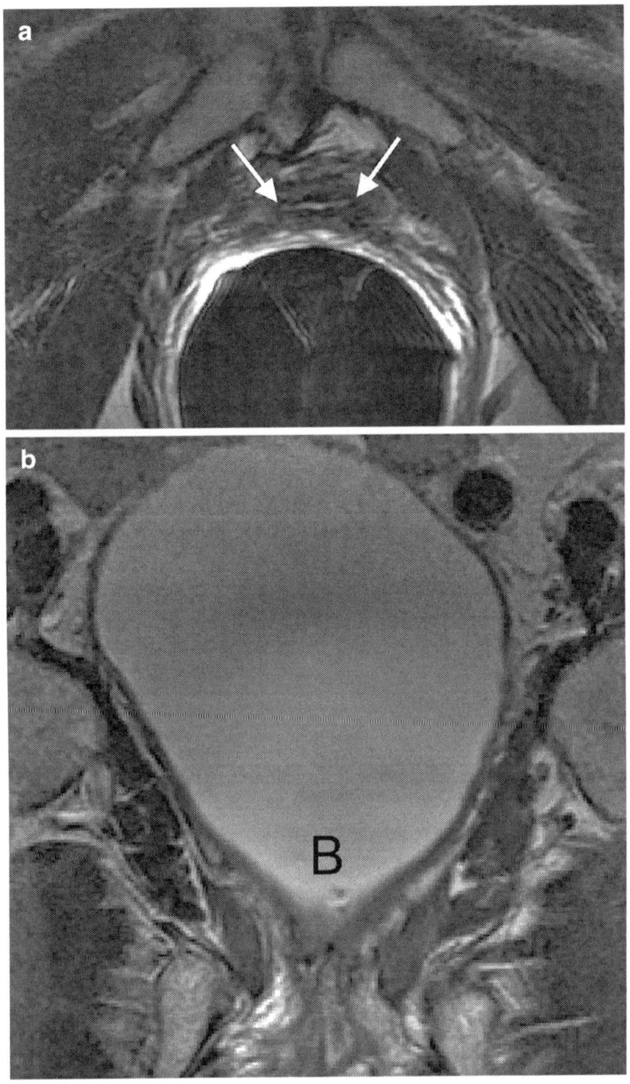

Fig. 4.16 Normal MRI appearance following radical prostatectomy. Axial T2-weighted image (**a**) demonstrates the typical low signal intensity surrounding the high signal intensity slit (*arrows*) in the normal vesicourethral anastomosis. Coronal T2-weighted image (**b**) showing the prostate bed occupied by the bladder (*B*)

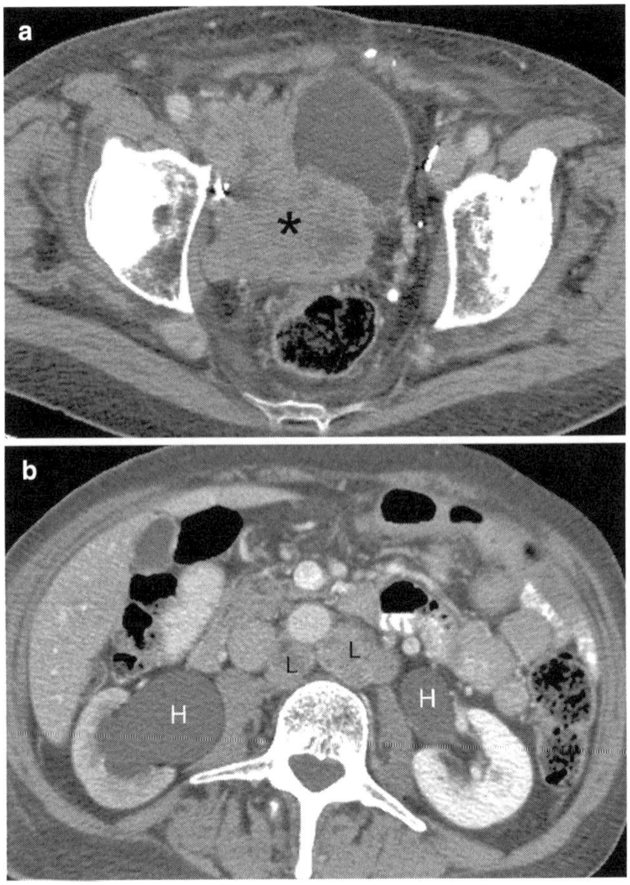

Fig. 4.17 Recurrence after radical prostatectomy. Axial CT images (**a**, **b**) demonstrating gross soft tissue in the pelvis (*asterisk*) representing prostate cancer recurrence that is causing ureteric obstruction and hydronephrosis (*H*). Retroperitoneal lymphadenopathy (*L*) is also shown

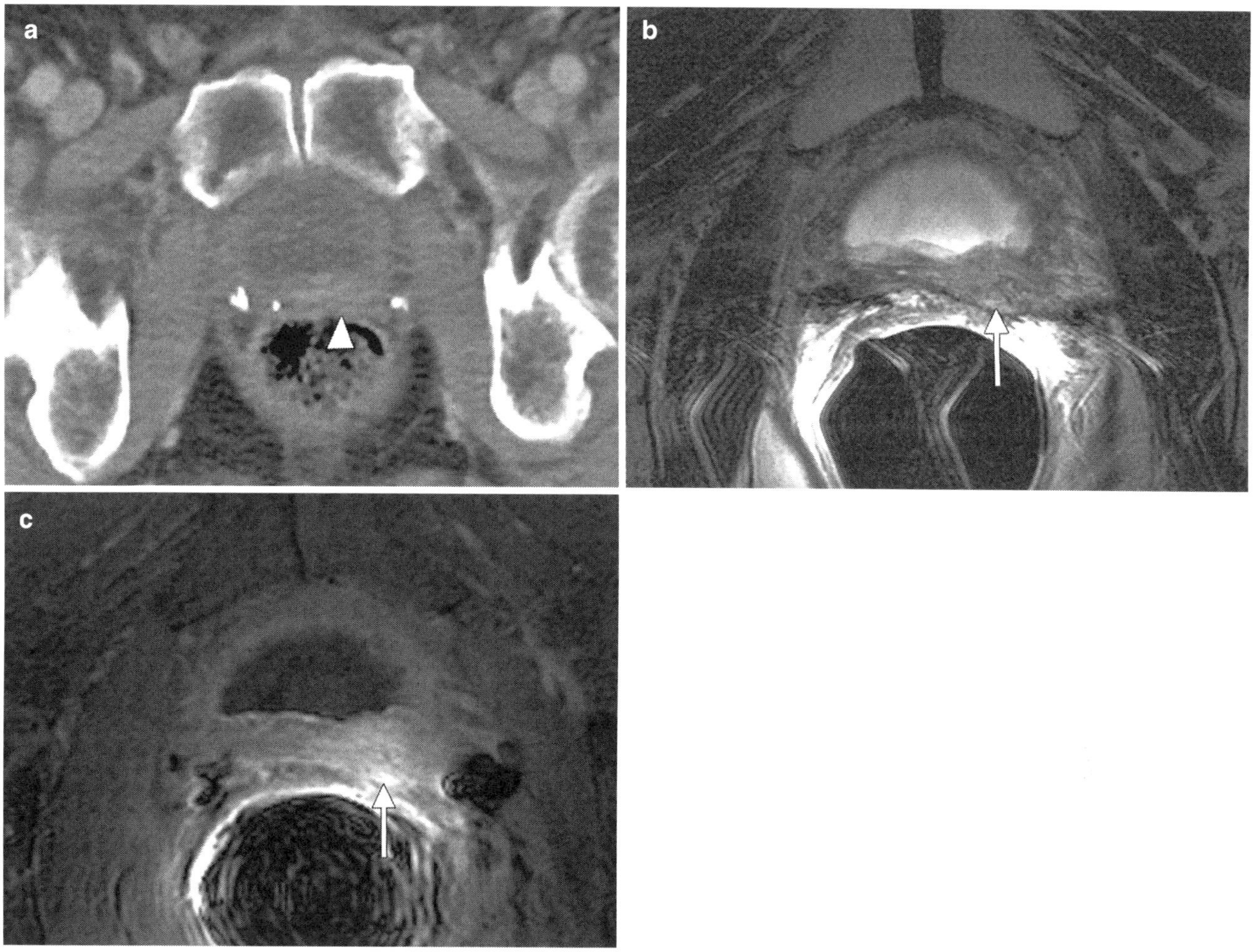

Fig. 4.18 Recurrence after radical prostatectomy. The improved soft tissue resolution of MRI better depicts prostate cancer recurrence. Axial CT (**a**) shows nonspecific thickening in the posterior bladder wall (*arrowhead*). Fat-suppressed T1-weighted image before (**b**) and after intravenous gadolinium (**c**) better delineates the enhancing soft tissue consistent with prostate cancer recurrence (*arrows*)

Table 4.13 Differential diagnosis of postprostatectomy fluid collections [11]

Lymphocele	Well-defined, thin walls, homogeneous contents, mild or no wall enhancement, no surrounding inflammatory changes
Abscess	Thick walls, internal septations, heterogeneous contents, marked wall enhancement, surrounding inflammatory changes
Hematoma	Contains blood degradation products
Bladder leak or urinoma	Contrast extravasation and direct contiguity with the urinary tract

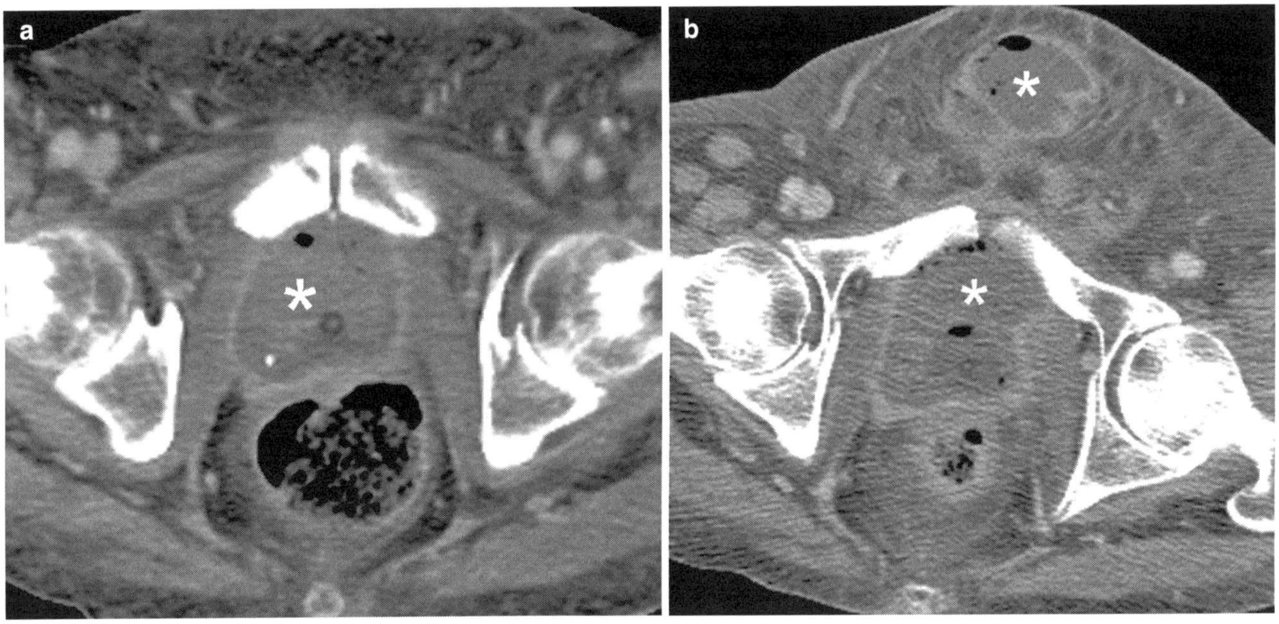

Fig. 4.19 Abscess following radical prostatectomy. Axial CT images (**a, b**) demonstrate air containing fluid collections (*asterisk*) with thick, irregular, enhancing walls in the prostatectomy bed and subcutaneous tissues

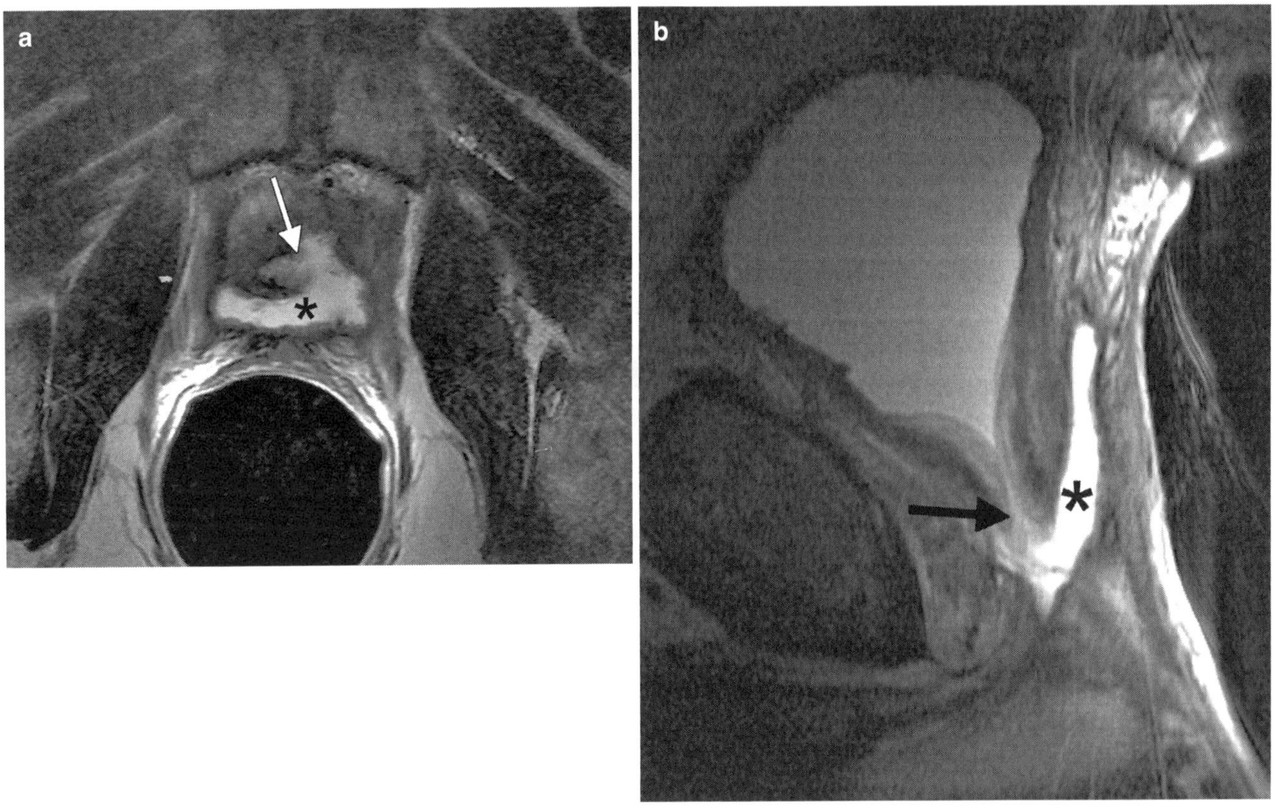

Fig. 4.20 Urinary leak following radical prostatectomy. Axial (**a**) and sagittal (**b**) T2-weighted images demonstrate a fluid collection (*asterisk*) in direct continuity with the vesicourethral anastomosis (*arrows*)

Table 4.14 Imaging after radiation therapy [12]

Normal post-treatment appearance:
Decrease in size and signal intensity on T2-weighted MRI
The prostatic zones appear less distinct from each other
Prostate tumors may decrease in size, capsular irregularity, or extracapsular extension
Clues to postpelvic radiotherapy status: high T2 signal and/or thickening of the bladder, rectal wall, perirectal fascia, and pelvic sidewall muscles
Typical appearance of recurrence:
Nodular lesion of lower signal intensity than the adjacent normal prostate on T2-weighted MRI, in the same location as the pre-radiotherapy tumor
Other identifying features: growth of the lesion and progressive bulging of the prostatic capsule over time
Restricted diffusion of DW-MRI and early enhancement and washout on DCE-MRI
Differential diagnosis and potential pitfalls:
Focal T2 hypointense regions in the prostate may represent treated tumor and not necessarily cancer recurrence
Recurrent tumors may not be apparent on T2-weighted MRI
Radiotherapy-induced capsular irregularity may hinder evaluation of extra-capsular extension

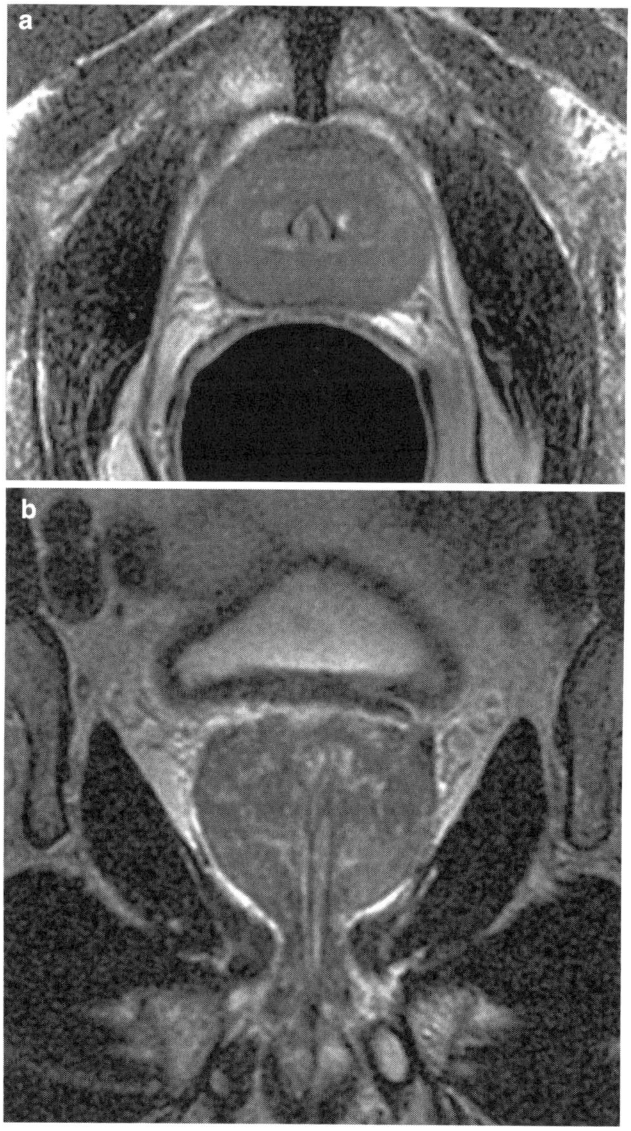

Fig. 4.21 Normal appearance after external-beam radiation therapy. Axial (**a**) and coronal (**b**) T2-weighted images demonstrating diffusely decreased signal intensity throughout the prostate with loss of zonal differentiation

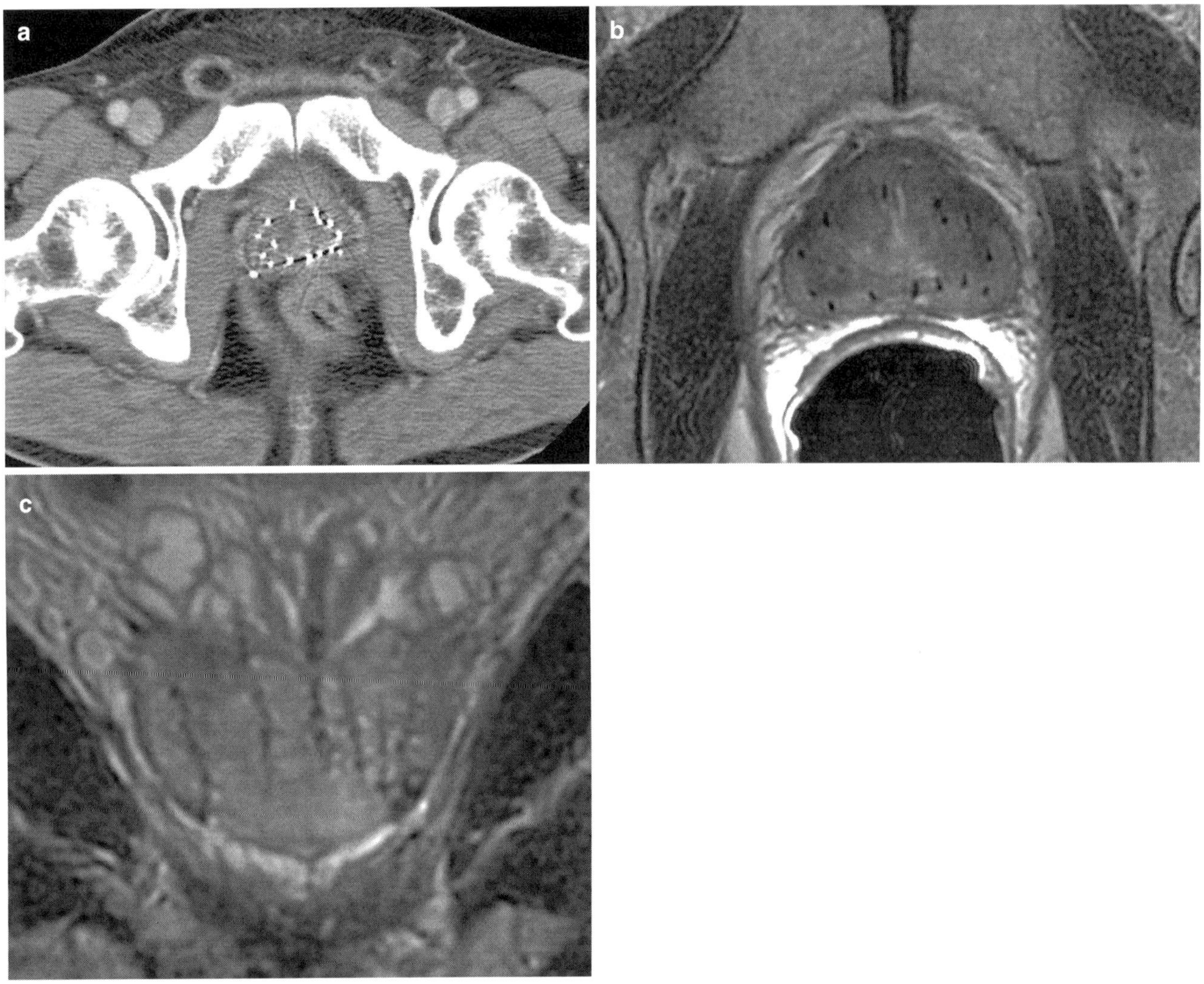

Fig. 4.22 Normal appearance after brachytherapy. Radioactive sources (seeds) are implanted directly into the prostate gland to deliver a high dose of radiation to the tumor while sparing the bladder and rectum as much as possible. The most commonly used permanent implants are iodine-125 or palladium-103 seeds. Axial CT (**a**) and axial (**b**) and coronal (**c**) T2-weighted MRI demonstrate multiple seeds implanted throughout the prostate

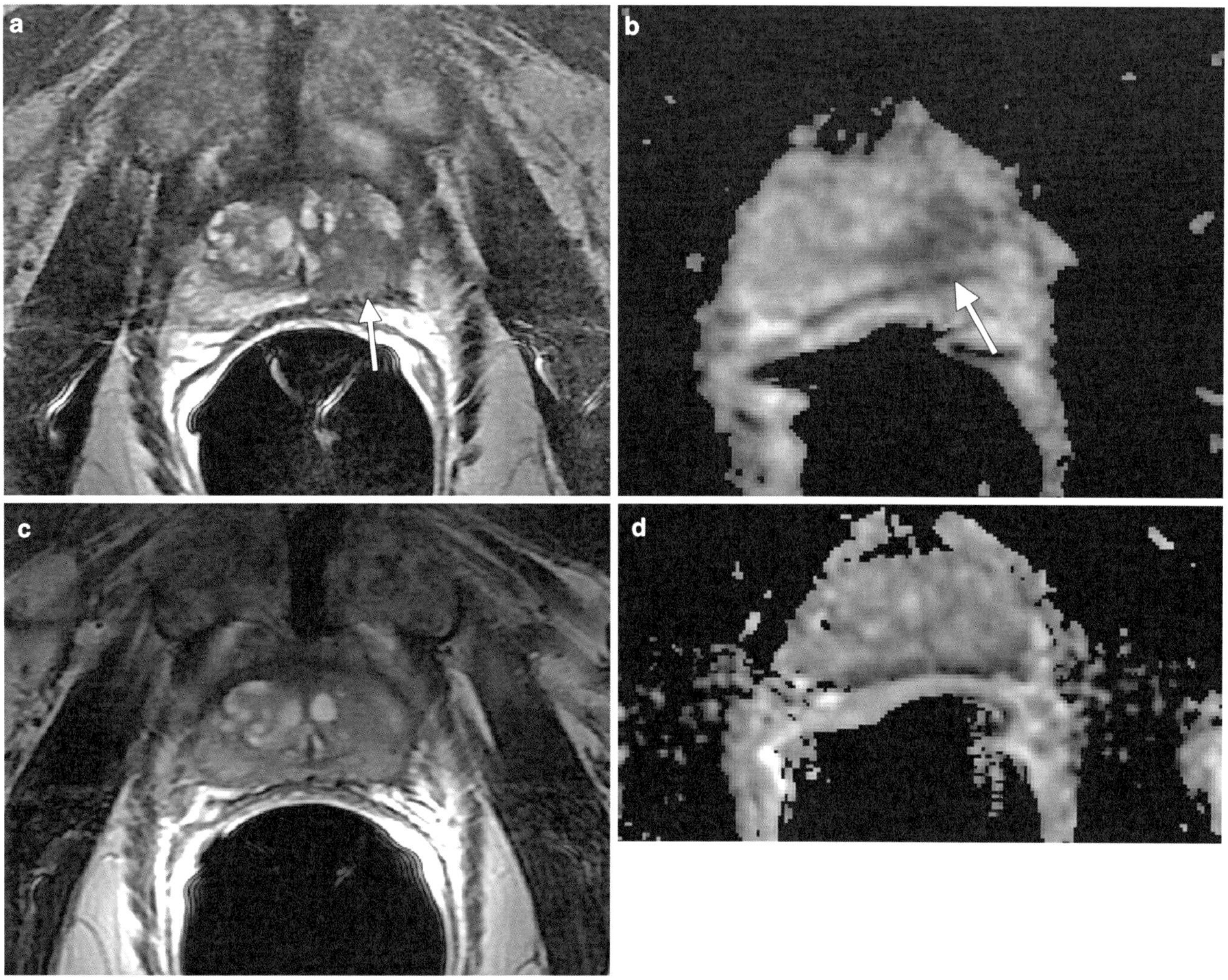

Fig. 4.23 Response to radiation therapy. Axial T2-weighted image (**a**) and ADC map (**b**) demonstrate a left peripheral zone tumor (*arrows*). One year after radiation, axial T2-weighted image (**c**) demonstrates loss of zonal differentiation. The left peripheral zone tumor is not discretely visualized on either T2-weighted image (**c**) or ADC map (**d**)

Table 4.15 Imaging after androgen deprivation therapy [11]

Normal post-treatment appearance:
Imaging features may be similar to those after radiotherapy (decreased volume, decreased signal intensity on T2-weighted MRI and loss of zonal differentiation); however radiotherapy-induced changes in adjacent structures are absent.
Typical appearance of recurrence:
Tumor is of low signal intensity on T2-weighted MRI, however because of therapy induced decreased signal intensity in the peripheral zone, differentiation between tumor and post-treatment change is difficult and the presence of tumor may be overestimated
Differential diagnosis and potential pitfalls:
Findings vary depending of the type and duration of androgen deprivation therapy
Differentiating between treated and recurrent tumor may be difficult after androgen deprivation therapy in the same way that it is difficult after radiotherapy

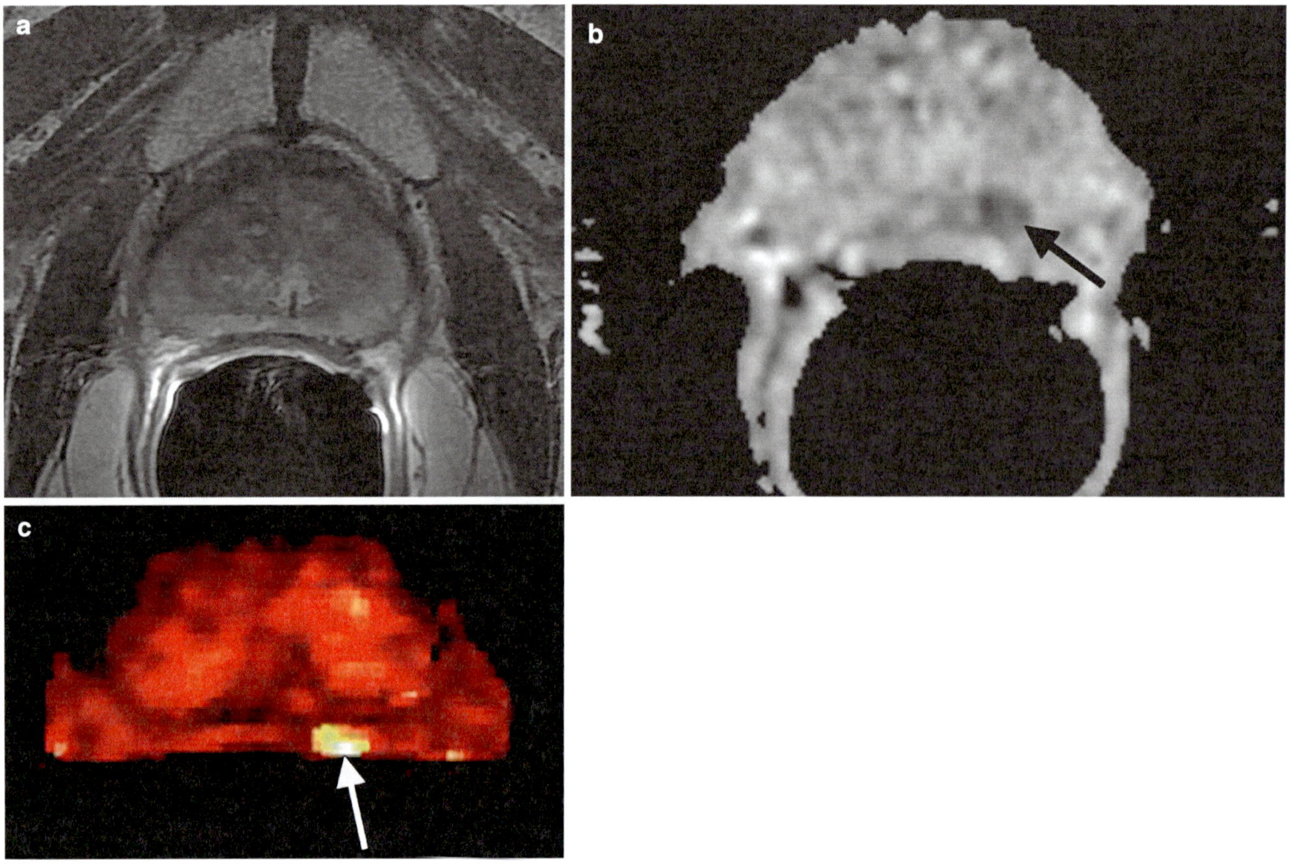

Fig. 4.24 Recurrence after radiation therapy and hormones. Multiparametric MRI is sometimes useful for the evaluation of suspected recurrence in the treated prostate [13]. In this patient with prostate cancer treated with external beam radiation therapy and hormones, axial T2-weighted images (**a**) did not demonstrate a significant abnormality. ADC map derived from diffusion-weighted MRI (**b**) and k^{trans} map derived from DCE-MRI (**c**) demonstrated a left peripheral zone tumor (*arrow*)

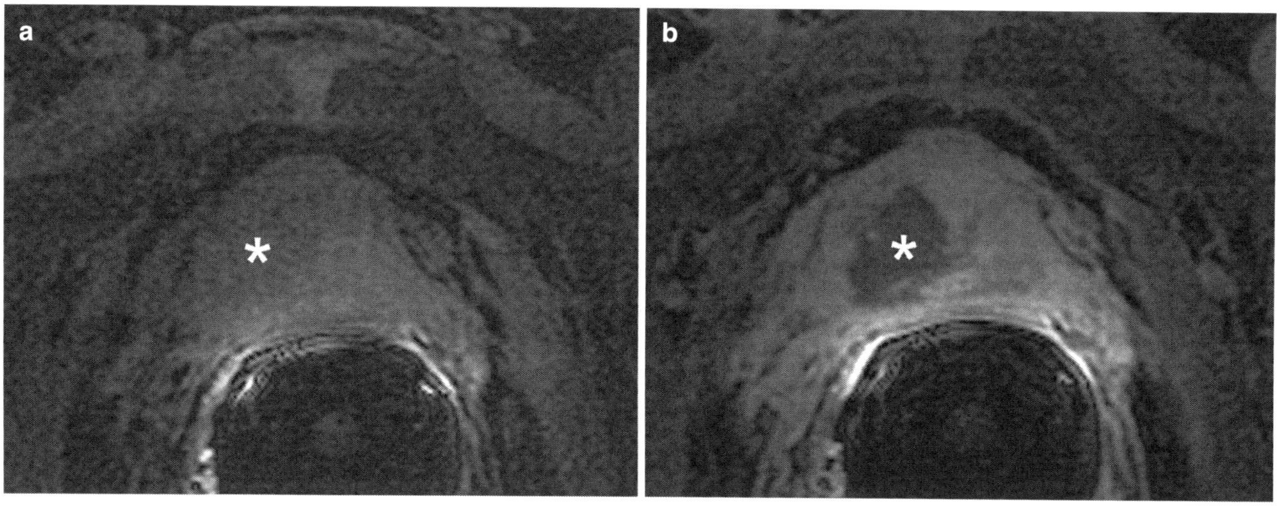

Fig. 4.25 Normal appearances following laser ablation therapy. Fat suppressed T1-weighted images before (**a**) and after (**b**) intravenous gadolinium demonstrate the normal necrotic cavity (*asterisk*) at the site of ablated tumor

Table 4.16 Focal therapies for prostate cancer

Type of therapy	Mechanism of action
Cryotherapy	Ablation of tissue by extremely cold temperatures
High-intensity focused ultrasound (HIFU)	Causes coagulation necrosis in the targeted tissue by converting mechanical energy into heat and generating a cavitation effect
Photodynamic therapy (PDP) and laser therapy	Enables destruction of targeted tissues using a light-sensitive agent (photosensitizer) and laser light of a specific wavelength in the presence of oxygen

Table 4.17 Imaging after focal treatments

Normal post-treatment appearance:
May be used to treat the entire prostate or target specific prostate regions, and may be delivered using a transrectal or transperineal approach
Depending on the extent of the treatment, loss of zonal differentiation, thickening of the prostatic capsule and periprostatic fibrosis and scarring may be present
Typical appearance of recurrence:
Soft tissue nodule. IV contrast is recommended for differentiating treatment-induced focal necrosis from viable tissue.
The site of treatment-related changes should correlate to the region of the prostate targeted by the focal therapy.
Differential diagnosis and potential pitfalls:
It may be difficult to differentiate viable tumor from reactive enhancing prostate tissue, particularly at the margins of the treated area.

Conclusion

Imaging plays an important role in every aspect of prostate cancer, from initial diagnosis and staging, to evaluation of residual or recurrent disease after treatment. Knowledge of the normal prostate anatomy and the typical imaging appearance of prostate cancer—as well as recognizing expected post-treatment imaging appearances and post-treatment complications and separating them from the imaging features indicative of recurrent cancer—are of paramount importance in order to adopt an appropriate management strategy.

References

1. Siegel R, Ward E, Brawley O, Jemal A. Cancer statistics, 2011. CA: Cancer J Clin. 2011;61:212–36.
2. McNeal JE, Redwine EA, Freiha FS, Stamey TA. Zonal distribution of prostatic adenocarcinoma. Correlation with histologic pattern and direction of spread. Am J Surg Pathol. 1988;12:897–906.
3. Edge SB, Byrd DR, Compton CC. American Joint Committee on Cancer: AJCC cancer staging manual. New York: Springer; 2010.
4. Beyersdorff D, Taupitz M, Winkelmann B, et al. Patients with a history of elevated prostate-specific antigen levels and negative transrectal US-guided quadrant or sextant biopsy results: value of MR imaging. Radiology. 2002;224:701–6.
5. Shukla Dave A, Hricak H, Moskowitz C, et al. Detection of prostate cancer with MR spectroscopic imaging: an expanded paradigm incorporating polyamines. Radiology. 2007;245:499–506.
6. Rosenkrantz A, Kopec M, Kong X, et al. Prostate cancer vs. post-biopsy hemorrhage: diagnosis with T2- and diffusion-weighted imaging. J Magn Reson Imaging. 2010;31:1387–94.
7. Akin O, Sala E, Moskowitz CS, et al. Transition zone prostate cancers: features, detection, localization, and staging at endorectal MR imaging. Radiology. 2006;239:784–92.
8. Bloch BN, Furman Haran E, Helbich T, et al. Prostate cancer: accurate determination of extracapsular extension with high-spatial-resolution dynamic contrast-enhanced and T2-weighted MR imaging—initial results. Radiology. 2007;245:176–85.

9. Wang L, Hricak H, Kattan MW, et al. Prediction of seminal vesicle invasion in prostate cancer: incremental value of adding endorectal MR imaging to the Kattan nomogram. Radiology. 2007;242:182–8.
10. Lawrentschuk N, Klotz L. Active surveillance for low-risk prostate cancer: an update. Nat Rev Urol. 2011;8:312–20.
11. Vargas HA, Wassberg C, Akin O, Hricak H. Magnetic resonance imaging of the treated prostate. Radiology. 2012;262:26–42.
12. Westphalen A, McKenna D, Kurhanewicz J, Coakley F. Role of magnetic resonance imaging and magnetic resonance spectroscopic imaging before and after radiotherapy for prostate cancer. J Endourol. 2008;22:789–94.
13. Akin O, Gultekin DH, Vargas HA, et al. Incremental value of diffusion weighted and dynamic contrast enhanced MRI in the detection of locally recurrent prostate cancer after radiation treatment: preliminary results. Eur Radiol. 2011;21:1970–8.

Imaging of Adrenal Neoplasms

5

Asim A. Afaq and Robert A. Lefkowitz

Lesions of the adrenal glands rarely present clinically and are usually detected as incidental findings on imaging. The incidence of adrenal masses found at computed tomography (CT) or magnetic resonance (MR) imaging of the abdomen has been reported to be 4–6 % [1–3], with the overall number of lesions having increased significantly in recent years given the rapid expansion of abdominal imaging in clinical practice. This incidence varies greatly with age: patients between 20 and 29 years of age, for example, have a 0.2 % incidence of adenomas detected on CT, compared with 7–10 % in elderly patients [4–6].

Incidental adrenal lesions are usually nonfunctioning and, therefore, asymptomatic. Very rarely, however, even nonfunctioning lesions can present with symptoms due to mass effect, necrosis, or hemorrhage [7]. Between 5 and 23 % of incidental adrenal lesions are functioning, with detectable levels of cortisol, aldosterone, or catecholamines [8–11]. Adenomas with sufficient functional activity can present clinically with Cushing syndrome (including hypertension, moon-shaped face, proximal myopathy, easy bruising, truncal obesity) or Conn syndrome (hypertension, hypokalemia, hypernatremia). Rarely, adenomas may also secrete sex hormones, but the incidence of androgen secretion is higher in adrenocortical carcinomas (ACC) than in adenomas [12]. On average, 55 % ACC are hormonally active; and, if enough hormone is produced, these patients can present with Cushing syndrome virilization syndromes, or a combination of both; only rarely do these patients present with feminization or hyperaldosteronism [7, 13, 14]. Approximately half of adults with nonfunctioning ACC present with abdominal pain or a palpable mass and, unfortunately, a high proportion of these patients (approximately 30 % of all nonfunctioning ACC) present with nodal or distant metastatic disease [14–16]. Patients with pheochromocytomas, which arise from the adrenal medulla, usually present with headache, palpitations, diaphoresis, and/or hypertension due to their production of excessive catecholamines [17].

Rarely, adrenal lesions can present with adrenal insufficiency. The most common infectious cause is tuberculosis, followed by histoplasmosis and blastomycosis, and less frequently opportunistic infections in the immunocompromised patient [18]. Primary adrenocortical tumors and metastatic disease are less common causes.

Work-Up of the Incidental Adrenal Lesion

Lesions that are less than 1 cm in size are rarely investigated further due to the very high likelihood of being benign. Size and rate of growth are two of the most important features in distinguishing benign from malignant lesions. For example, the incidence of metastasis has been reported to be 71 % in lesions greater than 4 cm or those that demonstrate significant size increase within a year [19]. Benign lesions rarely increase in size and those that do, such as the occasional adenoma, increase only very slowly. There are some exceptions, however. For example, acute hemorrhage can occur within some benign lesions or within normal adrenal glands after trauma, causing the gland to increase rapidly in size. Due to the importance of growth rate in evaluating incidental adrenal lesions, comparison with prior examinations is essential. When these are unavailable and the suspicion of malignancy is low, follow-up cross-sectional imaging in 4–6 months is generally recommended.

The likelihood of metastasis is significantly influenced by the presence or absence of underlying malignant disease. In one study of 1,049 incidentally detected adrenal lesions in patients with no known primary tumor, 75 % were adenomas, and the remaining were benign lesions including myolipomas, hematomas, and cysts; none of the lesions were malignant [20]. However, in the presence of a primary malignancy, the likelihood of an adrenal nodule representing metastatic disease ranges from 25 to 72 %, with the most common

A.A. Afaq, M.B.B.S., FRCR (✉) • R.A. Lefkowitz, M.D.
Department of Radiology, Memorial Sloan-Kettering Cancer Center, 1275 York Avenue, New York, NY 10065, USA
e-mail: asimafaq@doctors.org.uk; lefkowir@mskcc.org

A.M. Bach, J. Zhang (eds.), *Atlas of Genitourinary Oncological Imaging*, Atlas of Oncology Imaging,
DOI 10.1007/978-1-4614-4872-3_5, © Springer Science+Business Media New York 2013

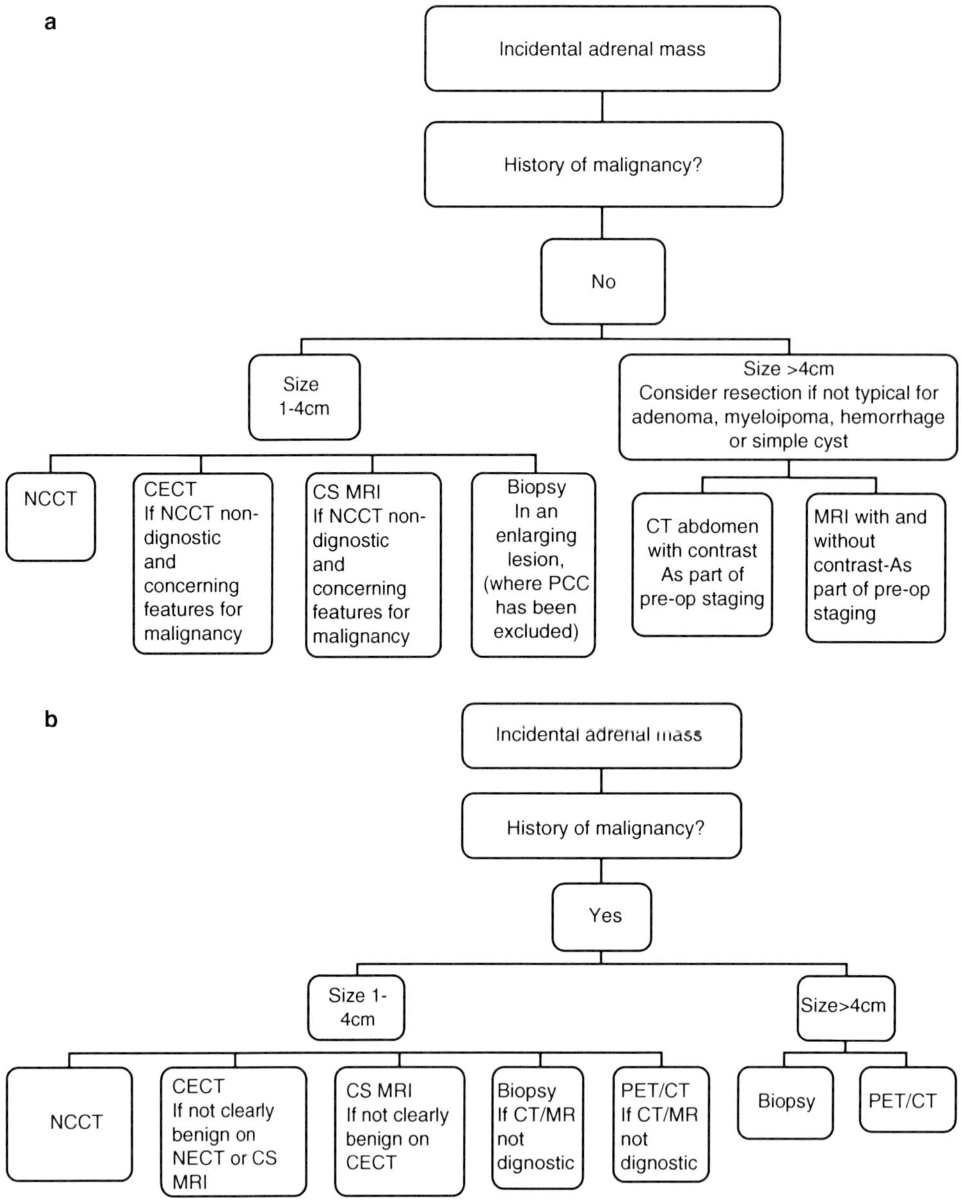

Fig. 5.1 American College of Radiology (ACR) appropriateness criteria. The ACR recently updated the appropriateness criteria for the investigation of incidental adrenal lesions. A summary from the recommendations is shown in the flow charts (**a** and **b**) [26]. The two main features in risk stratification are history of prior malignancy and the size of the adrenal lesion (1–4 cm vs >4 cm). Change in size of the lesion is the other major feature that alters decision-making once the lesion has been stratified. (**a**) In a patient with no history of malignancy presenting with a 1–4 cm adrenal mass, most lesions will turn out to be benign. If the lesion has been stable for at least 1 year (based on prior available studies) or has classic benign features (*e.g.*, fat in a myelolipoma), no additional follow-up is needed. If the lesion has enlarged, then biopsy or resection is an appropriate next step. If no prior studies are available and the lesion has no suspicious features, it may be safe to follow-up in 1 year with a non-contrast *CT* (*NCCT*) or chemical shift MRI (*see* Figs. 5.4 and 5.5). However, if suspicious features (*e.g.*, heterogeneity or lobulation) are present, a *NCCT* or chemical shift *MRI* should be performed immediately to determine if it represents an adenoma (*see* Fig. 5.4). If the lesion remains indeterminate, contrast-enhanced *CT* using washout technique (*see* Fig. 5.7) should be the next step. If the lesion does not meet imaging criteria for a benign lesion at this point, a biopsy may be appropriate after a pheochromocytoma has been excluded with biochemical work-up. An incidentally discovered adrenal mass measuring greater than 4 cm in a patient with no history of malignancy, is generally resected if it is not consistent with an adenoma, myelolipoma, hematoma, or simple cyst. In this situation, *CT* or *MRI* with contrast is recommended for staging purposes only. (**b**) In a patient with a history of malignancy and an incidental 1–4 cm adrenal nodule, the nodule need not be worked-up further if the patient has metastatic disease elsewhere and the presence of an additional metastasis in the adrenal gland would not alter therapy. However, in the absence of metastatic disease elsewhere, this nodule should be worked-up further with *PET-CT*, *NCCT*, or chemical shift *MRI* if the lesion does not have imaging features that are diagnostic for a benign lesion. If the lesion does not behave like a typical adenoma on any of these studies, then an adrenal *CT* with washout should be performed. At this point if the lesion does not behave like an adenoma, a biopsy should be performed. In a patient with a history of cancer and an adrenal mass greater than 4 cm, a biopsy or *PET-CT* should be performed

primary tumors being bronchogenic carcinoma, renal cancer, melanoma, breast cancer, gastrointestinal cancers, and pancreatic cancer [21–25].

This chapter will discuss both common and uncommon adrenal masses in adults (pediatric tumors are discussed in Chap. 10). Adenoma is by far the most common benign tumor of the adrenal gland. Although uncommon, myelolipoma is the next most frequent benign tumor of the adrenal gland. Pheochromocytoma and hemangioma are rare benign tumors. Hyperplasia and cysts are benign non-neoplastic entities that will also be discussed. Metastatic disease is by far the most common malignant tumor of the adrenal gland, although less common than adenoma, even in patients with known primary malignancy. Adrenal cortical carcinoma is the most common primary malignant tumor of the adrenal gland in adults, but is still rare, with an annual incidence of approximately 1–2 cases per million [24, 27, 28]. Although up to 4 % of patients with non-Hodgkin lymphoma have adrenal involvement [28], primary adrenal lymphoma is extremely rare. Other extremely rare, primary malignant adrenal tumors include sarcoma (the few reported cases including leiomyosarcoma and angiosarcoma) and melanoma.

Normal Anatomy and Imaging Techniques

Anatomy

The right adrenal gland is located superior to the upper pole of the right kidney, lateral to the crus of the diaphragm, medial to the right lobe of the liver, and just posterior to the inferior vena cava. The left adrenal gland is located anteromedial to the upper pole of the left kidney, lateral to the crus of the diaphragm, and lateral or slightly posterior to the abdominal aorta.

Each gland has two main components with different embryologic origins: the inner core, or adrenal medulla, which is thinner and arises from the neural crest, and the outer adrenal cortex, which is thicker and arises from the mesothelium. The cortex has three distinct divisions with separate functions: the zona glomerulosa, zona fasciculata, and zona reticularis secrete aldosterone, cortisol, and androgens, respectively. Catecholamines are secreted by the adrenal medulla. Eighty percent of the adrenal medulla secretes adrenaline (epinephrine) and 20 % secretes noradrenaline (norepinephrine). The adrenal glands have a very rich arterial supply: the superior adrenal artery arising from the inferior phrenic artery, the middle adrenal artery arising from the abdominal aorta, and the inferior adrenal artery arising from the renal artery. The suprarenal veins drain directly to the inferior vena cava (IVC) on the right and to either the left renal vein or the left inferior phrenic vein on the left.

On cross-sectional imaging, the shape of the adrenal glands is quite variable [29]. The right adrenal gland typically has an inverted V or Y shape in the axial plane (with symmetric or asymmetric limbs), and less often horizontal or K-shaped. The left adrenal gland tends to be more variable in shape, appearing like an inverted V, an inverted Y, linear, or triangular [30]. However, it is usually an abnormal increase in thickness of the adrenal gland on axial images, rather than length, that triggers further investigation.

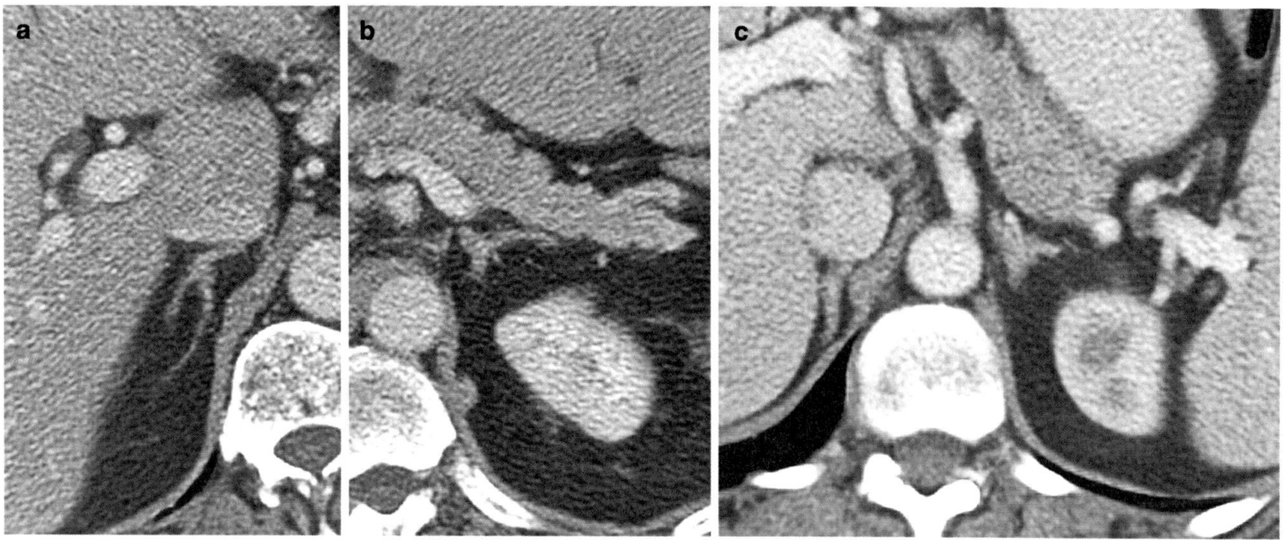

Fig. 5.2 Normal anatomy. (**a**, **b**) Contrast-enhanced CT demonstrates the classic appearance of the adrenal glands, which are seen at the same level in this case. (**c**) Contrast-enhanced CT in a different patient demonstrates a triangular-shaped left-adrenal gland, which is one of a number of normal variants in the shape of the left adrenal gland

Imaging Techniques

CT and MRI are the primary imaging modalities used to evaluate adrenal lesions. Depending on the clinical scenario, CT can be performed as a non-contrast study, a contrast study (with images acquired 80 seconds post contrast injection), or a combination of the two with additional delayed acquisition at 15 min post contrast (a three-phase study). If the entire abdomen is scanned, oral contrast is generally utilized; if the examination is limited to the adrenal glands only, oral contrast is generally unnecessary. Images can be reconstructed at 5 mm intervals for a general abdomen, or at 2.5 mm intervals for a dedicated adrenal imaging study. Sagittal and coronal reconstructed images are also generated. The dedicated adrenal MR protocol at our institution includes high-resolution axial and coronal spoiled gradient-echo T1-weighted in-phase (TE 4.2 ms at 1.5 T) and out-of-phase images (TE 1.2 ms at 1.5 T) with a 4 mm slice thickness and 1 mm gap. We also perform axial T2 fast spin-echo images with fat saturation and coronal single-shot fast spin echo (SSFSE) images. Gadolinium is not necessary for the work-up of adenomas, which represent the majority of adrenal masses.

Pathology

Benign Tumors

When drawing a ROI to measure attenuation, the following key technical points should be noted. The ROI must be drawn on a noncontrast-enhanced CT study; the size of ROI should be representative of the whole lesion (*e.g.*, >50 % surface area included on an axial image)—this will also reduce noise artifact; the ROI should be placed in the center of the lesion to avoid measuring adjacent retroperitoneal fat. In addition, areas of hemorrhage or necrosis should be avoided. The most commonly used cutoff to diagnose a lipid-rich adenoma is 10 HU, such that those lesions measuring less than 10 HU are consistent with lipid-rich adenomas whereas those measuring more than 10 HU can represent either lipid-poor adenomas or nonadenomas. Using a value of 10 HU to make the diagnosis of adenoma has a sensitivity of 71 % and specificity of 98 % [32]. If a cutoff value of 0 HU is used, the specificity becomes 100 %, but the sensitivity drops to 47 % [31]. Alternatively, a cutoff value of 20 HU would have a higher sensitivity (88 %), but would result in an unacceptably high false-positive rate, with a specificity of only 84 %.

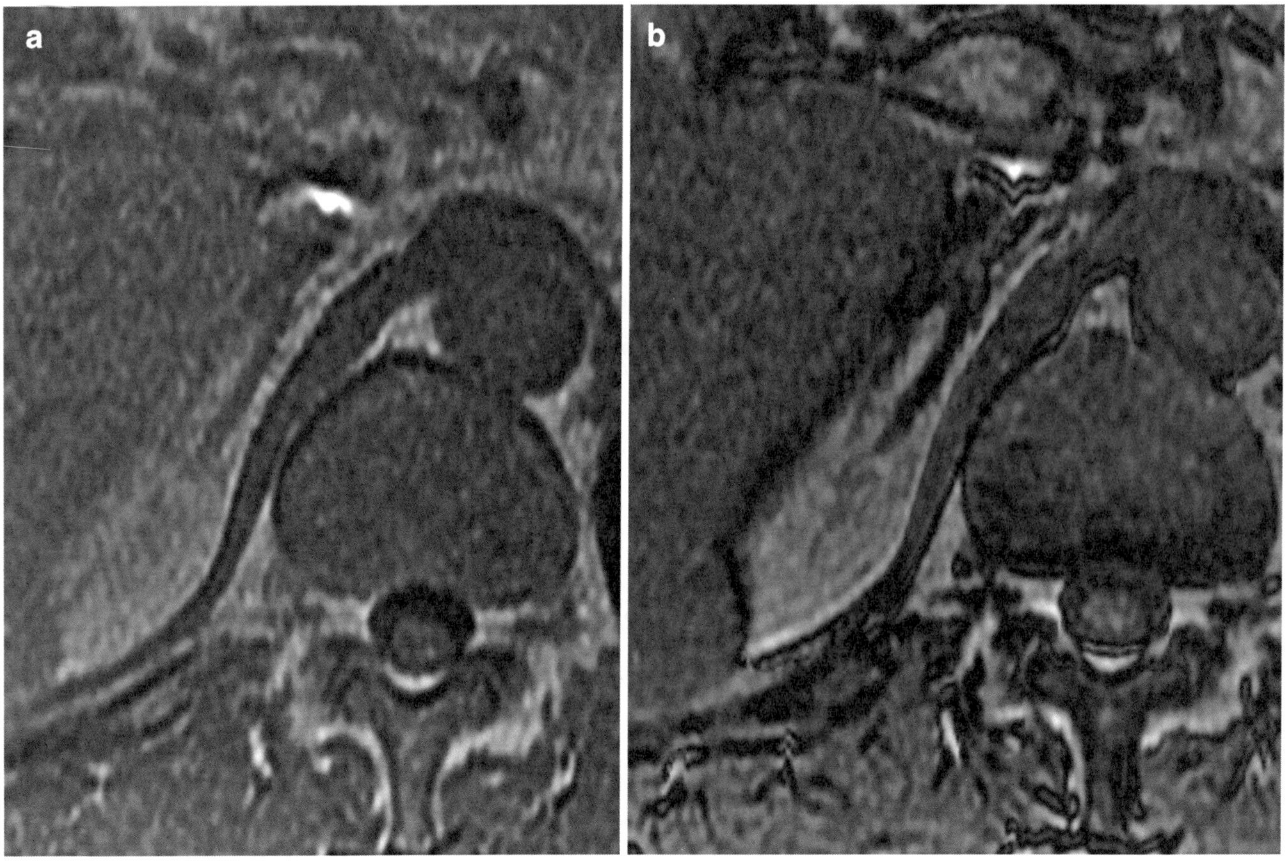

Fig. 5.3 MR imaging technique. (**a**, **b**) These are high-resolution axial in-phase (**a**) and opposed-phase (**b**) gradient-echo T1WI images through the right adrenal gland, which are the critical images needed to diagnose adrenal adenomas

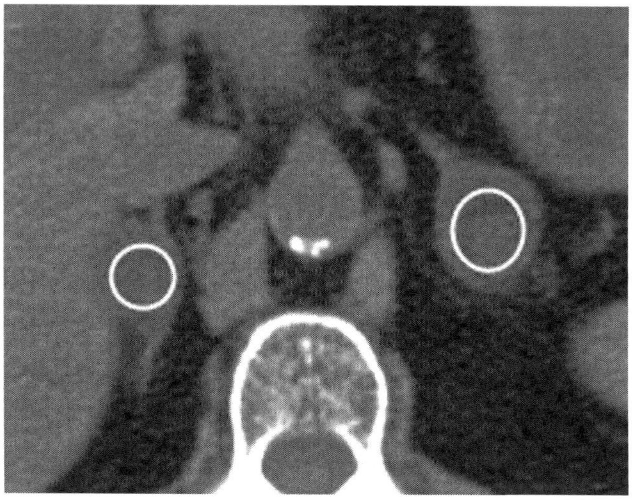

Fig. 5.4 Adrenal adenoma: NCCT. This NCCT demonstrates bilateral adrenal nodules (shown with *circular regions* of interests [ROIs]) measuring 1 HU on the right and −17 HU on the left, consistent with adenomas. Due to the presence of intracellular lipid within these lesions, the mean attenuation of adenomas is significantly lower on NCCT than nonadenomatous lesions [31]. Given this fact, many adenomas, specifically those that are lipid-rich, can be confidently diagnosed by CT-densitometry

In-phase (ip) and opposed-phase (or out-of-phase [op]) sequences are based on the principles of chemical shift imaging, which relies on differences in resonance frequencies within a given voxel between fat and water, with fat protons processing at a lower frequency than water protons. Thus, at certain times (TE of 4.2 ms on 1.5 T magnets), water and fat protons are in-phase and their signals will add together. At a time halfway between each in-phase time (TE of 2.1 ms with 1.5 T magnet), the fat and water protons will be out of phase within a given voxel, thus cancelling or demonstrating signal loss on opposed-phase sequences. Since lipid-rich adenomas contain both microscopic fat and lipid within the same voxel, these lesions demonstrate signal loss from the in-phase images to the out-of-phase images. With lipid-rich adenomas, this method can usually be performed qualitatively by visually determining if there is signal drop-out on opposed phase images. However, in cases where the signal loss is not so obvious, the lesions may also be evaluated quantitatively by placing ROI cursors over representative portions of the lesion and calculating the ratio of the in-phase signal (SI[ip]) of the lesion to the opposed-phase signal (SI[op]) at the same location. The spleen should be used to standardize the signal intensities between the two phases (the spleen should theoretically have the same SI value on in-phase and out-of-phase images, and thus, is used as the reference standard) such that: **adrenal lesion to spleen SI ratio (op)/adrenal lesion to spleen SI ratio (ip) ≤0.71** is consistent with a lipid-rich adenoma [33].

It can be assumed that adrenal adenomas, which contain sufficient lipid to measure less than 10 HU on noncontrast CT, will also have sufficient lipid to demonstrate qualitative signal loss with chemical shift imaging. However, for adenomas that measure more than 10 HU on NCCT, at what threshold will these lesions have insufficient lipid to be detected with chemical shift MRI? A study by Haider et al. [34], answered this question: for those adenomas measuring between 10 and 20 HU on NCCT, 100 % of these lesions demonstrated sufficient signal loss on chemical shift imaging to be confidently diagnosed as adenomas. For adenomas measuring 20–30 HU on NCCT, 75 % demonstrated significant signal loss on opposed phase images. However, for adenomas measuring more than 30 HU on NCCT, only 13 % demonstrated signal loss on opposed phase images [34]. Thus, they concluded that chemical shift MRI can still be of value for adrenal lesions that measure between 10 and 30 HU. The sensitivity of chemical shift imaging in distinguishing benign from malignant lesions has been reported to be 81–100 %, with the specificity ranging from 94 to 100 % [35]. Signal loss on chemical shift imaging is pathognomonic for the presence of lipid and water in same voxel, thus, indicating an adenoma or, much less frequently, a myelolipoma (also a benign lesion), the latter of which can contain trace amounts of fat mixed with soft tissue in the same voxel. Some ACCs also contain enough lipid to demonstrate signal loss with chemical shift imaging; however, ACC is a rare lesion, is generally large and heterogenous compared to adenomas, and demonstrates patchy areas of signal loss on the opposed phase images, in contrast to adenomas, which demonstrate uniform signal loss [36].

The key limitation of using NCCT alone to evaluate lipid content is that approximately 30 % of adenomas are lipid poor and will demonstrate an attenuation more than 10 HU on NCCT [32]. Given this limitation, an alternative technique has been developed that relies on the following principle: although both adenomas and malignant lesions enhance rapidly after IV contrast administration, the rate of washout is faster in adenomas than malignant lesions due to the presence of leaky capillaries in the latter [37]. As a result, measuring the percentage washout of contrast material on delayed images (different studies have used delayed imaging times ranging from 10 to 15 min) has been shown to be both a sensitive and specific method to identify adenomas. The washout method is only valid for lesions that are relatively homogenous in attenuation. The diagnosis of an adenoma cannot be made in lesions that contain large areas of low attenuation (often representing hemorrhage and/or necrosis) because these areas generally do not enhance significantly [3].

Myelolipoma is one of the most common adrenal neoplasms (following adenoma and metastasis). In one large series of patients without known malignancy, myelolipomas represented 6 % of all adrenal masses [20]. They are usually clinically silent with no known malignant potential and are

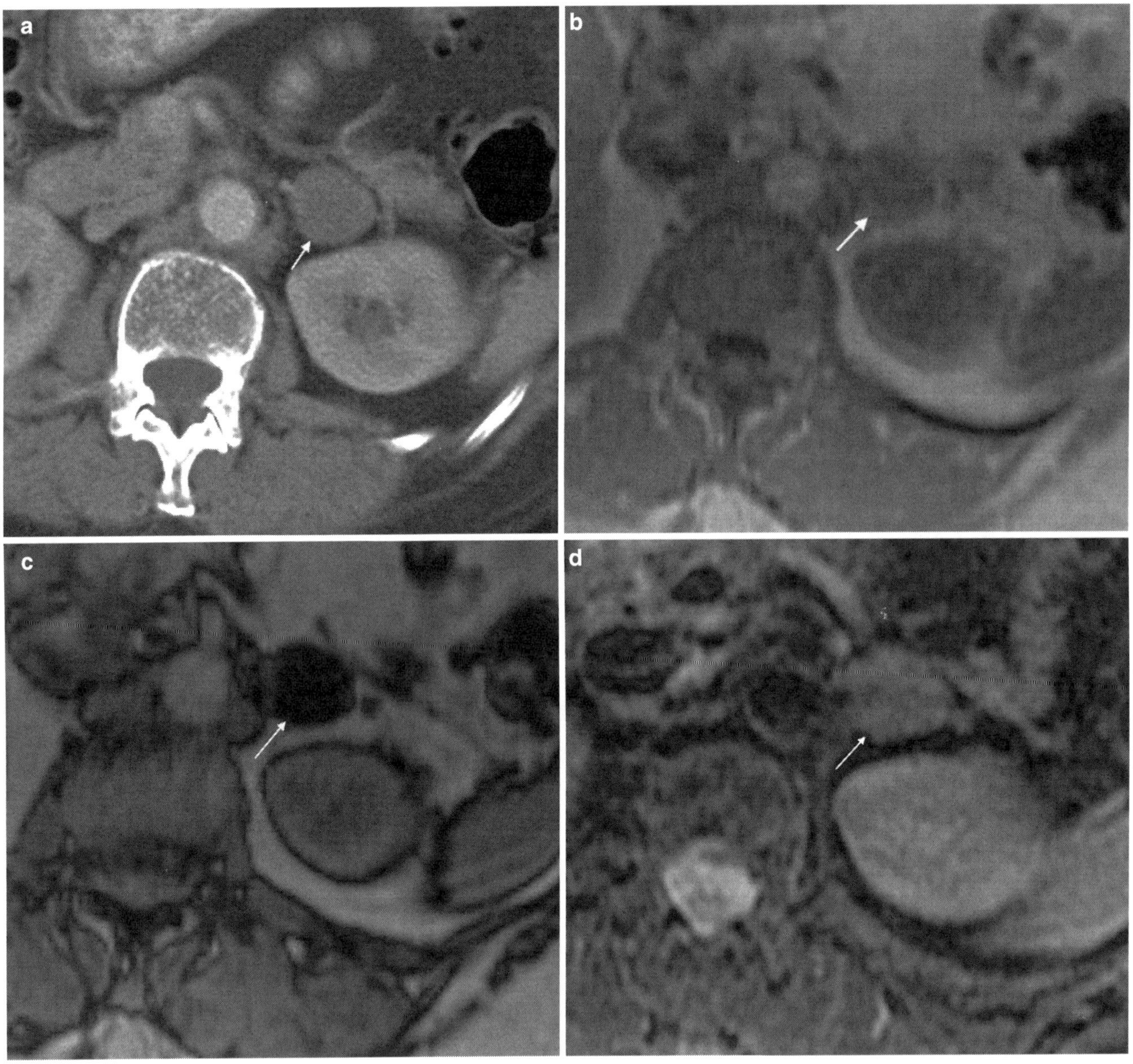

Fig. 5.5 Adrenal adenoma: MRI. (**a**) Contrast-enhanced CT in this patient with breast cancer demonstrates an incidentally detected 2.7 cm left adrenal nodule (*arrow*). A dedicated adrenal MRI was subsequently performed to determine if this nodule represents an adenoma. (**b**) Axial T1-weighted in-phase gradient-echo (GRE) image demonstrates that the adrenal nodule (*arrow*) is intermediate in signal (relative signal intensity of 75 [not shown]; this represents a unit-less number used for comparison purposes only). (**c**) Opposed-phase GRE sequence through the same lesion (*arrow*) demonstrates that the lesion is now very low in signal (relative signal intensity dropped from 75–17) consistent with a lipid-rich adenoma. (**d**) The same lesion (*arrow*) on this T2FS sequence demonstrates intermediate T2 signal, which is not specific for an adenoma

usually discovered incidentally. Occasionally, large myelolipomas may cause pain due to hemorrhage, necrosis, or compression of adjacent structures [28, 40]. Myelolipomas are composed of mature adipose tissue with variable amounts of hematopoietic tissue (erythroid and myeloid) [28, 40]. Often one component can predominate over the other, but only a small amount of gross fat is required to make the diagnosis; in fact, the presence of macroscopic fat (measuring between −30 and −100 HU) within an adrenal mass on cross-sectional imaging is virtually diagnostic of myelolipoma because adrenal lipomas and liposarcomas are extremely rare, and adenomas and ACC contain microscopic (rather than macroscopic) intracellular lipid [28, 40]. Up to 20 % of myelolipomas contain calcifications from prior hemorrhage [41]. Myelolipoma can occasionally be confused with a retroperitoneal liposarcoma that arises adjacent to the adrenal gland or an angiomyolipoma arising in the upper pole of the kidney; however, if one can confirm that the lesion actually

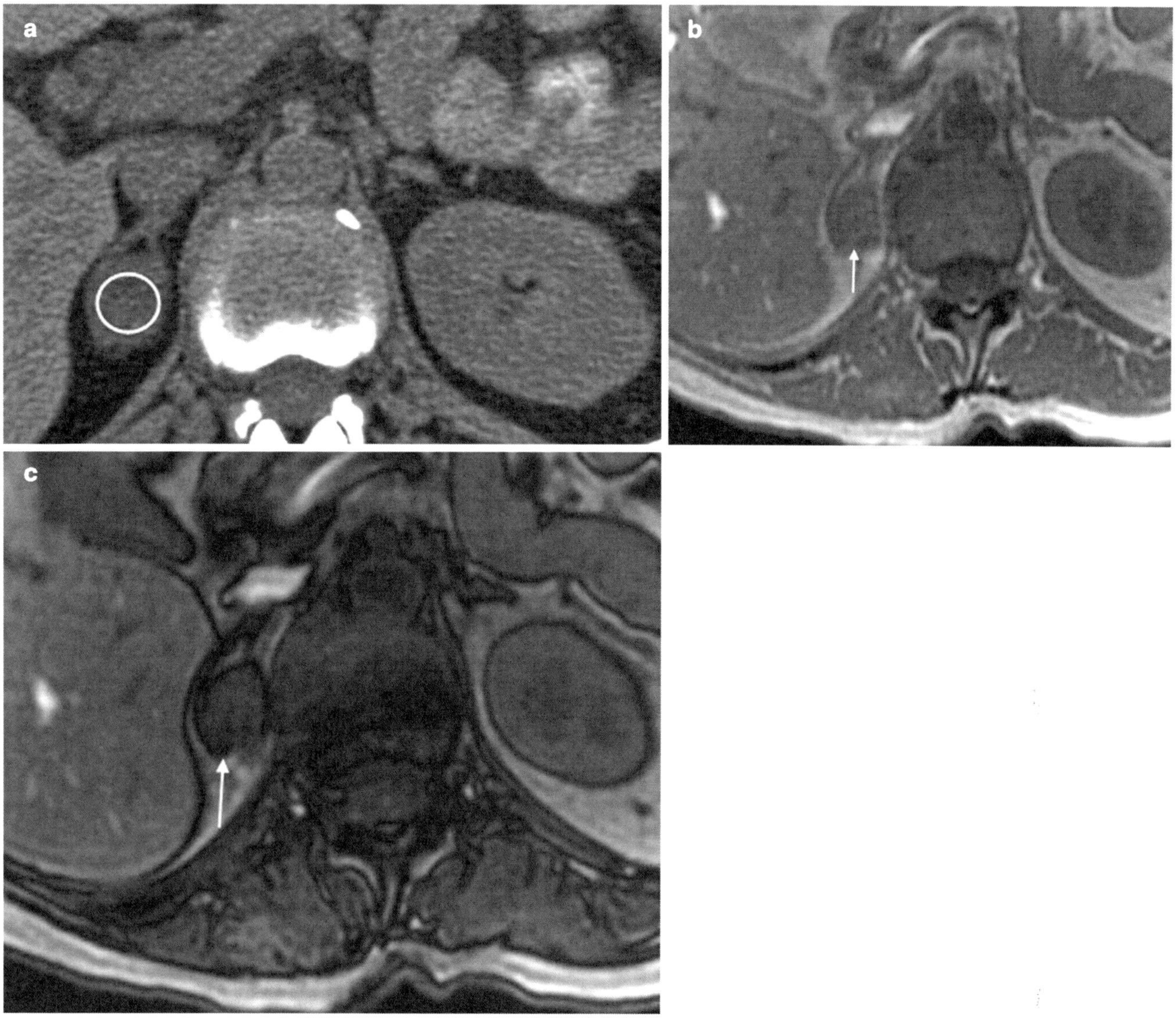

Fig. 5.6 Adrenal adenoma: NCCT versus MRI. (**a**) NCCT demonstrates a right adrenal nodule that measures 23 HU (circular ROI on adrenal nodule), not consistent with a lipid-rich adenoma. (**b**, **c**) Chemical shift MRI with in-phase (**b**) and opposed phase (**c**) sequences demonstrating mild signal loss on opposed phase image (approximately 20 % dropout) indicating the presence of some intracellular lipid, and thus, consistent with an adenoma (*arrows* on adrenal nodule in **b**, **c**)

arises from the adrenal gland, the diagnosis of myelolipoma should be made.

Unlike adenomas, myelolipomas do not typically demonstrate signal loss on opposed-phase sequences because the lipomatous components are usually "bulk" fat, rather than the microscopic intracellular fat seen with adenomas. As a result, myelolipomas demonstrate "India ink" artifact at the interface between the bulk fat and soft tissue components. A minority myelolipomas, however, will show some signal loss on opposed phase sequences if small fatty components are mixed with non-fatty components in the same voxel.

Pheochromocytoma is a catecholamine-secreting tumor arising from neuroectodermal tissue in the adrenal medulla. Common symptoms that suggest the diagnosis include paroxysmal (episodic or sporadic) hypertension, palpitations, tachycardia, headaches, anxiety, diaphoresis, flank pain, pallor, and weight loss, among other symptoms. The diagnosis is confirmed by the presence of elevated plasma or urinary catecholamines. Thus, cross-sectional imaging (CT and MRI, less often metaiodobenzylguanidine [MIBG] scan) is not generally used to make the diagnosis but rather to localize a known pheochromocytoma. CT demonstrates a mass that usually measures between 2 and 5 cm. Solid (noncystic) pheochromocytomas are classically hypervascular in both the arterial and portal venous phases following contrast administration with slow washout. The enhancement pattern can be quite variable, however; some tumors can demonstrate hypervascularity in the arterial phase with early washout, whereas others can demonstrate moderate or slow enhancement with early or delayed washout. Small tumors

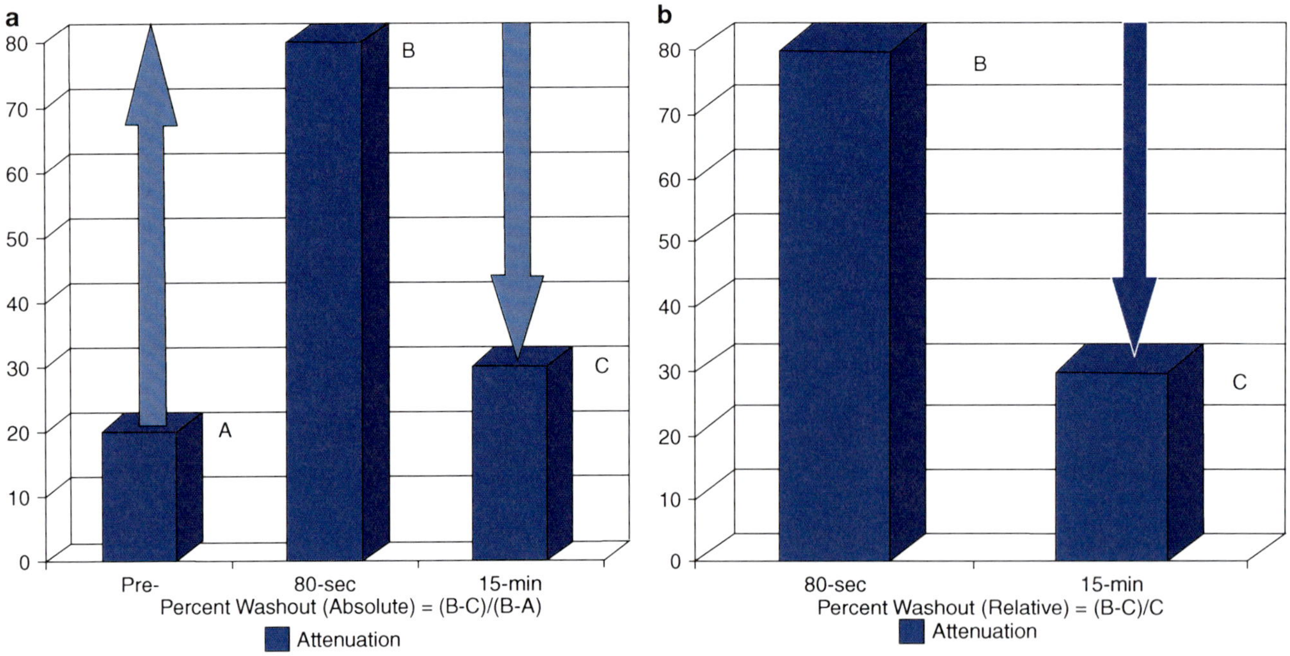

Fig. 5.7 Adrenal adenoma: CT washout technique. (**a**) Absolute washout technique: this protocol uses unenhanced, portal venous phase (approximately 70 or 80 s post injection) and 15-min delayed post-contrast images. The mean attenuation of the lesion is measured at each phase, and the resultant measurements are applied to the following formula yielding the absolute percentage washout (*APW*):

$$\mathbf{APW} = (\mathbf{HU}_{\text{portal venous}} - \mathbf{HU}_{15\,\text{min}})/(\mathbf{HU}_{\text{portal venous}} - \mathbf{HU}_{\text{preconstrast}}) \times 100$$

If the APW equals 60 % or greater, then the lesion is consistent with an adenoma (sensitivity and specificity of 89 and 95 %, respectively, for lipid-poor adenomas) [38]. (**A**) This bar graph demonstrates a theoretical example of a lipid poor adenoma with a precontrast attenuation of 20 HU. The attenuation of the lesion is 80 HU in the portal venous phase (**B**) and 30 HU at 15 min (**C**). Utilizing the above formula, the calculated washout percentage equals 50/60, or 83 %, consistent with an adenoma. When one uses this technique to characterize an adrenal lesion, the images should be checked immediately after the precontrast images are performed, because if the lesion measures less than 10 HU, confirming the presence of a lipid-rich adenoma, the study can be terminated before the contrast injection. (**b**) Relative washout: the absolute washout method requires that a noncontrast CT be performed first, which is not routinely performed in most abdominal CT protocols. Therefore, if an adrenal lesion is incidentally detected at the time of a contrast-enhanced study while the patient is still on the table, delayed images can still be performed and the relative percentage washout (RPW) can be calculated (without precontrast images) as follows: $\text{RPW} = (\text{HU}_{\text{portal venous}} - \text{HU}_{15\,\text{min}})/(\text{HU}_{\text{portal venous}}) \times 100$. If RPW is greater than or equal to 40 %, then the lesion is consistent with an adenoma with sensitivity and specificity of 93 and 98 %, respectively for lipid-rich adenomas, and 83 and 93 % for lipid poor adenomas [38]. The bar graph demonstrates the relative washout calculation for the same theoretical lesion: 50/80 = 63 %. Since this value is greater than 40 %, the lesion is consistent with an adenoma. *A* precontrast attenuation; *B* attenuation at portal venous phase; *C* attenuation at 15 min

are typically homogeneous in attenuation whereas larger tumors frequently demonstrate areas of cystic degeneration due to hemorrhage and necrosis, which appear as areas of lower attenuation on contrast-enhanced CT. Small, homogenous pheochromocytomas typically measure between 40 and 50 HU on NCCT. However, noncontrast images alone can be deceiving if the tumor is predominantly necrotic, because necrotic areas can measure less than 10 HU, mimicking an adenoma (pheochromocytoma is one cause of false positives when utilizing CT-densitometry to make the diagnosis of an adenoma). Nevertheless, when contrast-enhanced images are also performed and the appropriate clinical and laboratory data are available, pheochromocytoma should rarely be mistaken for an adenoma.

The solid components of pheochromocytomas are moderately hyperintense in T2 signal, whereas the cystic, necrotic components are very bright on T2WI. These lesions are low to intermediate signal on T1WI but can contain areas of high T1 signal if hemorrhage is present. As with CT, noncystic components of pheochromocytomas are frequently hypervascular on post-contrast MR images.

Pheochromocytomas are known to follow the "10 % rule;" that is, approximately 10 % are malignant and can metastasize, 10 % are bilateral, 10–15 % are extra-adrenal (extra-adrenal pheochromocytomas, also called *paragangliomas*, can arise anywhere from the neck to the pubis where neuroectodermal tissue is found, although most occur in the abdomen, especially in the retroperitoneum), 10 % occur in children, and 10 % are associated with heritable syndromes [28]. These syndromes include MEN II (*see* Fig. 5–13), Von Hippel-Lindau, and neurofibromatosis type 1. Recently, Welander [42] reviewed the literature on these syndromes

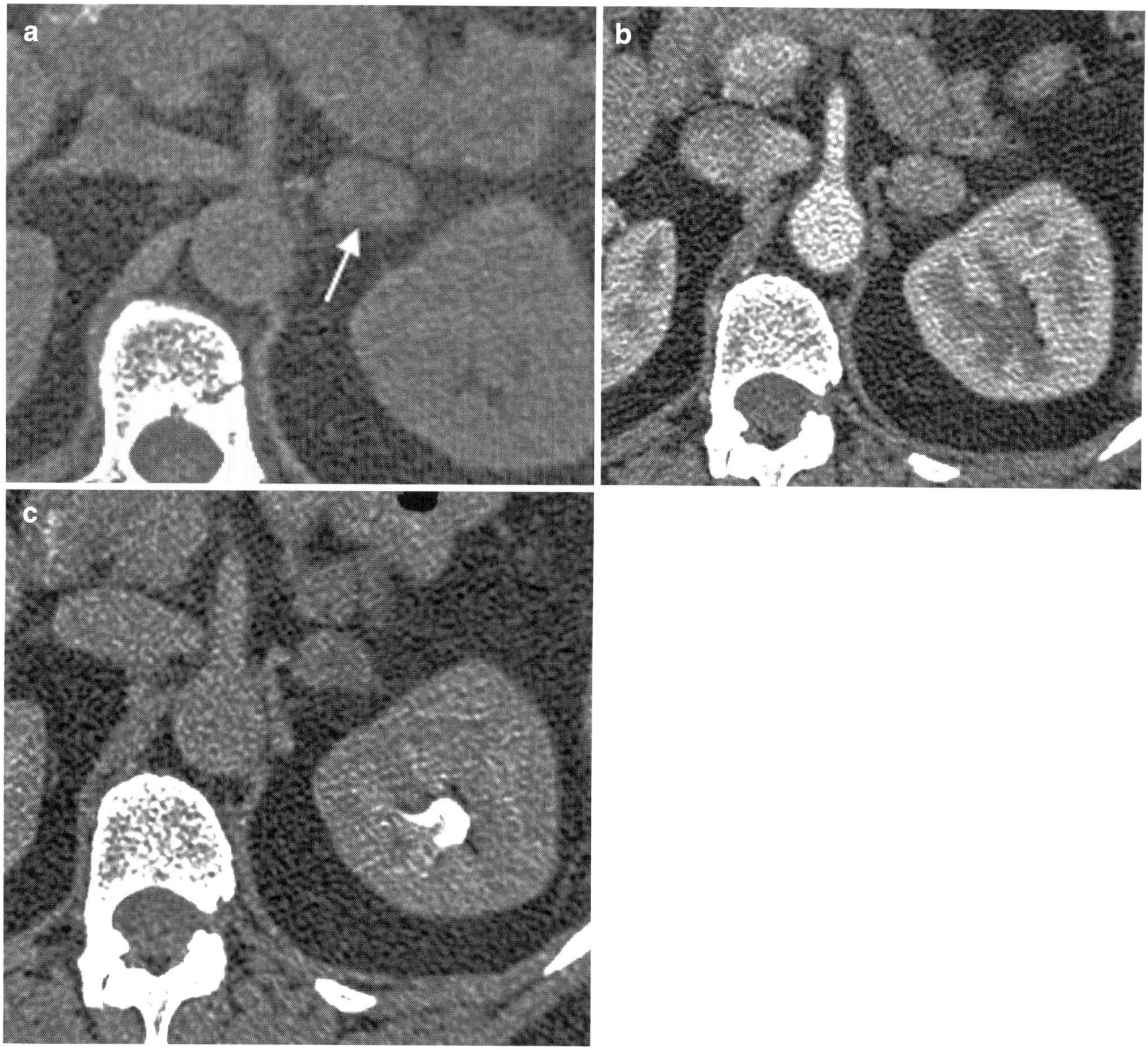

Fig. 5.8 Lipid poor adrenal adenoma: absolute CT washout. These images are from a patient with breast cancer with an incidentally detected indeterminate adrenal nodule on contrast-enhanced chest CT (*not shown*). A dedicated adrenal protocol CT was subsequently performed to work-up this lesion. (**a**) NCCT from this study demonstrates that the nodule (*arrow*) measures 25 HU, not consistent with a lipid-rich adenoma. The portal venous phase (**b**) and 15-min delayed image (**c**) demonstrates that the nodule measures 98 HU and 46 HU, respectively. The APW is calculated as follows: (98–46)/(98–25) = 52/73 = 71 % absolute washout. Thus, this lesion is consistent with a lipid-poor adenoma by CT criteria. Park et al. [39] compared CT washout with quantitative chemical shift imaging and found the sensitivity, specificity, and accuracy using absolute washout to diagnose adenomas to be 100 % (37 of 37), 83 % (5 of 6), and 98 % (42 of 43), respectively, versus 41 % (15 of 37), 100 % (6 of 6), and 49 % (21 of 43), for chemical shift MRI. This study and others suggest that CT washout is superior to chemical shift MRI for diagnosing adrenal adenomas [39]

and summarized the results (*see* Table 5.1). Notable features of hereditary pheochromocytoma include an earlier onset compared to the sporadic form and a predilection for multifocal and bilateral tumors. Pheochromocytoma can also occur in up to 6 % of patients with a very rare syndrome called Carney's triad (paragangliomas/pheochromocytoma, gastrointestinal stromal tumor, and pulmonary chondromas) [43]. Even more rarely, pheochromocytoma can occur in association with MEN 1 syndrome [42].

The high metabolic activity of pheochromocytoma allows detection with functional imaging. Because the diagnosis of pheochromocytoma is usually suggested by clinical symptomatology and laboratory data, PET is generally used for localizing site(s) of tumor rather than for diagnostic purposes.

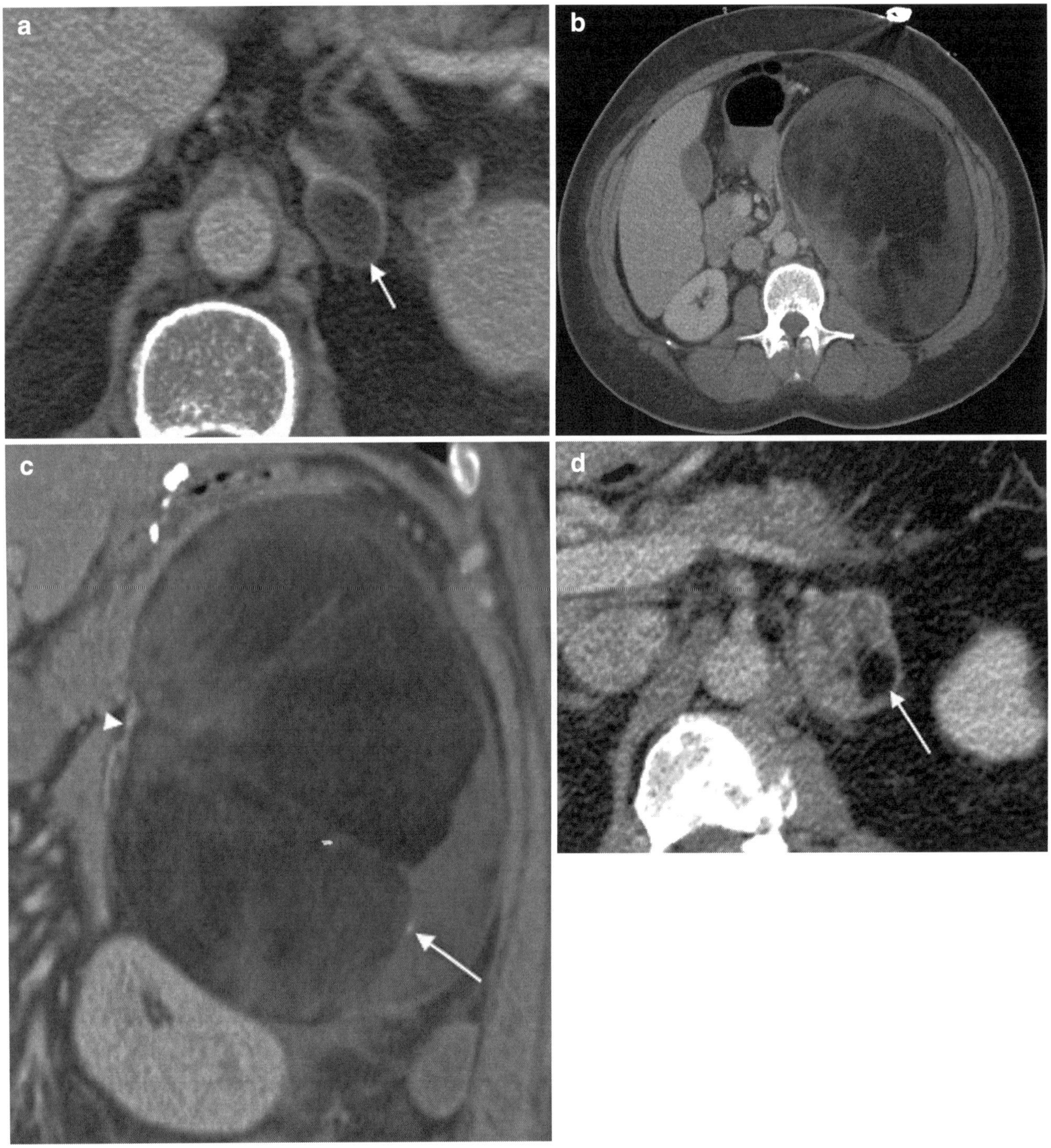

Fig. 5.9 Myelolipoma: CT. (**a**) This contrast-enhanced CT demonstrates a small fat attenuation nodule (*arrow*) in the left adrenal gland consistent with a classic myelolipoma. Axial (**b**) and coronal reconstruction (**c**) images from a contrast-enhanced CT on a different patient demonstrate an 18 cm left adrenal mass containing large areas of gross fat intermixed with areas of soft tissue, also consistent with a myelolipoma. This lesion could potentially be confused with a retroperitoneal liposarcoma. The key distinguishing feature, however, is that this mass is inseparable from the left adrenal gland in (**c**) (*arrowhead*), and consequently, displaces the kidney inferiorly. This lesion is also very well-circumscribed, a feature that is more typical of myelolipoma than liposarcoma. Note the small calcification within the lesion (arrow). (**d**) This contrast-enhanced CT demonstrates a 5 cm left adrenal mass composed predominantly of soft tissue, but with a small focus of gross fat (*arrow*), also consistent with a myelolipoma

A higher percentage of malignant pheochromocytomas demonstrate increased uptake on fluorodeoxyglucose (FDG) PET than benign pheochromocytomas (82 % vs. 58 % sensitivity, respectively) [44]. However, radioiodinated MIBG is actually more sensitive than FDG PET in detecting both benign (83 % vs. 58 %) and malignant pheochromocytoma (88 % vs. 82 %), as demonstrated in a study by Shulkin et al. [45]. Of note, all the pheochromocytomas that failed to concentrate MIBG in this study actually demonstrated FDG avidity, indicating that FDG PET should play a major role in staging this subset of patients [45]. More recently, FDG PET using agents such as 6-[^{18}F]fluoro-l-dopa (^{18}F-DOPA) and ^{18}F-fluorodopamine have yielded impressive results in the detection of both primary tumors and metastatic disease [46– 48]. Radiolabeled octreotide analogues may also be of use in detecting extra-adrenal or metastatic pheochromocytoma. ^{68}Ga-DOTOTATE-PET has been shown to identify pheochromocytoma not detected with MIBG [49, 50]. Overall, it is likely that a combination of anatomic imaging (to assess local disease involvement) and functional imaging (to detect extra-adrenal and distant metastatic disease) is the optimal method to stage pheochromocytoma.

Hyperplasia is defined as diffuse adrenal thickening, most often bilateral, and is usually due to hyperstimulation by excessive ACTH, which results in Cushing syndrome. Excluding exogenous hormone administration for medical purposes, Cushing syndrome is caused by ACTH overproduction in 80–85 % of cases, 85 % of which are caused by a pituitary adenoma (also known as Cushing disease) whereas the other 15 % are caused by an ectopic ACTH-secreting tumor. Fifteen to twenty percent of Cushing syndrome cases are non-ACTH dependent and are caused by primary adrenal overproduction from hyperplasia, adenoma, or adrenal cortical carcinoma [30]. A less common manifestation of hyperplasia than Cushing syndrome, Conn syndrome, or hyperaldosteronism can be caused by idiopathic bilateral adrenal hyperplasia, idiopathic unilateral adrenal hyperplasia, adrenal adenoma, or adrenal cortical carcinoma [30]. On CT, adrenal enlargement associated with these syndromes is most often diffuse, but can also be nodular or mixed [30]. Smooth, diffuse enlargement of both adrenal glands is the most common abnormality seen in Cushing disease, although 30–52 % of patients with Cushing disease have normal-appearing adrenal glands [30, 51]. In contrast, ectopic ACTH-secreting tumors more commonly present with nodular or lobular enlargement [51]. On MRI, adrenal hyperplasia can also be smooth or nodular and is frequently the same signal intensity as normal adrenal gland on all sequences. However, hyperplastic adrenal glands may demonstrate signal loss on opposed phase images, particularly in the presence of nodular thickening [24].

Adrenal cysts are rare, with a reported incidence of 0.064 and 0.18 % on autopsy series. They represent approximately 5 % of incidentally detected adrenal lesions [40]. Adrenal cysts are classified as endothelial cysts (45 %), pseudocysts (39 %), epithelial cysts (9 %), and parasitic cysts (7 %) [28, 40].

Endothelial cysts, also known as simple cysts, are usually asymptomatic unless they undergo hemorrhage or infection, or if they are large enough to cause mass effect upon adjacent structures [24]. More than 90 % of endothelial cysts are lymphangiomatous cysts, whereas the remaining are hemangiomatous. On CT, they are fluid-attenuation structures measuring less than 20 HU with smooth borders and thin walls that measure less than 3 mm [52]. Punctate or curvilinear calcifications are occasionally seen [40]. On MRI, these lesions are identical to fluid on all sequences: homogenously low in T1 signal and very high in T2 signal with no internal enhancement. Lymphangiomatous cysts can occasionally contain enhancing septations [40]. If hemorrhage or infection occurs within a cyst, the diagnosis will be difficult to make on single phase CT due to the increased attenuation. However, the diagnosis is more obvious on MRI, which will demonstrate increased T1 signal without enhancement, confirming the cystic nature.

Pseudocysts are usually the result of old hemorrhage and, thus, are more likely to be symptomatic than endothelial cysts. They contain a fibrous wall that lacks an epithelial or endothelial lining. On CT, most pseudocysts are similar to other adrenal cysts in that they are unilateral, well-defined, fluid-density masses. However, since they are usually the result of old hemorrhage, pseudocysts are more likely than endothelial cysts to contain septations, blood products, and soft tissue nodules [40]. Pseudocysts are also more likely to contain calcifications (20–56 % incidence) than endothelial cysts (9.5 %); the calcifications are usually located within the cyst wall and can be very thick [40, 52, 53]. Since pseudocysts contain hemorrhage of varying ages, the imaging appearance on MRI is quite variable.

Epithelial cysts have a nonspecific imaging appearance that is similar to other simple adrenal cysts.

Parasitic cysts are usually caused by echinococcus and are called hydatid cysts. These cysts can appear simple early in their development, in which case they are indistinguishable from other simple cysts. However, as they evolve, characteristic "daughter" cysts are often seen in the lumen on cross-sectional imaging, suggesting the diagnosis [40].

The diagnosis of adrenal cysts is usually straightforward but when large, they can be mistaken for hepatic, renal, pancreatic, or splenic cysts. Coronal and sagittal images are often helpful in determining the adrenal origin. Another potential diagnostic dilemma is encountered with NCCT: simple (noncalcified) cysts are indistinguishable from lipid-rich adenomas because both entities are equivalent to fluid in attenuation (−20–20 HU). However, the distinction can easily be made with IV contrast administration because adenomas enhance whereas cysts do not. Adrenal cysts are usually treated conservatively when the diagnosis is clear; however, if a thick or irregular wall is present, they can be difficult to distinguish from a malignant lesion in which case surgical treatment should be considered [40].

The most common cause of adrenal hemorrhage is blunt trauma (80 % of cases), which more commonly involves the right than the left adrenal gland (80 % are unilateral) due to the shorter right adrenal vein, which drains directly into the IVC and thus is more susceptible to changes in pressure caused by trauma [54, 55]. Other less common causes include neonatal stress, stress in adults (related to surgery, sepsis, burns, hypotension), bleeding diathesis, anticoagulation, adrenal vein thrombosis, underlying adrenal tumors, or unknown causes (idiopathic) [41, 54, 55]. Clinical symptoms of adrenal hemorrhage include abdominal or back pain and fever, although many cases are clinically inapparent [41, 52]. In severe cases of bilateral hemorrhage, when at least 90 % of the adrenal glands have been destroyed, acute primary adrenal insufficiency (addisonian crisis) can result. The most common cause of addisonian crisis is hemorrhage related to stress or bleeding diathesis [41]. On cross-sectional imaging, adrenal hemorrhage presents with mass-like enlargement of the adrenal gland (sometimes marked enlargement), frequently with infiltration in the surrounding fascial planes. On NCCT, acute adrenal hemorrhage measures between 50 and 90 HU, gradually decreasing in attenuation and size over weeks to months as the hematoma evolves [32]. If contrast-enhanced images alone are performed, adrenal hemorrhage can appear indistinguishable from a solid neoplasm. Both pre- and post-contrast images are necessary to rule out enhancement, and thus, a solid mass. If CT is equivocal, MR can be used to confirm the presence of a hematoma. Within the first 7 days, known as the acute phase, hematomas are typically isointense or slightly hypointense on T1-weighted images (T1WI) and markedly hypointense on T2-weighted images (T2WI) due to the presence of intracellular deoxyhemoglobin [52]. In the subacute phase (7 days to 7 weeks after the initial event), free methemoglobin predominates, resulting in a lesion that is hyperintense on T1WI due to T1 shortening. This increase in T1 signal begins in the periphery of the lesion (*see* Fig. 5.17c) at 7 days and progressively fills in over the course of several weeks [41, 52]. At the same time, the lesion becomes bright on T2WI, in part due to the presence of blood serum. Hematomas can sometimes be multilocular, with different signal intensities in each component due varying amounts of methemoglobin [41]. During the chronic stage, which generally begins after 7 weeks, a characteristic low T1, low T2 signal rim develops around the hematoma, which is due to the presence of hemosiderin and a fibrous capsule. The presence of hemosiderin can be confirmed by the observation of "blooming" on gradient echo sequences due to magnetic susceptibility of iron [41]. The evolution of a hematoma is generally slower with larger lesions compared with smaller ones [41]. Eventually, most hematomas will resolve, occasionally with residual calcifications. In a minority of cases, however, the hematoma will liquefy and persist as a pseudocyst, which sometimes contains a thick calcified wall (*see* Fig. 5.15) [52].

When adrenal hemorrhage is seen in a patient without a history of trauma or other risk factors, CT or MRI should be performed to search for an underlying mass. In a study by Swift et al. [56] adrenal cysts or tumors were found to be the fourth most common cause of spontaneous retroperitoneal hemorrhage. Patients with adrenal masses are also more susceptible to hemorrhage following trauma than patients with normal adrenal glands. Pheochromocytoma is the tumor most likely to be associated with massive adrenal hemorrhage as these lesions are quite vascular and frequently demonstrate cystic change, hemorrhage, and necrosis [41]. Up to 20 % of myelolipomas at histologic analysis demonstrate

Fig. 5.10 Myelolipoma: MRI. (**a**) NCCT on a patient with a 7 cm left adrenal myelolipoma. Note that the lesion is predominantly fatty in attenuation with a small focus of soft tissue (*arrow*) and punctate calcifications (*arrowhead*). (**b**) Axial T1WI in-phase without fat saturation demonstrates that the same lesion is predominantly high in signal except for the small focus of non-fatty tissue (*arrow*). (**c**) This T1 out-of-phase image demonstrates a band of low signal (*arrow*) at the interface between fat and soft tissue caused by the cancellation of lipid and water protons in the same voxel (the so-called "India ink" artifact because it appears as if someone has outlined these structures with ink). (**d**) This T2WI with fat-saturation (same lesion) demonstrates that the majority of the lesion is low in signal due to saturation of the fat. However, the non-fatty soft tissue component (*arrow*) is high in signal. (**e, f**) This 18 cm left adrenal myelolipoma (same patient as in Fig. 5.9b and c) is shown on T1-weighted fat-suppressed spin-echo (T1FS) pre- (**e**) and post- (**f**) gadolinium. Note that the non-fatty component (*arrow* in **f**) demonstrates a greater degree of enhancement than the fatty component. The MR features of myelolipomas vary depending upon the amount of fat within the lesion. The fatty components of these lesions are bright on T1WI, intermediate signal on T2WI, and low in signal on fat-saturated sequences (both T1 and T2). In fact, loss of signal in an adrenal mass on fat-saturated sequences confirms the presence of fat, and thus, the diagnosis of myelolipoma [28]. The non-fatty soft tissue components are low to intermediate signal on T1WI and heterogeneously hyperintense on T2WI [28]. The solid components enhance more than the fatty components

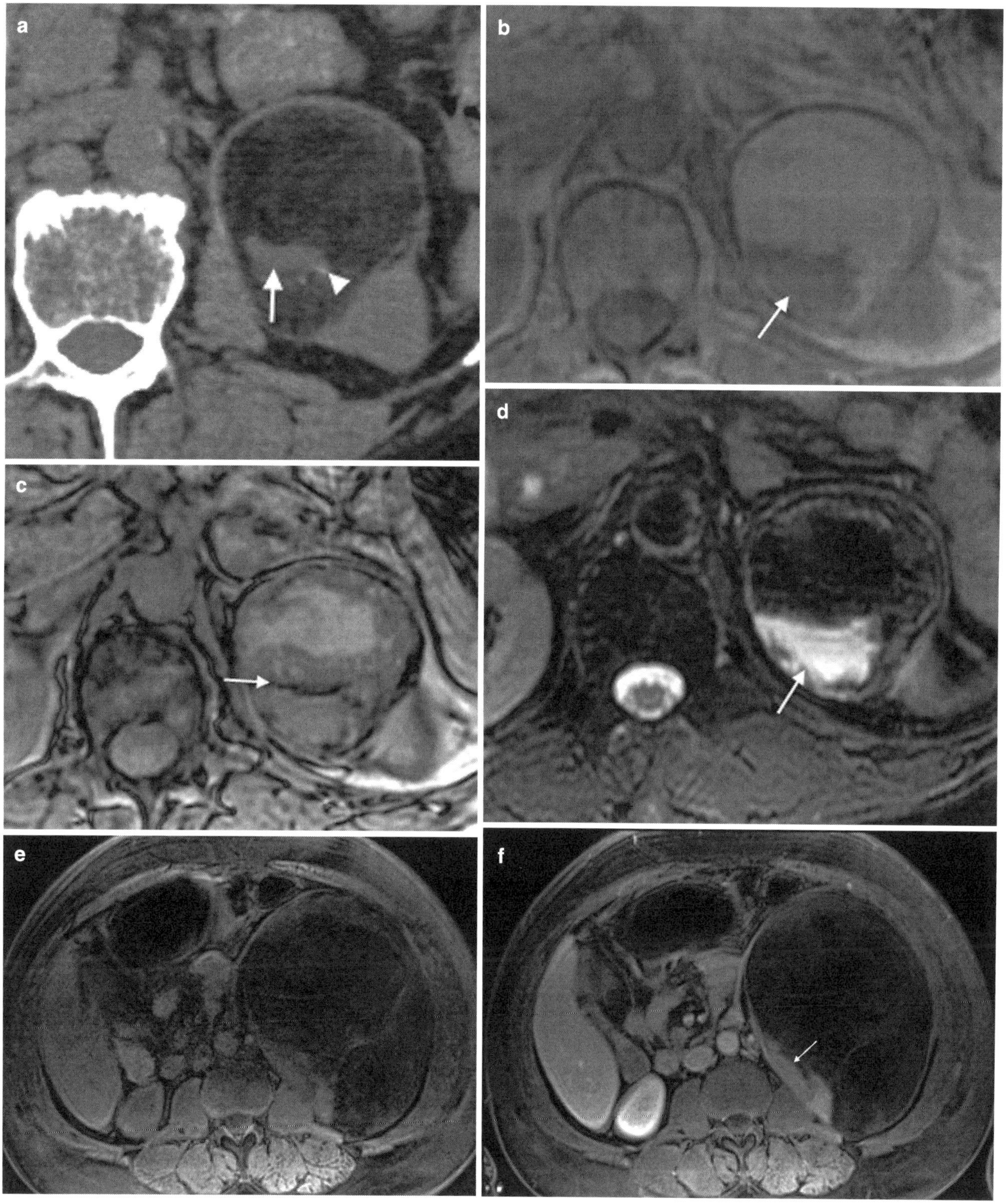
a
b
c
d
e
f

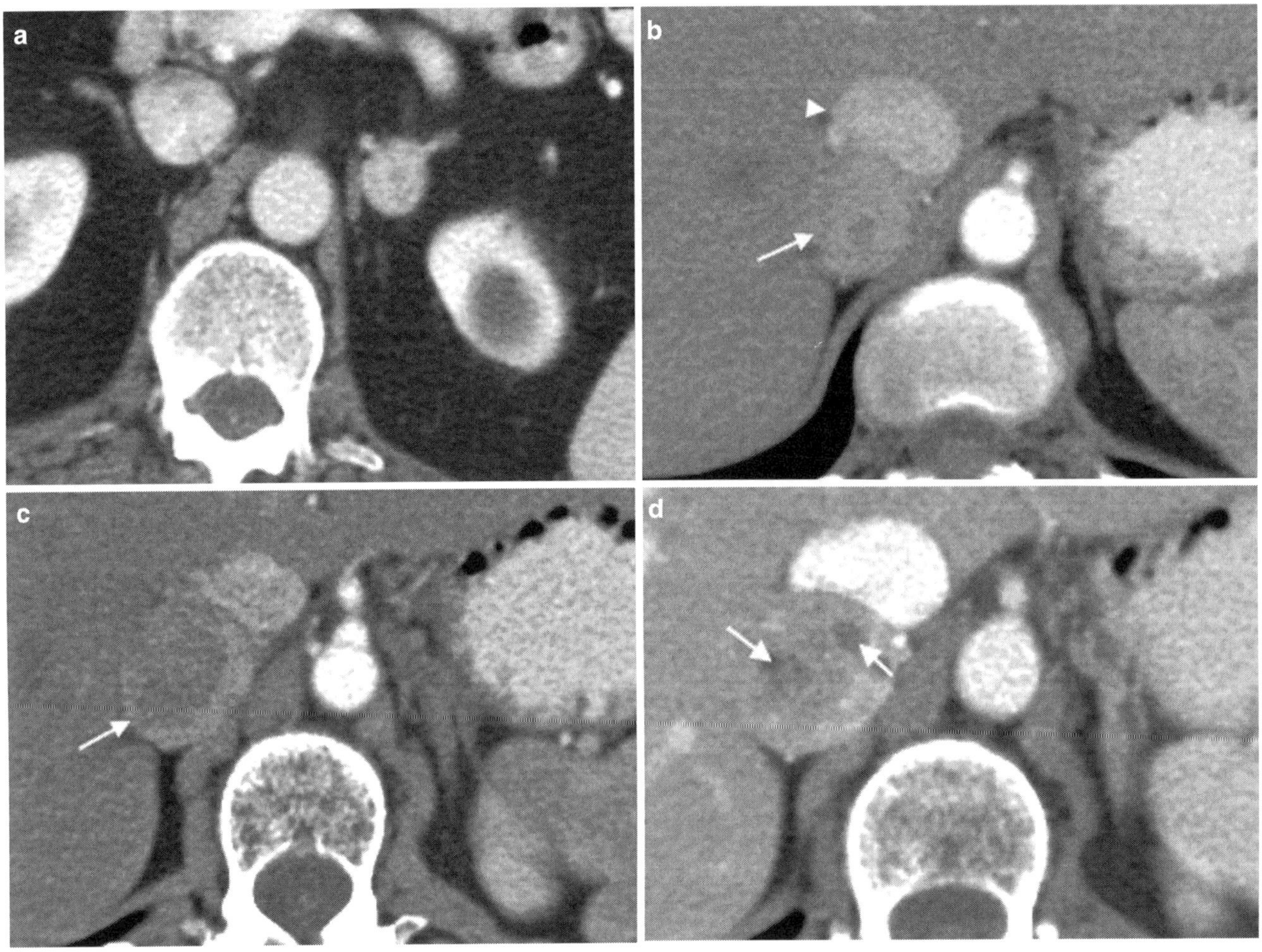

Fig. 5.11 Pheochromocytoma: CT. (**a**) This portal venous phase contrast-enhanced CT in a 67-year-old man with melanoma demonstrates a hypervascular 2 cm left adrenal mass that proved to be a pheochromocytoma at pathology. The imaging features are typical of a small pheochromocytoma, but are nonspecific, and the lesion was thought to represent metastatic melanoma prior to biopsy. The patient had hypertension but no other symptoms typically seen with pheochromocytoma. (**b**, **c**) This contrast-enhanced CT demonstrates a 3.5 cm right adrenal mass (*arrows*) that is hypervascular in both the arterial (**b**) and portal venous phases (**c**) in a patient who presented with headaches, diaphoresis, chest pain, and markedly elevated catecholamines (although only mild hypertension). Note that the mass lies just posterior to the IVC (*arrowhead*). (**d**) Slightly more inferiorly, the mass contains foci of low attenuation (*arrows*) consistent with necrosis. A hypervascular adrenal mass in a patient with elevated catecholamines is pathognomonic for pheochromocytoma

calcifications related to prior hemorrhage, although only a small percentage of myelolipomas present clinically with hemorrhage [41]. Adrenal hemangiomas bleed frequently, but are extremely rare tumors. In contrast, adrenal adenomas are very common lesions but only rarely bleed [41]. Among the malignant etiologies, adrenal cortical carcinomas are large masses that commonly contains hemorrhage but are rare lesions overall. Adrenal metastases, while common, are rarely associated with hemorrhage; when hemorrhage does occur with metastases, however, the most common primary tumor is bronchogenic carcinoma followed by melanoma [41]. In the absence of an underlying solid mass, hematomas are complex fluid collections that do not enhance after IV contrast administration. However, if solid, nodular areas of enhancement are seen (either on MRI or CT performed with pre- and post-contrast images) an underlying tumor should be suspected. MRI is probably superior to CT in detecting subtle areas of enhancement, in part because subtraction images are routinely performed, which facilitate detection of subtle changes in T1 signal due to gadolinium uptake (pre-contrast signal subtracted from post-contrast should equal zero in the absence of enhancement). MRI is also more sensitive for detecting focal areas enhancement within a calcified pseudocyst (related to chronic hemorrhage) because calcifications are much more prominent on CT, and thus, can obscure underlying enhancing components. Pseudocysts can also develop a thickened irregular, enhancing wall that can be mistaken for a cystic neoplasm [41].

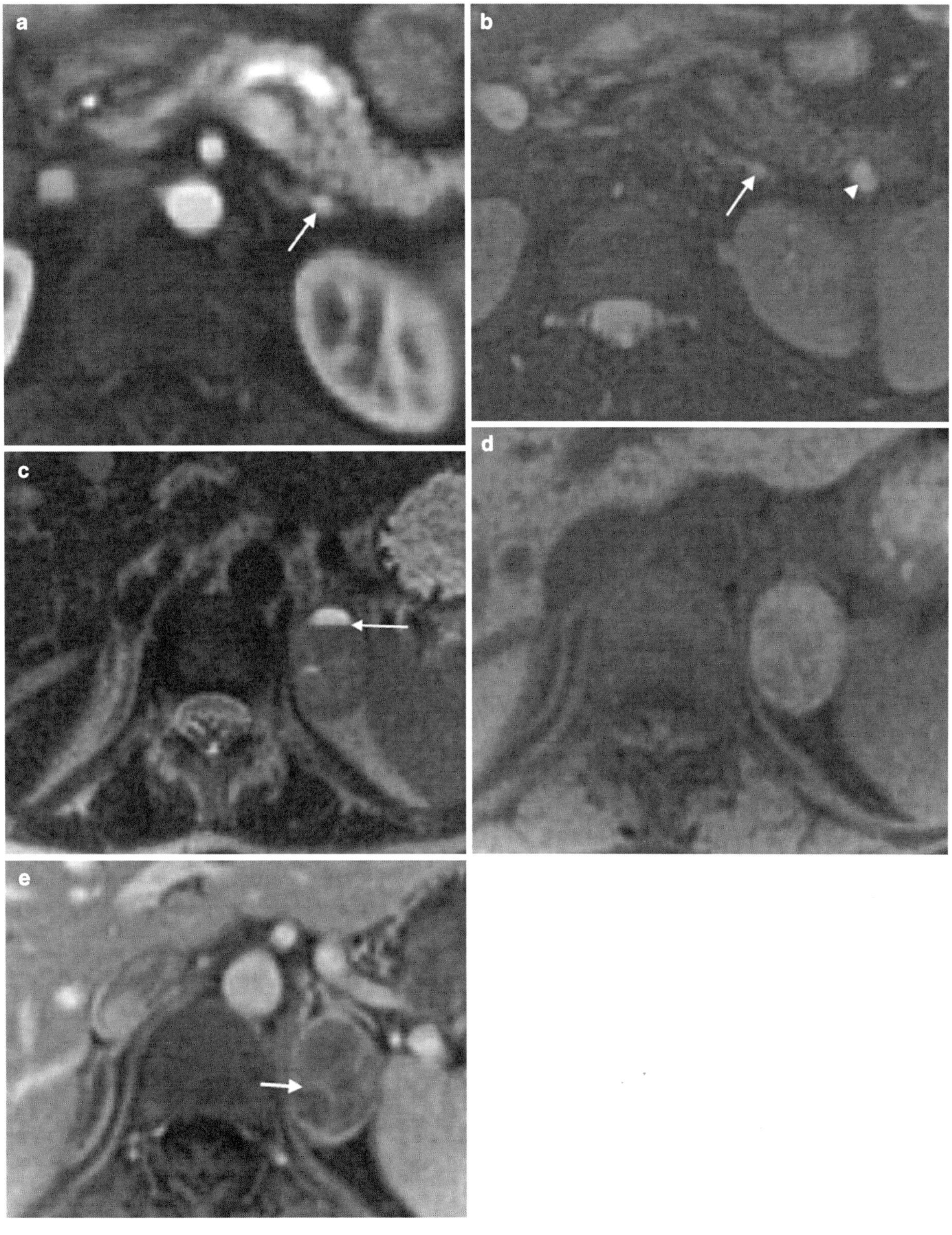

Fig. 5.12 Pheochromocytoma: MRI. (**a**) Arterial phase post-contrast image in this patient with Von Hippel-Lindau syndrome (VHL) demonstrates a 7 mm homogenously hypervascular nodule (*arrow*) in the lateral limb of the left adrenal gland consistent with a pheochromocytoma. There is no associated necrosis with this small nodule. (**b**) The same lesion (*arrow*) on this T2FS image is mildly hyperintense, yet lower in signal than the fluid seen in an adjacent pancreatic tail cyst (*arrowhead*). (**c**) This SSFSE T2WI without fat saturation demonstrates a 3.5 cm left adrenal nodule that proved to be a pheochromocytoma. Note the fluid–fluid level (*arrow*) indicating a cystic, necrotic component which is very high in T2 signal. (**d**) This T1FS precontrast image of the same lesion demonstrates that the mass is mildly hyperintense due to hemorrhage. (**e**) Post-contrast T1WI in the portal venous phase shows that the mass is largely necrotic with multiple enhancing septations consistent with small areas of viable tumor (*arrows*)

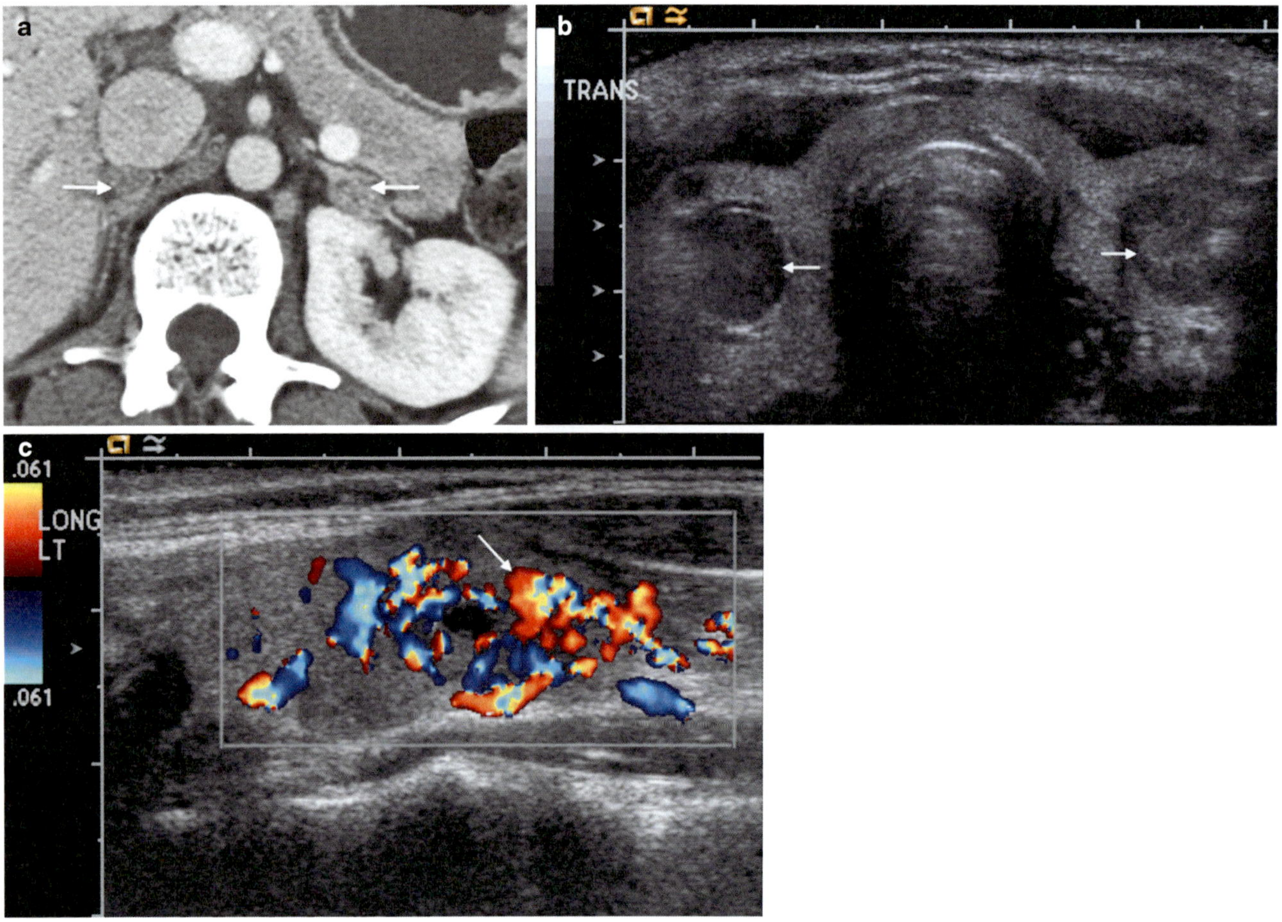

Fig. 5.13 Pheochromocytoma: hereditary. (**a**) This contrast-enhanced CT scan demonstrates small enhancing bilateral adrenal nodules (*arrows*) in a 32-year-old female who presented with elevated urinary catecholamines, consistent with multifocal pheochromocytomas. (**b**) A thyroid ultrasound on the same patient demonstrates bilateral heterogenous solid thyroid nodules that proved to be medullary carcinoma at pathology. (**c**) Note the marked hypervascularity of one of the nodules on color Doppler imaging (*arrow*). This patient originally presented with elevated serum calcium levels and was subsequently shown to have a parathyroid adenoma. The triad of parathyroid adenoma, medullary carcinoma of the thyroid, and pheochromocytoma is known as multiple endocrine neoplasia type 2B (MEN IIB)

Table 5.1 Hereditary pheochromocytoma syndromes [42]

Syndrome	Genetic defect	Incidence of syndrome	Incidence of pheochromocytoma in this population (%)	Mean age of onset of pheochromocytoma, *y*	Bilateral (%)	Malignant (%)
MEN 2A and MEN 2B pheochromocytoma, medullary carcinoma of thyroid, and either parathyroid tumor (2A) or mucocutaneous neuroma (2B)	RET (autosomal dominant)	1/40,000	50	36	63	3
VHL hemangioblastomas, pheochromocytoma, pancreatic islet cell tumors, renal tumors, lymphatic sac tumors	VHL (autosomal dominant)	1/36,000	10–20 (PCC or paragangliomas)	29	44	3
NF1 neurofibromas, café au lait patches, skin fold freckling, iris Lisch nodules, optic gliomas, bone dysplasias, pheochromocytoma	NF1 (autosomal dominant, but up to 50 % can be sporadic)	1/3,500	5.7 (up to 13 % at autopsy)	42	14	9

MEN multiple endocrine neoplasia, *NF1* neurofibromatosis type 1, *VHL* von Hippel-Lindau

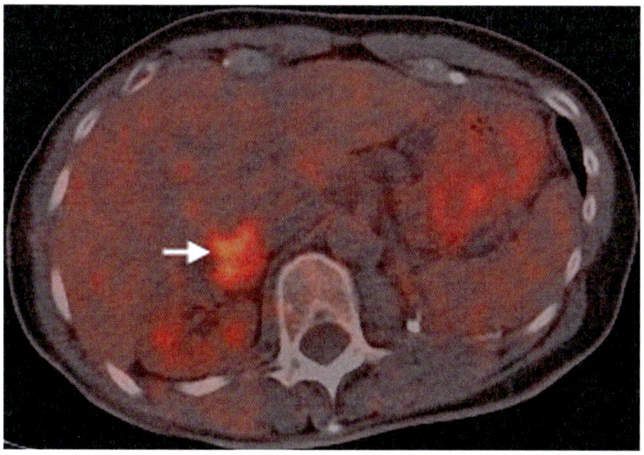

Fig. 5.14 Pheochromocytoma: PET. This fused PET-CT image demonstrates a 3 cm right adrenal mass (*arrow*) with a standardized uptake value (SUV) of 5

Malignant Adrenal Neoplasms

Metastases

The most common tumor to metastasize to the adrenal glands is lung cancer, followed by breast cancer and melanoma. Other common primary tumors include bowel, pancreas, and kidney cancers [24, 25]. The adrenal gland is the fourth-most common site of distant metastatic disease, exceeded only by the lungs, bones, and liver. Adrenal metastases are reportedly seen at autopsy in up to 27 % of patients with malignant epithelial tumors [24, 28, 57]. In fact, metastatic disease is by far the most common malignant tumor of the adrenal gland since primary malignant adrenal neoplasms are rare. However, adrenal metastases are much less common than adrenal adenomas (the most common of all adrenal tumors)

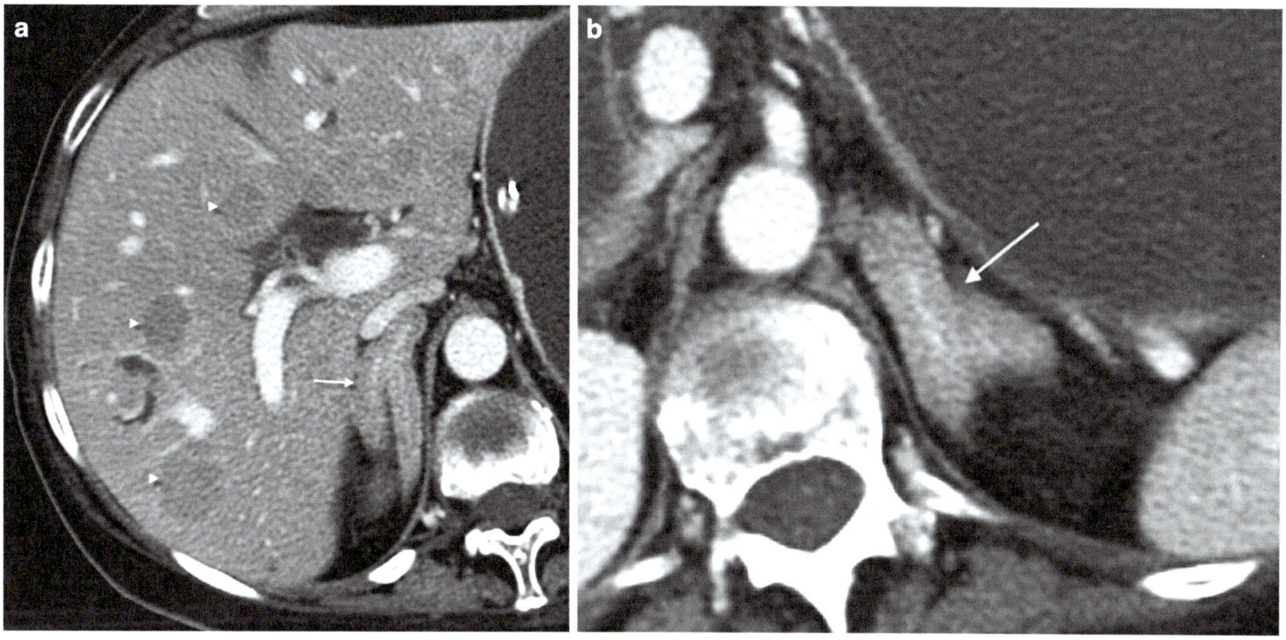

Fig. 5.15 Adrenal hyperplasia. (**a**, **b**) This contrast-enhanced CT in a patient with Cushing syndrome demonstrates marked diffuse thickening of both adrenal glands consistent with hyperplasia (*arrows*). Both adrenal glands were subsequently resected revealing diffuse adrenocortical hyperplasia. The cause of the hyperplasia in this case was an adrenocorticotropic hormone (ACTH)-secreting neuroendocrine tumor of the pancreas that metastasized to the liver (*arrowheads* on metastases in **a**)

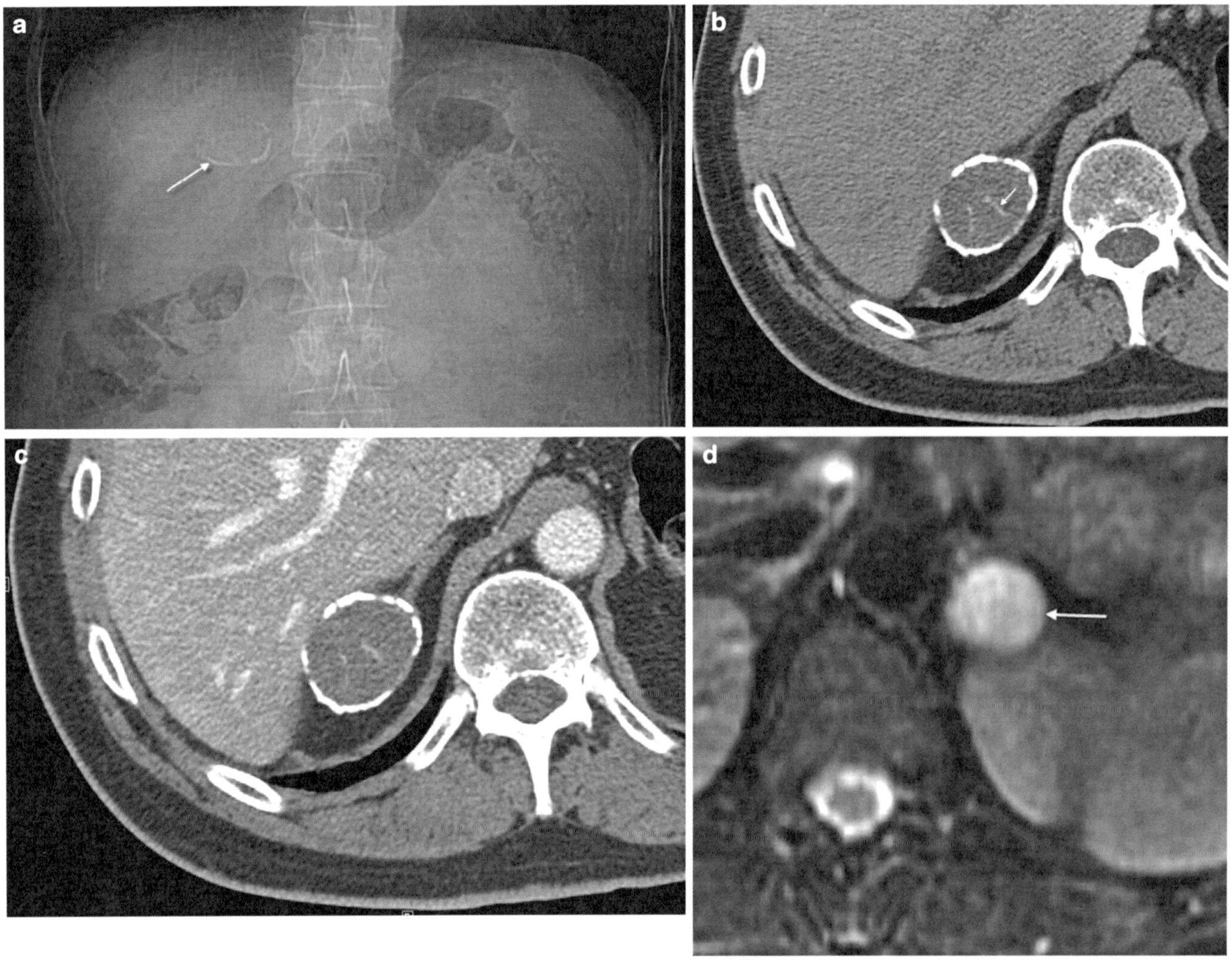

Fig. 5.16 Adrenal cysts. (**a**) Scout radiograph from CT in a 61-year-old man with a history of lung cancer demonstrates a 3.5 cm rim calcified mass in the right upper quadrant (*arrow*). (**b**, **c**) NCCT and contrast-enhanced CT, respectively, demonstrate a right adrenal mass with rim calcification and a few thin calcified septations (*arrow*). The noncalcified portion of the mass measures between 35 and 40 HU on both the pre- and post-contrast images consistent with a cystic, hemorrhagic lesion. No solid, enhancing component is identified. However, due to the complex nature of the lesion, it was resected and pathology confirmed a pseudocyst with extensive fibrosis and calcification. (**d**) This T2WI demonstrates a 2 cm left adrenal mass, which is very high in signal consistent with a cyst (*arrow*)

in the general population. Even in patients with known primary malignancies, an incidental adrenal nodule is more likely to be an adenoma than metastatic disease [28]. Adrenal metastases are more often bilateral than unilateral [24]. They are more likely to be large, heterogenous (due to necrosis), and irregular in contour than adenomas, but many metastatic lesions, particularly smaller ones, are homogenous and smooth in contour and thus cannot be reliably distinguished from adenomas by their morphologic appearance on imaging alone [3, 28]. On NCCT, almost all adrenal metastases measure greater than 10 HU. After contrast, they generally demonstrate heterogenous enhancement, but this appearance is nonspecific. On MRI, adrenal metastases are usually low in T1 signal and high in T2 signal with progressive enhancement after gadolinium administration, all which are nonspecific [24]. The imaging appearance of metastases tends to resemble that of the primary tumor (*i.e.*, hypervascular with renal cancer; hypovascular with most lung metastases) [25] but the morphology alone cannot be reliably used to distinguish metastases from adenomas because significant overlap does occur, particularly with small lesions.

Since morphologic features of metastases and adenomas overlap considerably on cross-sectional imaging, the only reliable methods to distinguish these entities are CT densitometry, MR chemical-shift imaging, and CT washout imaging. Diffusion imaging has thus far proven ineffective at distinguishing benign from malignant adrenal lesions, with

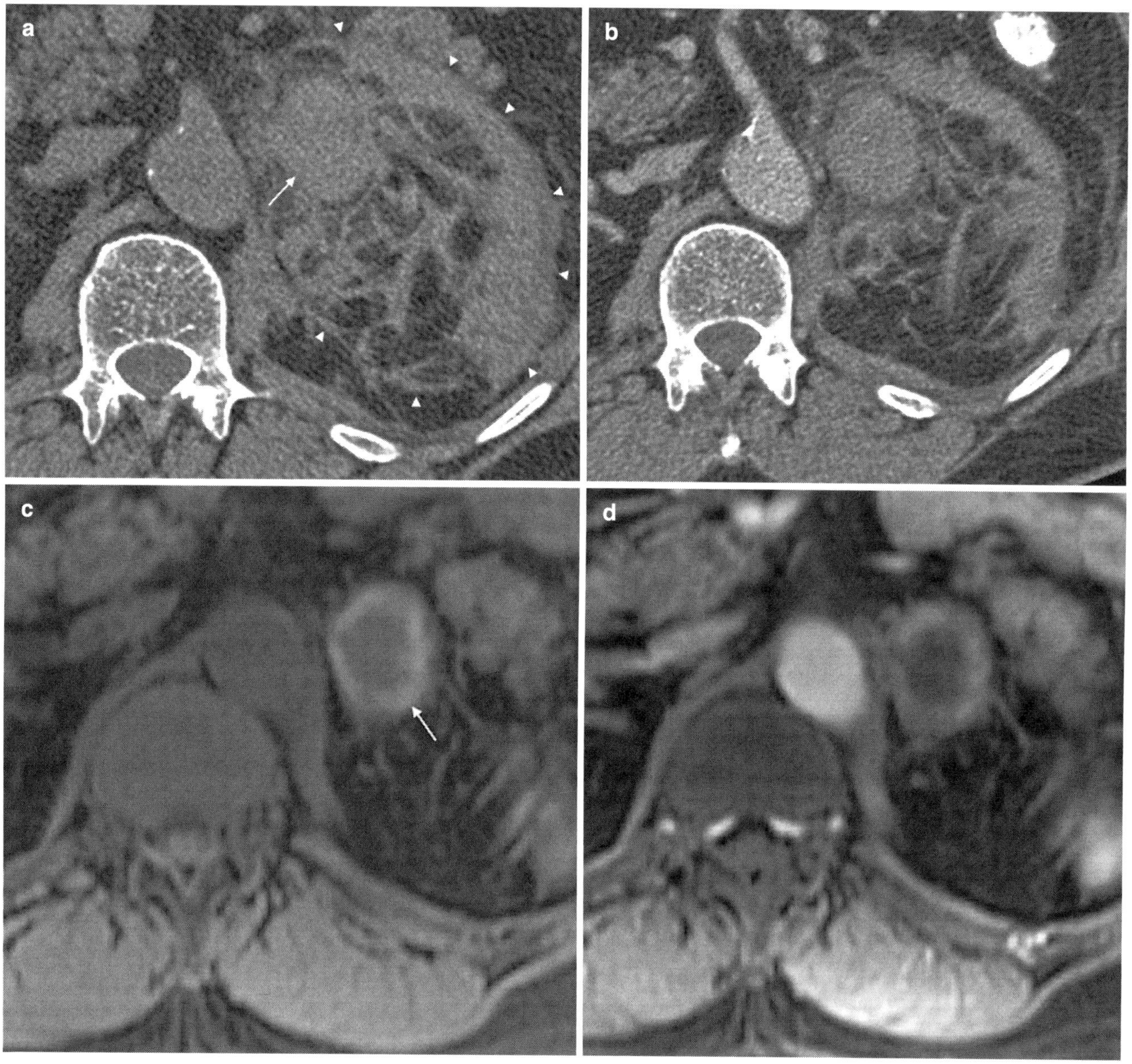

Fig. 5.17 Adrenal hematoma. A 71-year-old man who presented to the emergency room with severe acute left-sided abdominal pain, which radiated to the chest. (**a**) NCCT demonstrates a 4 cm high attenuation left renal mass measuring 65 HU (*arrow*). Note extensive infiltration of the adjacent perinephric fat suspicious for hemorrhage (*arrowhead*). (**b**) A contrast-enhanced CT performed later the same day demonstrates that the mass again measures 65 HU, indicating a lack of enhancement. (**c**) Two weeks later, an MR was performed. Axial T1FS image demonstrates that the mass (*arrow*) has a rim of high signal consistent with hemorrhage. (**d**, **e**) Post-contrast (**d**) and subtraction image (**e**) demonstrate lack of central or nodular enhancement confirming the absence of an underlying solid mass. The thin rim of peripheral enhancement (*arrow*) probably represents a combination of normal adrenal tissue and a fibrous wall surrounding the hematoma. (**f**) Follow-up MR 1-year later demonstrates near-complete resolution of the hematoma (*arrow*)

no significant difference in ADC values [58]. Adrenal metastases are histologically similar to the primary tumor, and, thus, rarely contain intracytoplasmic lipid [28]. On the other hand, most adenomas contain significant amounts of intracellular lipid that causes their attenuation on NCCT to be lower than that of metastases [3]. Using a value of 10 HU or less to diagnose an adenoma yields a specificity of 98 %. Thus, fewer than 2 % of lesions measuring 10 HU or less on CT densitometry will represent malignancies [32]. If CT densitometry is inconclusive, chemical shift MRI or the CT

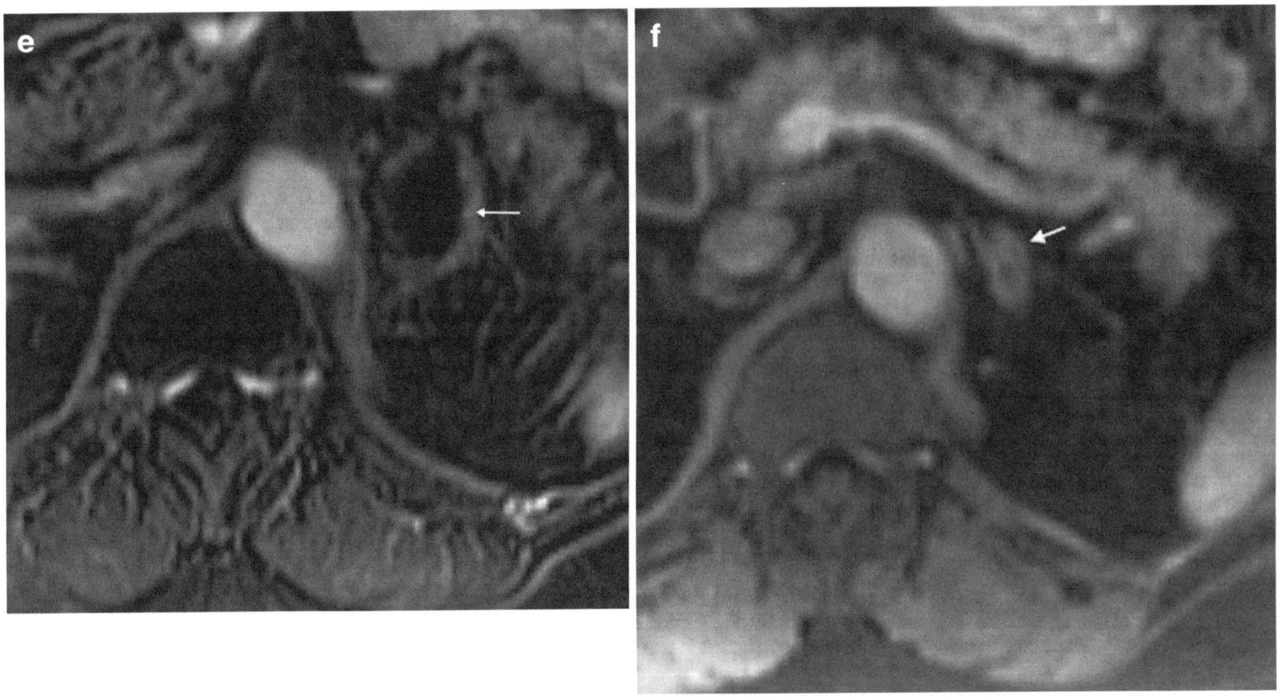

Fig. 5.17 (continued)

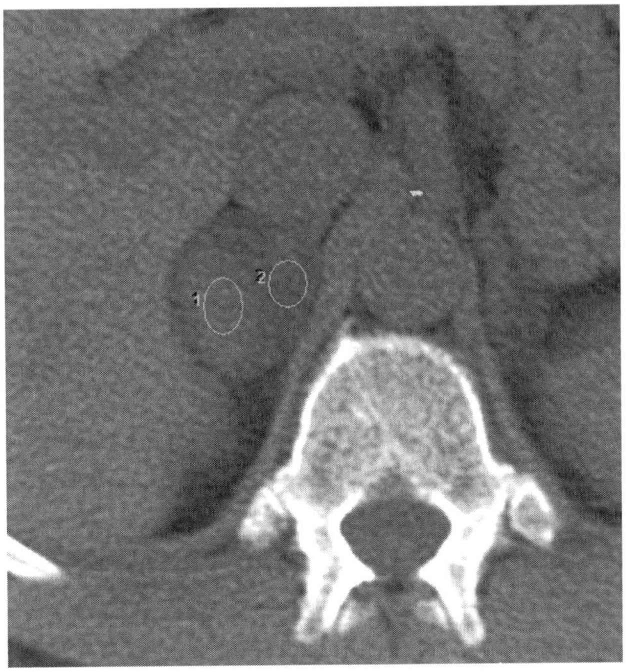

Fig. 5.18 Adrenal hemorrhage due to underlying mass. This NCCT demonstrates an incidentally detected, heterogenous right adrenal mass in a 50-year-old male with flank pain. ROI #2 is placed on the lower attenuation region, which measures −2 HU, suggesting an adenoma. ROI #1 is placed on the higher attenuation region, giving a value of 40 HU, suggesting the possibility of a collision tumor (two coexisting lesions within the same organ). Surgical pathology revealed an adrenal adenoma containing hemorrhage, but no evidence of malignancy or collision tumor

washout technique should be employed for further work-up, the latter of which has been shown to have superior sensitivity and overall accuracy [39]. Using chemical shift MRI to diagnose an adenoma is very specific because the presence of intracellular lipid within a lesion effectively rules out metastatic disease (specificity of nearly 100 %; metastases rarely contain enough intracytoplasmic lipid to lose signal on out-of-phase images); however, the sensitivity of this test is low. Since many adenomas contain insufficient lipid to cause noticeable signal loss on opposed phase images. The absolute washout method (*see* Fig. 5.7) is much more sensitive (100 %) with very good specificity, and thus is the preferred method [39]. For patients with a known primary malignancy, an absolute washout value of 60 % or less in an adrenal nodule is suspicious for metastatic disease [38]. For some patients, including those with an allergic history to iodinated contrast or with concerns about ionizing radiation, MRI may still be preferred over CT. If these tests are inconclusive, PET imaging can be helpful, but ultimately a core biopsy may be needed to make a definitive diagnosis.

Adrenal Cortical Carcinoma

Although rare compared to metastatic disease, primary ACC is the most common primary malignant tumor of the adrenal gland with a reported incidence of 1–2 cases per million and a peak incidence between 30 and 70 years of age [24, 27, 28]. Because these tumors are usually large at presentation,

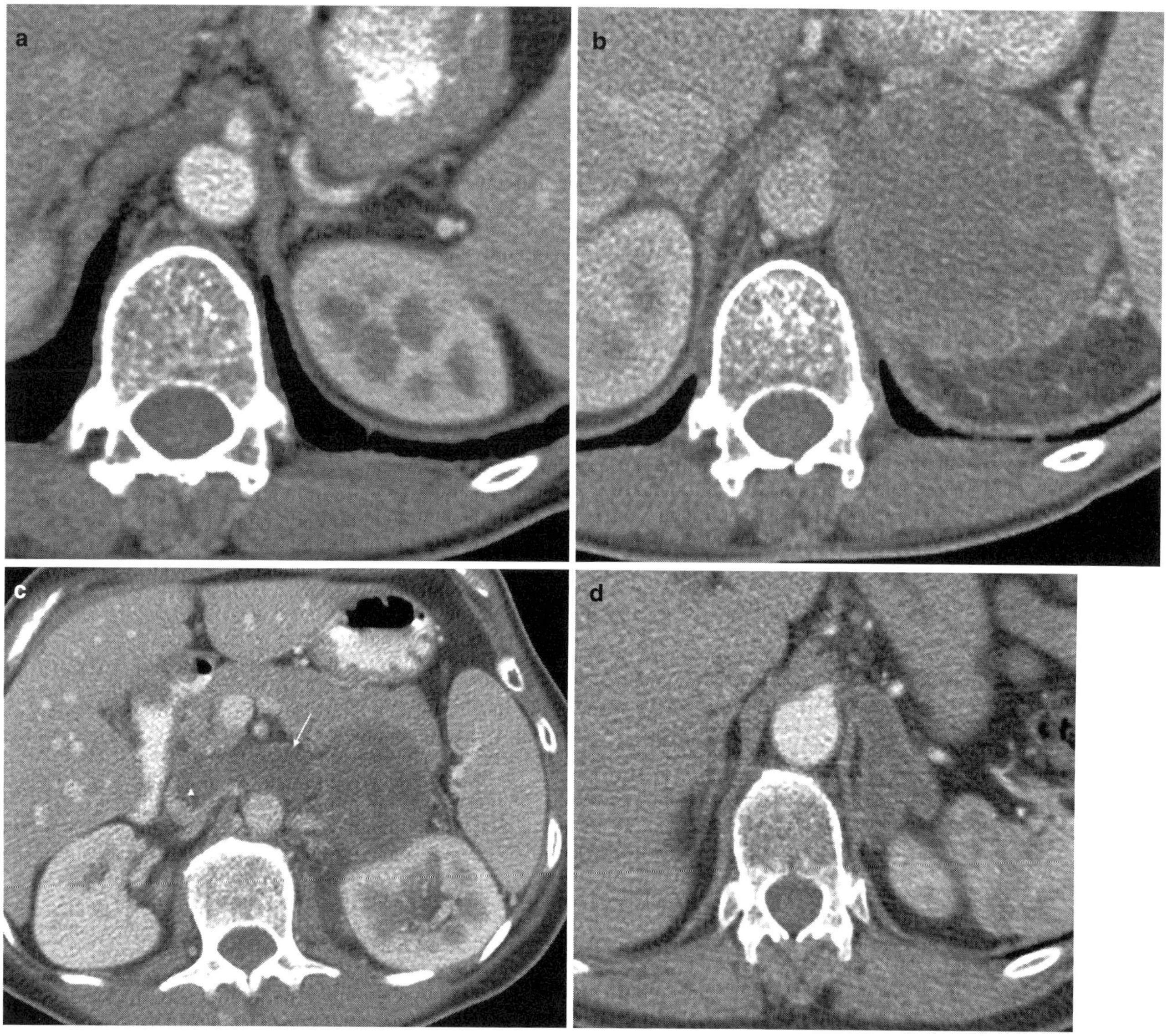

Fig. 5.19 Metastatic disease: general CT and MR appearance. (**a**) Contrast-enhanced CT on a 49-year-old woman demonstrating a normal left adrenal gland. (**b**) A contrast-enhanced CT performed 5 months later demonstrates a new 8 cm heterogeneously enhancing left adrenal mass which, on biopsy, proved to be a metastatic poorly differentiated adenocarcinoma, most likely originating from the lung. (**c**) On a lower slice extensive tumor thrombus originating from the adrenal mass is seen throughout the left renal vein (*arrow*), partially extending into the IVC (*arrowhead*). (**d**) This contrast-enhanced CT in a different patient demonstrates diffuse enlargement of the left adrenal gland, which maintains it adeniform shape. Occasionally, metastatic disease can diffusely involve the adrenal gland, causing enlargement with some preservation of the normal shape. (**e**) Contrast-enhanced CT in a 67-year-old man with melanoma demonstrates an indeterminate 1 cm right adrenal nodule. (**f**) CT performed 9 months later demonstrates marked interval increase in size of the nodule, now measuring 5 cm, consistent with metastatic melanoma. The mass in this case is relatively homogenous. Note that the tumor is focally growing into the IVC (*arrow*) via the short right adrenal vein. (**g**) Contrast-enhanced CT in this 38-year-old man demonstrates a 5 cm hypervascular right renal mass consistent with clear cell carcinoma. The patient subsequently underwent a partial nephrectomy. (**h**) This CT performed 5 years later on the same patient demonstrates a new 2 cm hypervascular right adrenal nodule (*arrow*), which resembles the primary renal tumor, consistent with metastatic renal carcinoma

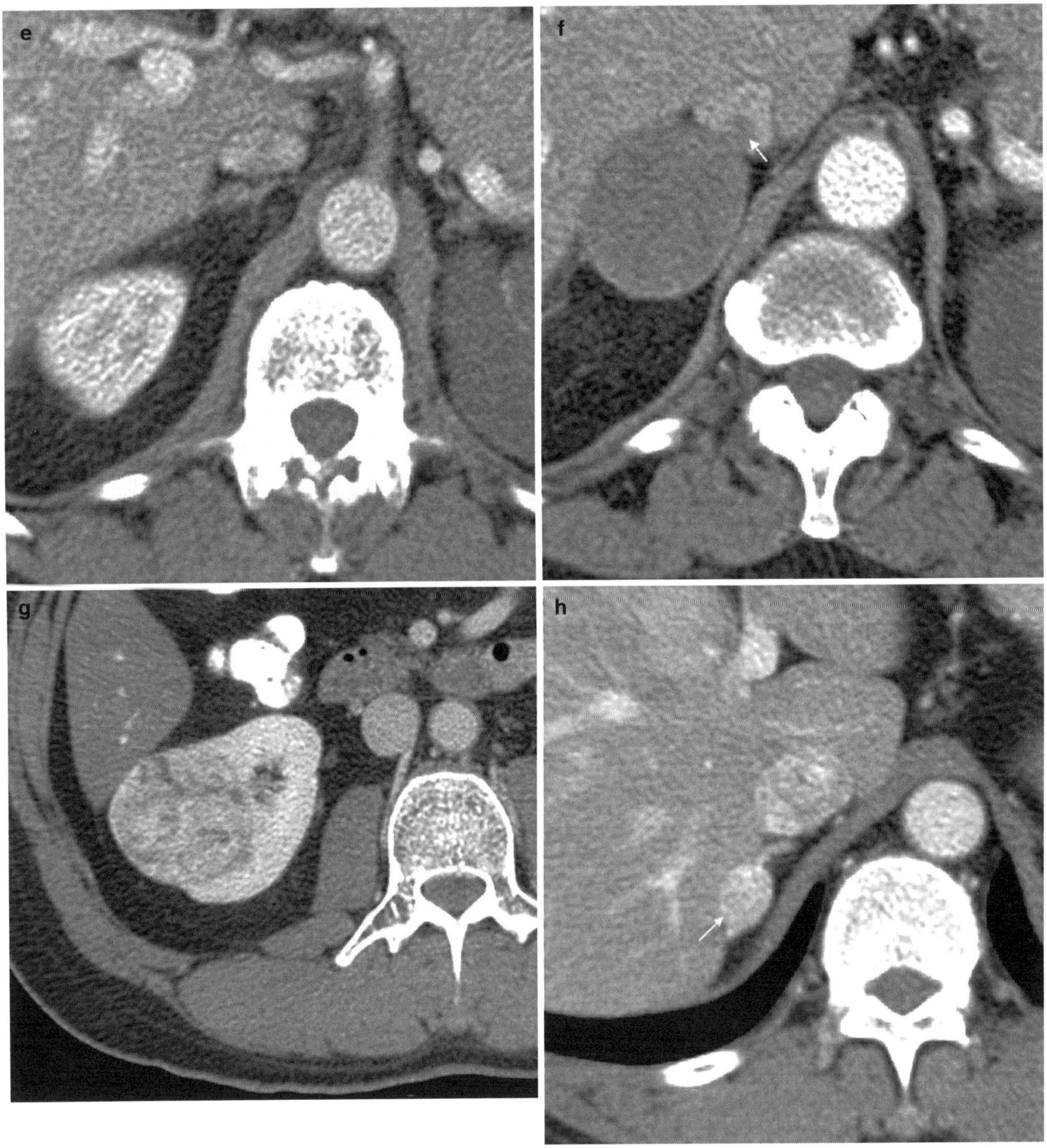

Fig. 5.19 (continued)

patients may present with abdominal pain or a palpable mass. Because ACC arise from the adrenal cortex, like adenomas, they can be associated with excess production of steroids. On average, 55 % (range 26–94 % in multiple series) of ACC are functional [7]. However, hormone production in ACC is less efficient than in normal adrenal tissue, and thus, not all tumors produce enough steroids to cause clinical syndromes. For those patients in whom excessive hormones are produced, the most common clinical syndrome produced is Cushing, followed by virilization or a combination of the two. Other endocrine manifestations, including Conn syndrome and feminization, are rare [3, 7, 13, 14, 28]. Since hormonal production in ACC is inefficient, by the time these patients present clinically, the tumors are often very large, usually between 4 and 20 cm [24, 35]. Ten percent of cases have been reported to be bilateral [35]. Table 5.2 lists relevant information to include in the radiology reports for patients with ACC.

Table 5.2 Important information to include in the radiology report for patients with adrenal cancer [36]

Reporting features	Comments
Size	Maximal transverse, longitudinal, and cranio–caudal dimensions
Capsular integrity	Extension into surrounding fat/breach of capsule indicates stage 3 or higher and increases likelihood of metastatic disease
Kidney involvement	Does tumor infiltrate the ipsilateral kidney?
	Is there evidence of altered perfusion to the kidney?
	Is there evidence of mass effect/hydronephrosis
Adjacent structures	Right: liver, diaphragm
	Left: diaphragm, aorta, lesser sac, stomach, pancreas
	Is there left renal vein or IVC extension?
Tumor description	Heterogeneity, necrosis, calcification
Contralateral adrenal gland	Bilateral disease?
Contralateral kidney	Treatment may involve ipsilateral nephrectomy; therefore, commenting on enhancement and morphology of contralateral kidney is helpful
Lymph nodes	Size and presence of lymph nodes in retroperitoneum and retrocrural space
Metastases	Lung, liver, bone

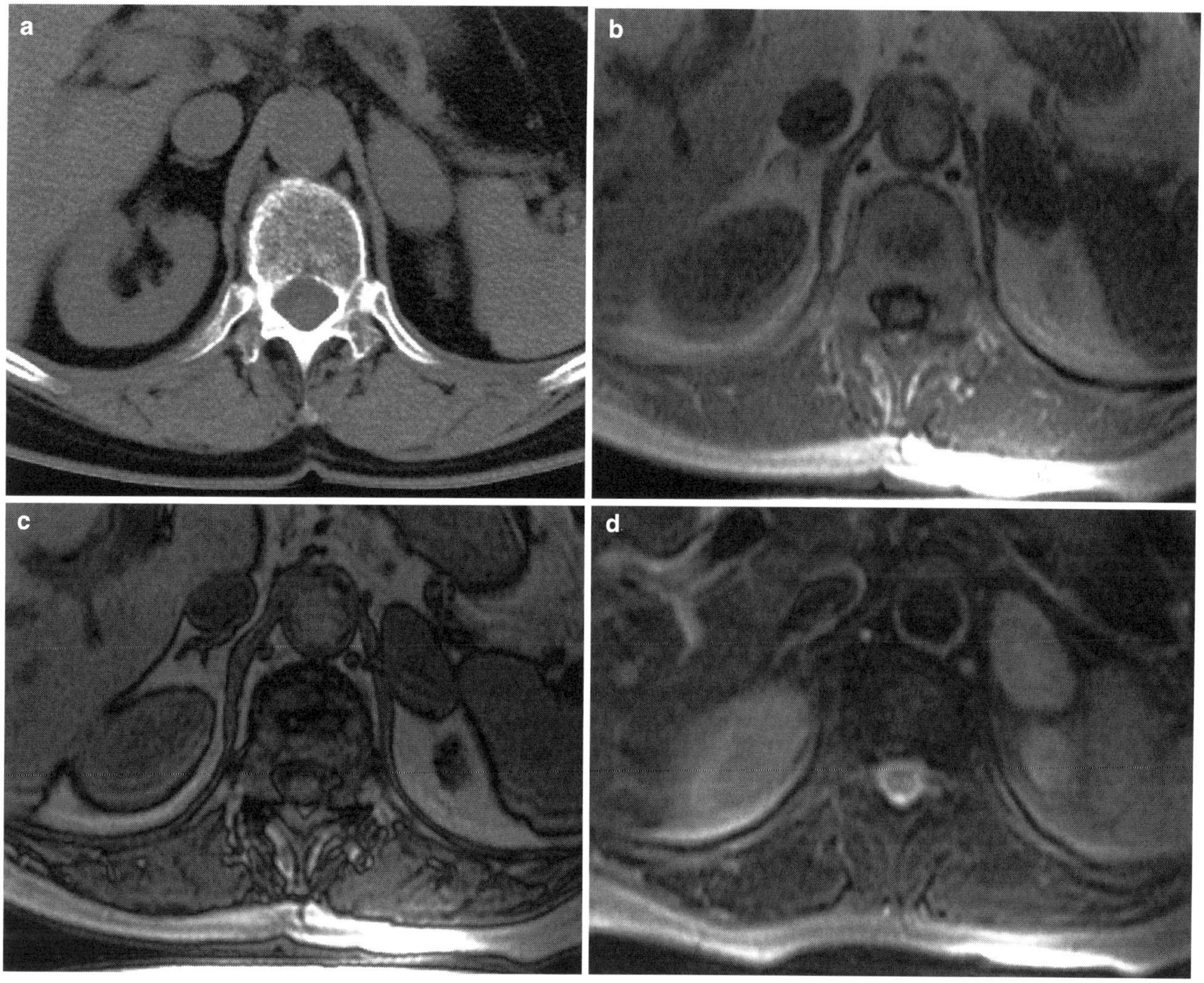

Fig. 5.20 Distinguishing metastases from adenomas on CT and MRI. (**a**) NCCT in this patient with non–small cell lung cancer demonstrates a 4 cm left adrenal mass that measures 26 HU. (**b**, **c**) Axial T1-weighted MR images demonstrate no significant signal loss from the in-phase (**b**) to out-of-phase (**c**) images, indicating the absence of significant intracellular lipid. (**d**) Axial T2FS MR image demonstrates that the lesion is mildly hyperintense (*arrow*). (**e**) PET scan from the same patient reveals marked FDG avidity (*arrow*) consistent with metastatic disease, which was subsequently confirmed by surgical pathology

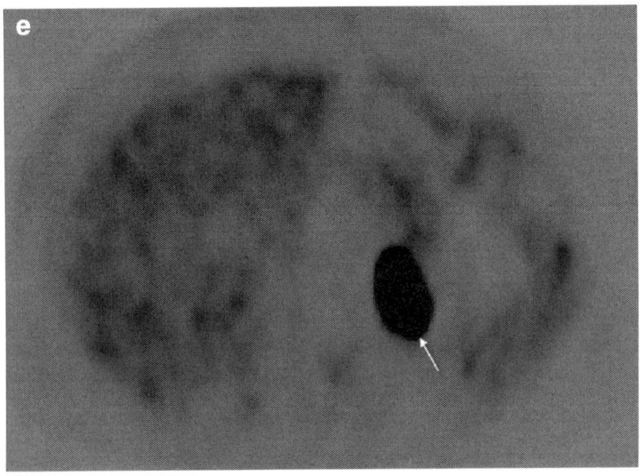

Fig. 5.20 (continued)

The typical appearance of ACC on CT is that of a large (>4 cm) lobulated mass with irregular margins, which displaces the kidney inferiorly (sometimes posteriorly for left-sided tumors) from its normal position. They are typically heterogenous in attenuation and often contain large areas of central necrosis, hemorrhage, and cystic change. Enhancement is seen in the solid, mostly peripheral, viable components whereas the necrotic central areas do not enhance. Central calcifications are seen in up to 20–30 % of cases [3, 16, 35]. Fishman et al. [59] reported a thin, enhancing capsule-like rim in 7 of 38 patients on CT. Prominent tumor vascularity is often seen within or around large ACC. Similar to renal carcinoma, tumor extension into the left renal vein or IVC is common and is best appreciated on post-contrast images [3]. Additional features that suggest malignancy are invasion of adjacent organs, retroperitoneal adenopathy, and distant metastatic disease.

Due to the large areas of central necrosis, ACC is usually very heterogenous on MR imaging. The solid, non-necrotic portions of the tumor, typically in the periphery of the mass, are low to intermediate signal on T1WI, although foci of high signal are frequently seen in areas of hemorrhage. The solid areas demonstrate intermediate to high signal on T2WI. The necrotic portions of the tumor are very high in T2 signal, and can vary from low to high signal on T1WI depending on the amount of hemorrhage that is present. The solid components demonstrate nodular areas of intense enhancement with delayed washout whereas the necrotic components do not enhance [3, 28]. Venous invasion is well-depicted on the multiplanar sequences, particularly the T2-weighted and post-contrast images.

In the absence of a known primary extra-adrenal malignancy, almost all adrenal masses smaller than 3 cm are adenomas, and most of these lesions can be confirmed as adenomas with the CT and MR imaging technique previously described, requiring no additional follow-up after confirmation [3]. However, if a unilateral adrenal mass greater than 4 cm without specific imaging features such as those seen with

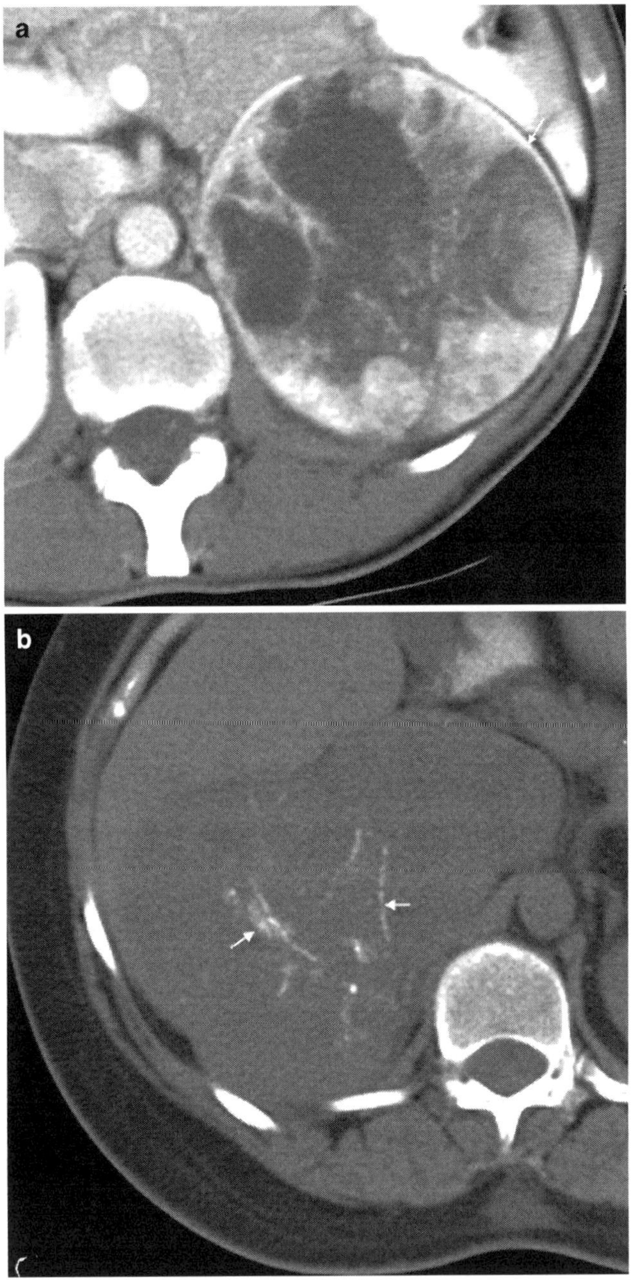

Fig. 5.21 Adrenal cortical carcinoma: CT. (**a**) This contrast-enhanced CT in a 42-year-old woman demonstrates a markedly heterogenous 9 cm left adrenal mass consistent with ACC. The imaging features of this mass are typical for ACC, including the large areas of low attenuation centrally consistent with necrosis. The periphery of the mass demonstrates areas of hypervascularity consistent with viable tumor. Also note the thin-enhancing pseudocapsule around the mass (*arrow*). (**b**) This NCCT in a 32-year-old female demonstrates a 13 cm right adrenal mass with central amorphous and linear calcifications (*arrows*). (**c**) Post-contrast CT in the same patient demonstrates a heterogeneously enhancing, lobulated right adrenal mass consistent with ACC. This patient presented with Cushing syndrome, indicating that the tumor was metabolically active. (**d**) This arterial phase CT in a 55-year-old man with a 15 cm left ACC demonstrates multiple prominent arteries (*arrows*) in the mass consistent with tumor vascularity. (**e**) The same mass imaged during the portal venous phase demonstrates multiple prominent draining veins surrounding the tumor (*arrow*)

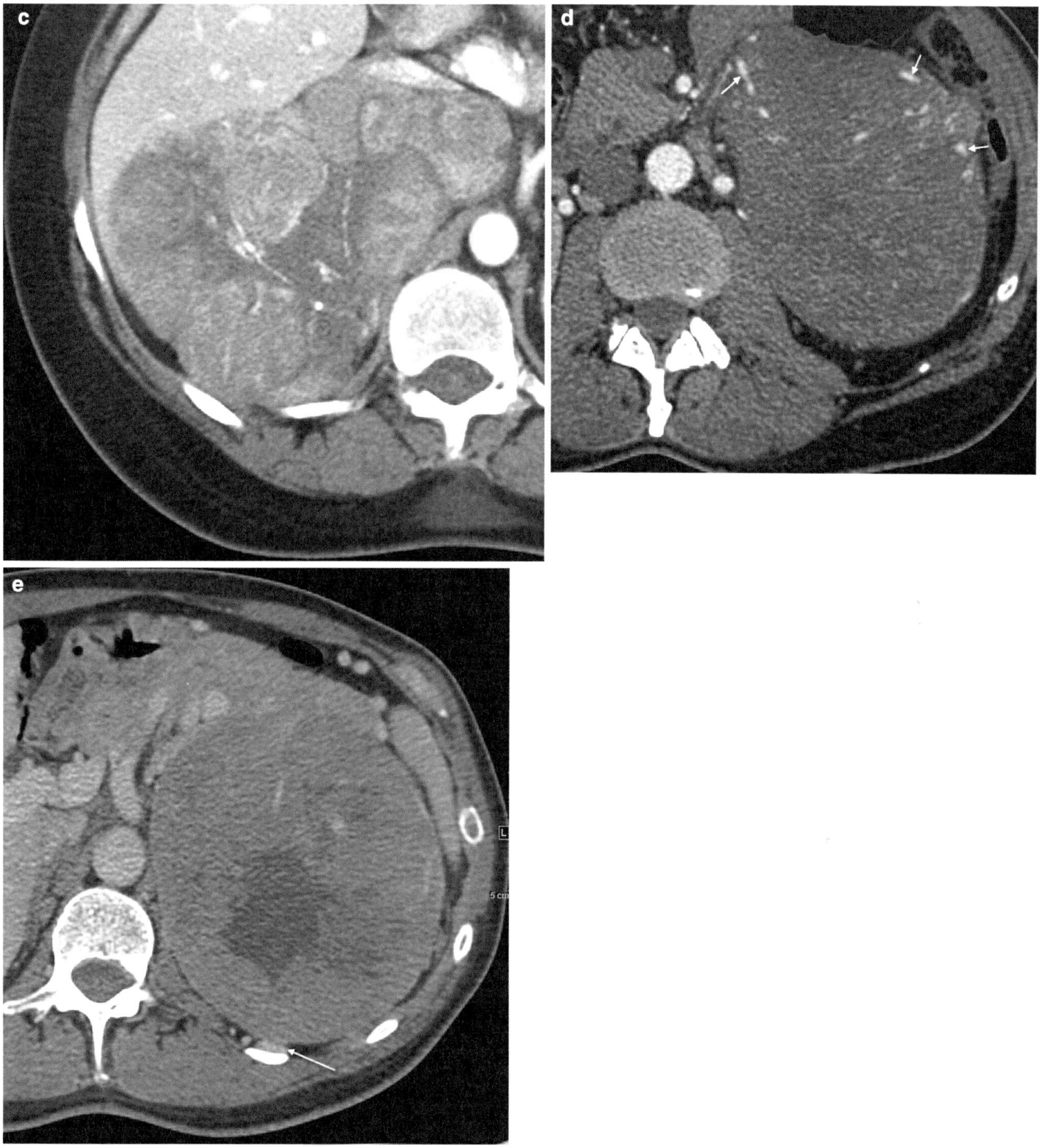

Fig. 5.21 (continued)

myelolipoma, hematoma, or cyst, is encountered, ACC should be suspected [3, 16]. Many of these lesions will be associated with obvious metastatic disease elsewhere, further supporting the diagnosis. However, in the absence of obvious metastatic disease, adenoma will remain in the differential diagnosis. The larger the lesion, the more likely it is to represent ACC. The presence of heterogenous enhancement, hemorrhage, necrosis, and calcification also favors the diagnosis of ACC, although on rare occasions, these features can also be seen in large adenomas [3]. Smooth, well-defined margins favor a benign diagnosis, but these features are also unreliable because they can occasionally be seen in ACC [59]. A study by Hussain et al. [60] demonstrated that tumor size greater than 4 cm and heterogenous enhancement were the most important predictors of malignancy [60]. Unlike adenomas, the solid portions of ACC rarely have attenuation measurements less than

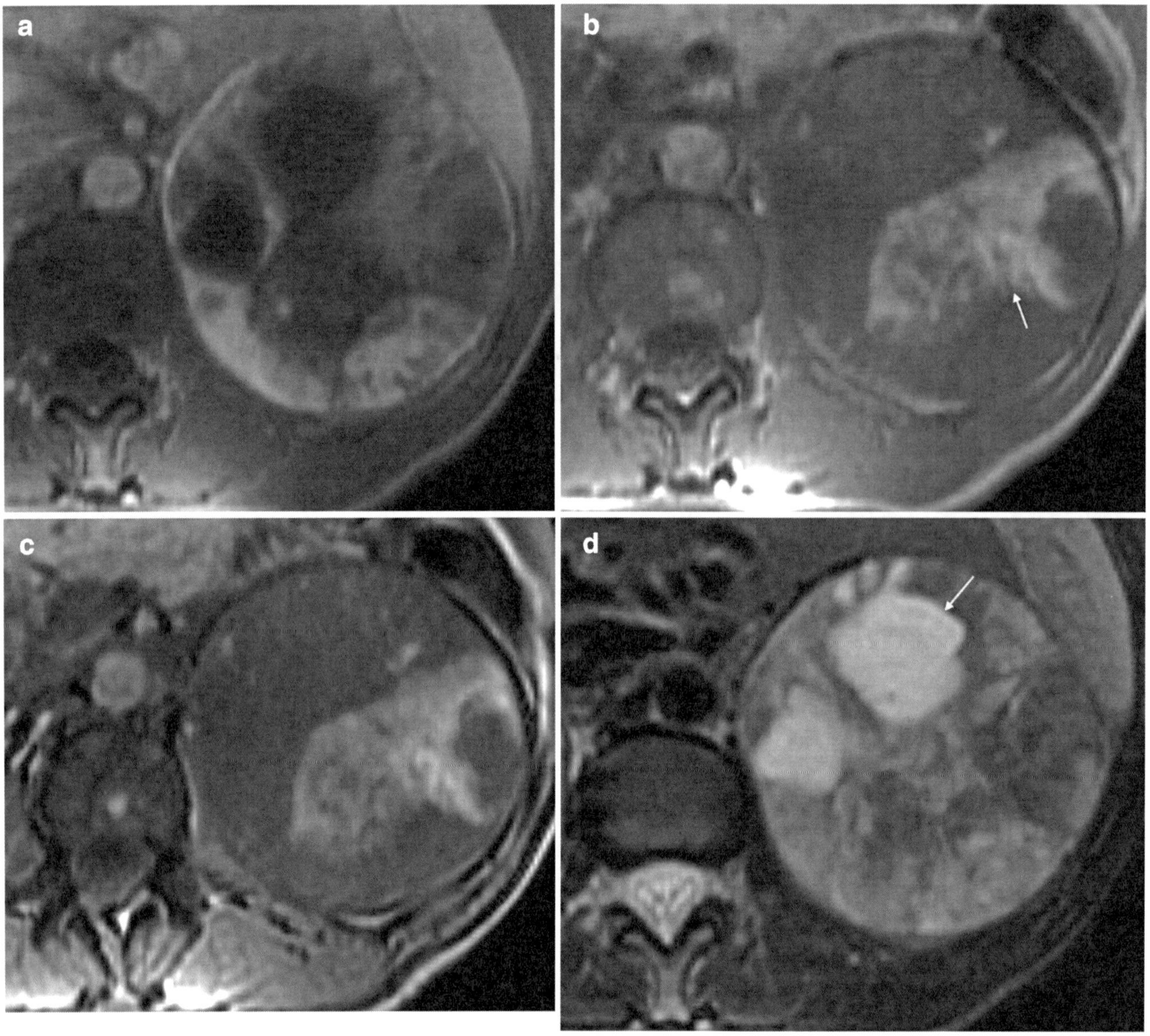

Fig. 5.22 Adrenal cortical carcinoma: MRI. (**a**) This portal venous phase post-contrast MR image performed in the same patient as Fig. 5.21a demonstrates markedly heterogenous enhancement within the large left adrenal mass. The high signal, enhancing peripheral areas are consistent with viable tumor whereas the central low signal areas are consistent with tumor necrosis. (**b**) Axial in-phase T1WI in the same patient demonstrates that the mass is mostly low in T1 signal but does contain large areas of hemorrhage (*arrow*). (**c**) The corresponding opposed phase image does not demonstrate any signal loss within the lesion, indicating lack of significant intracellular lipid. Incidentally, the patient did not present with any symptoms of excess adrenocortical hormone production. (**d**) Axial T2WI with fat saturation demonstrates that the mass is heterogenous with areas of fluid signal consistent with cystic change (*arrow*). (**e**) Coronal T2 SSFSE image again demonstrates areas of very high T2 signal consistent with cystic change, as well as areas of low T2 signal (*arrowhead*) due to hemorrhage. Note that the mass displaces the left kidney inferiorly (*long arrow*). (**f**) Post-contrast T1FS image in a different patient with ACC demonstrates a 14 cm right adrenal mass with moderate enhancement, with relatively small areas of necrosis. Note, the intact fat plane between the liver and the mass, which is dark on this sequence due to fat saturation (*arrow*). Also note prominent peritumoral vascularity commonly seen with large ACC (*arrowhead*)

10 HU, and tend to retain contrast on delayed images, resulting in absolute and relative washout percentages of less than 60 and 40 %, respectively, at 15 min [16]. When using CT densitometry and CT washout techniques on suspected ACC, care must be taken to avoid necrotic components that can result in invalid results. Due to their hormonal production, a minority of ACC, particularly well-differentiated ones, can contain enough intracytoplasmic lipid to lose signal on chemical shift MRI. Thus, if an adrenal mass measuring greater than 5 cm loses signal on out-of-phase images one should remain suspicious for ACC, especially if the mass contains areas of necrosis, hemorrhage, and calcification. A study by

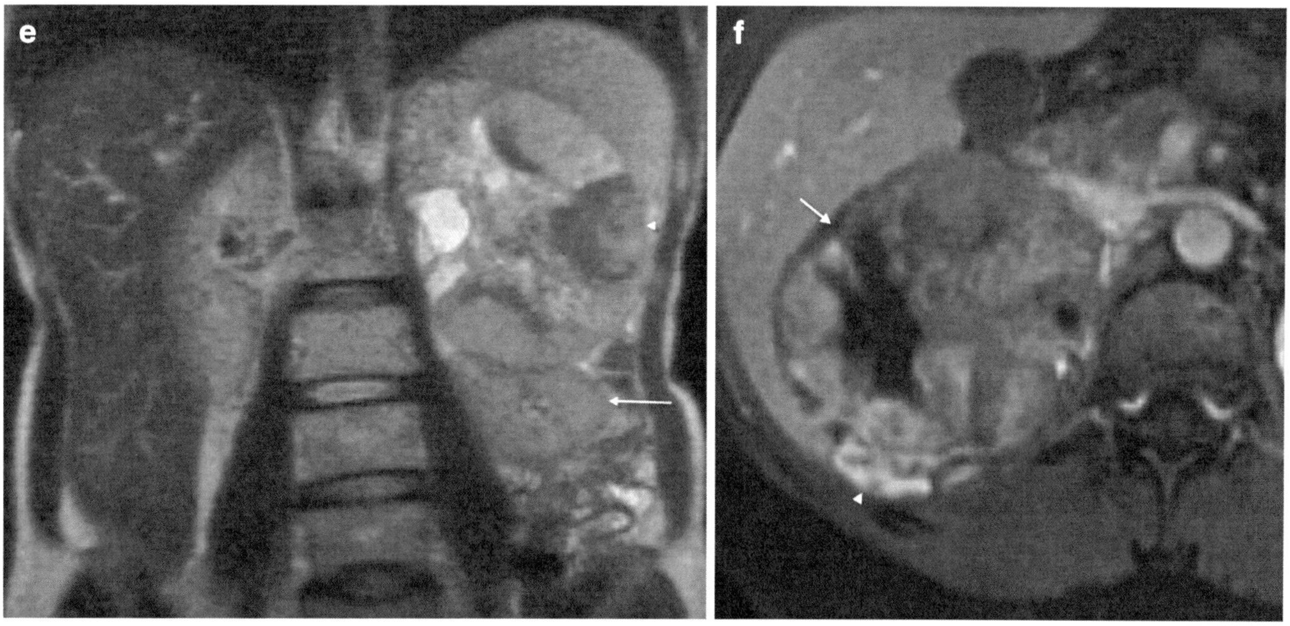

Fig. 5.22 (continued)

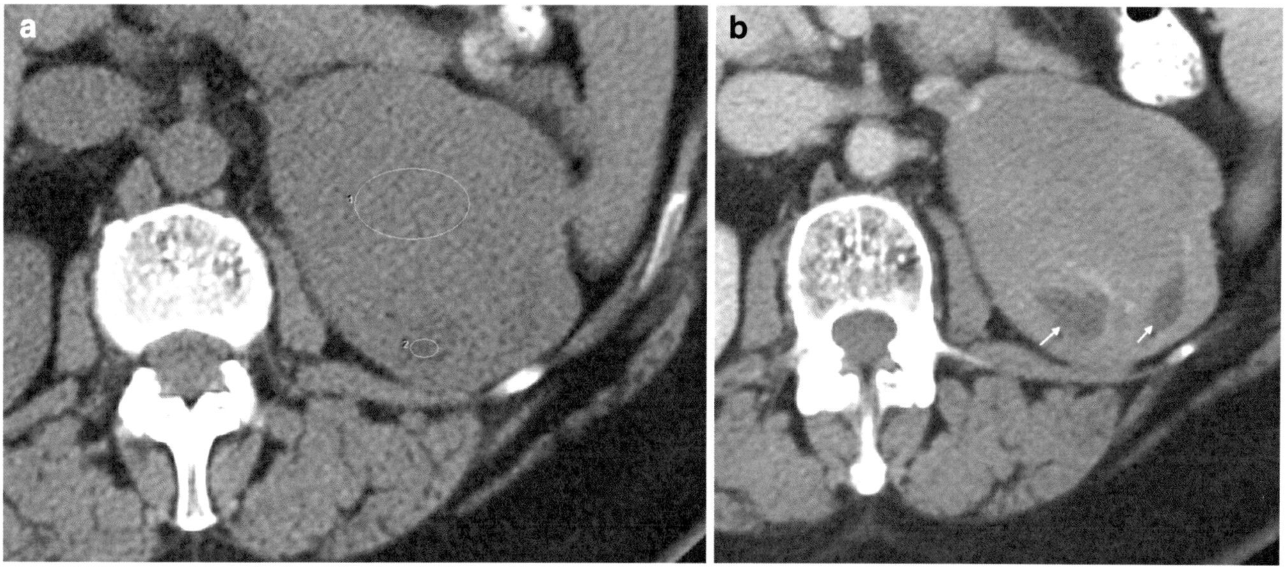

Fig. 5.23 Adrenal cortical carcinoma versus adenoma. (**a**) This NCCT performed in a 68-year-old woman with abdominal pain demonstrates an 8.5 cm left adrenal mass. The circular ROI #1 has an attenuation measurement of 31 HU (*not shown*). ROI #2 on a small focus of necrosis has a reading of 13 HU. (**b**) Contrast-enhanced images in the portal venous phase demonstrate that the mass is almost completely homogenous, except for small foci of low attenuation in the periphery (*arrows*). Fifteen-minute delayed images (*not shown*) demonstrate absolute washout value of less than 60 %, which is not consistent with an adenoma. A PET scan (*not shown*) demonstrated a maximum SUV of 2.3, which is borderline between a benign and a malignant lesion. This mass is very unusual in that it has features of both a benign (very homogenous) and malignant lesion (large size and lobulated border). Due to its large size, the mass was resected and pathology demonstrated a very low-grade malignancy, which focally invaded the adrenal capsule but demonstrated a complete absence of nuclear atypia. The patient has remained disease free for at least 2 years

Faria et al. [61] evaluating MR spectroscopy showed promising early results in distinguishing adenomas and pheochromocytomas from metastases and ACC with high sensitivity and specificity when using choline–creatinine and choline–lipid ratios [61]. Lesions that have grown over serial examinations, especially those which have grown rapidly, are also suspicious for malignancy. Rarely, adenomas and myelolipomas can increase in size slowly on serial examinations.

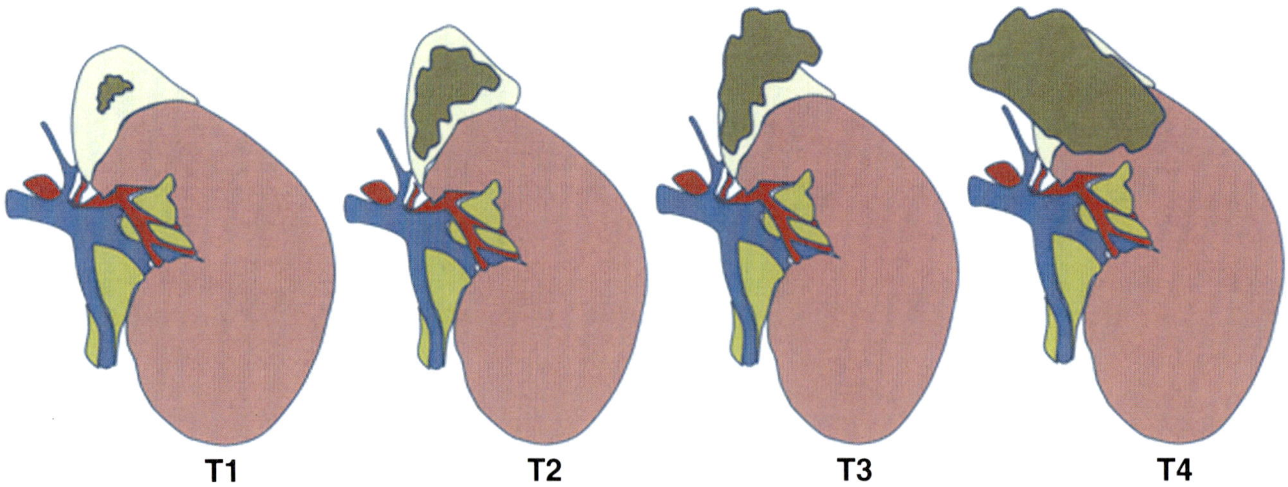

Fig. 5.24 Schematic representation of stages *T1–T4* ACC

Sudden hemorrhage into a benign lesion is an uncommon cause of rapid enlargement. On the other hand, lesions that have remained stable for at least 6 months are almost always benign, since untreated malignant adrenal tumors almost always grow within that time period [37]. Ultimately, percutaneous biopsy or adrenalectomy (open or laparoscopic) should be performed for lesions measuring greater than 6 cm if a specific diagnosis cannot be achieved with imaging [3]. Making the distinction between adenoma and ACC is critical because, if left untreated, the median survival of patients with ACC is 6 months. If detected early, however, they are potentially curable with resection [59].

The modified McFarlane system (*see* Table 5.3) is often used to stage ACC, as the American Joint Committee on Cancer and International Union Against Cancer does not have a formal staging system [36]. The European Network for the Study of Adrenal Tumors is similar to the modified McFarlane system but, in addition, includes venous invasion as Stage III disease.

CT and MR are the primary imaging modalities used to stage adrenal cancer. T1 and T2 tumors are distinguished by size only, the latter being greater than 5 cm. However, distinguishing T1 and T2 tumors from T3 tumors can be more challenging because adrenal capsular invasion can be difficult to assess radiologically. However, this distinction is not critical because T1,T2, and T3 lesions are all amenable to surgery in the absence of distant metastatic disease. The liver and the ipsilateral kidney are the organs most commonly invaded by ACC [28]. Preservation of fat planes around the tumor indicates that it has not invaded adjacent organs, indicating stage T3 or less. However, in patients with little retroperitoneal fat, this distinction can be difficult to make [16]. Left renal vein and IVC invasion are common with ACC, the latter is more often seen with right-sided tumors due to their proximity to the IVC (the right adrenal vein drains directly into the IVC, whereas the left adrenal vein drains directly into the left renal vein before draining into the IVC) [7]. MRI is superior to CT in delineating both the presence and extent of IVC invasion [3, 16]. In a review of the literature by Chiche [62], 51 % of patients with IVC invasion had tumor extension at least as far as the suprahepatic IVC, with some extending into the right atrium [62]. When ACCs become very large and invade the IVC, it can difficult to determine the origin of the tumor because renal carcinoma, hepatocellular carcinoma, and IVC leiomyosarcoma can also extend into the IVC [7].

Table 5.3 Staging of adrenal cancer [26]

T-stage			
T1	T2	T3	T4
Tumor <5 cm Confined within capsule	Tumor >5 cm Confined within capsule	Tumor extends beyond adrenal capsule (extends into surrounding fat)	Tumor invades adjacent organ/ kidney
Nodal Staging (N)			
N0: No positive lymph nodes			
N1: Positive lymph nodes			
Metastasis Staging (M)			
M0: No metastases			
M1: Metastases present			
The above stages can be grouped as follows [36]			
Stage grouping	T stage	N stage	M stage
I	T1	N0	M0
II	T2	N0	M0
III	T1	N1	M0
	T2	N1	M0
	T3	N0	M0
IV	Any T	Any N	M1
	T3	N1	M0
	T4	N1	M0

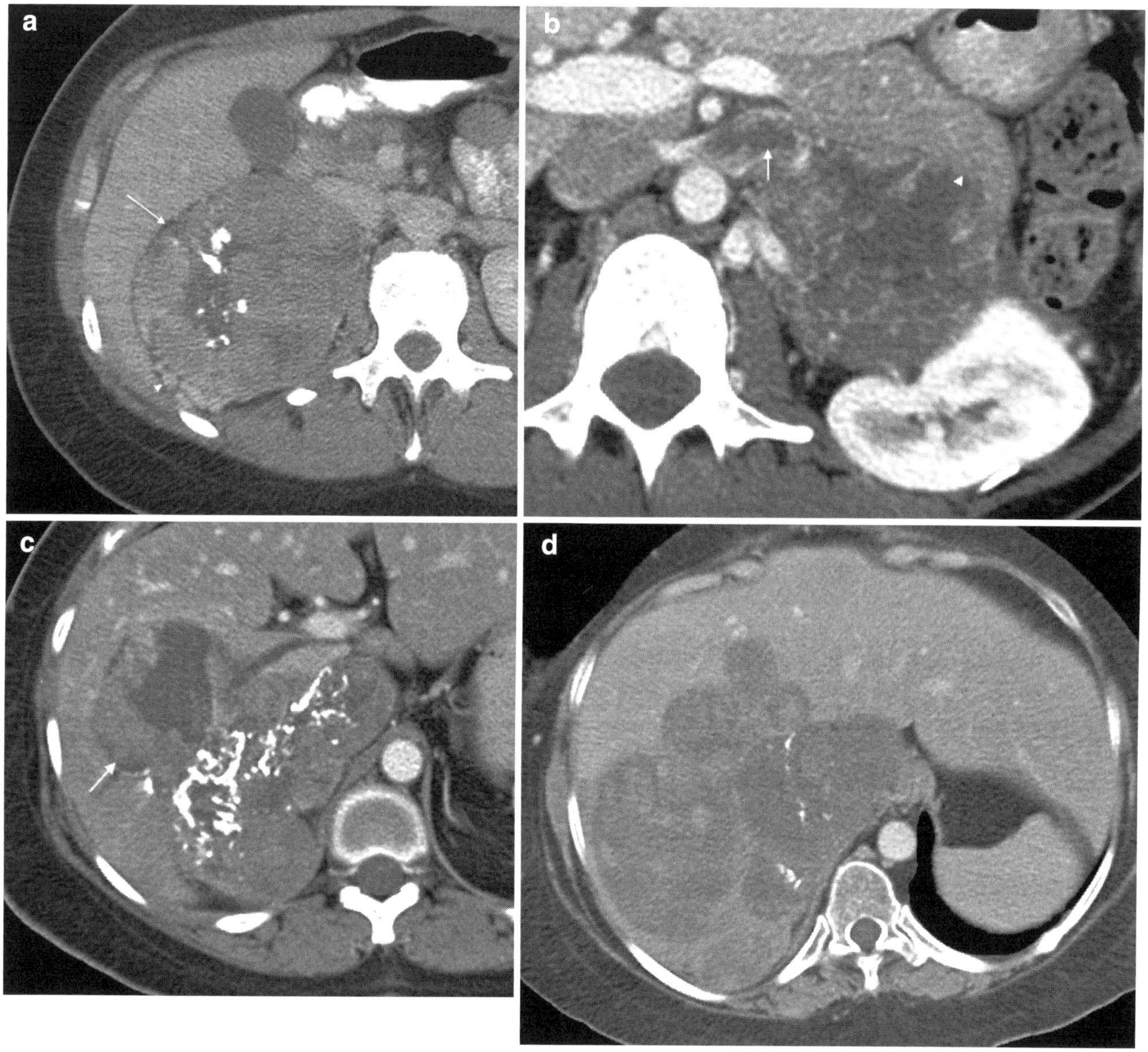

Fig. 5.25 T-staging of adrenal cortical carcinoma. (**a**) Contrast-enhanced CT scan in a 30-year-old woman (same patient as in Fig. 5.22f) demonstrates a 14 cm right adrenal mass with central calcifications and necrosis. Note the intact fat plane between the mass and the liver (*arrow*) indicating the absence of hepatic invasion. Prominent draining veins are also noted around the tumor (*arrowheads*). The mass was subsequently resected and the tumor proved to represent a T3 adrenal cortical carcinoma with negative surgical margins. The patient remained disease free for at least 5 years after surgery. (**b**) Contrast-enhanced CT in this 33-year-old woman who presented with abdominal pain demonstrates a 10 cm heterogeneously enhancing left adrenal mass consistent with ACC. Tumor invades the left renal vein (*arrow*) and displaces the left kidney posteriorly without invasion. Tumor also contacts the pancreatic tail (*arrowhead*), as well as the spleen and stomach more superiorly (*not shown*) without invasion. This tumor qualifies as a T3 lesion by virtue of renal vein invasion, but was not resected because the patient also had hepatic and pulmonary metastases at the time of presentation (M1), thus making this Stage IV disease (T3N0M1). (**c**) Contrast-enhanced CT in a 37-year-old woman with features of Cushing syndrome demonstrates a calcified right ACC that grossly invades the right hepatic lobe (*arrow*), consistent with T4 disease. (**d**) One year later, hepatic invasion has increased significantly. (**e**) This left-sided ACC in a 53-year-old man demonstrates gross splenic (*arrow*) and probable gastric wall invasion (*arrowhead*), consistent with T4 disease. Left renal and pancreatic tail invasion were also present (*not shown*). (**f**) Coronal CT image in a 42-year-old woman with partially imaged right-sided ACC (*short arrow*) demonstrates extensive tumor thrombus in the IVC extending to the junction with the right atrium (*long arrow*)

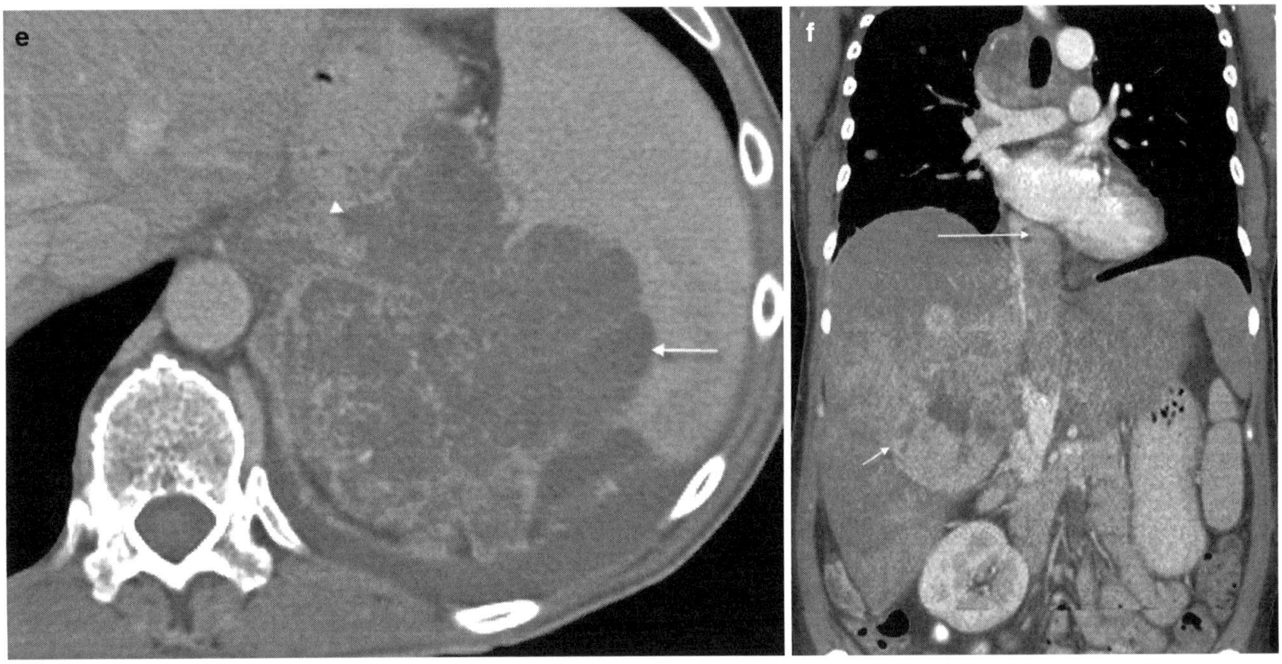

Fig. 5.25 (continued)

Treatment of Adrenal Cortical Carcinoma

There are three main treatment options in adrenocortical carcinoma: surgery, medical therapy, and radiotherapy. Radical adrenalectomy is the treatment of choice for localized ACC as this is the only option to achieve a long-term cure [28, 63]. Lymphadenectomy, in addition to adrenalectomy, has been shown to significantly reduce the risk of disease recurrence and disease-related death [64]. IVC invasion is not a contraindication to surgery provided that the tumor can be removed in its entirety both within the IVC and at its primary location [62]. Surgery can even be performed in some cases if the tumor extends into the right atrium. Tumor thrombus is usually well-encapsulated and can often be removed from the vein intact [16]. Identifying the exact level of IVC extension on imaging is critical for surgical planning as this defines the location where the surgeon must gain vascular control of the tumor for resection [3]. Occasionally, patients with Stage IV disease and IVC invasion may be candidates for palliative resection in order to improve symptoms from mass effect, to alleviate hormonal symptoms in functioning ACC, or to prevent tumor embolism [62]. Potential complications of adrenalectomy include infection, hematoma, pulmonary embolism, pneumothorax, adrenal insufficiency in patients with Cushing syndrome (because the opposite adrenal gland has been suppressed by the excess hormones), injury to the spleen and pancreas on the left-sided resections, and duodenum and liver on the right-sided resections. Despite the ease of recovery and reduced morbidity associated with laparoscopy, the value of the laparoscopic adrenalectomy as applied to ACC has been controversial for several years [65, 66]. However, more recent studies evaluating minimally invasive techniques have shown outcomes comparable to open surgery [65]. However, laparoscopic adrenalectomy is likely best reserved for experienced centers performing more than 20 procedures per year and in tumors smaller than 10 cm without invasive disease [63, 65].

In an adjuvant setting, postoperative radiotherapy can prevent local recurrence in the majority of patients and therefore has been proposed for use in the resection bed in high-risk patients. [67]. Palliative radiotherapy can be helpful in patients with symptomatic lesions (*e.g.*, bone metastases), with some response having been achieved in up to 57 % of patients [68].

For those cases not amenable to compete resection, medical therapy with mitotane is the preferred treatments, either alone or in combination with cytotoxic therapies. A partial response can be achieved in 25 % of cases although it is usually of a relatively short duration and complete responses are rare [69]. Work is currently being done to evaluate cytotoxic agents in combination with targeted therapies, with IGF-1 receptor inhibitors being of most interest.

There are no strict guidelines regarding imaging surveillance for patients with ACC following adrenalectomy, but CT, MRI, and PET/CT are the modalities of choice [16]. Among patients having undergone complete surgical resection, 35–85 % will eventually develop local tumor recurrence or distant metastatic disease [70, 71]. Local recurrence manifests as an enhancing nodule in the retroperitoneum anywhere within the surgical bed. The recurrent mass has similar imaging features as the original tumor, such as marked enhancement, except that the degree of necrosis is generally less than the original tumor because the recurrent tumor

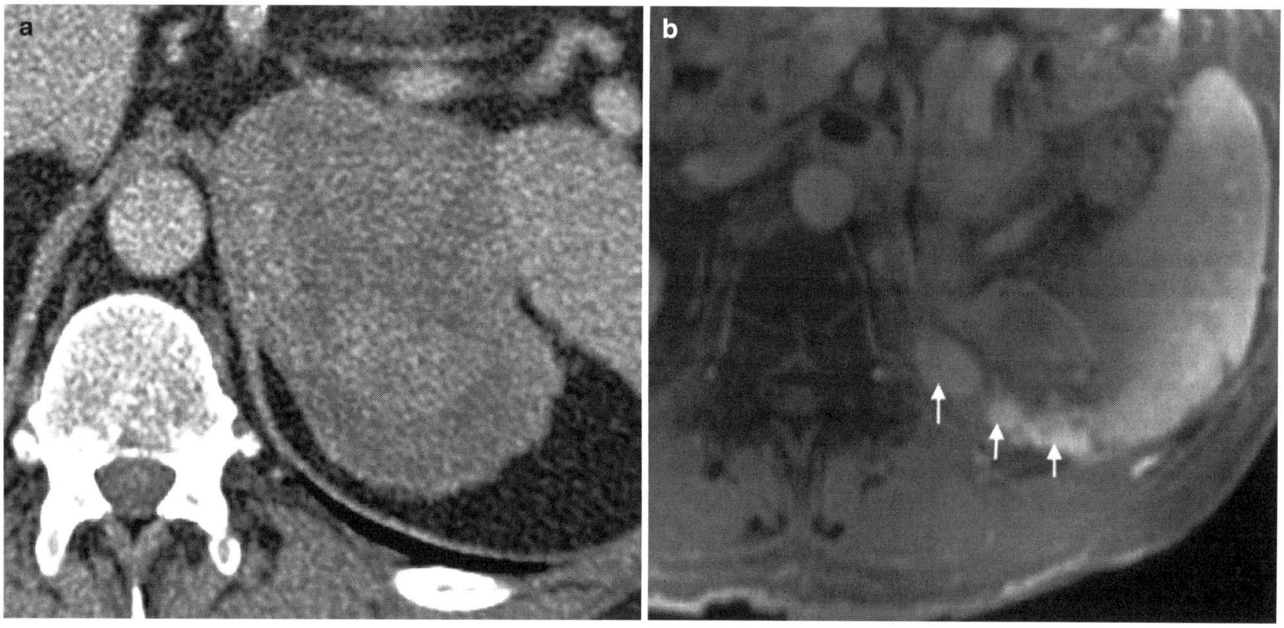

Fig. 5.26 Recurrent adrenal cortical carcinoma. (**a**) This contrast-enhanced CT in a 65-year-old man demonstrates an 11 cm left adrenal mass consistent with ACC. The lesion broadly contacts the spleen but there is a smooth interface between these structures indicating that there is probably no gross invasion. Pathology confirmed a T3 high-grade adrenocortical carcinoma with positive surgical margins medially. (**b**) MRI performed 5 months after resection demonstrates three hypervascular nodules in the resection bed (*vertical arrows*) consistent with local tumor recurrence

nodules are generally small when first discovered. The overall 5-year survival rate for patients with ACC is 38 %. When Stage I and II disease is treated aggressively with surgery, this rate is approximately 65 %, but falls to 40 % with Stage III disease and 10 % with Stage IV disease [16].

The liver is the most common site of metastatic disease in ACC (48–96 % in various series) [7, 16]. The hepatic metastases are usually hypervascular and are often best seen on arterial phase images [16]. Other common sites of metastatic disease are the lungs (45–97 %), regional/paraortic lymph nodes (25–46 %), and bone (11–33 %) [16]. Patients frequently have radiologic evidence of metastatic disease at presentation.

Lymphoma

Primary adrenal lymphoma is extremely rare with only 70 cases having been reported in the English medical literature [72]. Secondary involvement of the adrenal glands is more frequent with a reported incidence of 1–4 % in patients with non-Hodgkin lymphoma (NHL) involving other sites [37]. NHL is more likely to involve extralymphatic sites than Hodgkin lymphoma, and thus, involves the adrenal gland more often [73]. Bilateral involvement of the adrenal glands is seen in approximately 50 % of cases and occasionally may cause adrenal insufficiency due to extensive replacement of normal adrenal tissue [24, 31, 74]. On CT, early in the course of the disease, the adrenal glands may appear normal or diffusely thickened while maintaining their adeniform shape, often mimicking hyperplasia [28, 37]. As the disease progresses, the adrenal glands become more nodular in appearance, eventually becoming discrete, rounded, homogenous, well-circumscribed masses [3, 28, 31]. Other evidence of retroperitoneal disease, including adenopathy, is frequently present. In some cases of lymphomas, the adrenal glands may become engulfed by extensive retroperitoneal adenopathy [3]. The enhancement pattern of lymphoma on CT is classically homogenous and less than that of the aorta and IVC [3]. On MRI, adrenal lymphoma is typically heterogeneously low in signal on T1WI, and heterogeneously high in signal on T2WI, while showing minimal progressive enhancement after the administration of gadolinium [3, 24, 37]. PET/CT can be useful in distinguishing lymphoma from other adrenal tumors and hyperplasia because the FDG-avidity of the adrenal lymphoma should parallel that of lymphoma elsewhere in the body [37]. Likewise, if extraadrenal sites of lymphoma demonstrate decreased FDG uptake due to treatment response, the adrenal activity should decrease in parallel fashion [37]. Thus, PET may be a valuable noninvasive imaging method for diagnosis, staging, and evaluation of treatment response in patients with adrenal lymphoma [72]. In summary, the presence of a nonadenomatous adrenal mass in a patient with known NHL should be regarded as suspicious for lymphoma [73]. Only if the adrenal mass differs in its imaging appearance from tumor at other known sites of disease or does not show a similar response to treatment as disease at other sites should an alternative diagnosis be suspected [73].

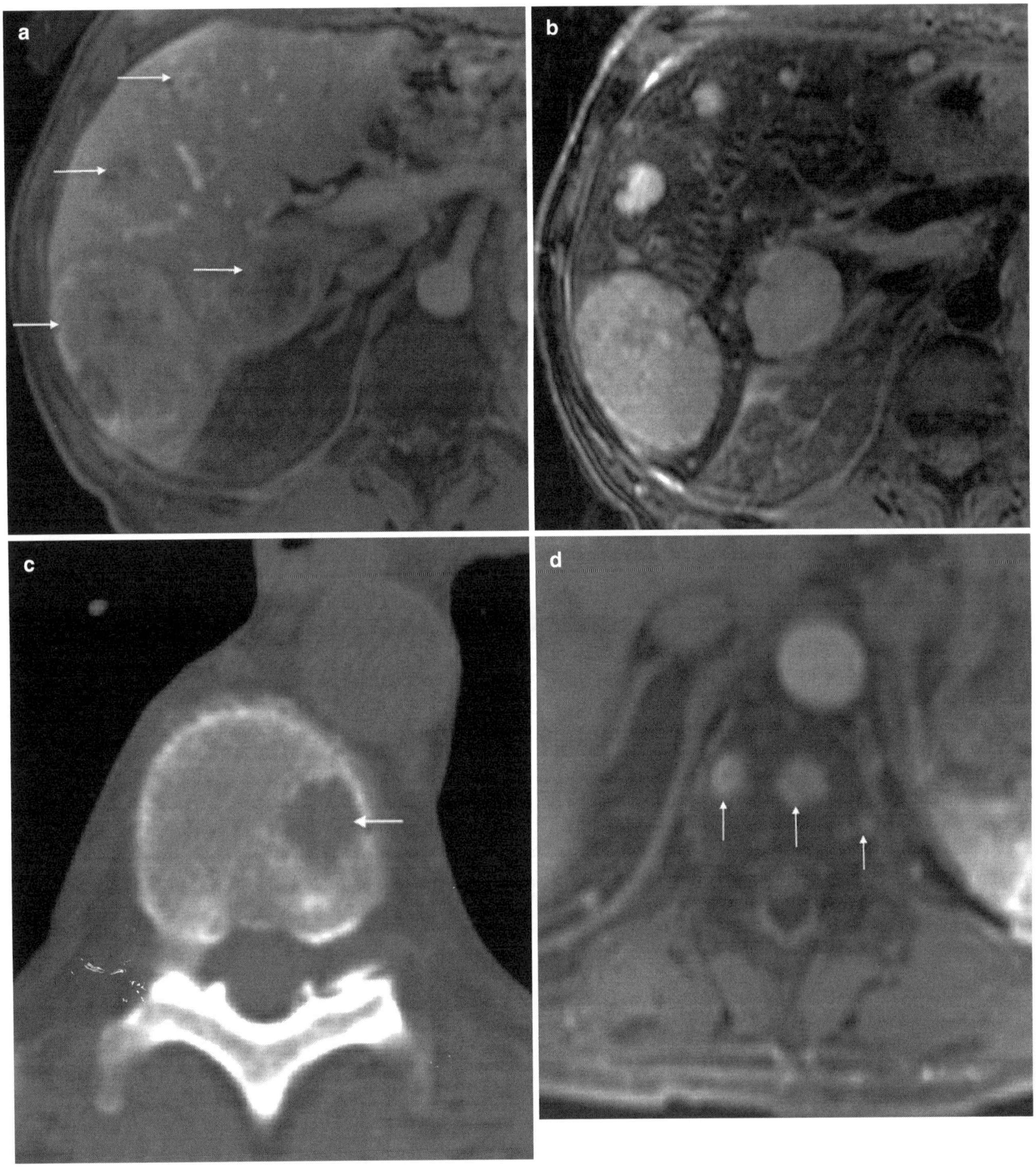

Fig. 5.27 Metastatic adrenal cortical carcinoma. (**a**) This post-contrast T1WI in the arterial phase (same patient as Fig. 5.26) demonstrates multiple hypervascular hepatic masses (*arrows*) consistent with metastatic ACC. (**b**) Corresponding T2WI with fat saturation demonstrates that the masses are T2 hyperintense. (**c**) Chest CT in same patient demonstrates a lytic lesion (*arrow*) in the T10 vertebral body consistent with metastatic disease. (**d**) Arterial phase T1WI with fat saturation through T12 vertebra in same patient demonstrates multiple small enhancing lesions (*arrows*) consistent with bone metastases. (**e**) T1WI from a lumbar spine MR in same patient demonstrates a low T1 signal metastasis (*arrow*) involving the first and second sacral segments. (**f**) Chest CT with lung windows in this 42-year-old man with ACC demonstrates extensive bilateral pulmonary metastases. (**g**) Soft tissue windows at a different level demonstrate mediastinal and bilateral hilar nodal metastases (*arrows*) in addition to the lung metastases. (**h**) This 57-year-old man had a 15 cm left ACC resected 1 year earlier. This image demonstrates a normal right hepatic lobe. (**i**) 6 months later, a 9.5 cm centrally necrotic mass with irregular peripheral enhancement has developed, consistent with metastatic disease

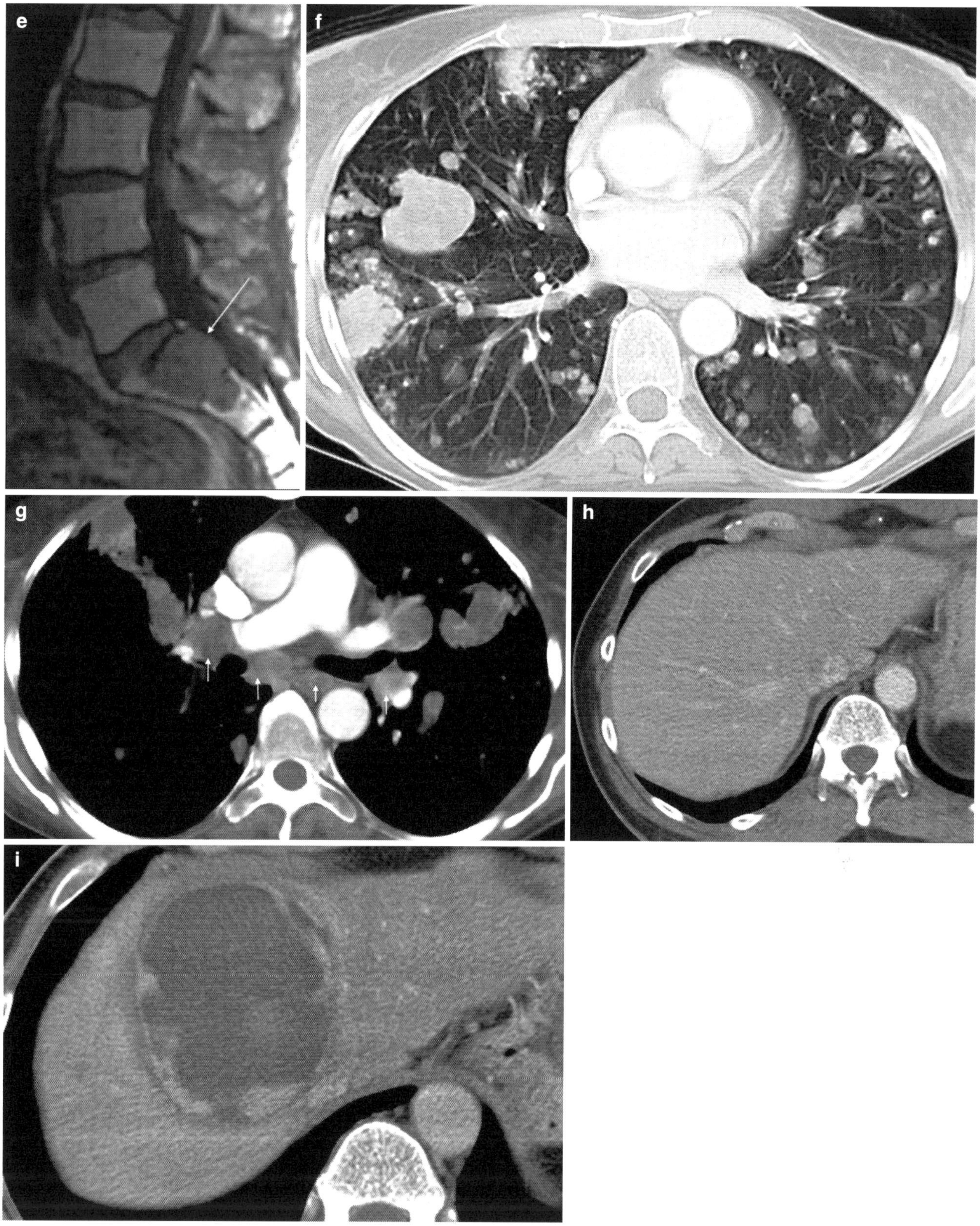

Fig. 5.27 (continued)

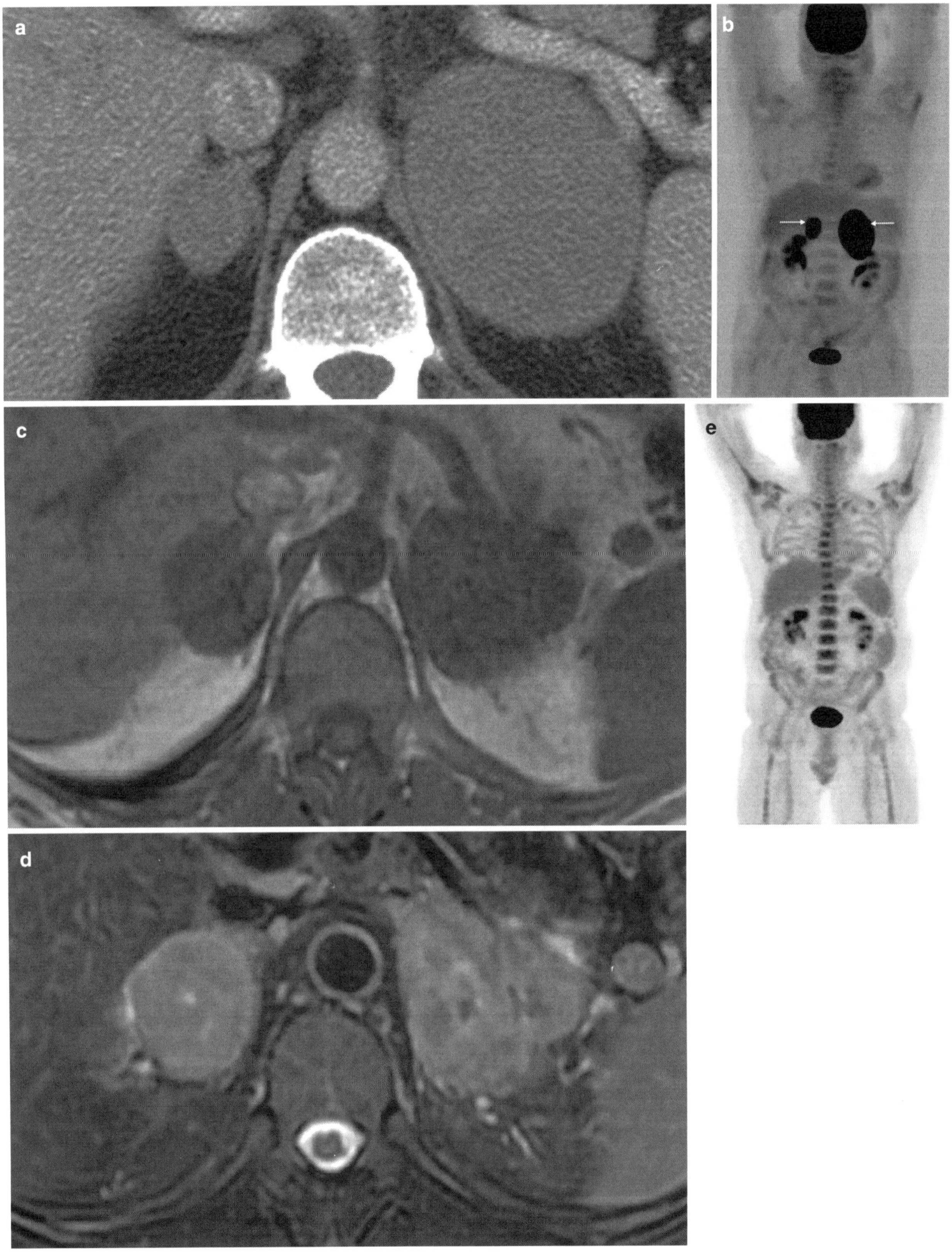

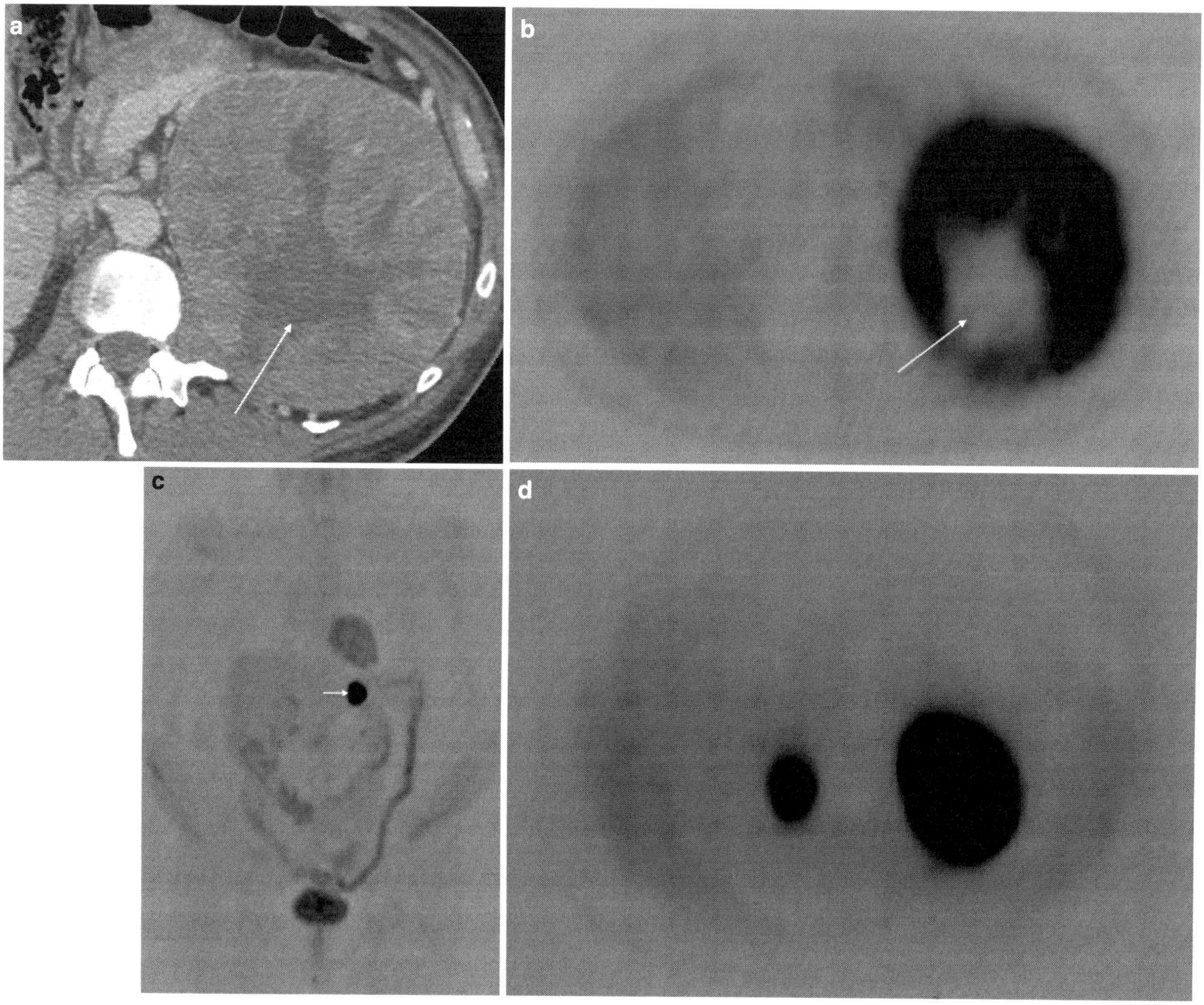

Fig. 5.29 Accuracy of PET-CT in distinguishing benign from malignant adrenal masses. (**a**) This CT scan in a patient with adrenocortical carcinoma demonstrates a 16 cm left adrenal mass with central necrosis (*arrow*). (**b**) PET image at the same level demonstrates that the mass is markedly FDG avid (SUV, 15.7) except for the central area (*arrow*) that corresponds to the region of necrosis on the corresponding CT. (**c**) This PET scan from the same patient as Fig. 5.20E with lung cancer demonstrates marked FDG avidity (SUV, 30) in the left adrenal gland (*arrow*) consistent with metastatic disease. (**d**) This PET scan from the same patient as Fig. 5.28 with bilateral adrenal lymphoma demonstrates marked FDG uptake in both adrenal glands (SUV up to 31) consistent with malignancy

Fig. 5.28 Adrenal lymphoma. (**a**) This contrast-enhanced CT scan was performed on a 63-year-old man with a history of rectal cancer that was treated 12 years earlier. The image demonstrates bilateral adrenal masses measuring 8 cm on the left and 3 cm on the right. The masses demonstrate mild, homogenous enhancement (60 HU post-contrast, 40 HU pre-contrast [*not shown*]). Metastatic rectal cancer was thought to be unlikely given the lack of metastatic disease elsewhere for the past 12 years. In addition, the striking homogeneity of these masses would be atypical for metastases of that size. (**b**) This maximum-intensity projection (MIP) from a PET scan demonstrates extremely intense activity in bilateral suprarenal masses (*arrows*; SUV of 31 on the left). No other abnormal activity is seen. (**c**) This T1 in-phase MR image acquired 3 weeks after the CT in (**a**) demonstrates bilateral low signal adrenal masses. (**d**) Corresponding T2WI demonstrates slightly heterogenous, intermediate to high signal bilateral adrenal masses. Subsequent biopsy demonstrated diffuse large B-cell lymphoma. (**e**) PET scan performed 1 month after initiation of chemotherapy demonstrates no residual abnormal uptake in either adrenal gland consistent with treatment response. CT images from same examination (*not shown*), demonstrated marked reduction in the size of the masses

PET-CT Evaluation of Adrenal Tumors

Due to the increased metabolic activity of malignant adrenal lesions, 18 F FDG is retained intracellularly and therefore demonstrates increased uptake on PET. This increased uptake can be evaluated qualitatively by visual assessment or quantitatively by measurement of the maximum SUV. An adrenal lesion is generally considered malignant if FDG uptake is greater than that of the liver (normal SUV, 1.5–2). However, physiologic adrenal uptake can vary, with SUVs ranging from 0.95 to 2.46, thus overlapping to some extent with malignant lesions [74]. However, using an SUV of 3.1 to distinguish benign from malignant lesions, Mester et al. [75] reported PET/CT to have sensitivity of 99 % and specificity of 92 % in a study analyzing 175 adrenal masses. A recent meta-analysis of 21 studies involving 1,391 adrenal lesions in 1,217 patients showed that malignancy could be on PET imaging with a sensitivity of 97 % and specificity of 91 % and that there was no significant difference in accuracy between visual assessment and quantitative methods using SUV values or standardized uptake ratio [76]. Studies that combined PET/CT with other CT methods—including CT densitometry, CT histogram analysis (an analysis of individual pixel attenuation which has been used in some studies to identify adenomas), and CT washout techniques—demonstrated higher sensitivities and specificities than studies using PET/CT alone [77, 78]. However, FDG PET cannot differentiate between the different types of malignant adrenal lesions, including metastases, ACC, lymphoma, and malignant pheochromocytoma, all of which can have similar SUV values. False-negative results can be found in malignant lesions that contain large areas of necrosis or hemorrhage, and thus, do not take up sufficient FDG. Malignant lesions which have undergone successful therapy typically show reduced FDG uptake as well, and it is this phenomenon that renders PET/CT useful for monitoring treatment response. In addition, certain types of metastases characteristically have very low FDG avidity, the most notable of which are bronchoalveolar carcinoma (well-differentiated adenocarcinoma of the lung) and carcinoid tumors, leading to false-negative results on PET/CT [79]. False-positive rates of up to 5 % have been reported in adrenal lesions (benign lesions with increased FDG uptake). Possible causes include granulomatous diseases such as sarcoidosis and tuberculosis, endothelial cysts, adrenal cortical hyperplasia and a small percentage of adrenal adenomas [80]. FDG uptake in adrenal adenomas does correlate with the degree of lipid content (both lipid-rich and lipid-poor adenomas can show increased uptake) [76].

In addition to its complementary role in distinguishing benign from malignant lesions, PET/CT plays a valuable role in staging and monitoring disease status in patients with ACC because it is sensitive in identifying sites of metastatic disease [37]. PET/CT is extremely valuable for monitoring patients with adrenal lymphoma because FDG uptake is usually quite high in untreated disease, whereas SUV values typically decrease significantly following successful therapy, demonstrating good correlation with treatment response. However, there are certain subtypes of lymphoma, including marginal zone, peripheral T-cell, and low-grade lymphomas, which demonstrate variable FDG uptake that can often be quite low; PET/CT less useful in these patients [37].

Other Rare Adrenal Neoplasms

Other very rare adrenal neoplasms in adults include hemangioma, schwannoma, and mature teratoma in the benign category and primary sarcoma and primary melanoma in the malignant category. Hemangiomas are usually of the cavernous type, can be very large and frequently contain calcifications [28]. Contrast-enhanced CT and MRI may demonstrate peripheral pooling of contrast material that persists on delayed images similar to hemangiomas in other organs. These lesions are hyperintense on T2WI [28]. Schwannoma, a type of benign peripheral nerve sheath tumor representing 5 % of retroperitoneal tumors, can occasionally mimic adrenal tumors when they arise in the periadrenal region. However, primary adrenal schwannomas are exceedingly rare, with only a few cases having been reported in the literature [40]. Teratomas most commonly arise from the gonads but can also occur in many other locations throughout the body, almost all of which are in the midline. Only a few cases of adrenal teratomas have been reported. On imaging these lesions demonstrate various tissue components arising from ectoderm, mesoderm, and endoderm, including fat, fluid, soft tissue, and calcifications [40]. Of the few reported cases of adrenal sarcoma, most have been angiosarcomas and leiomyosarcomas [81]. The expected appearance of adrenal sarcoma is one of a large mass with heterogenous enhancement and prominent areas of necrosis. The primary diagnostic difficulty is in distinguishing the exceedingly rare primary adrenal sarcoma from a much more common retroperitoneal sarcoma that secondarily involves the adrenal gland [81]. Melanoma is one of the most common tumors to metastasize to the adrenal glands, but primary adrenal melanoma is extremely rare; however, melanoma can arise from neuroectodermal cells in the adrenal medulla (chromaffin cells and melanocytes have a common embryogenesis) [81] with imaging features identical to that of melanomas elsewhere, which can include hemorrhage, necrosis, and the presence of melanin, which is high in T1 signal on MR. The diagnosis of primary adrenal melanoma can only be made if there is no prior history of cutaneous, mucosal, or ocular melanoma; the adrenal mass contains melanin; is unilateral; and is the only site of disease detected at autopsy [81]. One final rare lesion of note is a "collision tumor," which is defined as two independently coexisting neoplasms in the same organ without significant admixture of the tissues from each tumor [81]. Some of the more commonly encountered collision tumors include an adrenal metastasis next to a preexisting adenoma and an adenoma and myelolipoma in the same adrenal gland. Imaging of an adrenal collision tumor demonstrates features of both tumors, juxtaposed to each other. For example, in a patient with a coexisting lipid-rich adrenal adenoma and metastasis, the adenoma will demonstrate signal loss on the opposed phase images, whereas the metastatic component will not [82].

References

1. Bovio S, Cataldi A, Reimondo G, et al. Prevalence of adrenal incidentaloma in a contemporary computerized tomography series. Endocrinol Invest. 2006;29:298–302.
2. Mansmann G, Lau J, Blak E, et al. The clinically inapparent adrenal mass: update in diagnosis and treatment. Endocr Rev. 2004; 25:309–40.
3. Dunnick NR, Korobkin M. Imaging of adrenal incidentalomas. AJR Am J Roentgenol. 2002;179:559–68.
4. Young Jr WF. The incidentally discovered adrenal mass. N Engl J Med. 2007;356:601–10.
5. Kloos RT, Gross MD, Francis IR, et al. Incidentally discovered adrenal masses. Endocr Rev. 1995;16:460–84.
6. Young Jr WF. Management approaches to adrenal incidentalomas: a view from Rochester, Minnesota. Endocrinol Metab Clin North Am. 2000;29:159–85.
7. Johnson PT, Horton KM, Fishman EK. Adrenal mass imaging with multidetector CT: pathologic conditions, pearls and pitfalls. Radiographics. 2009;29:1333–51.
8. Bülow B, Ahrén B. Swedish research council study group of endocrine abdominal tumours. Adrenal incidentaloma—experience of a standardized diagnostic programme in the Swedish prospective study. J Intern Med. 2002;252:239–46.
9. Caplan RH, Strutt PJ, Wickus GG. Subclinical hormone secretion by incidentally discovered adrenal masses. Arch Surg. 1994;129:291–6.
10. Reincke M, Nieke J, Krestin GP, et al. Preclinical Cushing's syndrome in adrenal "incidentalomas": comparison with adrenal Cushing's syndrome. J Clin Endocrinol Metab. 1992;75:826–32.
11. Bernini GP, Vivaldi MS, Argenio GF, et al. Frequency of pheochromocytoma in adrenal incidentalomas and utility of the glucagon test for the diagnosis. J Endocrinol Invest. 1997;20:65–71.
12. Mannelli M, Colagrande S, Valeri A, Parent G. Incidental and metastatic adrenal masses. Semin Oncol. 2010;37:649–61.
13. Wooten MD, King DK. Adrenal cortical carcinoma: epidemiology and treatment with mitotane and a review of the literature. Cancer. 1993;72:3145–55.
14. Nader S, Hickey RC, Sellin RV, Samaan NA. Adrenal cortical carcinoma: a study of 77 cases. Cancer. 1983;52:707–11.
15. Luton JP, Cerdas S, Billaud L, et al. Clinical features of adrenocortical carcinoma, prognostic factors, and the effect of mitotane therapy. N Engl J Med. 1990;322:1195–201.
16. Bharwani N, Rockall A, Sahdev A, et al. Adrenocortical carcinoma: the range of appearances on CT and MRI. AJR Am J Roentgenol. 2011;196:W706–14.
17. Willatt JM, Francis IR. Radiologic evaluation of incidentally discovered adrenal masses. Am Fam Physician. 2010;81:1361–6.
18. Patnaik MM, Deshpande AK. Diagnosis: Addison's disease secondary to tuberculosis of the adrenal glands. Clin Med Res. 2008;6:29.
19. Frilling A, Tecklenborg K, Weber F, et al. Importance of adrenal incidentaloma in patients with a history of malignancy. Surgery. 2004;136:1289–96.
20. Song JH, Chaudhry FS, Mayo-Smith WW. The incidental adrenal mass on CT: prevalence of adrenal disease in 1,049 consecutive adrenal masses in patients with no known malignancy. AJR Am J Roentgenol. 2008;190:1163–8.
21. Bernardino ME, Walther MM, Phillips VM, et al. CT-guided adrenal biopsy: accuracy, safety, and indications. AJR Am J Roentgenol. 1985;144:67–9.
22. Francis IR, Smid A, Gross MD, et al. Adrenal masses in oncologic patients: functional and morphologic evaluation. Radiology. 1988;166:353–6.
23. McGahan JP. Adrenal gland: MR imaging. Radiology. 1988;166: 284–5.
24. Elsayes KM, Mukundan G, Narra VR, et al. Adrenal masses: MR imaging features with pathologic correlation. Radiographics. 2004;24:S73–86.
25. Zornoza J, Bracken R, Wallace S. Radiologic features of adrenal metastases. Urology. 1976;8:295–9.
26. Dighe M, Francis IR, Casalino DD, et al. ACR appropriateness criteria on obstructive voiding symptoms secondary to prostate disease. J Am Coll Radiol. 2010;7:255–9.
27. Hedican SP, Marshall FF. Adrenocortical carcinoma with intracaval extension. J Urol. 1997;158:2056–61.
28. Krebs TL, Wagner BJ. MR imaging of adrenal gland: radiologic pathologic correlation. Radiographics. 1998;18:1425–40.
29. Wilms G, Baert A, Marchal G, Goddeeris P. Computed tomography of the normal adrenal glands: correlative study with autopsy specimens. J Comput Assist Tomogr. 1979;3:467–9.
30. Johnson PT, Horton KM, Fishman EK. Adrenal imaging with MDCT: nonneoplastic disease. AJR Am J Roentgenol. 2009;193:1128–35.
31. Lee MJ, Hahn PF, Papanicolaou N, et al. Benign and malignant adrenal masses: CT distinction with attenuation coefficients, size, and observer analysis. Radiology. 1991;179:415–8.
32. Boland GW, Lee MJ, Gazelle GS, et al. Characterization of adrenal masses using unenhanced CT: an analysis of the CT literature. AJR Am J Roentgenol. 1998;171:201–4.
33. Boland GW, Blake MA, Hahn PF, Mayo-Smith WW. Incidental adrenal lesions: principles, techniques and algorithms for imaging characterization. Radiology. 2008;249:756–75.
34. Haider MA, Ghai S, Jhaveri K, Lockwood G. Chemical shift MR imaging of hyperattenuating (> 10 HU) adrenal masses: does it still have a role? Radiology. 2004;231:711–6.
35. Mayo-Smith WW, Boland GW, Noto RB, Lee MJ. State-of-the-art adrenal imaging. Radiographics. 2001;21:995–1012.
36. Hricak H, Husband J, Panicek DM. Oncologic imaging: essentials of reporting common cancers. Philadelphia: Saunders/Elsevier; 2007.
37. Blake MA, Cronin CG, Boland GW. Adrenal imaging. AJR Am J Roentgenol. 2010;194:1450–60.
38. Caoili EM, Korobkin M, Francis IR, et al. Delayed enhanced CT of lipid-poor adrenal adenomas. AJR Am J Roentgenol. 2000;175: 1411–5.
39. Park BK, Kim CK, Kim B, Lee JH. Comparison of delayed enhanced CT and chemical shift MR for evaluating hyperattenuating incidental adrenal masses. Radiology. 2007;243:760–5.
40. Guo YK, Yang ZG, Li Y, et al. Uncommon adrenal masses: CT and MRI features with histopathologic correlation. Eur J Radiol. 2007;62:359–70.
41. Kawashima A, Sandler CM, Ernst RD. Imaging of nontraumatic hemorrhage of the adrenal gland. Radiographics. 1999;19:949–63.
42. Welander J, Söderkvist P, Gimm O. Genetics and clinical characteristics of hereditary pheochromocytomas and paragangliomas. Endocr Relat Cancer. 2011;18:R253–76.
43. Carney JA. Gastric stromal sarcoma, pulmonary chondroma, and extra-adrenal paraganglioma (Carney triad): natural history, adrenocortical component, and possible familial occurrence. Mayo Clin Proc. 1999;74:543–52.

44. Yun M, Kim W, Alnafisi N, et al. 18 F-FDG PET in characterizing adrenal lesions detected on CT or MRI. J Nucl Med. 2001;42: 1795–9.
45. Shulkin BL, Thompson NW, Shapiro B, et al. Pheochromocytomas: imaging with 2-[fluorine-18]fluoro-2-deoxy-D-glucose PET. Radiology. 1999;212:35–41.
46. Wong KK, Arabi M, Bou-Assaly W, et al. Evaluation of incidentally discovered adrenal masses with PET and PET/CT. Eur J Radiol. 2012;81:441–50.
47. Gross MD, Gauger PG, Djekidel M, Rubello D. The role of PET in the surgical approach to adrenal disease. Eur J Surg Oncol. 2009;35:1137–45.
48. Imani F, Agopian VG, Auerbach MS, et al. 18 F-FDOPA PET and PET/CT accurately localize pheochromocytomas. J Nucl Med. 2009;50:513–9.
49. Win Z, Al-Nahhas A, Towey D, et al. 68 Ga-DOTATATE PET in neuroectodermal tumours: first experience. Nucl Med Commun. 2007;28:359–63.
50. Naji M, Zhao C, Welsh SJ, et al. 68 Ga-DOTA-TATE PET vs. 123I-MIBG in identifying malignant neural crest tumours. Mol Imaging Biol. 2011;13:769–75.
51. Sohaib SA, Hanson JA, Newell-Price JD, et al. CT appearance of the adrenal glands in adrenocorticotrophic hormone-dependent Cushing's syndrome. AJR Am J Roentgenol. 1999;172:997–1002.
52. Rozenblit A, Morehouse HT, Amis ES. Cystic adrenal lesions: CT features. Radiology. 1996;201:541–8.
53. Asbeshouse GA, Goldstein RB, Asbeshouse BS. Adrenal cysts: review of literature and report of three cases. J Urol. 1959;81: 711–9.
54. Peppercorn PD, Reznek RH. State-of-the-art CT and MRI of the adrenal gland. Eur Radiol. 1997;7:822–36.
55. Burks DW, Mirvis SE, Shanmuganathan K. Acute adrenal injury after blunt abdominal trauma: CT findings. AJR Am J Roentgenol. 1992;158:503–7.
56. Swift DL, Lingeman JE, Baum WC. Spontaneous retroperitoneal hemorrhage: a diagnostic challenge. J Urol. 1980;123:577–82.
57. Abrams HL, Spiro R, Goldstein N. Metastases in carcinoma: analysis of 1000 autopsied cases. Cancer. 1950;3:74–85.
58. Tsushima Y, Takahashi-Taketomi A, Endo K. Diagnostic utility of diffusion-weighted MR imaging and apparent diffusion coefficient value for the diagnosis of adrenal tumors. J Magn Reson Imaging. 2009;29:112–7.
59. Fishman EK, Deutch BM, Hartman DS, et al. Primary adrenocortical carcinoma: CT evaluation with clinical correlation. AJR Am J Roentgenol. 1987;148:531–5.
60. Hussain S, Belldegrun A, Seltzer SE, et al. Differentiation of malignant from benign adrenal masses: predictive indices on computed tomography. AJR Am J Roentgenol. 1985;144:61–5.
61. Faria JF, Goldman SM, Szejnfeld J, et al. Adrenal masses: characterization with in vivo proton MR spectroscopy–initial experience. Radiology. 2007;245:788–97.
62. Chiche L, Dousset B, Kieffer E, Chapuis Y. Adreno-cortical carcinoma extending into the inferior vena cava: presentation of a 15-patient series and review of the literature. Surgery. 2006;139: 15–27.
63. Zini L, Porpiglia F, Fassnacht M. Contemporary management of adrenocortical carcinoma. Eur Urol. 2011;60:1055–65.
64. Reibetanz J, Jurowich C, Erdogan I, et al. Impact of lymphadenectomy on the oncologic outcome of patients with adrenocortical carcinoma. Ann Surg. 2012;255:363–9.
65. Porpiglia F, Fiori C, Daffara F, et al. Retrospective evaluation of the outcome of open versus laparoscopic adrenalectomy for stage I and II adrenocortical cancer. Eur Urol. 2010;57: 873–8.
66. Porpiglia F, Miller BS, Manfredi M, et al. A debate on laparoscopic versus open adrenalectomy for adrenocortical carcinoma. Horm Cancer. 2011;2:372–7.
67. Fassnacht M, Hahner S, Polat B, et al. Efficacy of adjuvant radiotherapy of the tumor bed on local recurrence of adrenocortical carcinoma. J Clin Endocrinol Metab. 2006;91:4501–4.
68. Polat B, Fassnacht M, Pfreundner L, et al. Radiotherapy in adrenocortical carcinoma. Cancer. 2009;115:2816–23.
69. Hahner S, Fassnacht M. Mitotane for adrenocortical carcinoma treatment. Curr Opin Investig Drugs. 2005;6:386–94.
70. Ng L, Libertino JM. Adrenocortical carcinoma: diagnosis, evaluation and treatment. J Urol. 2003;169:5–11.
71. Pommier RF, Brennan MF. Management of adrenal neoplasms. Curr Probl Surg. 1991;28:657–739.
72. Paes FM, Kalkanis DG, Sideras PA, Serafini AN. FDG PET/CT of extranodal involvement in non-Hodgkin lymphoma and Hodgkin disease. Radiographics. 2010;30:269–91.
73. Paling MR, Willimason BRJ. Adrenal involvement in non-hodgkins lymphoma. AJR Am J Roentgenol. 1983;141:303–5.
74. Mester U, Goor O, Lerman H, et al. PET–CT of extranodal lymphoma. AJR Am J Roentgenol. 2004;182:1579–86.
75. Blake MA, Prakash P, Cronin CG. PET/CT for adrenal assessment. AJR Am J Roentgenol. 2010;195:W91–5.
76. Mester U, Miller E, Lerman H, et al. 18 F-FDG PET/CT in the evaluation of adrenal masses. J Nucl Med. 2006;47: 32–7.
77. Boland GW, Dwamena BA, Jagtiani Sangwaiya M, et al. Characterization of adrenal masses by using FDG PET: a systematic review and meta-analysis of diagnostic test performance. Radiology. 2011;259:117–26.
78. Blake MA, Slattery JM, Kalra MK, et al. Adrenal lesions: characterization with fused PET/CT image in patients with proved or suspected malignancy—initial experience. Radiology. 2006;238:970–7.
79. Perri M, Erba P, Volterrani D, et al. Adrenal masses in patients with cancer: PET/CT characterization with combined CT histogram and standardized uptake value PET analysis. AJR Am J Roentgenol. 2011;197:209–16.
80. Chong S, Lee KS, Kim HY, et al. Integrated PET-CT for the characterization of adrenal gland lesions in cancer patients: diagnostic efficacy and interpretation pitfalls. Radiographics. 2006;26:1811–24.
81. Otal P, Escourrou G, Mazerolles C, et al. Imaging features of uncommon adrenal masses with histopathologic correlation. Radiographics. 1999;19:569–81.
82. Schwartz LH, Macari M, Huvos AG, Panicek DM. Collision tumors of the adrenal gland: demonstration and characterization at MR imaging. Radiology. 1996;201:757–60.

Testicular Cancer Imaging

6

Harpreet K. Pannu, Ariadne M. Bach, and Jerrold B. Teitcher

Background and Presentation

Testicular cancer is the most common malignancy in young men 15–35 years old and is responsible for approximately 1 % of all cancers in men [1, 2]. Risk factors for its development include cryptorchidism or undescended testes, Klinefelter syndrome, family history of testicular tumor, presence of a contralateral tumor, and intratubular germ cell neoplasia (*see* Table 6.1). There is a high overall survival rate of more than 90 % with appropriate management [1]. Location of the primary tumor and disease extent determined by imaging, laboratory markers, and pathologic results classify patients as low, intermediate, or high risk. Although patients typically present with painless scrotal swelling, 10 % may have acute pain due to tumoral hemorrhage or infarction [1]. Approximately 20 % of patients may also present with distant symptoms such as back pain due to retroperitoneal adenopathy, respiratory complaints from pulmonary metastases, or breast enlargement secondary to hormone secretion by the testis tumor.

Table 6.1 Risk factors associated with testicular cancer [3,4]

Cryptorchidism	2.5–14× increased risk
Personal history of testicular cancer	20× increased risk of contralateral tumor
Intratubular germ cell neoplasia	Up to 50 % of patients develop invasive tumor
Genetic disorders	Klinefelter syndrome, Down syndrome, abnormal short arm of chromosome 12
Family history	6× increased risk if testicular cancer in first-degree relative
White race	5× increased risk compared with black individuals
Supernumerary nipples	4.5× increased risk

Histology and Tumor Markers

Germ cell tumors account for 95 % of testicular cancers and are divided into seminomatous or nonseminomatous subtypes, each comprising approximately 40–45 % of germ cell tumors, with the remaining being mixed [2]. Nonseminomatous tumors usually contain more than one cell type and may include seminoma mixed with other germ cell neoplasms such as embryonal cell carcinoma, choriocarcinoma, yolk sac tumor, and teratoma. Serum alpha fetoprotein (AFP) can help distinguish patients with pure seminoma from those with mixed tumors as it is only secreted by nonseminomatous tumors. AFP levels are elevated in 20 % of patients with clinical stage I disease and in more than 50 % of patients with metastases [1]. Human chorionic gonadotropin (hCG) is less specific as it can be elevated in both seminomatous and nonseminomatous tumors. Lactate dehydrogenase (LDH) levels are used in both tumor types as a marker of disease burden, as it is elevated in more than 50 % of patients with advanced disease. Non-germ cell tumors of the testis include lymphoma, Sertoli, and Leydig cell tumors [2]. Tumor histology is determined by radical orchiectomy, which involves resecting the testis and ligating the spermatic cord at the inguinal ring (*see* Table 6.2).

Testicular Cancer Staging

Testicular cancer staging is based on local tumor extent, presence and size of regional nodes, serum tumor marker levels, and distant metastases (*see* Table 6.3) [1]. Local disease is divided as limited to testis and epididymis (T1), involving testis and epididymis with vascular/lymphatic invasion or tumor extension through the tunica albuginea to tunica vaginalis (T2), tumor invading spermatic cord (T3),

H.K. Pannu, M.D. (✉) • A.M. Bach, M.D. • J.B. Teitcher, M.D.
Department of Radiology, Memorial Sloan-Kettering Cancer Center, 1275 York Avenue, New York, NY 10065, USA
e-mail: pannuh@mskcc.org; bacha@mskcc.org; teitchej@mskcc.org

A.M. Bach, J. Zhang (eds.), *Atlas of Genitourinary Oncological Imaging*, Atlas of Oncology Imaging,
DOI 10.1007/978-1-4614-4872-3_6, © Springer Science+Business Media New York 2013

Table 6.2 Neoplasms of the testis [2–4]

Germ cell tumors	95 % of testicular tumors	
	Seminoma 40–45 %	
	Nonseminomatous tumors* 40–45 %	
	Mixed malignant germ cell tumors† 10 %	
	Intratubular germ cell neoplasia–precursor lesion	
	*Embryonal carcinoma	Elevated AFP and/or β-hCG
	*Yolk sac carcinoma	Elevated AFP
	*Choriocarcinoma	Elevated β-hCG
	*Teratoma	Mature or immature elements
	†Mixed tumors	One or more histologic subtype of nonseminomatous tumor with or without seminoma
Sex cord and stromal tumors	90 % benign	
	Leydig cell tumor–stromal tumor	
	Sertoli cell tumor–sex cord tumor	
	Granulosa cell tumor	
	Fibroma–thecoma	
	Leydig cell tumor	Most common, 30 % hormonally active producing androgens or estrogens
Mixed germ cell and sex cord stromal tumor	Gonadoblastoma	
Lymphoid	Lymphoma ~4 % of testicular tumors	Patients >60 years old, B cell lymphoma
Other	Sarcoma	
	Metastasis	

Table 6.3 Staging of testicular tumors [4]

Highlights of testicular cancer staging	
Regional nodes	N1: <2 cm; N2: >2, >5 cm; N3: >5 cm
Stage I	Includes local T1-T4 disease. No nodal or distant metastases.
Stage II	Retroperitoneal (regional) adenopathy, N1–N3. No distant metastases.
Stage III	Nonregional nodes or other distant metastases
T staging	
T0	No primary tumor (may have fibrosis in testis)
T1	Limited to testis and epididymis No vascular, lymphatic, or tunica vaginalis invasion
T2	Limited to testis and epididymis
	Vascular, lymphatic, or tunica vaginalis invasion may be present
T3	Invasion of spermatic cord
	Vascular or lymphatic invasion may be present
T4	Invasion of scrotum
	Vascular or lymphatic invasion may be present
N staging	
N0	No regional node metastases
N1	Metastases to <5 regional nodes; each node <2 cm
N2	Metastases to more than 5 regional nodes (each <5 cm) or nodes >2 and <5 cm
N3	Metastases to regional nodes >5 cm
M staging	
M0	No distant metastases
M1a	Metastases to nonregional nodes or lungs
M1b	Metastases to other distant sites (besides nonregional nodes or lungs)
Serum tumor marker staging	
S0	Normal markers
S1	LDH <1.5 times normal
	hCG <5,000 mIU/mL
	AFP <1,000 ng/mL
S2	LDH 1.5–10 times normal
	hCG 5,000–50,000 mIU/mL
	AFP 1,000–10,000 ng/mL
S3	LDH >10 times normal
	hCG >50,000 mIU/mL
	AFP >10,000 ng/mL

and tumor invading scrotum (T4) [1]. Stage I tumors can range from T1 (stage Ia disease) to T4 (stage Ib or Is) but have no nodal or distant metastases. Stage Ib tumors have negative serum tumor markers whereas stage Is tumors are positive. These serum markers are also classified according to the degree of elevation of LDH, hCG, and AFP with S0 referring to normal markers, and S1, S2, and S3 are for increasing serum levels of these proteins. Regional nodes are staged both clinically and pathologically using size cut-offs of 2 and 5 cm. For clinical evaluation, regional nodes less than or equal to 2 cm are N1 disease, those greater than 2 cm but less than 5 cm are N2 disease, whereas nodes greater than 5 cm are N3 disease [1]. Pathologic assessment includes the number of positive nodes. Patients with stage II testicular cancer have retroperitoneal spread with stages IIa, IIb, and IIc having N1, N2, and N3 nodal disease, respectively. Distant metastases are stage III and are either M1a with nonregional (nonretroperitoneal) nodes or pulmonary spread, or M1b with nonpulmonary visceral metastases such as to the brain, bones, and liver. Staging of nodal and distant disease is typically performed with computed tomography (CT).

Nodal Disease

Regional nodes for testicular cancer are in the retroperitoneum following the primary drainage pathway of each testis. These sites are precaval, paracaval, and interaortocaval nodes for right-sided testicular tumors, and paraaortic and preaortic

Table 6.4 Key differences between seminoma and nonseminomatous tumors

Seminoma	Nonseminomatous germ cell tumor (NSGCT)
No elevation of serum AFP	Serum AFP can be elevated
Surveillance or radiation for clinical stage I disease	Retroperitoneal node dissection, surveillance or chemotherapy for clinical stage I disease
Teratomatous change rare	Teratomatous change seen in nodes after chemotherapy
Resection considered for FDG avid residual retroperitoneal mass >3 cm	Residual retroperitoneal mass >1 cm resected regardless of activity on PET as teratoma is not FDG avid

Table 6.5 Imaging evaluation of testicular cancer

Diagnosis	Primary modality: testicular ultrasound Problem solving: testicular MRI
Staging	Nodal or visceral metastases: CT chest, abdomen, pelvis Brain metastases in high-risk or symptomatic patients: CT brain Brain or bone metastases: MRI
Post-treatment evaluation	Pulmonary recurrence: chest radiograph Abdominal recurrence in first 3 years: CT or MRI Assessment for tumor in residual mass, or for evaluating patients with normal CT/MRI but elevated serum tumor markers: FDG-PET

nodes for left-sided tumors [1, 2]. Contralateral nodes are usually seen with large volume disease and right-sided tumors but are rare without ipsilateral adenopathy. Metastatic nodes are of soft tissue density or are heterogeneous with mixed solid and cystic components, the latter usually seen with nonseminomatous tumors. Progressive spread occurs to retrocrural, subcarinal, and supraclavicular nodes. Pelvic nodes can become enlarged secondary to lymphatic obstruction by bulky abdominal adenopathy [2]. Inguinal adenopathy can also occur when the primary tumor involves the scrotal wall. Although a short axis diameter of 10 mm is typically used to assess nodes, smaller nodes in expected sites of lymphatic drainage can harbor metastases [5].

The management of retroperitoneal nodes in early-stage testicular cancer differs for seminomatous and nonseminomatous tumors, both at initial presentation and after treatment (*see* Table 6.4). Retroperitoneal node dissection is not performed in early-stage seminoma but can be considered in nonseminomatous tumors. Seminoma is radiosensitive, unlike nonseminomatous tumors, and patients with clinical stage I disease may receive radiation to the retroperitoneum or surveillance for recurrence, which typically occurs at a median of 15 months in 15 % of patients [1]. For patients with nonseminomatous tumors, approximately 30 % of those with clinical stage I disease have occult nodal metastases, and options include retroperitoneal node dissection, chemotherapy, or surveillance for recurrence, which typically occurs in the first year [1, 2]. Node dissection is considered in particular for patients with risk factors such as lymphovascular invasion, embryonal carcinoma, or scrotal extension of tumor [1].

Retroperitoneal lymph node dissection has been modified over time by limiting it to infrarenal nodes in low stage disease, as well as performing a unilateral dissection. The aim is to maximize the likelihood of resecting metastatic nodes while minimizing morbidity. If feasible, the sympathetic nerves are spared to preserve antegrade ejaculation. Based on studies mapping nodal stations, there are several side-specific templates for guiding dissection. For right-sided tumors, the precaval, paracaval, interaortocaval, and hilar gonadal vein nodes are resected and, in some templates, the preaortic and ipsilateral iliac nodes may also be included [6, 7]. For left-sided tumors, the preaortic, paraaortic, and hilar gonadal vein nodes are resected and the interaortocaval and ipsilateral iliac nodes may also be included depending on the template [6, 7].

Surveillance is included as a clinical option in patients with early-stage testicular cancer to avoid the complications of lymphadenectomy and the morbidity of radiation and chemotherapy, which carry the risk of long-term cardiovascular complications and second malignancy [8]. Patients are monitored by checking serum tumor markers, chest radiography or CT, and abdominal CT and this regimen is most intensive in the first year after treatment. Magnetic resonance imaging (MRI) is a nonradiation alternative to CT for surveillance of the retroperitoneum [9]. Chemotherapy is administered for advanced stages of both seminomatous and nonseminomatous tumors (*see* Table 6.5).

Once retroperitoneal nodes have been nonsurgically treated with radiation or chemotherapy, residual masses can be seen at imaging in up to 70 % of patients [10]. The majority of these masses in patients with seminoma consist of fibrotic tissue without active tumor or teratoma and are therefore observed [2]. Surgery is considered for masses larger than 3 cm with increased activity on positron emission tomography (PET) scans but complete resection can be challenging due to an appreciable desmoplastic reaction [1]. In contrast to seminoma, residual masses larger than 1 cm in patients with nonseminomatous tumors are resected as they have teratoma in 40 % of cases and viable tumor in 10 % [10]. Teratoma is seen either due to persistence of the original teratomatous component or due to transformation of the tumor with chemotherapy [3]. Change in the appearance of the mass to a simple-appearing cyst is seen with evolution to a differentiated mature teratoma. This is resected, as there is potential for growth with mass effect or malignant transformation in approximately 5 % of patients [1, 2, 8, 11].

A residual nodal mass with mixed solid and cystic appearance is also resected, as this can be seen with fibrosis, tumor, and/or necrosis. Increased ^{18}F-fluorodeoxyglucose (FDG) activity in the residual mass on PET imaging suggests viable tumor [12, 13].

Other Metastases and Relapse

Although metastases from testicular tumors are typically by the lymphatic route, hematogenous spread can also occur. This is more common with nonseminomatous tumors and is seen in the lungs, liver, brain, and bones. Late relapse of testicular cancer is defined as a recurrence occurring more than 2 years after completing initial therapy. It occurs in 2–6 % of patients at a median interval of 6 years at sites such as the retroperitoneum, lungs, and mediastinum [1, 14]. Prognostic indicators for patients with germ cell tumors at presentation are serum tumor marker levels, primary tumor location, and visceral metastases. Seminoma patients without nonpulmonary visceral metastases are considered at good risk, regardless of the primary tumor site or serum tumor marker levels. However, seminoma patients with nonpulmonary metastases are at intermediate risk [1]. For patients with nonseminomatous tumors, the presence of a gonadal or retroperitoneal primary tumor, absence of nonpulmonary visceral metastases, and normal or stage 1 elevation of tumor markers are considered good risk features. Stage 2 serum tumor markers put the patient at intermediate risk and presence of a mediastinal primary tumor or nonpulmonary visceral metastases are poor risk factors.

Risk Factors for Testicular Cancer

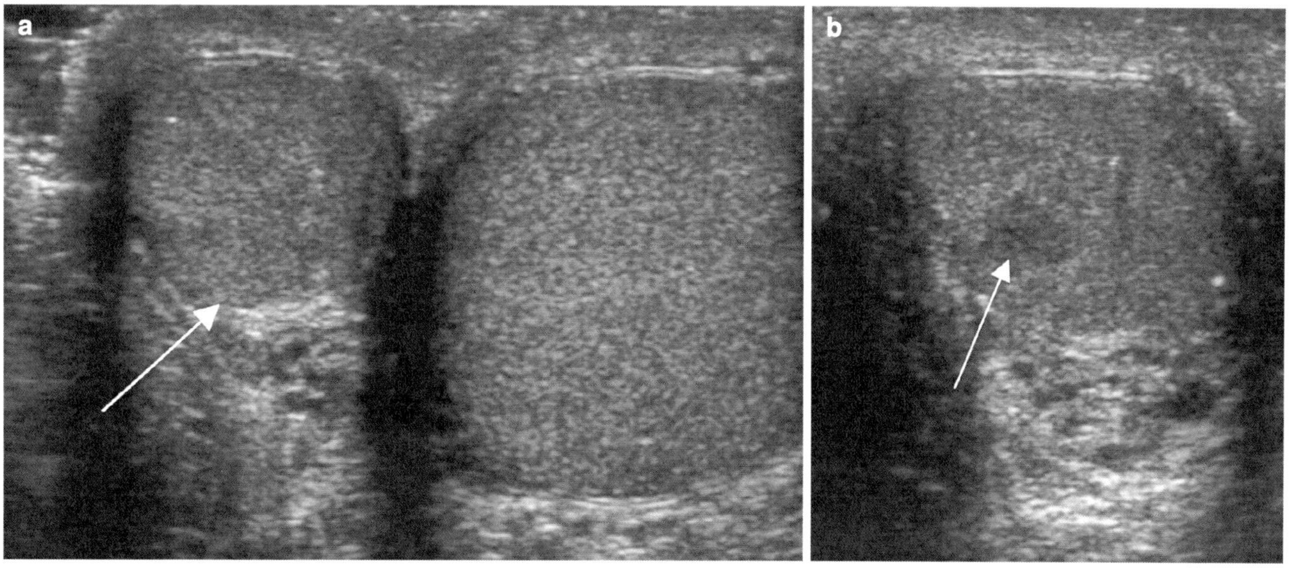

Fig. 6.1 Testicular atrophy. Ultrasound images of the scrotum in a 35-year-old man with right scrotal discomfort that was not alleviated by antibiotics. (**a**) Grayscale image of both testes shows asymmetry in testicular size with atrophy of the right testis (*arrow*). (**b**) Dedicated grayscale image of the right testis revealed a 5 mm hypoechoic mildly lobulated mass (*arrow*). The background parenchyma was mildly hypoechoic with scattered punctate calcifications. An atrophic testis is a risk factor for testicular cancer, rendering this lesion suspicious for malignancy. A 1 cm seminoma was diagnosed at orchiectomy

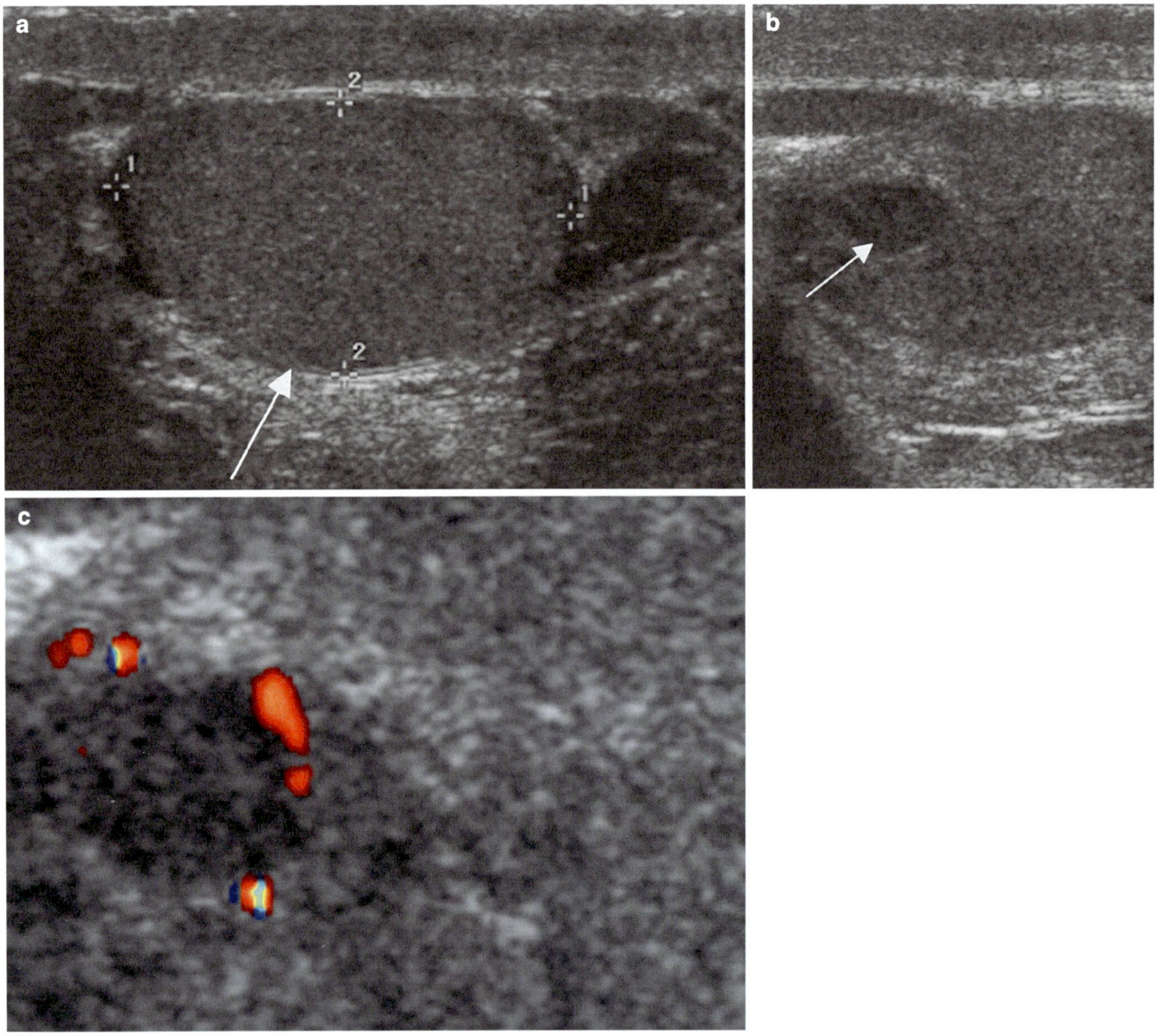

Fig. 6.2 Prior history of testicular cancer and testicular atrophy. Ultrasound images of the left testis from a patient with a history of right orchiectomy 12 years earlier for embryonal carcinoma and seminoma. (**a**) Grayscale image shows an atrophic left testis (*arrow*). Grayscale (**b**) and color Doppler (**c**) images reveal a well-circumscribed hypoechoic new lesion (*arrow* in **b**) in the left testis with peripheral vascularity. Pathology revealed a 2 cm mixed germ cell tumor composed of 65 % seminoma and 35 % embryonal carcinoma. This patient had two risk factors for testicular cancer: a prior personal history of testicular cancer and an atrophic remaining testis

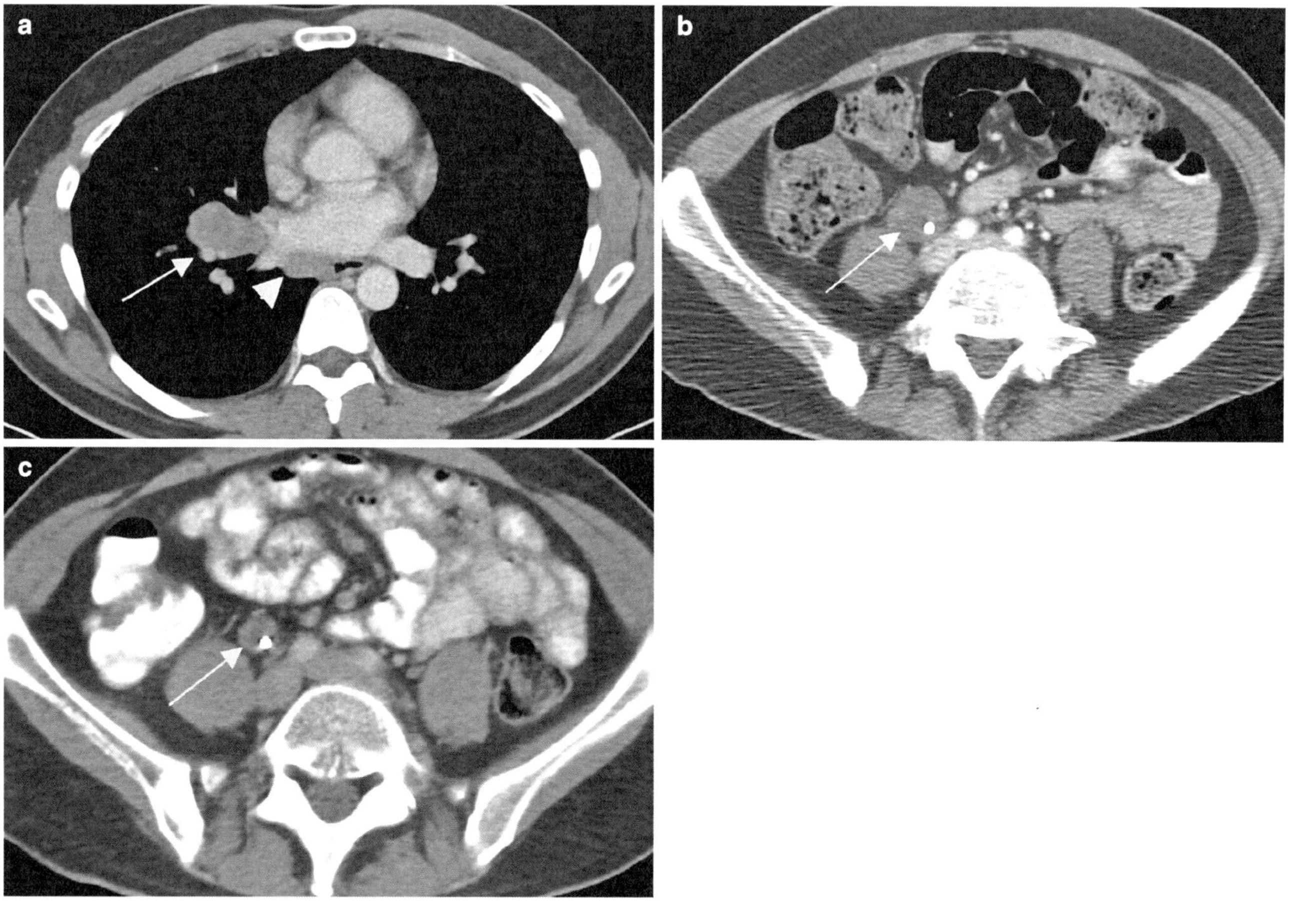

Fig. 6.3 Prior history of testicular cancer. Axial CT images with intravenous contrast in a 40-year-old patient with a previous history of left orchiectomy and retroperitoneal radiation therapy for seminoma. Fourteen years later the patient presents with new right testicular enlargement and a heterogeneous testis on ultrasound. (**a**) CT image of the chest shows right hilar (*arrow*) and paraesophageal (*arrowhead*) adenopathy. The patient also had a history of sarcoidosis so biopsy was performed and revealed non-necrotizing epithelioid granulomata without malignancy. A right radical orchiectomy was subsequently performed and was positive for seminoma in the testis. The patient received chemotherapy as he had already received radiation to the retroperitoneum. A few months later the patient presented with back pain and (**b**) CT of the abdomen showed a retroperitoneal mass (*arrow*) encasing the right ureter. Biopsy of this mass was positive for metastatic seminoma and chemotherapy was given. (**c**) CT 3 months after chemotherapy shows the retroperitoneal mass (*arrow*) has decreased in size

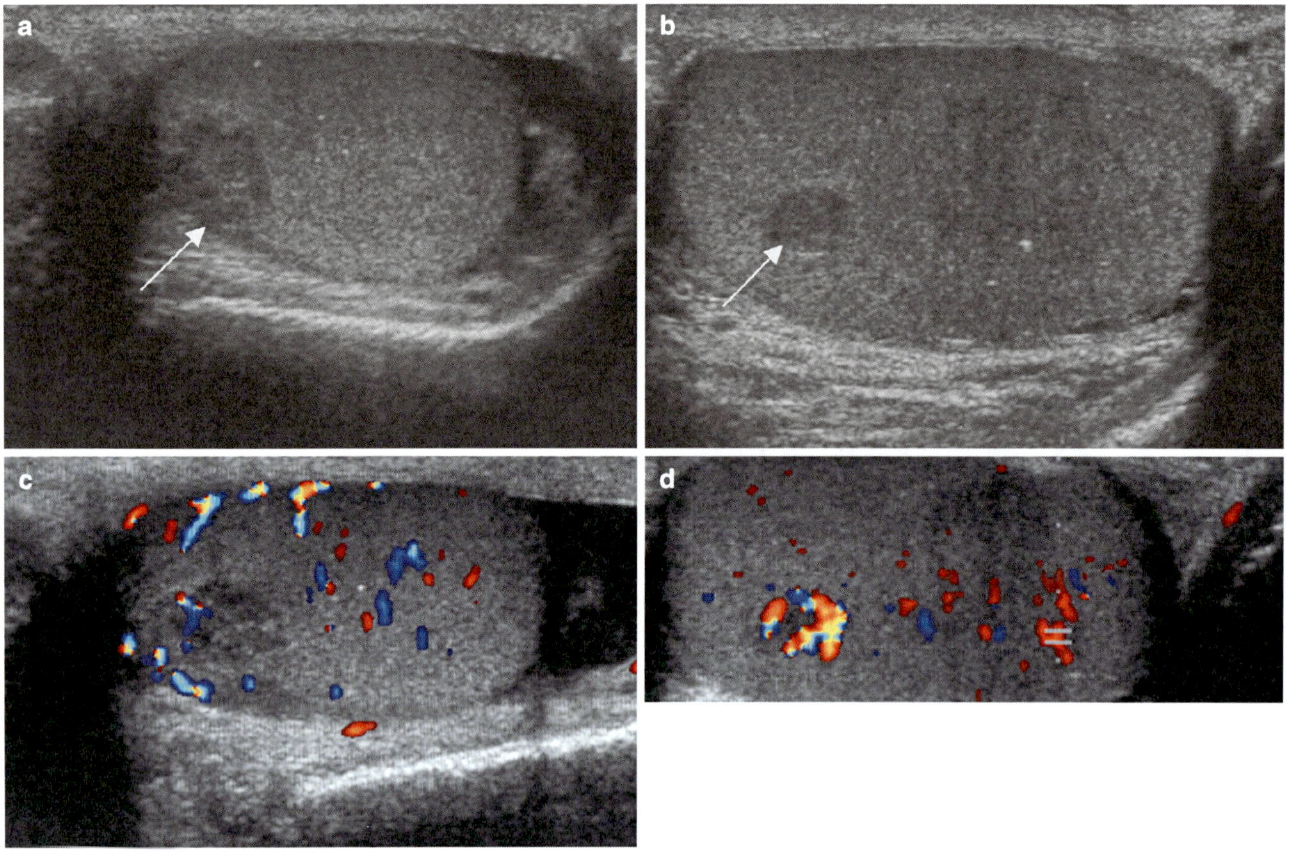

Fig. 6.4 Undescended testis. Ultrasound images of the testis from a 25-year- old man with history of undescended testis and prior orchiopexy who now presented with vague scrotal swelling. Grayscale images of the left (**a**) and right (**b**) testes show a hypoechoic mass (*arrow*) in each testis and scattered punctate calcifications. The mass in the left testis is lobulated and larger. Color Doppler images of left (**c**) and right (**d**) testes show internal vascularity in the lesions, greater on the right. The patient's serum tumor markers were normal. The patient desired intraoperative testicular biopsy prior to orchiectomy for positive biopsy. A left testicular biopsy followed by orchiectomy revealed a 0.9 cm mixed germ cell tumor, mainly embryonal subtype, with vascular invasion. A biopsy of the right testicular lesion revealed Leydig cell hyperplasia

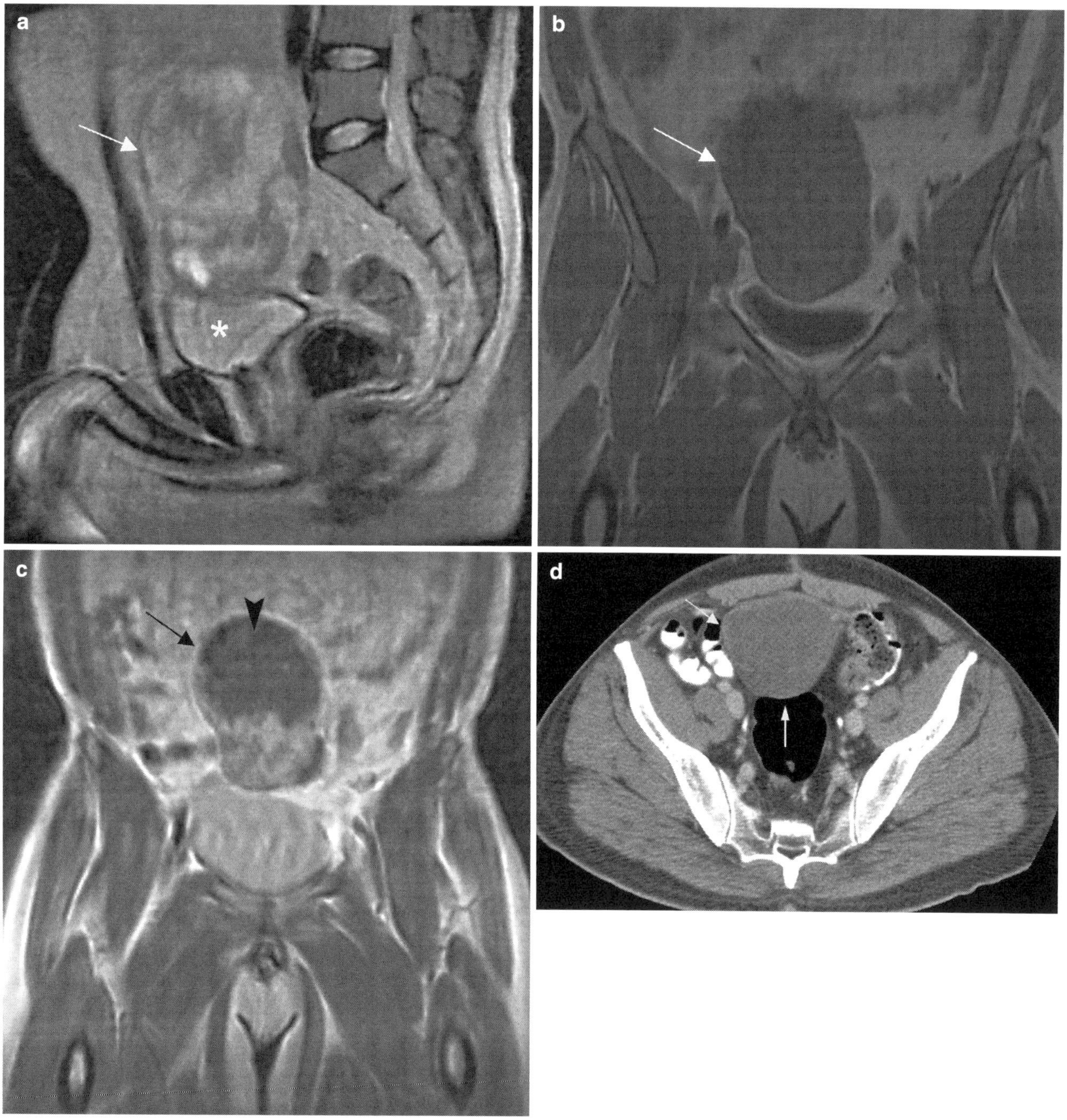

Fig. 6.5 Undescended testis. MR and CT images of the pelvis in a 40-year-old patient who presented with a sensation of pressure in the suprapubic region. (**a**) Sagittal T2-weighted MR image of the pelvis shows a heterogeneous hyperintense mass (*arrow*) superior to the bladder (*asterisk*). Pre- (**b**) and post-contrast (**c**) T1-weighted coronal MR images of the pelvis show an enhancing soft tissue component in inferior aspect of mass (*arrow*) and necrosis (*arrowhead*) in the superior aspect of mass. Biopsy of the pelvic mass showed a poorly differentiated yolk sac tumor. Ultrasound (*not shown*) revealed a normal right testis but no convincing evidence of a left testis. Surgical exploration of the scrotum also did not reveal any left testicular tissue in the resected specimen. The patient was given chemotherapy and a follow-up CT was performed. (**d**) CT image of the upper pelvis shows a hypodense mass (*arrows*) in the midline. (**e**) A more inferior CT image shows the mass (*arrow*) is adjacent to the bladder (*asterisk*) and also has soft tissue (*arrowhead*) extending toward the left inguinal canal. (**f**) CT image of the lower pelvis shows absence of the left spermatic cord (*arrow*). A right spermatic cord is present (*arrowhead*). (**g**) CT at the level of the scrotum shows a solitary testis (*arrow*) with a small hydrocele. (**h**) Coronal CT reconstruction shows the mass (*arrow*), bladder (*asterisk*), and solitary testis (*arrowhead*) in the scrotum. The pelvic mass was resected after chemotherapy and consisted of testicular tissue with marked parenchymal atrophy and necrotic tissue without residual viable tumor

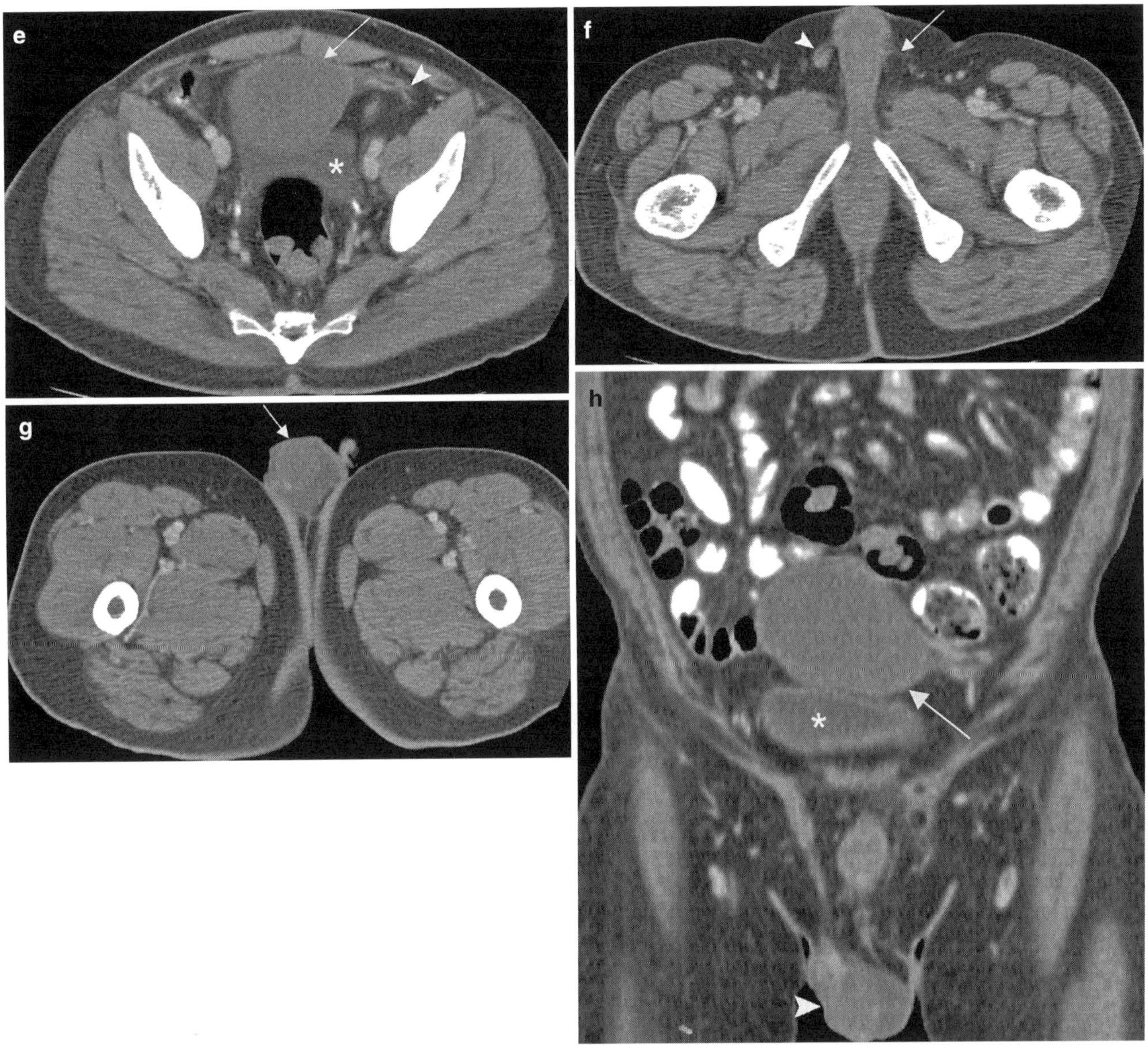

Fig. 6.5 (continued)

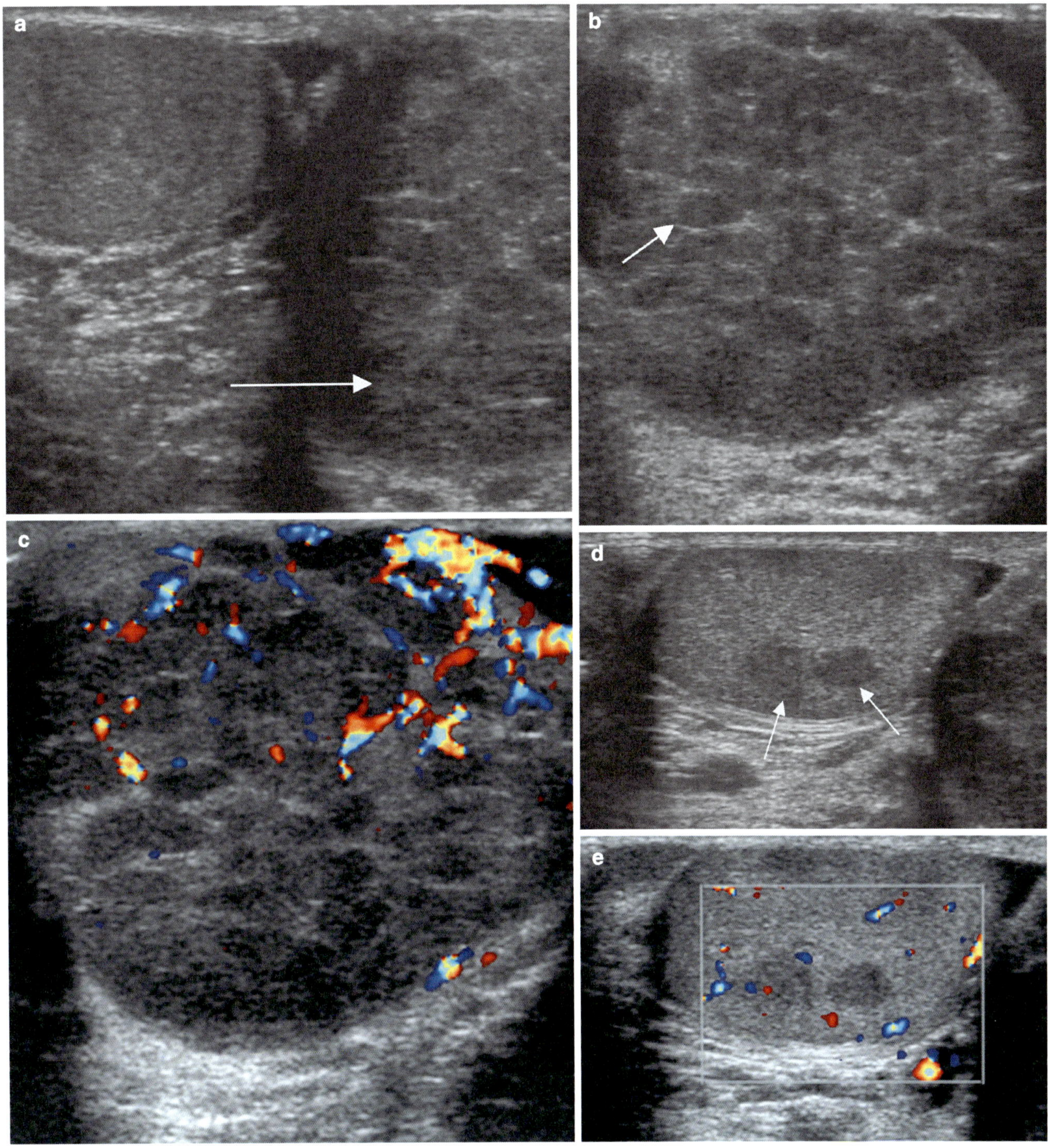

Fig. 6.6 Intratubular germ cell neoplasia. Ultrasound images of the scrotum from a 30-year-old man with a palpable left testicular mass. (**a**) Grayscale midline image shows asymmetric testicular size (*arrow*) with enlargement of the left testis. Grayscale (**b**) and color Doppler (**c**) images of the left testis show the parenchyma is replaced by multiple hypoechoic confluent nodules (*arrow*). Grayscale (**d**) and color Doppler (**e**) images of the right testis show two focal hypoechoic nodules (*arrows*) that are relatively well circumscribed. Bilateral orchiectomies revealed a 5.5 cm seminoma in the left testis and intratubular germ cell neoplasia. The right testicular parenchyma was atrophic with foci of intratubular germ cell neoplasia

Modes of Presentation of Testicular Cancer

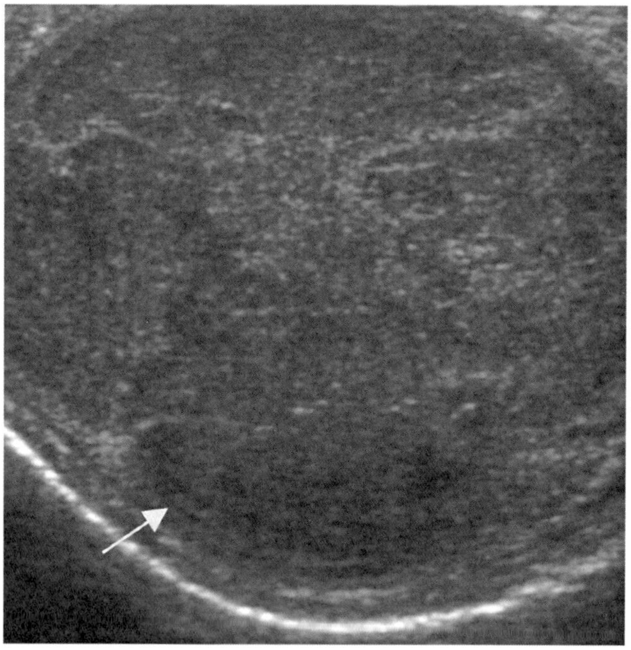

Fig. 6.7 Palpable scrotal mass. A patient in his early twenties who presented with a palpable scrotal mass and weight loss. Grayscale ultrasound image of the left testis shows the testis is enlarged by a hypoechoic mass (*arrow*). Orchiectomy revealed seminoma. A palpable mass is a common presentation of testicular cancer

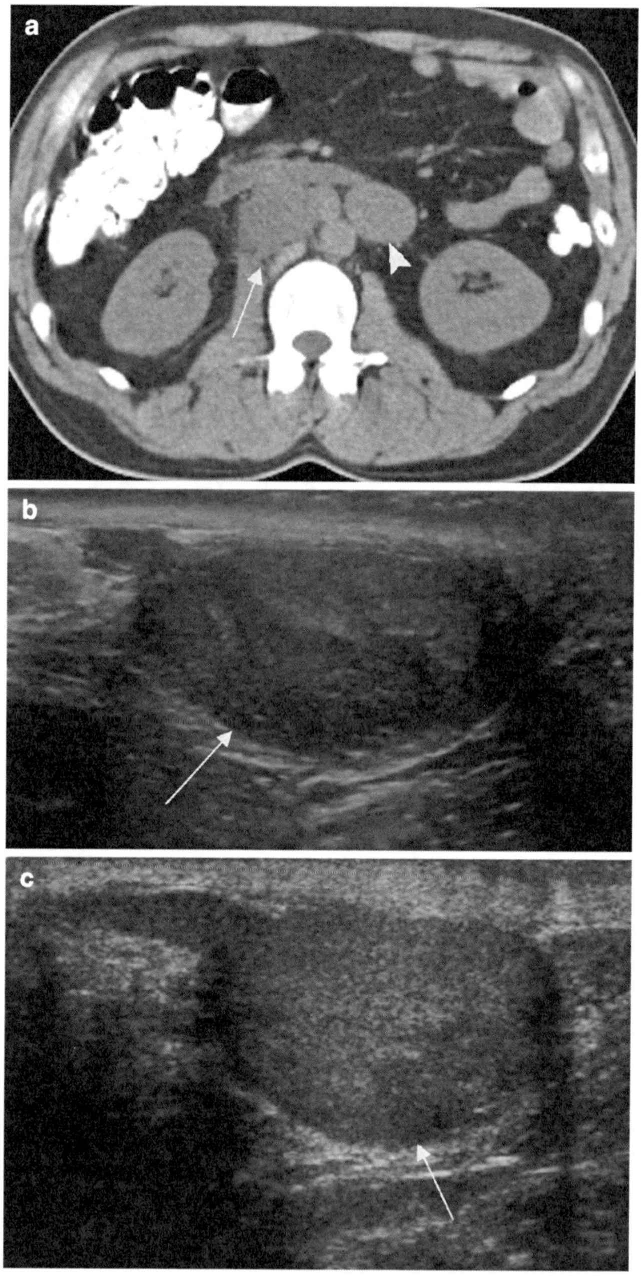

Fig. 6.8 Flank pain as presentation of stage II seminoma. A 35-year-old patient presented with flank pain and CT was performed to evaluate for renal stone. (**a**) Scans of the abdomen and pelvis showed no urinary tract calculi or hydronephrosis. However, retroperitoneal adenopathy is noted in the retrocaval (*arrow*) and left paraaortic regions (*arrowhead*). As the adenopathy is in the nodal drainage pathway of the testis, ultrasound was performed to evaluate for a possible testicular lesion as the primary source. (**b**) Grayscale ultrasound image of the right testis demonstrates a hypoechoic mass (*arrow*) replacing most of the parenchyma suspicious for malignancy. Biopsy of a retroperitoneal node revealed seminoma and the patient was treated with chemotherapy. (**c**) Grayscale ultrasound image of the right testis 3 months after chemotherapy shows decreased size of the testicular mass (*arrow*). The residual hypoechoic parenchyma demonstrated fibrosis at orchiectomy without viable tumor. Post-treatment fibrosis without viable tumor is a common pathologic finding in treated seminoma

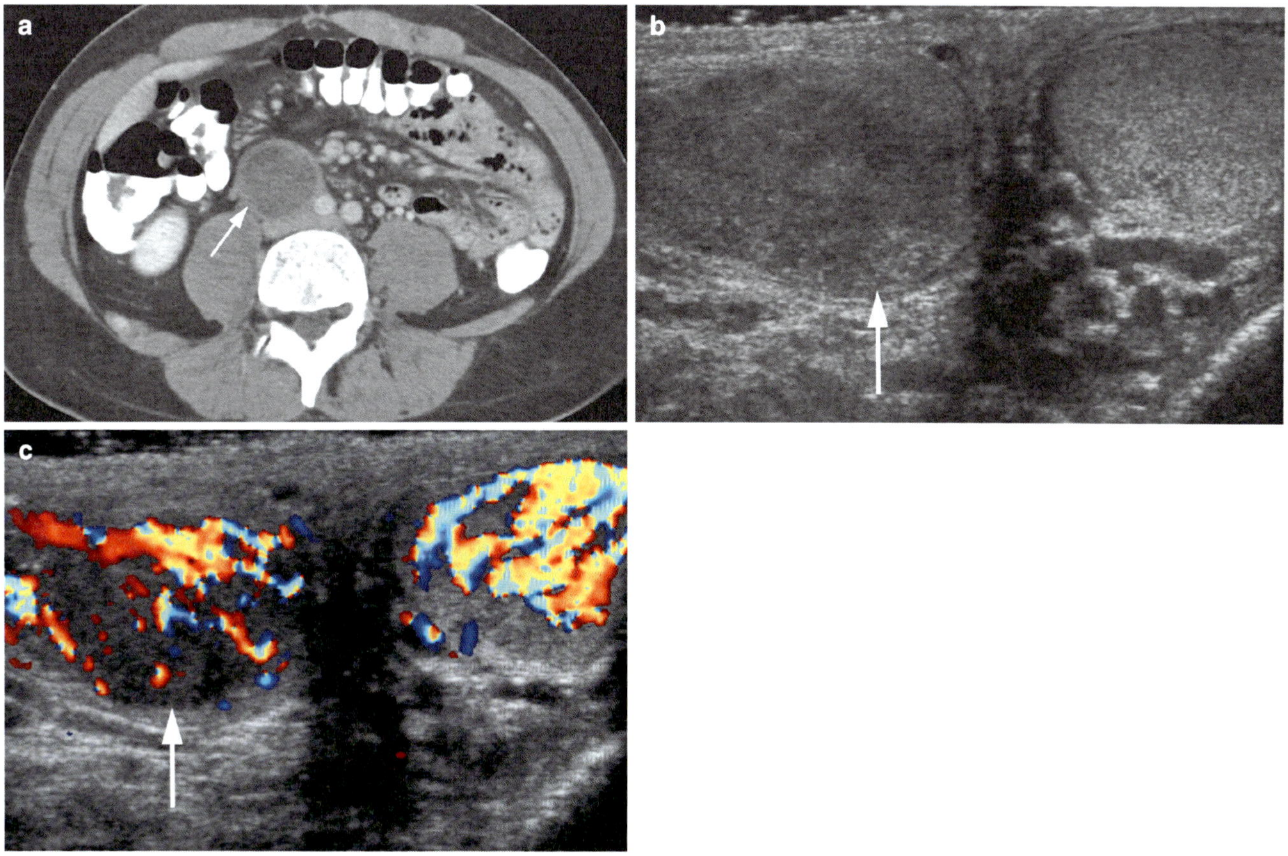

Fig. 6.9 Abdominal pain as presentation of stage II seminoma. A 40-year-old male with history of inflammatory bowel disease presented with abdominal pain. (**a**) Axial CT image of the abdomen with oral and intravenous contrast CT showed a cystic thick-walled retroperitoneal mass (*arrow*). Biopsy of this mass revealed a necrotic, poorly differentiated neoplasm, possibly lymphoma, but the specimen was insufficient for further classification. A testicular ultrasound was performed as part of the workup of this retroperitoneal mass. Grayscale (**b**) and color (**c**) Doppler ultrasound images show a right testicular mass (*arrow*), which proved to be a seminoma with a hyalinized scar at orchiectomy and was compatible with a partially regressed germ cell tumor

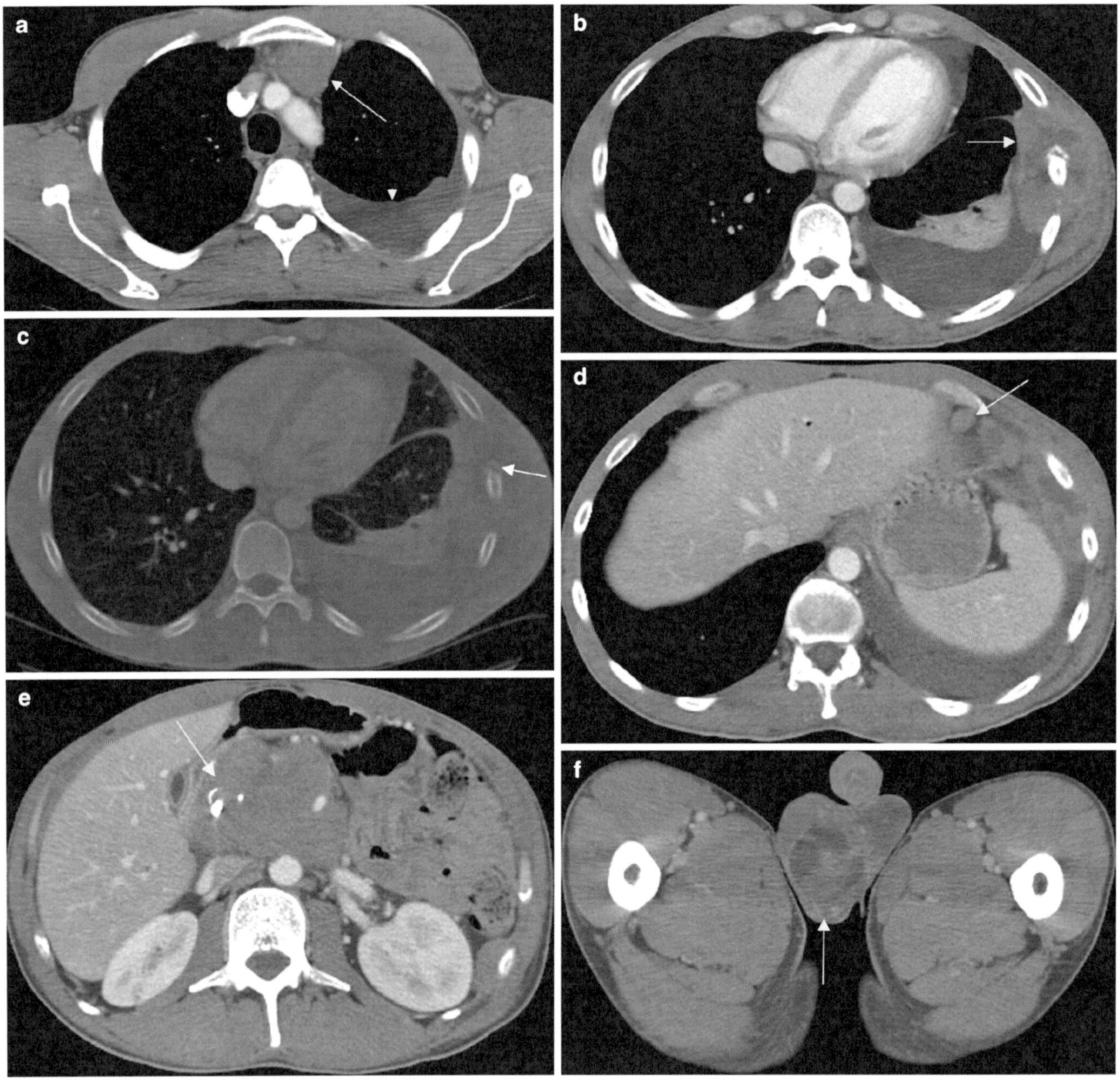

Fig. 6.10 Chest pain as presentation of stage III seminoma. A 30-year-old patient presented with chest pain and CT was performed for evaluation. (**a**) Axial CT image of the chest with intravenous contrast demonstrates anterior mediastinal adenopathy (*arrow*) and a left pleural effusion (*arrowhead*). Soft tissue (**b**) and bone (**c**) windows of the lower chest revealed a mass in the left chest wall (*arrow*) with destruction of the adjacent rib. (**d**) Enlarged anterior diaphragmatic nodes (*arrow*) were also seen in the lower chest. Laboratory tests at the time of presentation also showed the patient to have jaundice. A staging CT of the abdomen (**e**) revealed a large peripancreatic mass (*arrow*). (**f**) The right hemiscrotum (*arrow*) was also noted to be enlarged and heterogeneous. Biopsy of the rib lesion was not definitive in characterizing the type of tumor so orchiectomy was performed and revealed seminoma

Testicular Masses on Ultrasound

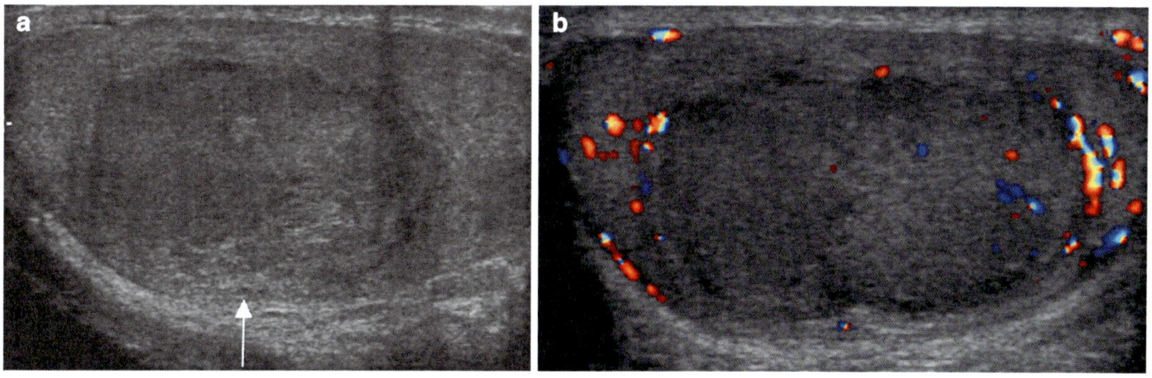

Fig. 6.11 Seminoma. A 25-year-old patient presented with a palpable testicular mass. Grayscale (**a**) and color Doppler ultrasound (**b**) images of the left testis show a well-defined solid testicular mass (*arrow*) with some internal vascularity. Orchiectomy revealed a pure seminoma. Seminoma is typically a hypoechoic homogenous mass

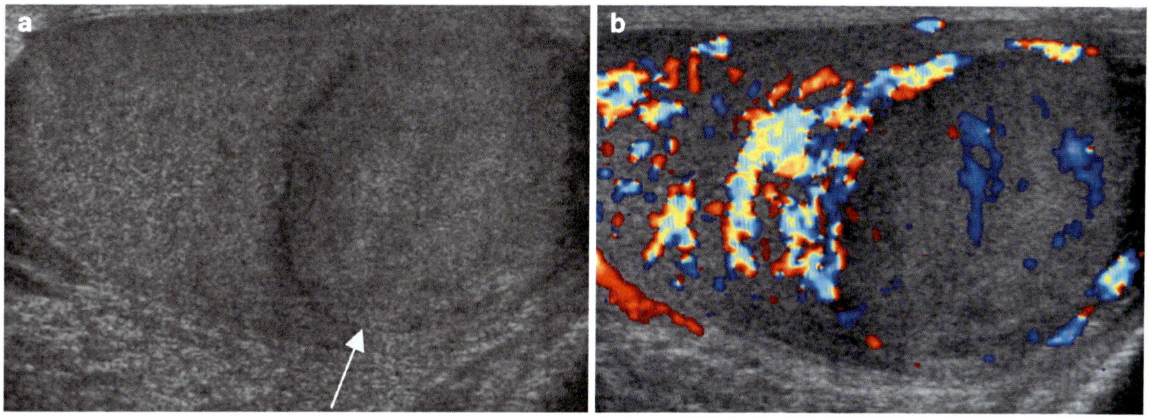

Fig. 6.12 Embryonal cell carcinoma. A 30-year-old patient presented with testicular pain. Grayscale (**a**) and color Doppler ultrasound (**b**) images of the right testis show a homogeneous isoechoic mass (*arrow*) in the right testis with some internal vascularity. Orchiectomy revealed a pure embryonal cell carcinoma. Pure embryonal cell carcinoma is uncommon, occurring in approximately 3 % of cases. Embryonal carcinoma is usually an ill-defined hypoechoic mass that is typically part of a mixed germ cell tumor [4, 15]

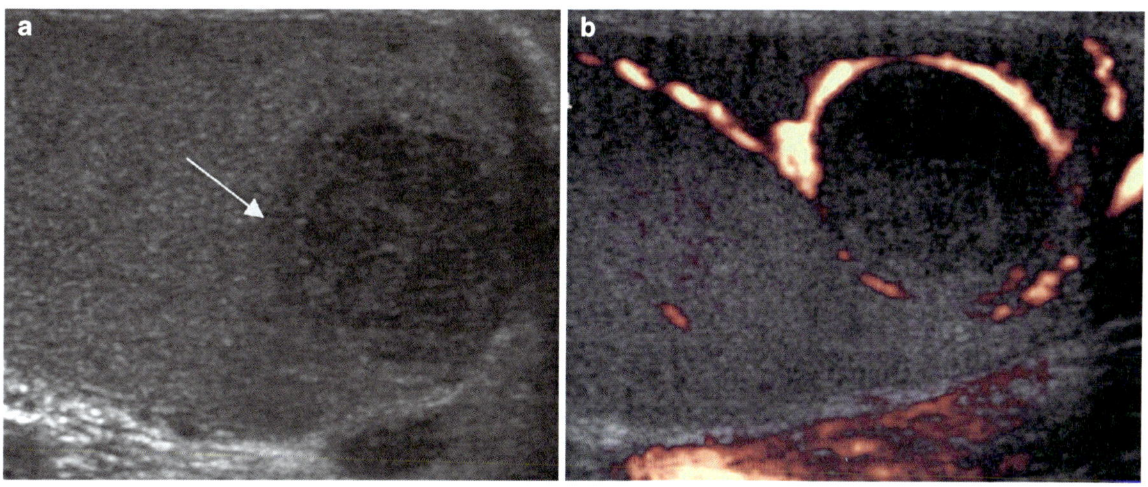

Fig. 6.13 Embryonal cell carcinoma. A 20-year-old patient presented with a palpable testicular mass. Grayscale (**a**) and color Doppler ultrasound (**b**) images of the right testis show a hypoechoic mass (*arrow* in **a**) in the right testis with peripheral vascularity. Orchiectomy revealed a 1.4 cm embryonal cell carcinoma with vascular invasion

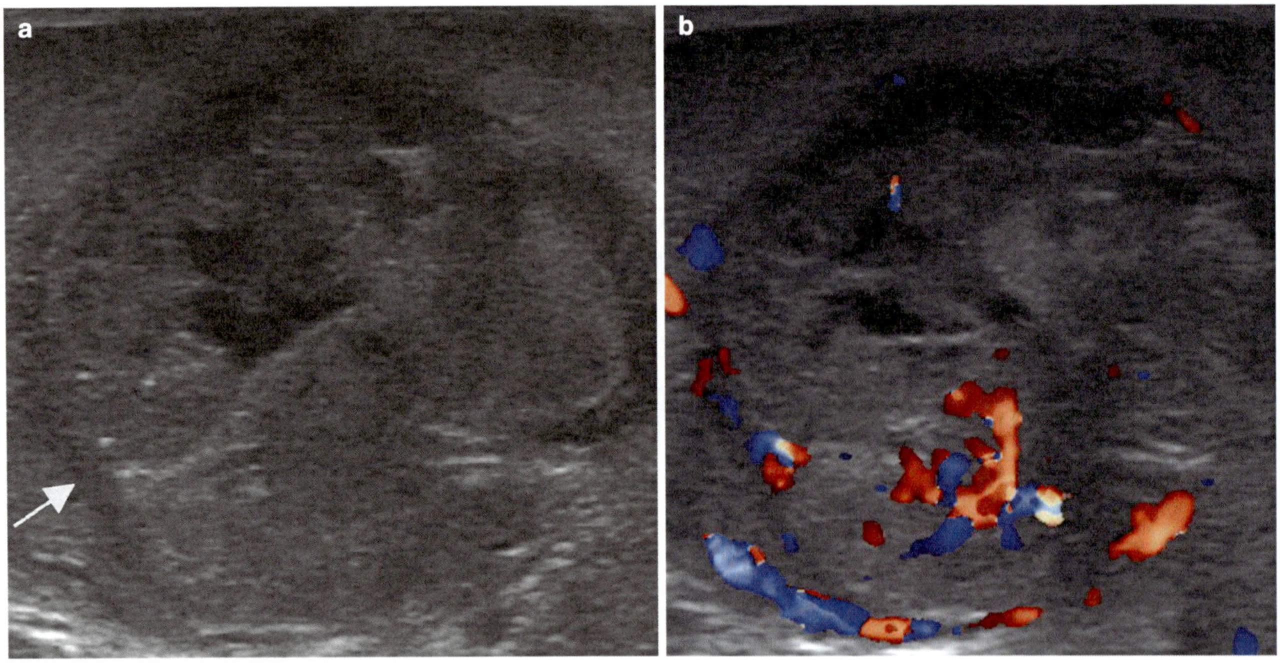

Fig. 6.14 Mixed germ cell tumor. A 20-year-old male presented with progressive back pain and emesis. The patient had enlarged retroperitoneal nodes on abdominal CT (*not shown*) and scrotal ultrasound was performed for further workup. Grayscale (**a**) and color Doppler ultrasound (**b**) images of the testis show a heterogeneous mixed solid and cystic mass (*arrow* in **a**) with internal vascularity. Pathologic examination of the orchiectomy specimen revealed a mixed germ cell tumor with a dominant embryonal carcinoma component, as well as smaller amounts of choriocarcinoma, yolk sac tumor, and mature teratoma. NGSCT are usually heterogeneous with cystic and echogenic components. The latter are due to calcification, fibrosis, or hemorrhage, whereas the former can be due to teratoma, necrosis, or dilated rete testes. Appreciable necrosis and hemorrhage can give choriocarcinoma the appearance of a mixed solid and cystic mass. Cystic regions are common in teratomas, which can also contain echogenic foci of bone and cartilage [4, 15]

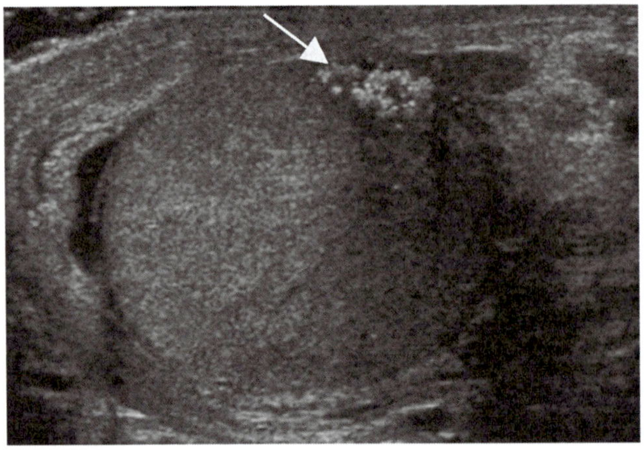

Fig. 6.15 Burned-out testicular tumor in a teenager who presented with flank pain and fatigue. The patient had retroperitoneal adenopathy on CT (*not shown*) and an elevated serum hCG level. Scrotal ultrasound was performed. A grayscale ultrasound image of the left testis demonstrated a cluster of coarse calcifications (*arrow*) without a discrete hypoechoic mass. Shadowing is evident from the calcifications. Calcified scar without viable tumor was seen at orchiectomy and findings were consistent with a regressed or burned-out tumor. Burned-out tumor occurs when the mass outgrows its blood supply and infarcts with resultant fibrosis. The residual mass in the testis can appear as echogenic foci or a small hypoechoic mass [4, 15]

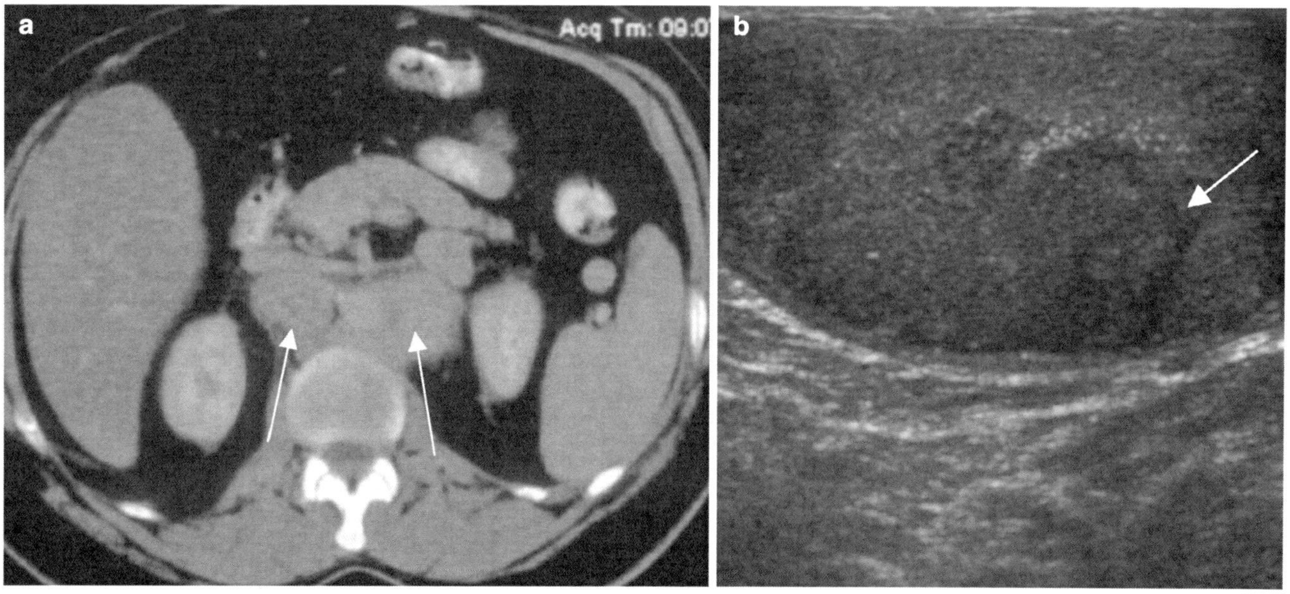

Fig. 6.16 Burned-out testicular tumor. A 50-year-old patient with a history of seminoma in the right testis 30 years earlier presented with abdominal pain and weight loss. (**a**) Axial CT image of the abdomen with oral and intravenous contrast showed retroperitoneal adenopathy (*arrows*) and biopsy revealed seminoma. (**b**) Grayscale ultrasound image of the left testis showed hypoechoic masses (*arrow*) with punctate calcifications. There was extensive scarring with hyalinization and focal microcalcification at orchiectomy consistent with a burned-out lesion

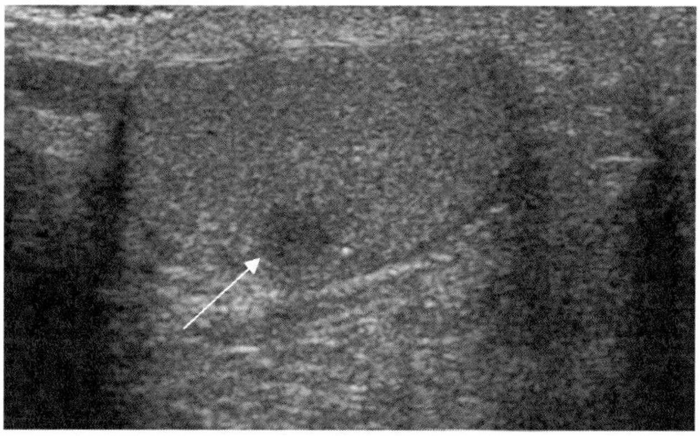

Fig. 6.17 Burned out testicular tumor. A 40-year-old man presented with back pain and had a large retroperitoneal mass on MRI of the spine (*not shown*). A biopsy of this mass revealed a poorly differentiated germ cell tumor and a testicular ultrasound was performed. Grayscale ultrasound image demonstrates a small hypoechoic well-defined testicular mass (*arrow*). Orchiectomy revealed intratubular germ cell neoplasia and scarring possibly due to regression of an invasive germ cell tumor

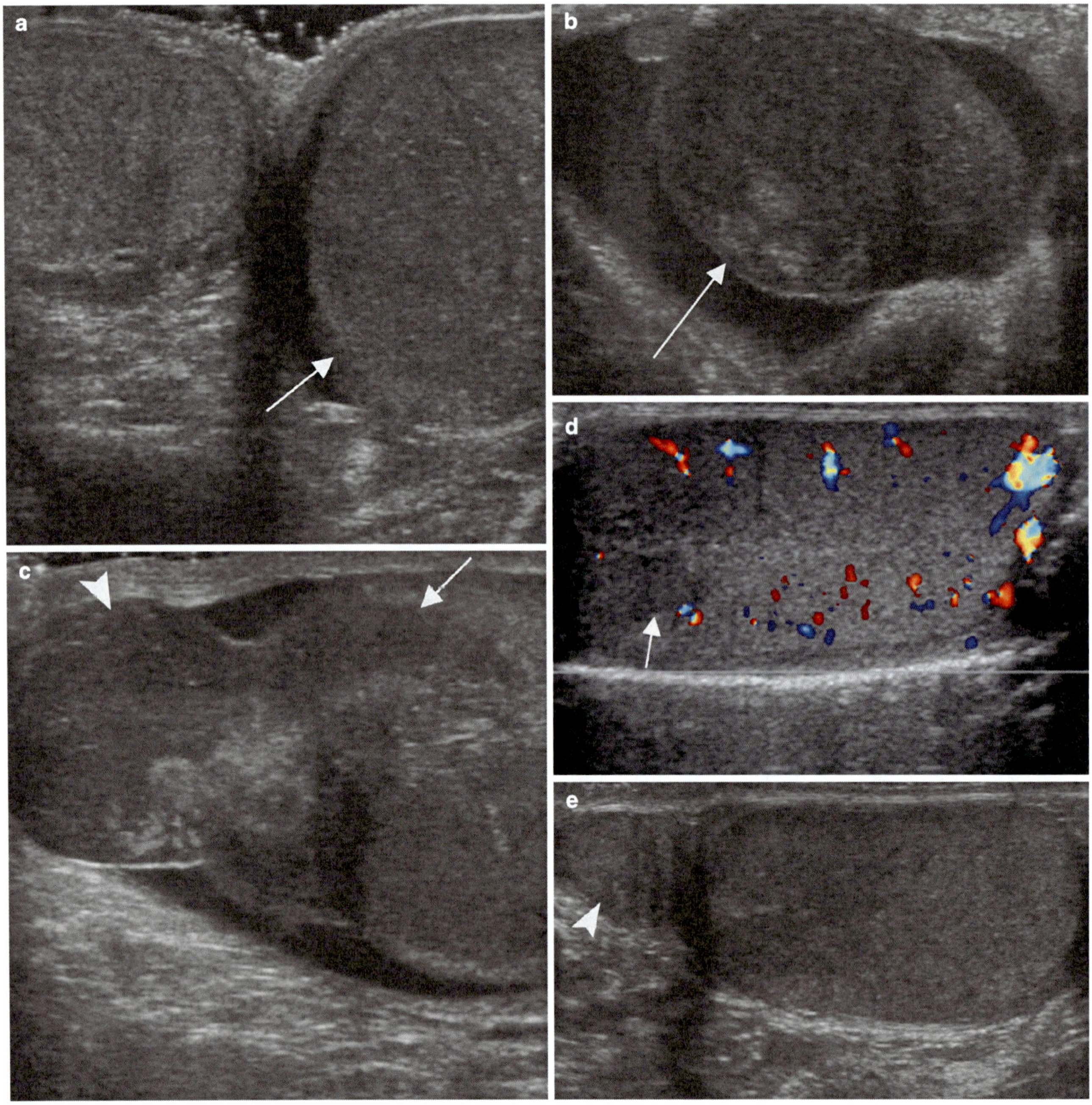

Fig. 6.18 Leukemic infiltration of the testis. A teenager with a recent systemic relapse of leukemia presented with an enlarged left testis. (**a**) Grayscale ultrasound image of both testes shows asymmetric testicular size with enlargement of the left testis (*arrow*). Grayscale images of the left testis (**b**) and left epididymis (**c**) show hypoechoic tissue infiltrating the testis (*arrow*) and enlarging the epididymis (*arrowhead*). (**d**, **e**) Follow-up ultrasound 2 weeks after chemotherapy showed significant improvement in the left testis. (**d**) Color Doppler image of the testis shows normal echogenicity of the parenchyma except for a small residual hypoechoic area around the mediastinum testis (*arrow*) consistent with resolving leukemic infiltration. (**e**) Grayscale image shows decreased swelling of the left epididymis (*arrowhead*) and normal contour of the testis

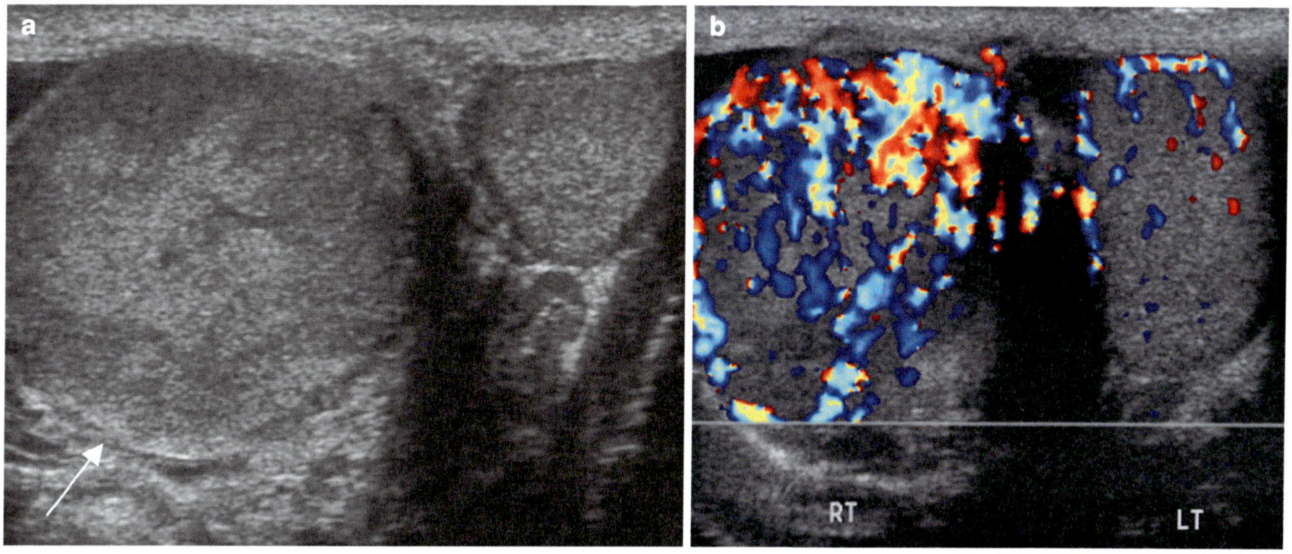

Fig. 6.19 Primary testicular lymphoma. A 60-year-old man presented with painless right testicular swelling and a palpable mass. Grayscale (**a**) and color Doppler ultrasound (**b**) images of both testes show asymmetric enlargement of the right testis (*arrow* in **a**), which is diffusely heterogeneous and has increased vascularity. Orchiectomy revealed a diffuse large B-cell lymphoma. There was no systemic adenopathy. Testicular lymphoma is invariably B-cell non-Hodgkin lymphoma. Single or multiple hypoechoic homogenous masses are typically present. The testis is enlarged and tumor can also infiltrate the epididymis. The tumor has increased vascularity on color Doppler ultrasound [4, 15]

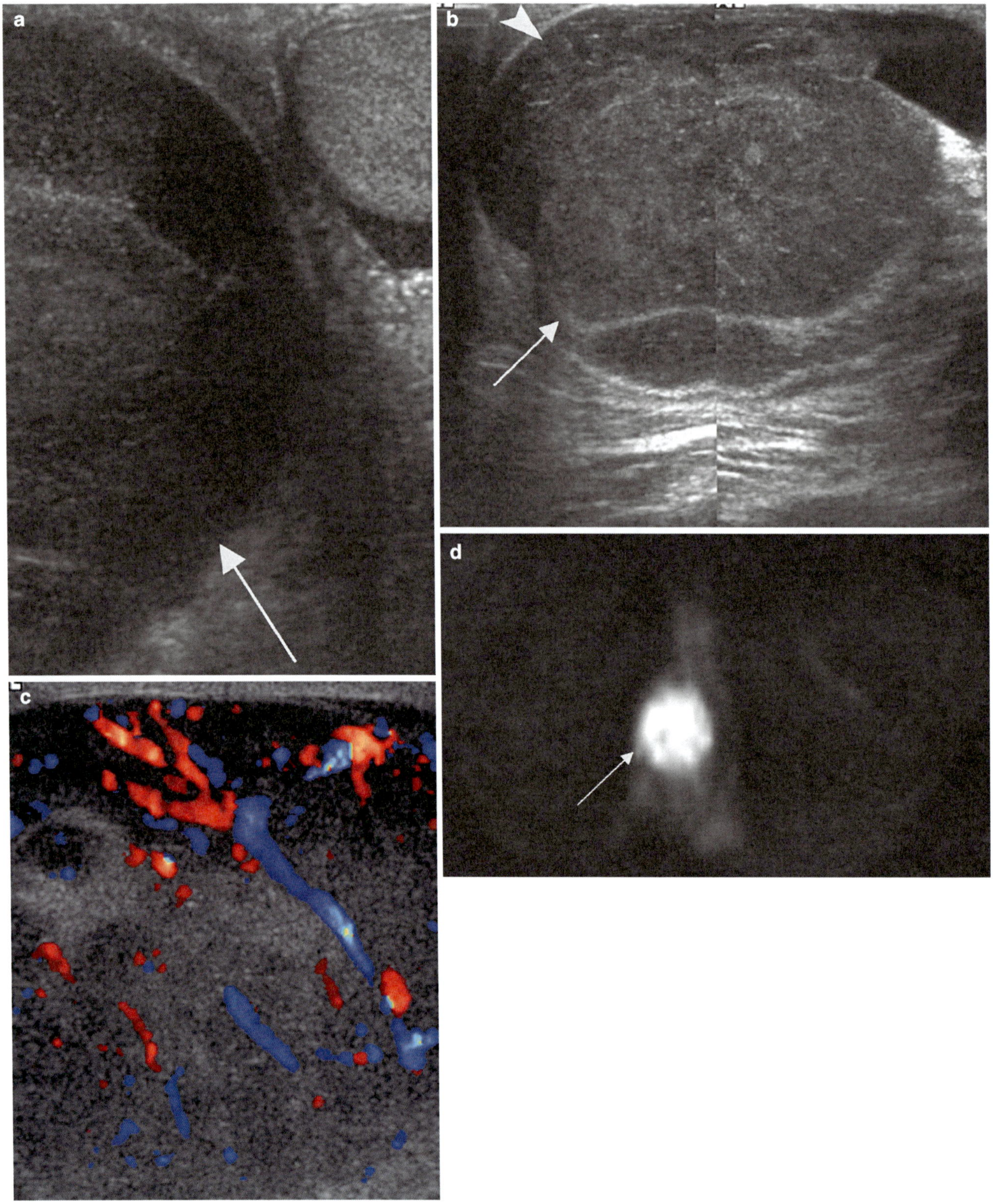

Fig. 6.20 Lymphoma relapse in testis. A 60-year-old patient with a history of treated primary central nervous system lymphoma now presents with an enlarged painless right testis. (**a**) Grayscale ultrasound image of both testes shows an asymmetrically enlarged right testis (*arrow*). Grayscale (**b**) and color Doppler (**c**) images of the right testis (*arrow* in **b**) show it is diffusely hypoechoic with increased vascularity. Infiltrating hypoechoic tumor is also seen in the right epididymis (*arrowhead* in **b**). (**d**) Axial image from a PET scan performed for staging demonstrated a hypermetabolic right testicular mass (*arrow*) with no evidence of recurrent hypermetabolic tumor in the brain or lymph nodes. Orchiectomy revealed a diffuse large B cell lymphoma in the testis and epididymis

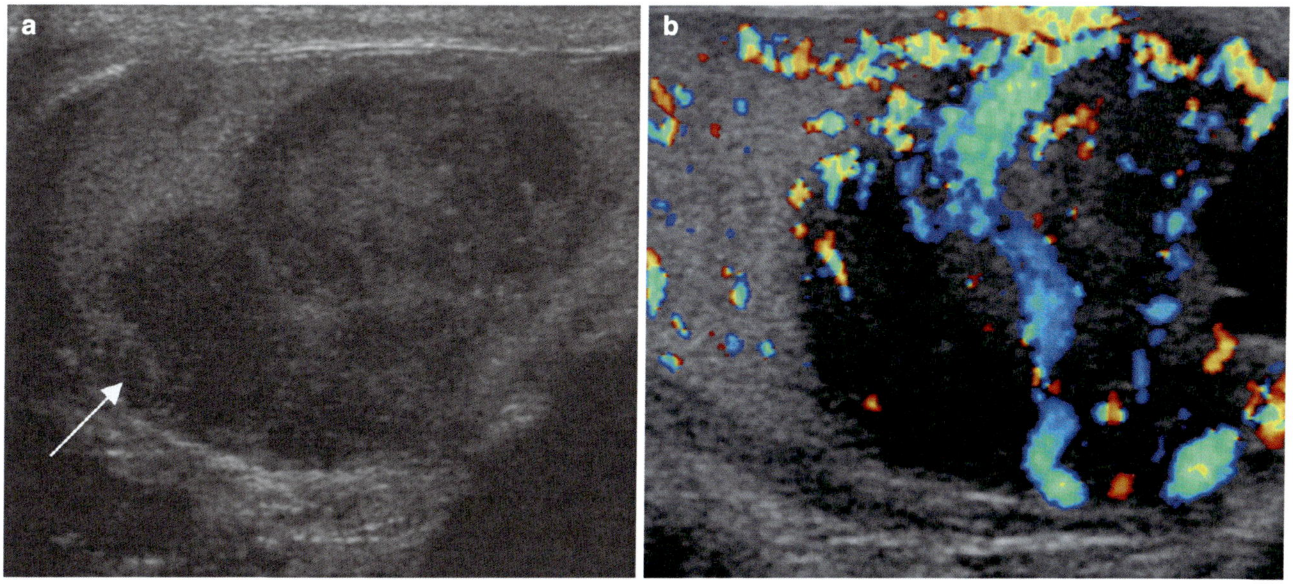

Fig. 6.21 Sex cord stromal tumor, unclassified type. A 75-year-old patient presented with a painless right testicular mass. Grayscale (**a**) and color Doppler (**b**) ultrasound images of the right testis show a lobulated hypoechoic testicular mass (*arrow* in **a**) with appreciable internal vascularity. Orchiectomy revealed an unclassified sex cord stromal tumor. No further treatment was given and the patient was disease free 4 years later

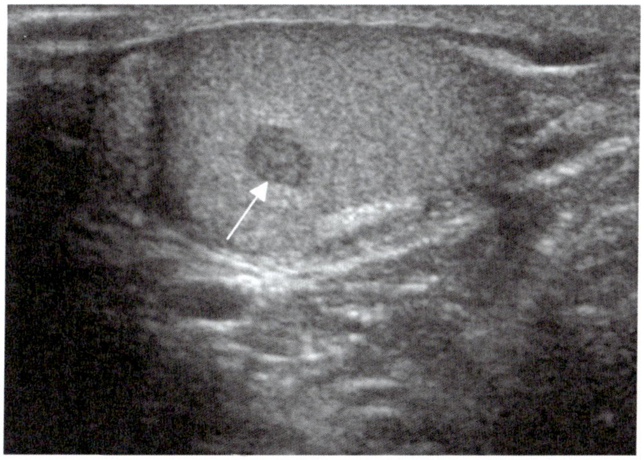

Fig. 6.22 Sex cord stromal tumor, Leydig cell type. A 25-year-old patient who had a scrotal ultrasound for testicular discomfort. Grayscale ultrasound image of the right testis shows a small hypoechoic mass (*arrow*) that proved to be a 0.6 cm Leydig cell tumor at pathology. Sex cord stromal tumors are usually hypoechoic masses that have well-defined margins. Leydig cell tumors have a variable appearance and may have hemorrhage and necrosis [4, 15]

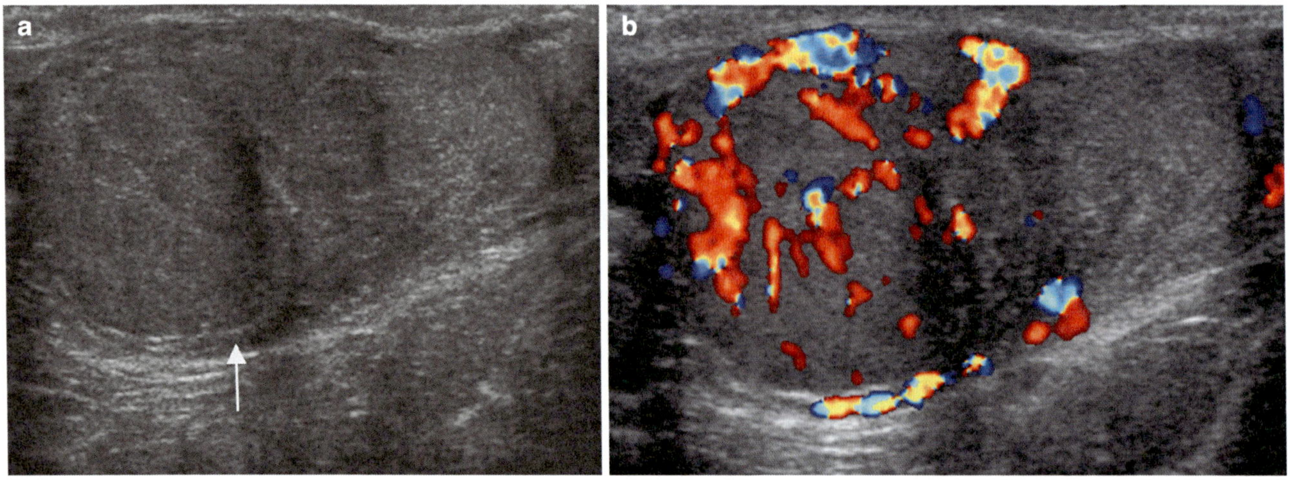

Fig. 6.23 Sex cord stromal tumor, Leydig cell type. A 55-year-old patient who presented with a firm palpable testicular mass. Grayscale (**a**) and color Doppler ultrasound (**b**) images of the right testis show a lobulated hypoechoic mass (*arrow* in **a**) with internal vascularity. The mass expanded the testicle and had echogenic bands probably due to fibrosis. Pathology showed Leydig cell tumor

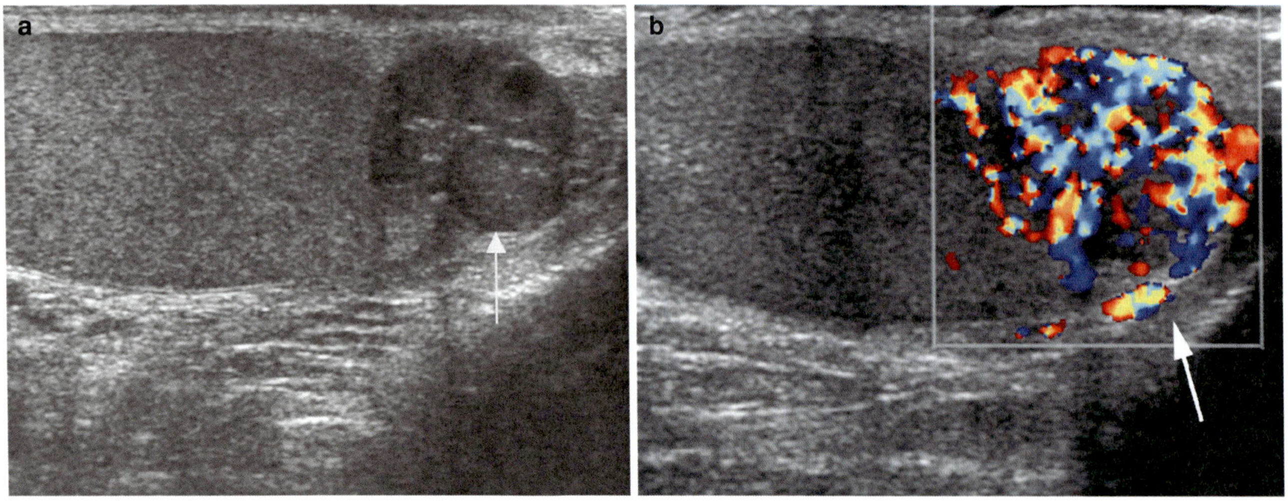

Fig. 6.24 Sex cord stromal tumor, Leydig cell type. A 60-year-old patient with a prior history of left orchiectomy for undescended testis now presents with a right testicular mass. Grayscale (**a**) and color Doppler ultrasound (**b**) images of the right testis show a well-defined hypoechoic exophytic right testicular mass (*arrow*) with significant internal vascularity. The mass was a 1.2 cm Leydig cell tumor at pathology that penetrated, but did not perforate, the tunica albuginea

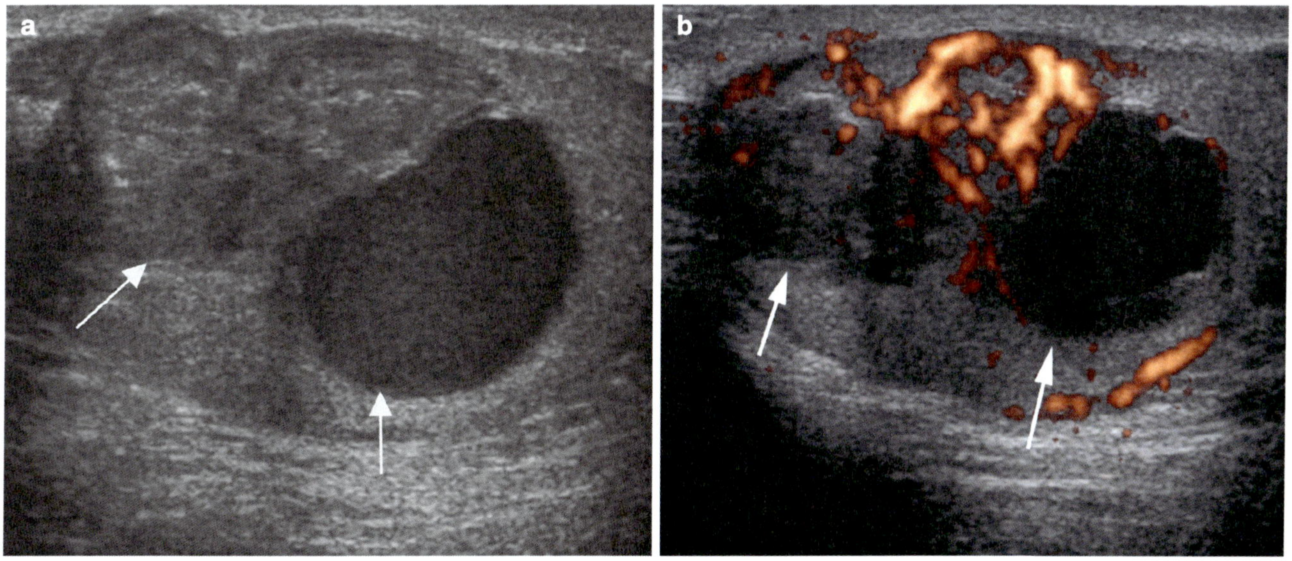

Fig. 6.25 Sex cord stromal tumor, Sertoli cell type. A 20-year-old patient presented with a palpable mass. Grayscale (**a**) and color Doppler ultrasound (**b**) images of the right testis show a lobulated mixed solid and cystic mass (*arrows*) replacing most of the right testis and distorting the capsule. Orchiectomy revealed a 3.2 cm Sertoli cell tumor with a solid component and a unilocular cyst with serous fluid. There was no extratesticular extension of the tumor

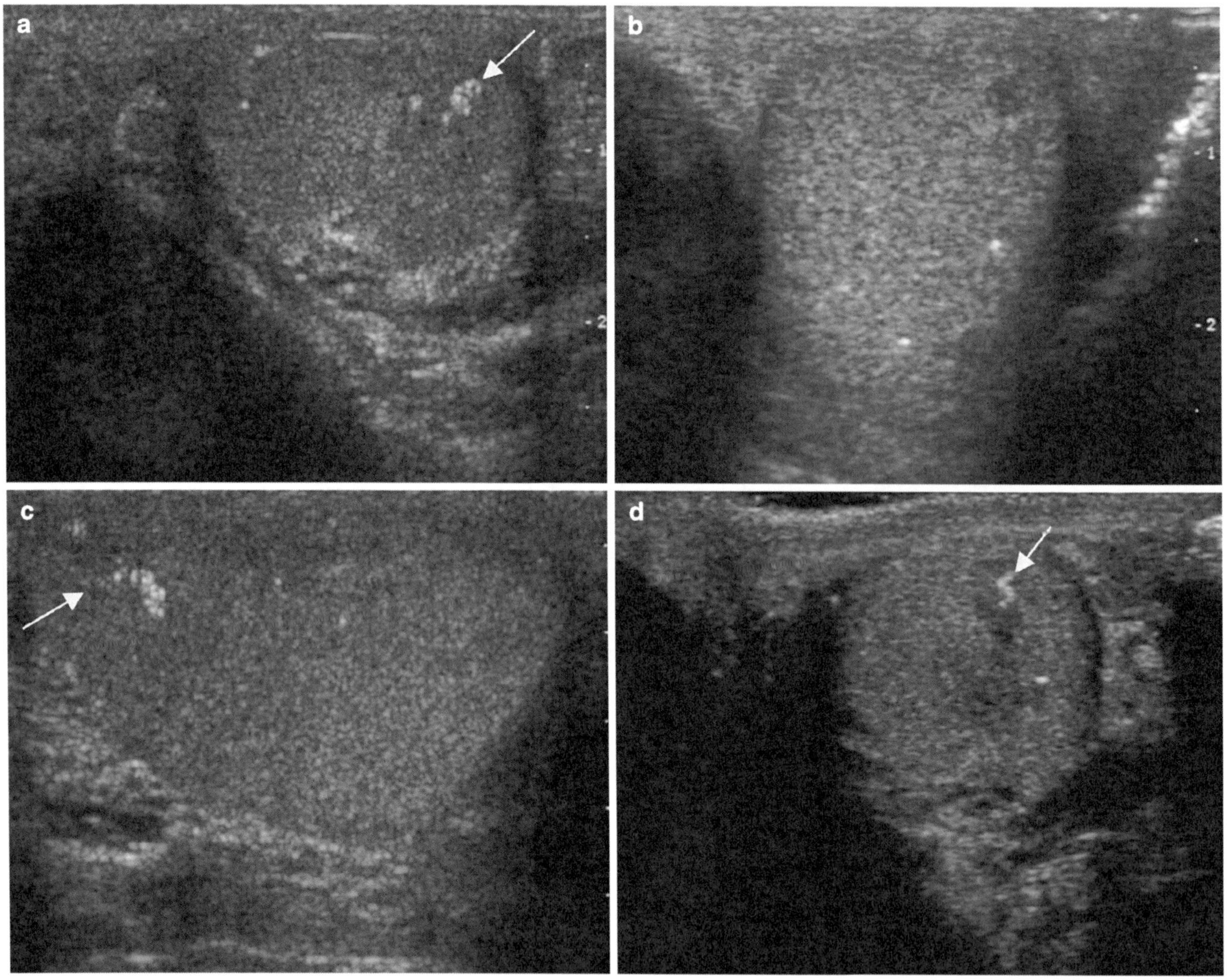

Fig. 6.26 Sex cord stromal tumor, large-cell calcifying Sertoli cell type. A teenager presented with an enlarged testis on physical examination. Ultrasound revealed bilateral calcified testicular masses, more numerous on the right (*not shown*). There was no evidence of metastatic disease at staging CT of the abdomen. The decision was made to perform a right orchiectomy, intraoperative biopsy of the left testicular masses, and left orchiectomy if malignancy was demonstrated at biopsy. Pathology from both testes revealed a Sertoli cell tumor of the large cell calcifying type. Grayscale ultrasound images of the left testis (**a–c**) show coarse calcifications and small hypoechoic masses of the biopsy proven calcifying Sertoli cell tumor (*arrows*) that were stable at 1-year follow-up (**d**). Large-cell calcifying Sertoli cell tumor usually appears as multiple bilateral masses with prominent calcifications. It is associated with Peutz-Jeghers Syndrome and Carney Syndrome. Benign tumors occur in pediatric age patients but can be malignant in older patients [4, 15]

Nodal Pathway of Disease

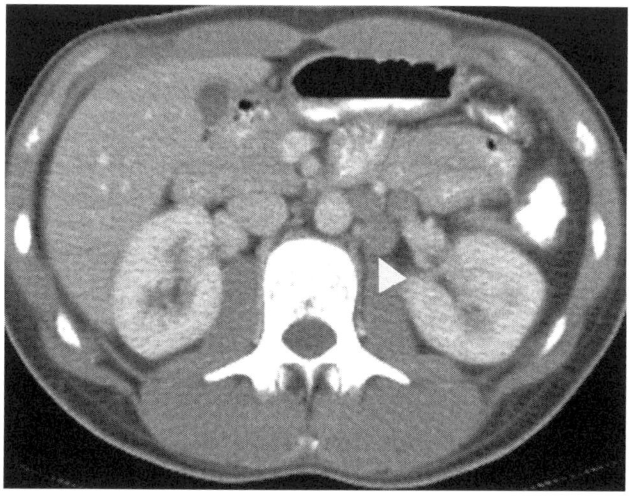

Fig. 6.27 Nodal landing site from a tumor of the left testis. Axial CT image of the abdomen with oral and intravenous contrast in a patient with a left testicular tumor shows adenopathy in the left paraaortic distribution (*arrowhead*) below the level of the left renal vessels. The left para-aortic and preaortic regions are the expected landing sites for a left testicular tumor

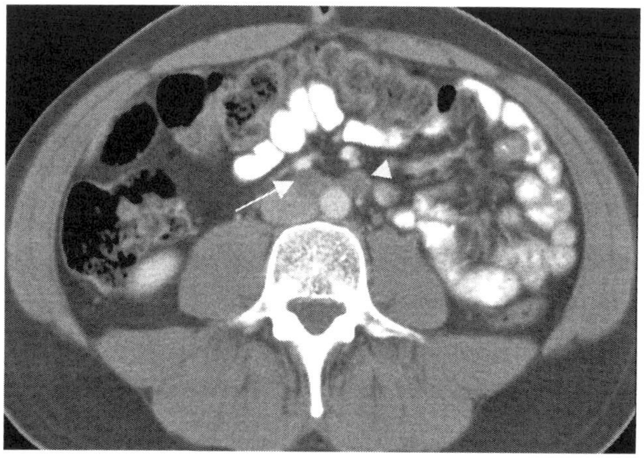

Fig. 6.29 Contralateral adenopathy from a tumor of the right testis. Axial CT image of the abdomen with oral and intravenous contrast in a patient with a right testicular tumor shows ipsilateral aortocaval node (*arrow*) and contralateral left para-aortic metastatic node (*arrowhead*)

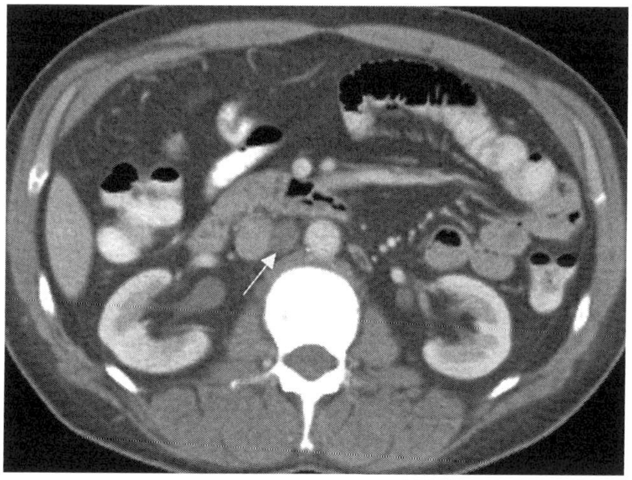

Fig. 6.28 Nodal landing site from a tumor of the right testis. Axial CT image of the abdomen with oral and intravenous contrast in a patient with a right testicular tumor shows adenopathy below the level of the renal vessels in the interaortocaval region (*arrow*). The aortocaval, precaval, and paracaval regions are the expected landing sites for a right testicular tumor

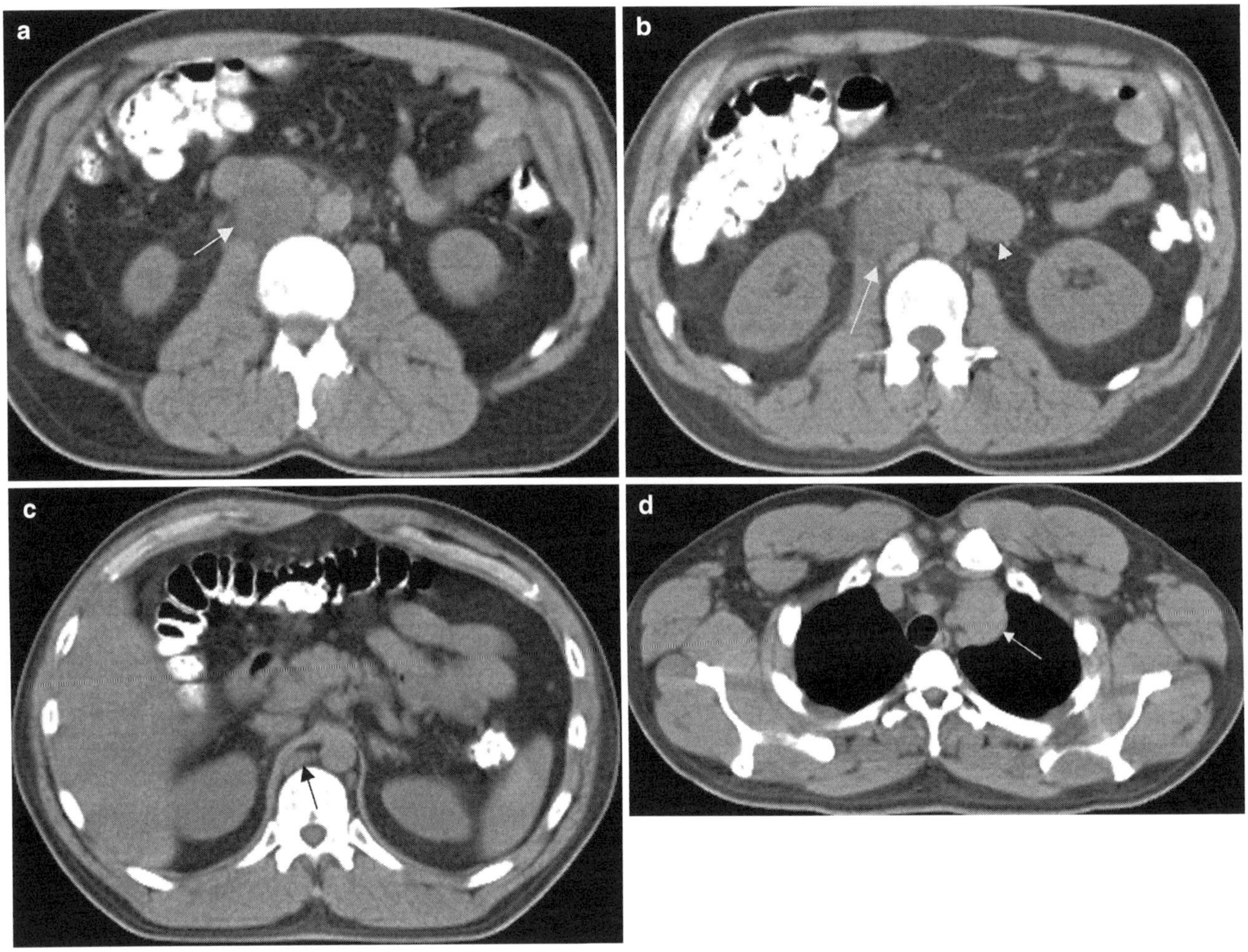

Fig. 6.30 Nodal landing site from a tumor of the right testis and nodal pathway of spread of disease. Cephalad extension of nodal disease is along the thoracic duct to the retrocrural, subcarinal, and prevascular regions of the chest. Axial CT images of the abdomen and chest with oral contrast in a patient with a right testicular tumor. (**a**) CT image at the level of the lower poles of the kidneys shows an enlarged ipsilateral retrocaval (*arrow*) node below the level of the renal vessels. (**b**) CT image at the level of the mid kidneys shows ipsilateral aortocaval (*arrow*) and contralateral left paraaortic (*arrowhead*) adenopathy. (**c**), CT image at the level of the diaphragm shows an enlarged retrocrural node (*arrow*). (**d**) Further superiorly, CT image at the level of the superior mediastinum shows an enlarged prevascular node (*arrow*)

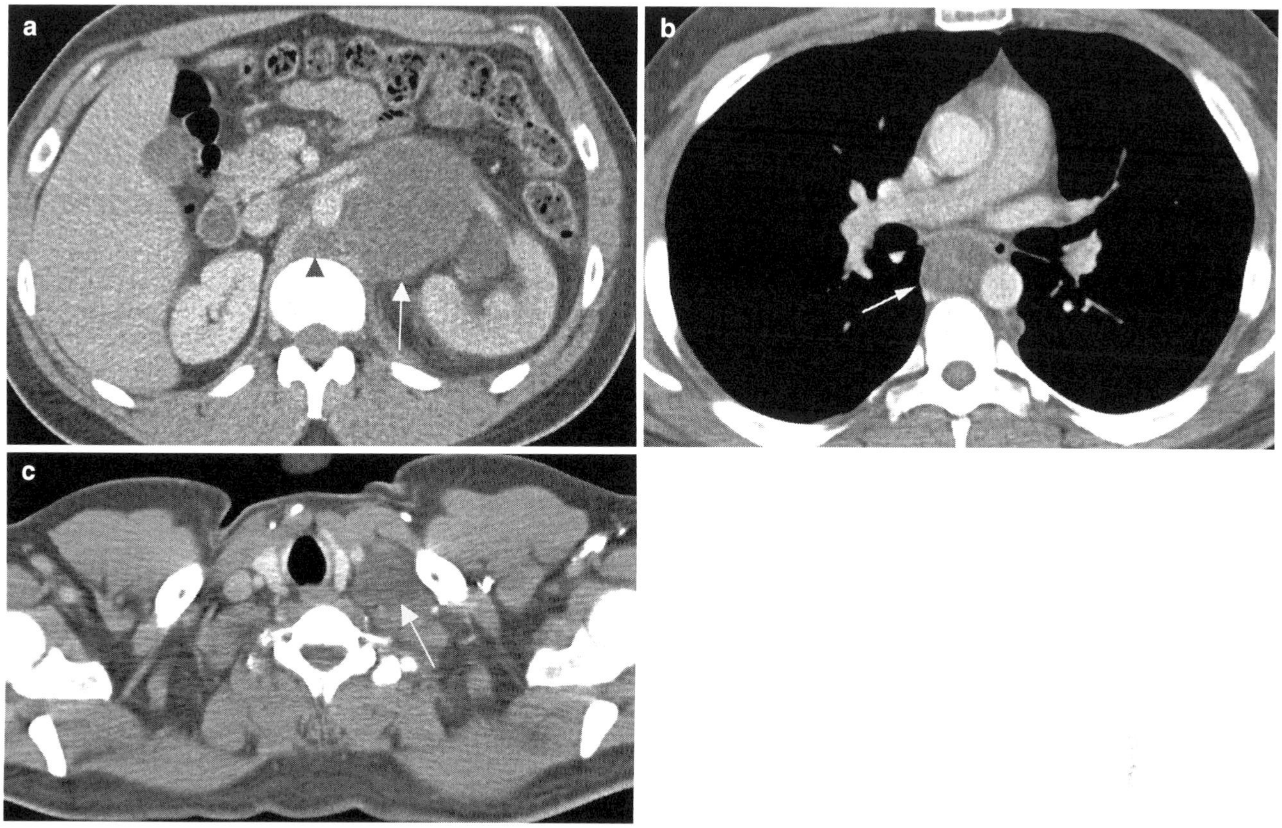

Fig. 6.31 Nodal pathway of spread of disease. Cephalad extension of nodal disease to the posterior mediastinal and left supraclavicular regions of the chest. Axial CT images of the chest and abdomen with intravenous contrast in a patient with a left testicular tumor. (**a**) CT image at the level of the kidneys shows left para-aortic adenopathy (*arrow*) extending into the retro-aortic region and posterior to the right crus of the diaphragm (*arrowhead*). (**b**) CT image below the level of the carina shows enlarged posterior mediastinal nodes (*arrow*). (**c**) CT image at the level of the upper thorax shows an enlarged left supraclavicular node (*arrow*)

Nodal Stages

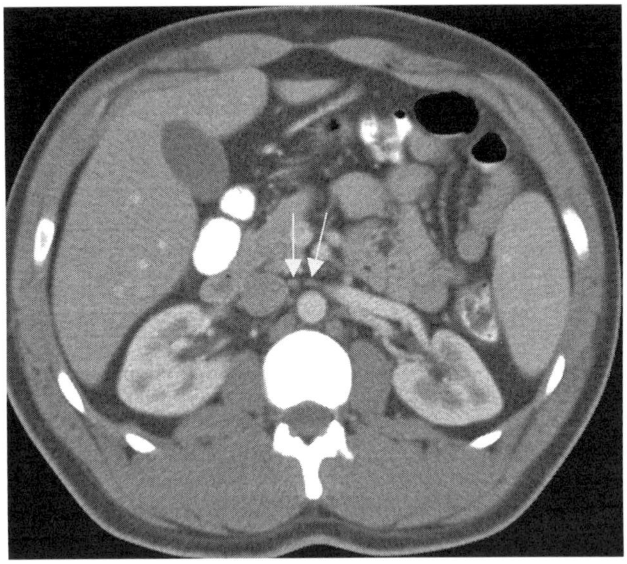

Fig. 6.32 N1 disease. Axial CT image of the abdomen with oral and intravenous contrast in a patient with a right testicular tumor shows subcentimeter aortocaval nodes (*arrows*) that were resected and positive for tumor at pathology. Nodes were less than 2 cm in size, meeting the criteria for N1 disease

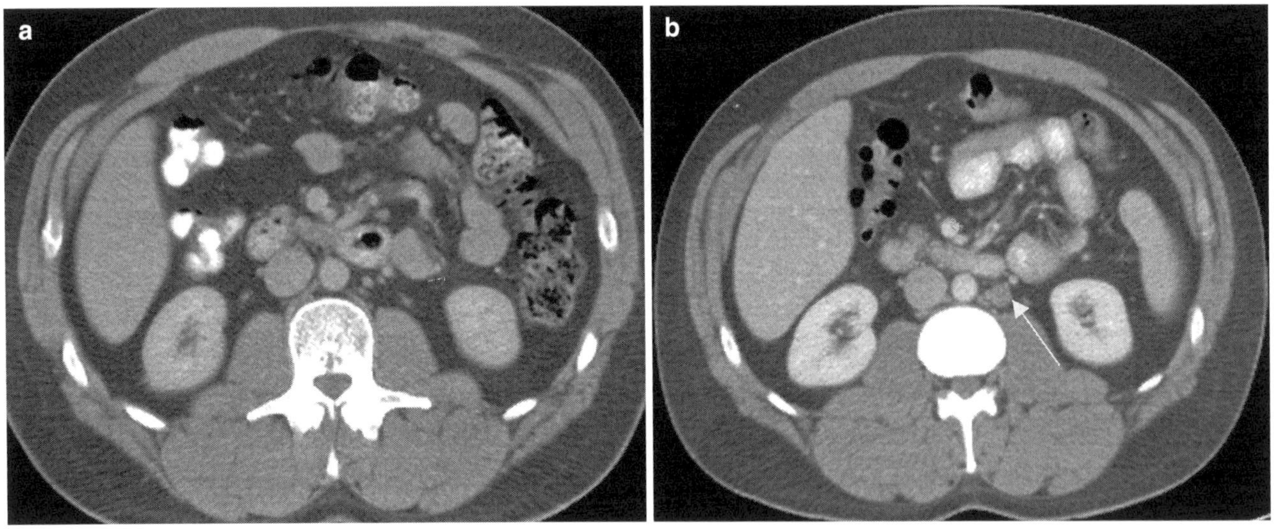

Fig. 6.33 N1 disease. Axial CT images of the abdomen with oral and intravenous contrast in a patient with a left testicular tumor. (**a**) Initial CT at the time of cancer diagnosis shows subcentimeter left paraaortic nodes that are normal by size criteria. (**b**) Follow-up CT 1 month later shows increased size of a left para-aortic node (*arrow*) that is suspicious for metastatic disease

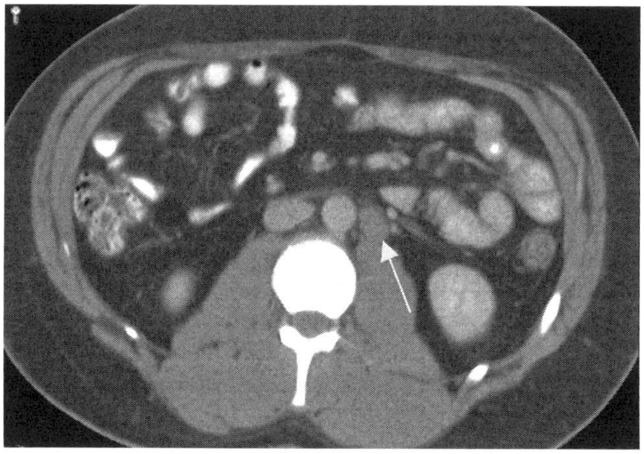

Fig. 6.34 N2 disease. Axial CT image of the abdomen with oral and intravenous contrast in a patient with a left testicular tumor. There is an enlarged left para-aortic node (*arrow*) suspicious for metastatic disease. The node is greater than 2 cm, but less than 5 cm in size, meeting the criteria for N2 disease

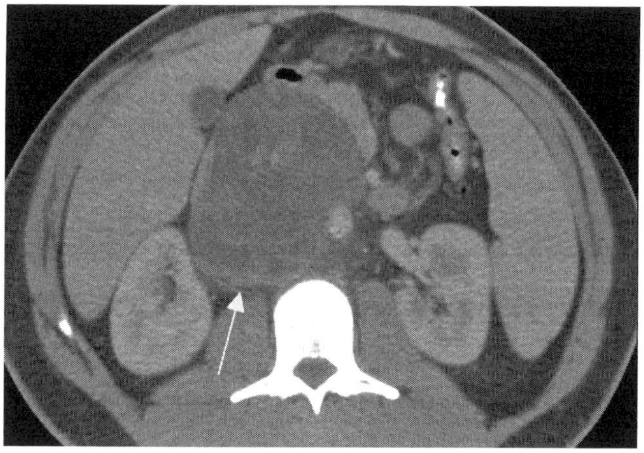

Fig. 6.35 N3 disease. Axial CT image of the abdomen with oral and intravenous contrast in a patient with a right testicular tumor. There is an enlarged paracaval node (*arrow*) suspicious for metastatic disease. The node is larger than 5 cm in size, meeting the criteria for N3 disease

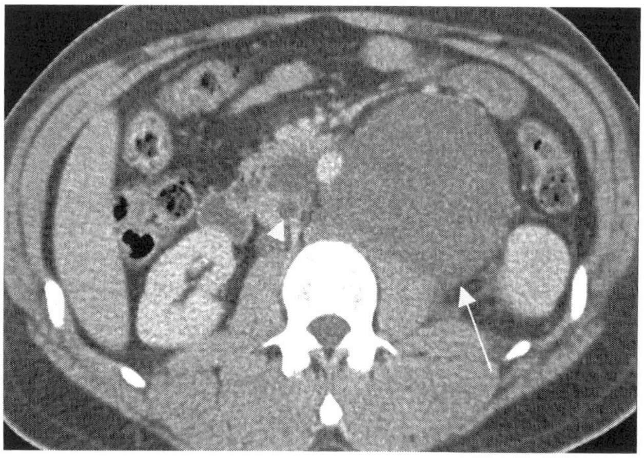

Fig. 6.36 Invasive nodes. Axial CT image of the abdomen with intravenous contrast in a patient with a left testicular tumor. There is an enlarged left para-aortic node (*arrow*) suspicious for metastatic disease. The node extends posterior to the aorta and invades the inferior vena cava (IVC), which has a nonocclusive hypodense thrombus (*arrowhead*). The caval mass was resected and proved to be metastatic mature teratoma

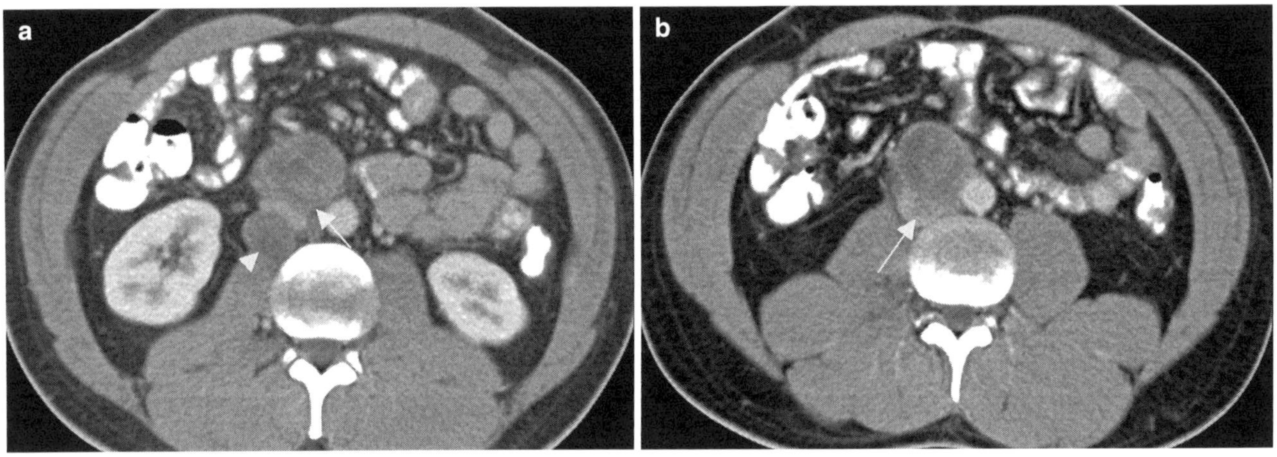

Fig. 6.37 Invasive nodes. Axial CT images of the abdomen with oral and intravenous contrast in a patient with a right testicular tumor. (**a**) There are enlarged paracaval (*arrow*) and retrocaval (*arrowhead*) nodes encasing the IVC. (**b**) CT image at a different level shows invasion of the IVC by the node. Tumor abuts the anterior margin of the IVC and there is low attenuation tumor (*arrow*) within the enhanced vessel lumen

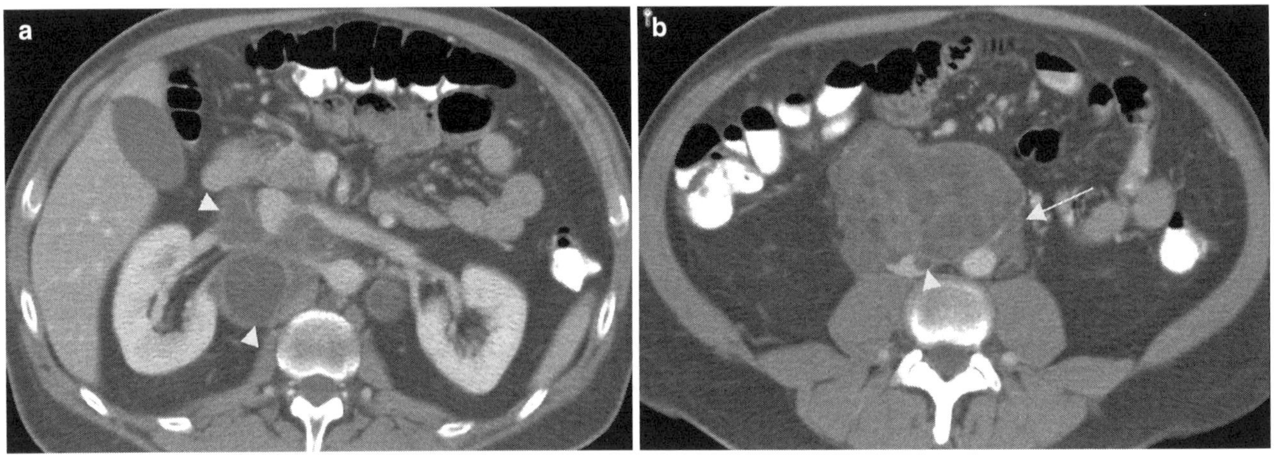

Fig. 6.38 Invasive nodes. Axial CT images of the abdomen with oral and intravenous contrast in a patient with a right testicular tumor. (**a**) Retrocaval (*arrowhead*) and paracaval (*arrowhead*) adenopathy encases the renal vessels. (**b**) Further inferiorly, there is bulky heterogeneous retroperitoneal adenopathy encasing the inferior mesenteric artery (*arrow*) and invading the IVC (*arrowhead*)

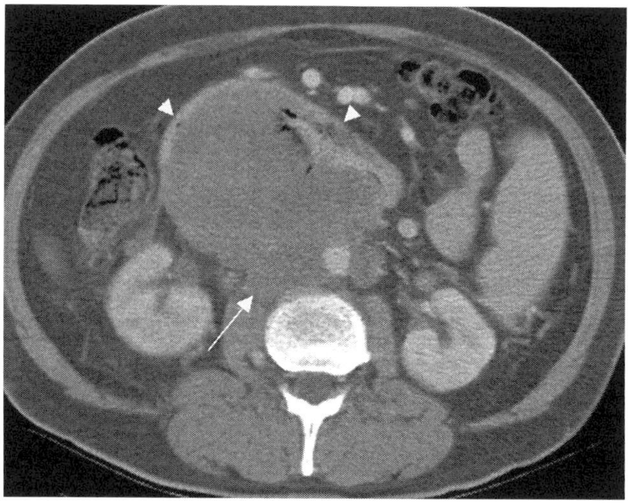

Fig. 6.39 Invasive nodes. Axial CT image of the abdomen with intravenous contrast in a patient with a right testicular tumor and bulky retroperitoneal adenopathy. The mass (*arrow*) encases and obliterates the IVC and is inseparable from the duodenum (*arrowheads*), which is displaced anteriorly. The patient developed an upper gastrointestinal bleed and endoscopy showed tumor infiltrating into, and obstructing, the duodenum. Biopsy of the mass demonstrated a poorly differentiated germ cell tumor with components of embryonal cell carcinoma and seminoma

Stages of Disease

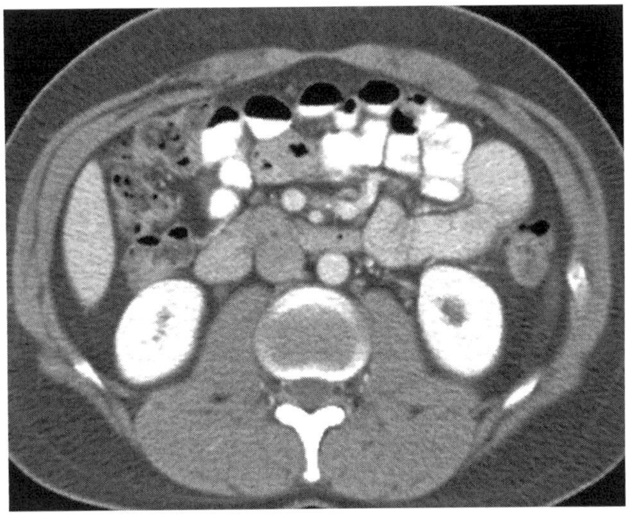

Fig. 6.40 Stage I seminoma. Axial CT image of the abdomen with oral and intravenous contrast in a patient with a 1 cm right testicular seminoma shows no adenopathy. The tumor was confined to the testis and meets the criteria for stage I disease

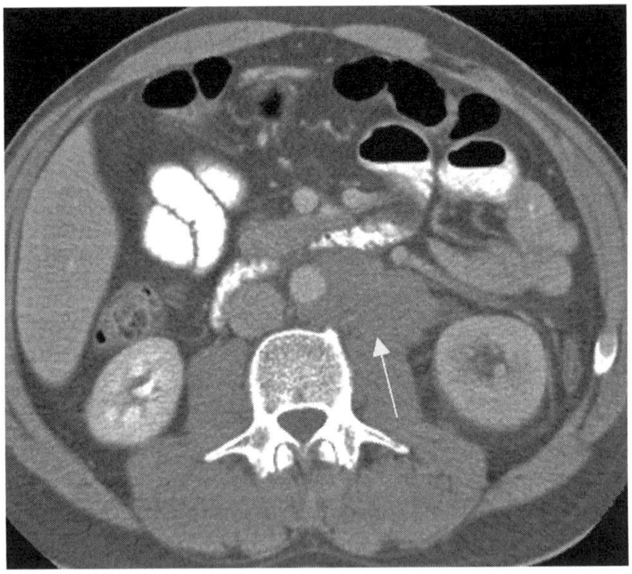

Fig. 6.41 Stage II seminoma. Axial CT image of the abdomen with oral and intravenous contrast in a patient with a left testicular seminoma shows an enlarged left para-aortic node (*arrow*). There was no nonregional adenopathy or distant metastatic disease and the patient met the criteria for stage II disease. The retroperitoneal node was larger than 5 cm and therefore was classified as stage IIC disease

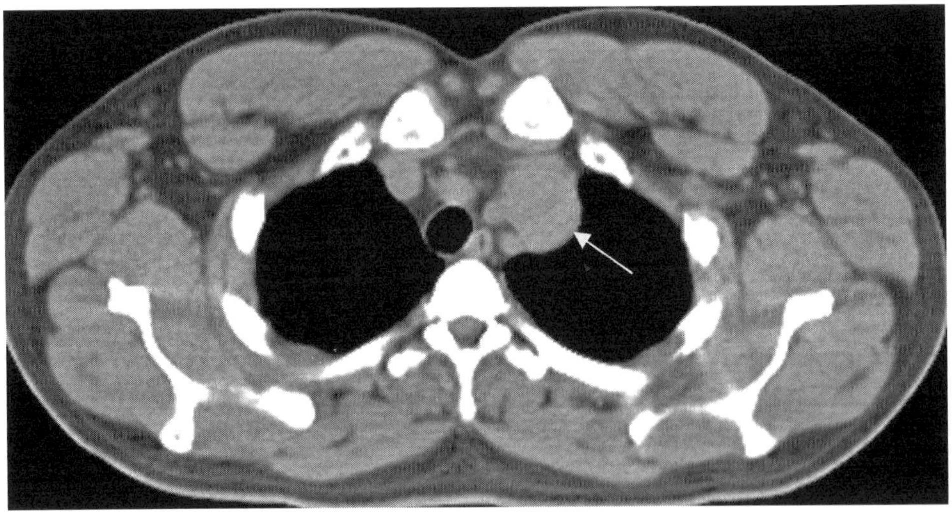

Fig. 6.42 Stage III seminoma. Axial CT image of the chest without intravenous contrast in a patient with a right testicular seminoma shows mediastinal adenopathy (*arrow*). Thoracic adenopathy is nonregional for testicular cancer and meets the criteria for stage III disease

Management of Stage I Disease

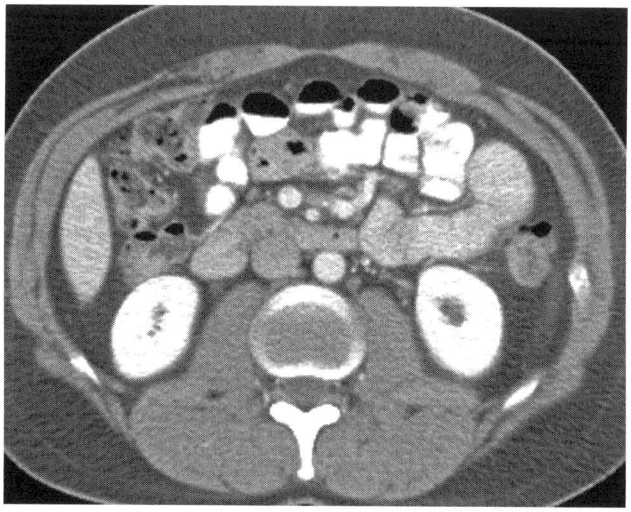

Fig. 6.43 Stage I seminoma managed with surveillance without recurrence. Axial CT image of the abdomen with oral and intravenous contrast in a patient with a 1 cm right testicular seminoma shows no adenopathy. The patient was considered low risk due to tumor subtype (seminoma), lack of vascular invasion at pathology, lack of elevation of tumor markers, and lack of symptoms. Follow-up was done with surveillance CT, which showed no development of adenopathy. Surveillance or radiation is performed for stage I seminoma rather than retroperitoneal node dissection. The majority (70–75 %) of patients with clinical stage I disease have no nodal metastases at retroperitoneal node dissection. A retroperitoneal relapse is rare in these patients [7]

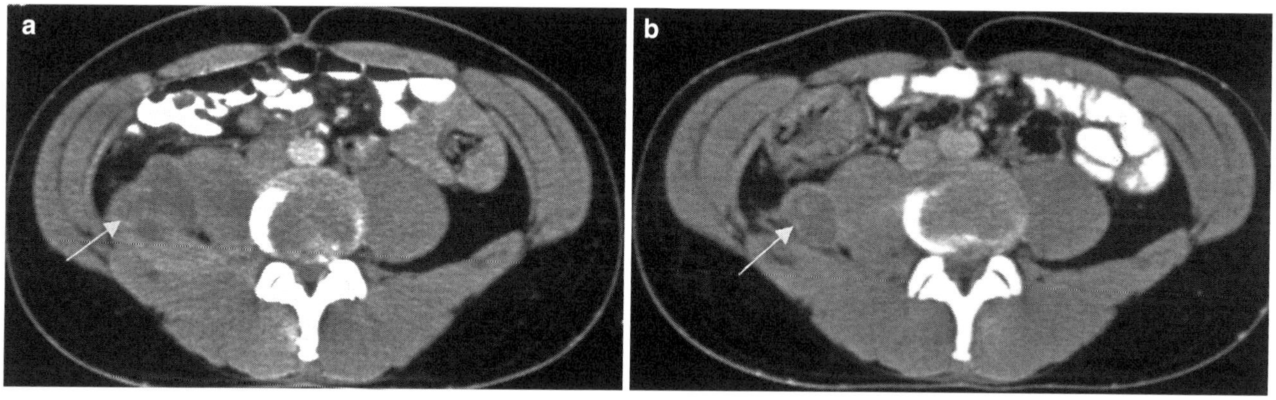

Fig. 6.44 Stage I seminoma managed with surveillance with retroperitoneal recurrence. Axial CT image of the abdomen with oral and intravenous contrast in a patient with a previous right orchiectomy for an 8 cm seminoma. The tumor had perforated the tunica albuginea and vascular invasion was also present. The patient was managed with surveillance and developed a para-aortic recurrence 1 year later for which he received radiation. Four years later, the patient had a rise in his tumor markers. CT (*not shown*) showed a mass adjacent to the right psoas muscle, which was metastatic seminoma at biopsy. The patient was given chemotherapy and the mass initially resolved but subsequently recurred 2 years later. (**a**) CT shows a necrotic recurrent tumor mass (*arrow*) adjacent to the right psoas. (**b**) Additional chemotherapy was given and the mass (*arrow*) decreased in size at follow-up CT. The residual mass was resected and consisted of necrotic tissue but no viable tumor

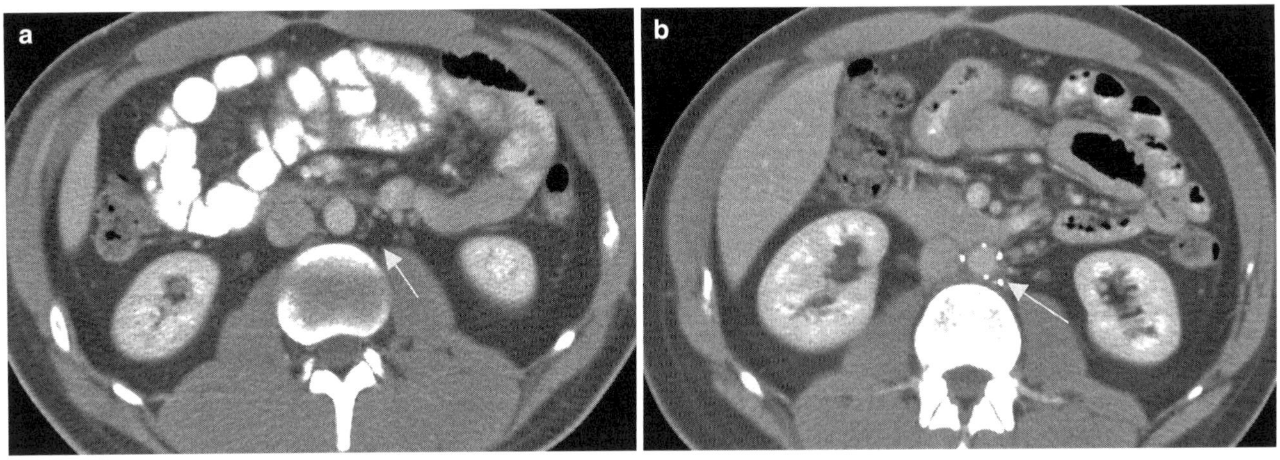

Fig. 6.45 Stage I NSGCT managed with retroperitoneal node dissection with benign nodes. Axial CT images of the abdomen with oral and intravenous contrast in a patient with a left testicular mixed germ cell tumor, mainly embryonal cell carcinoma subtype, with vascular invasion. (**a**) There were a few subcentimeter nodes (*arrow*) with fatty hila in the retroperitoneum. The patient was at high risk for recurrence (approximately 50 %) due to embryonal cell carcinoma subtype with vascular invasion and therefore elected to have a retroperitoneal node dissection in lieu of surveillance. All nodes were benign at surgery. (**b**) Postoperative CT shows left para-aortic (*arrow*), pre-aortic and aortocaval clips at the site of node resection, targeting nodes at the ipsilateral landing sites from a left testicular tumor. Approximately 20–30 % of patients who have clinical stage II A disease have negative nodes at pathology with a retroperitoneal node dissection. Retroperitoneal node dissection helps stratify patients for additional management. Patients with nodal metastases receive chemotherapy whereas those with negative nodes can have a less intensive follow-up regimen without the toxicity of chemotherapy [7]

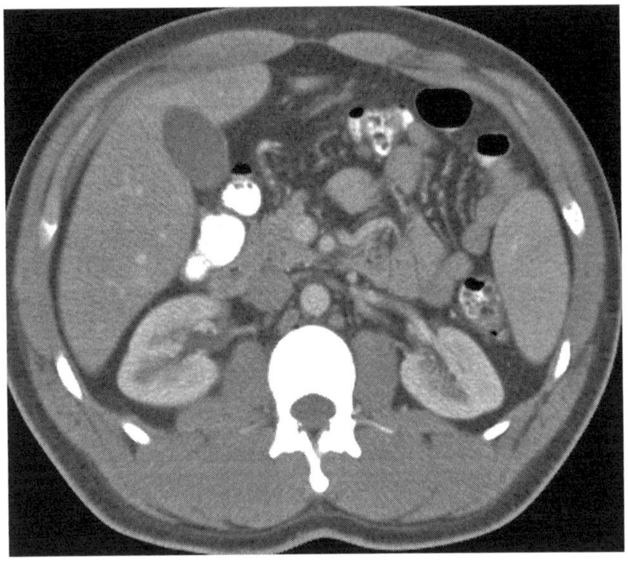

Fig. 6.46 Stage I NSGCT managed with retroperitoneal node dissection with malignant nodes. Axial CT image of the abdomen with oral and intravenous contrast in a patient with a right testicular pure embryonal cell carcinoma without vascular invasion. CT showed subcentimeter retroperitoneal nodes and the serum tumor marker levels were not elevated. However, the patient was at high risk for recurrence due to embryonal cell carcinoma subtype and therefore elected to have a retroperitoneal node dissection instead of surveillance. At pathology, one interaortocaval node was positive for tumor and the patient was subsequently also treated with chemotherapy. Approximately 20–30 % of patients are understaged by CT. For patients with clinical stage I disease who have nodal metastases at pathology, retroperitoneal node dissection is curative in the majority. If clinical stage I patients receive chemotherapy instead of retroperitoneal node dissection, a late relapse beyond 2 years occurs in a minority of patients [7]

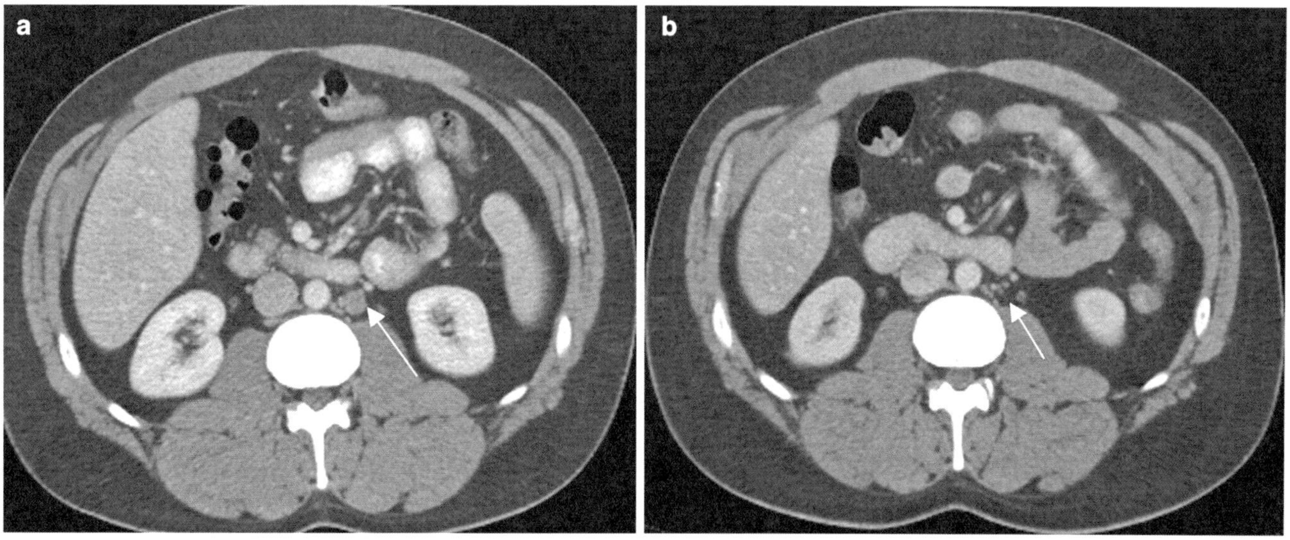

Fig. 6.47 Stage I NSGCT managed with surveillance with recurrence. Axial CT images of the abdomen with oral and intravenous contrast in a patient with a left testicular mixed germ cell tumor, mainly embryonal cell carcinoma subtype, with vascular invasion. (**a**) Surveillance CT less than 6 months after diagnosis shows a newly enlarged left para-aortic node (*arrow*). (**b**) Chemotherapy was administered and the node (*arrow*) decreased at follow-up CT 3 months later. Post-chemotherapy retroperitoneal node dissection showed fibrosis and necrosis in the nodes but no viable tumor. The patient had high-risk features for recurrence such as tumor subtype (embryonal cell carcinoma) and vascular invasion. For stage I patients who have a retroperitoneal node dissection, the risk of recurrent disease in the retroperitoneum is less than 2 %. In these patients, follow-up is focused on checking for lung metastases and serum tumor markers, with 90 % of recurrences occurring in the first year. If active surveillance is performed for clinical stage I disease, CT of the abdomen is included in the regimen, as approximately 25 % of patients will recur in the retroperitoneum [7]

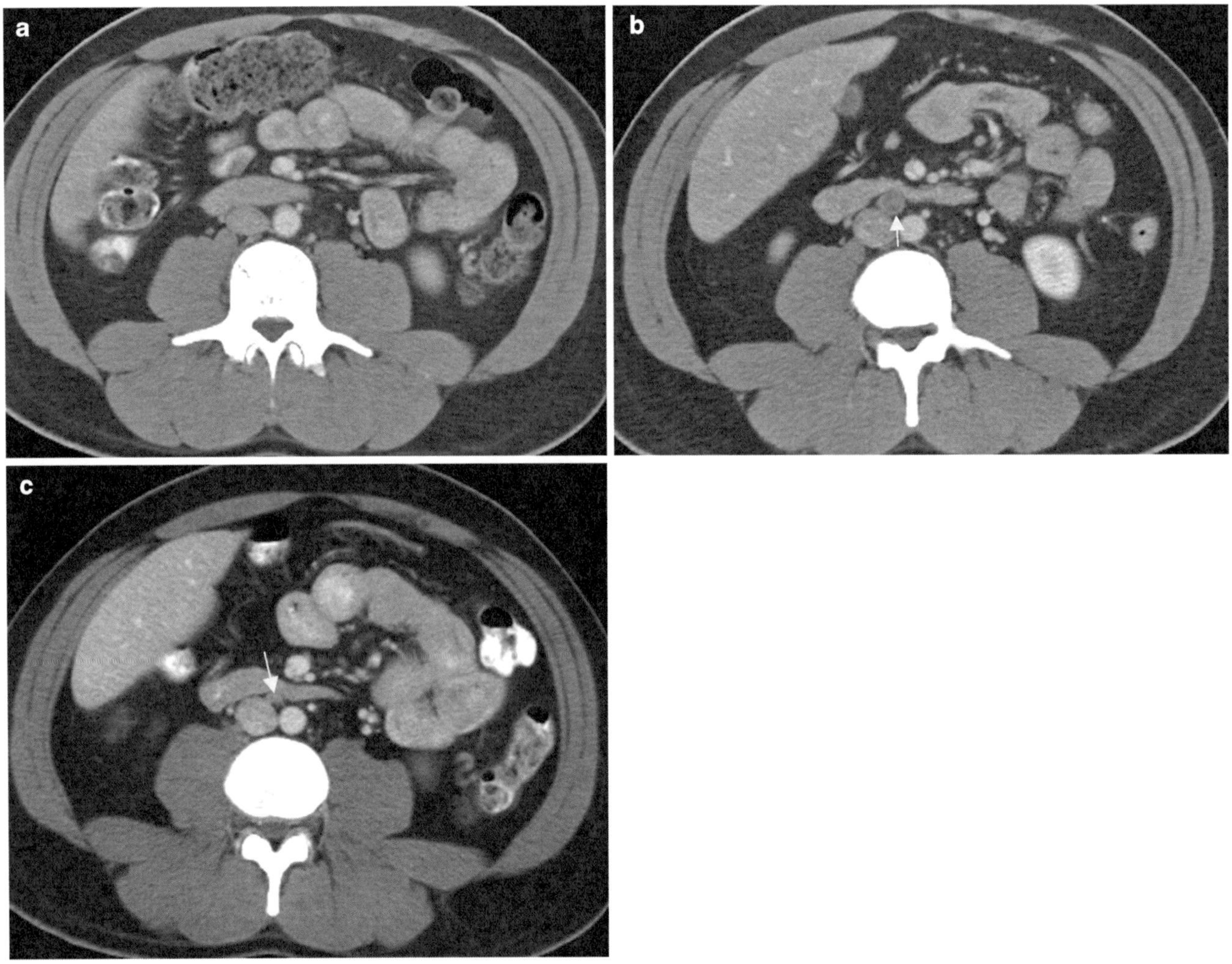

Fig. 6.48 Stage I NSGCT managed with surveillance with recurrence. Axial CT images of the abdomen with oral and intravenous contrast in a patient with a right testicular pure embryonal cell carcinoma with vascular invasion. Although the patient was at high risk for relapse, surveillance instead of retroperitoneal node dissection was performed as the patient had had previous inguinal surgery, which could have altered the lymphatic drainage pathway of the testis. (**a**) CT image at the time of diagnosis of testicular cancer showed no retroperitoneal adenopathy. (**b**) CT performed 1 year later showed a new aortocaval node (*arrow*). The patient also had elevated tumor marker levels at this time. Chemotherapy was given and follow-up CT (**c**) 2 months later showed the node (*arrow*) had decreased in size. A retroperitoneal node dissection was performed at this time and, at pathology, the nodes had mature teratoma and fibrosis

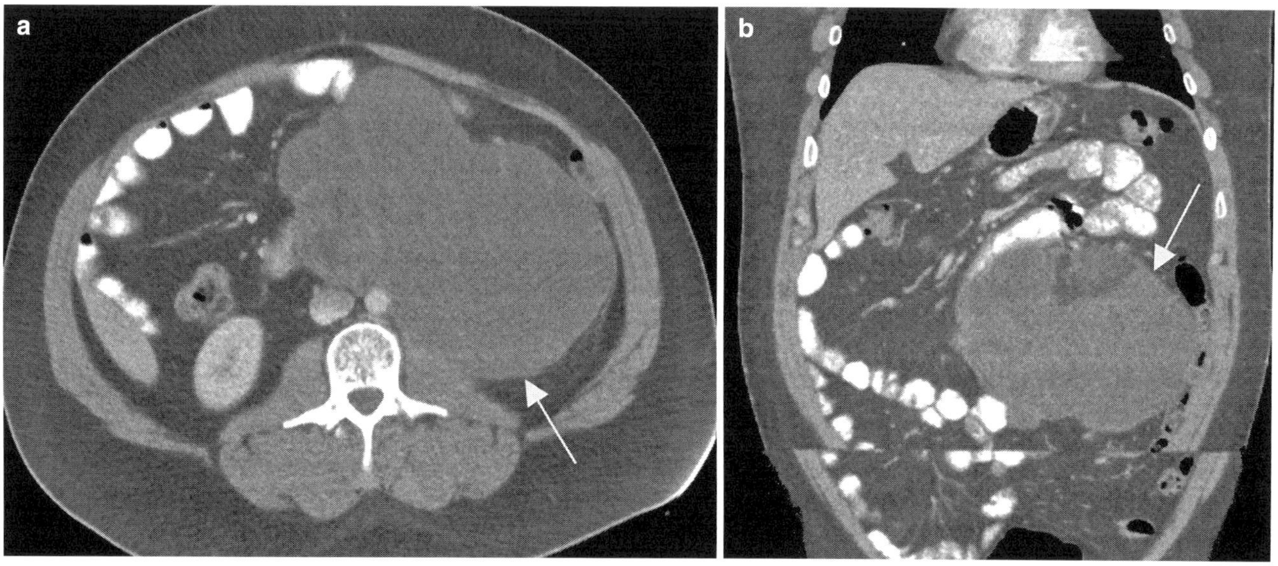

Fig. 6.49 Stage I NSGCT managed with surveillance with recurrence. CT images of the abdomen with oral and intravenous contrast in a patient with a history of bilateral testicular tumors. The patient had undergone left orchiectomy for a seminoma 5 years earlier followed by prophylactic radiation therapy to the retroperitoneum. Three years later, the patient had a right orchiectomy for a mixed germ cell tumor, predominantly embryonal cell carcinoma with vascular invasion. The patient was placed on surveillance and developed abdominal pain and elevated tumor markers 22 months later. CT (*not shown*) demonstrated a tumor recurrence with a 25 cm retroperitoneal mass and the patient was treated with chemotherapy. Post-therapy axial (**a**) and coronal (**b**) CT images demonstrated a large cystic residual mass (*arrows*) in the retroperitoneum. Resection of this residual mass showed metastatic germ cell tumor with a component of teratoma and a component of secondary somatic malignancy of rhabdomyosarcoma. The majority (90 %) of the mass was necrotic whereas the remainder contained viable tumor

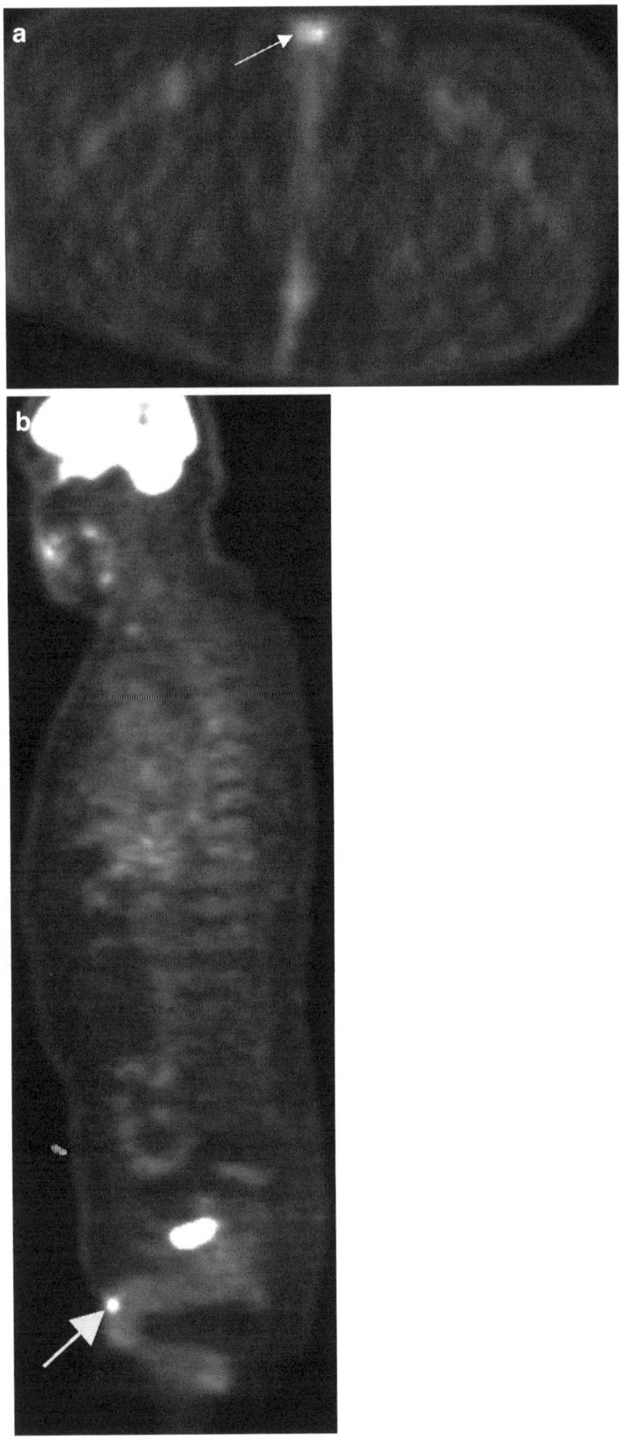

Fig. 6.50 Late recurrence of stage I seminoma in the penis. Axial and sagittal PET-CT images in a patient who underwent orchiectomy for seminoma 2 years earlier and received prophylactic radiation therapy to the retroperitoneum. He was doing well till he developed penile mass. Excisional biopsy revealed seminoma. PET-CT showed no other site of disease. Chemotherapy was administered and he has been free of disease for 3 years. PET-CT axial (**a**) and sagittal (**b**) images show focal increased uptake in the penile region (*arrows*)

Management of Stage II Disease

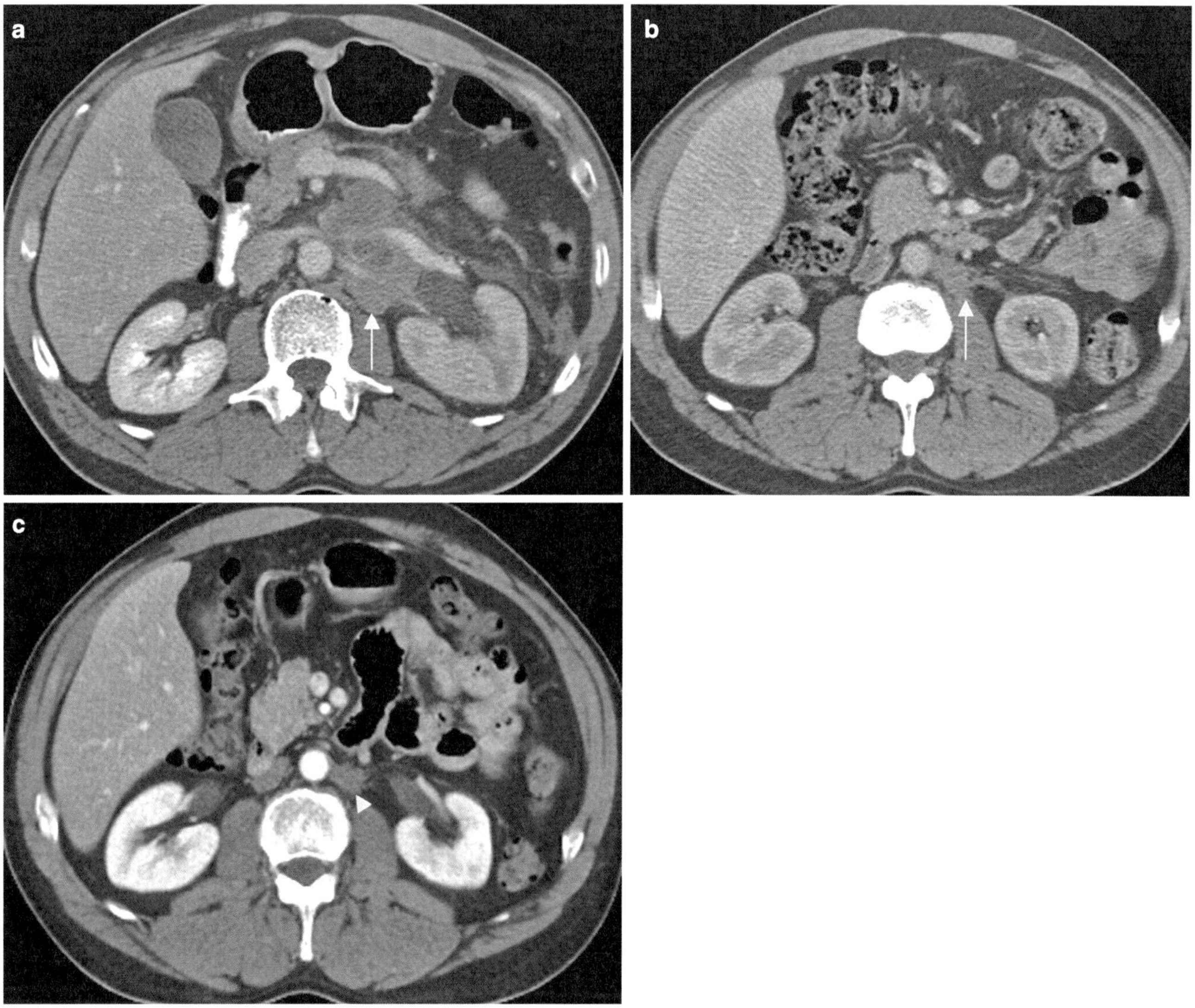

Fig. 6.51 Stage IIC seminoma with surveillance after chemotherapy. Axial CT images of the abdomen with oral and intravenous contrast in a patient with a left testicular seminoma and retroperitoneal metastasis. Pre-treatment scan (**a**) shows left para-aortic adenopathy (*arrow*) extending up to the level of the left renal hilum. The patient was given chemotherapy and the adenopathy has decreased. Post-therapy scans (**b**) and (**c**) show a small amount of residual soft tissue adjacent to the left renal vein (*arrow* in **B**) and in the left para-aortic region (*arrowhead* in **C**). This residual soft tissue was not FDG avid at PET-CT and remained unchanged at 1-year follow-up scan. The findings are probably due to a desmoplastic reaction without viable tumor and the patient is on continued surveillance. In contrast to patients with NSGCT, residual masses in patients with seminoma consist of necrotic tissue in 90 % of cases and a retroperitoneal node dissection is not particularly helpful. Surgery is also challenging as there is usually a significant desmoplastic reaction. Teratoma is rare in patients with seminoma, whereas viable tumor is found in 10 % of cases. Balancing the low likelihood of residual tumor with the difficulty of surgery, residual masses in patients with seminoma are typically observed unless the residual mass is large [7]

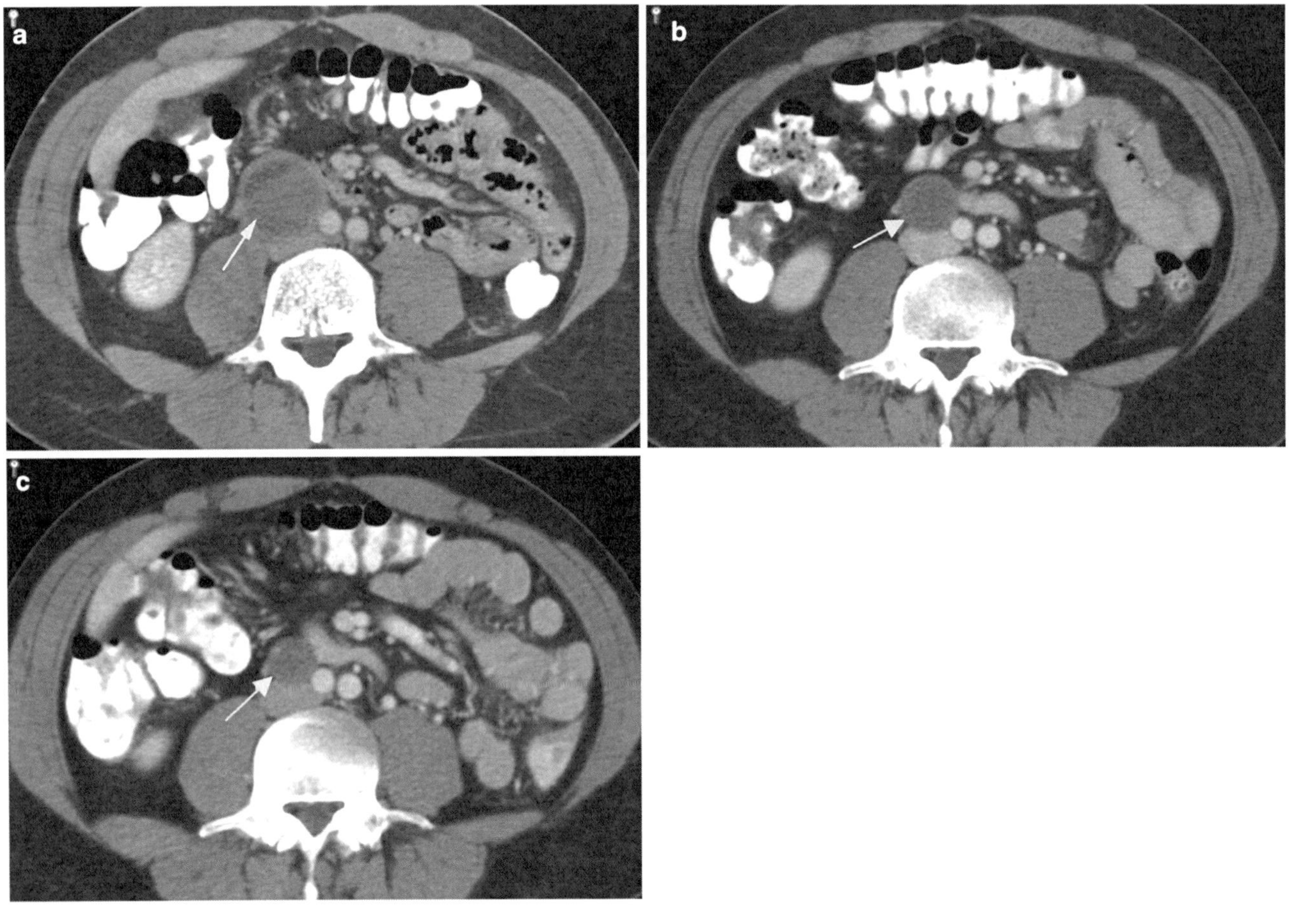

Fig. 6.52 Stage II seminoma with a stable residual retroperitoneal mass after chemotherapy. Axial CT images of the abdomen with oral and intravenous contrast in a patient with a right testicular seminoma and retroperitoneal metastasis at presentation. (**a**) CT at time of diagnosis shows a thick walled cystic precaval mass (*arrow*) that was metastatic germ cell tumor. Follow-up CT after completion of chemotherapy (**b**) and 2 years later (**c**) show the mass (*arrows*) decreased slightly in size and remained stable thereafter. There was no increased FDG activity noted at PET-CT (*not shown*). The majority of residual masses in patients with seminoma consist of fibrotic tissue without active tumor or teratoma and are therefore observed

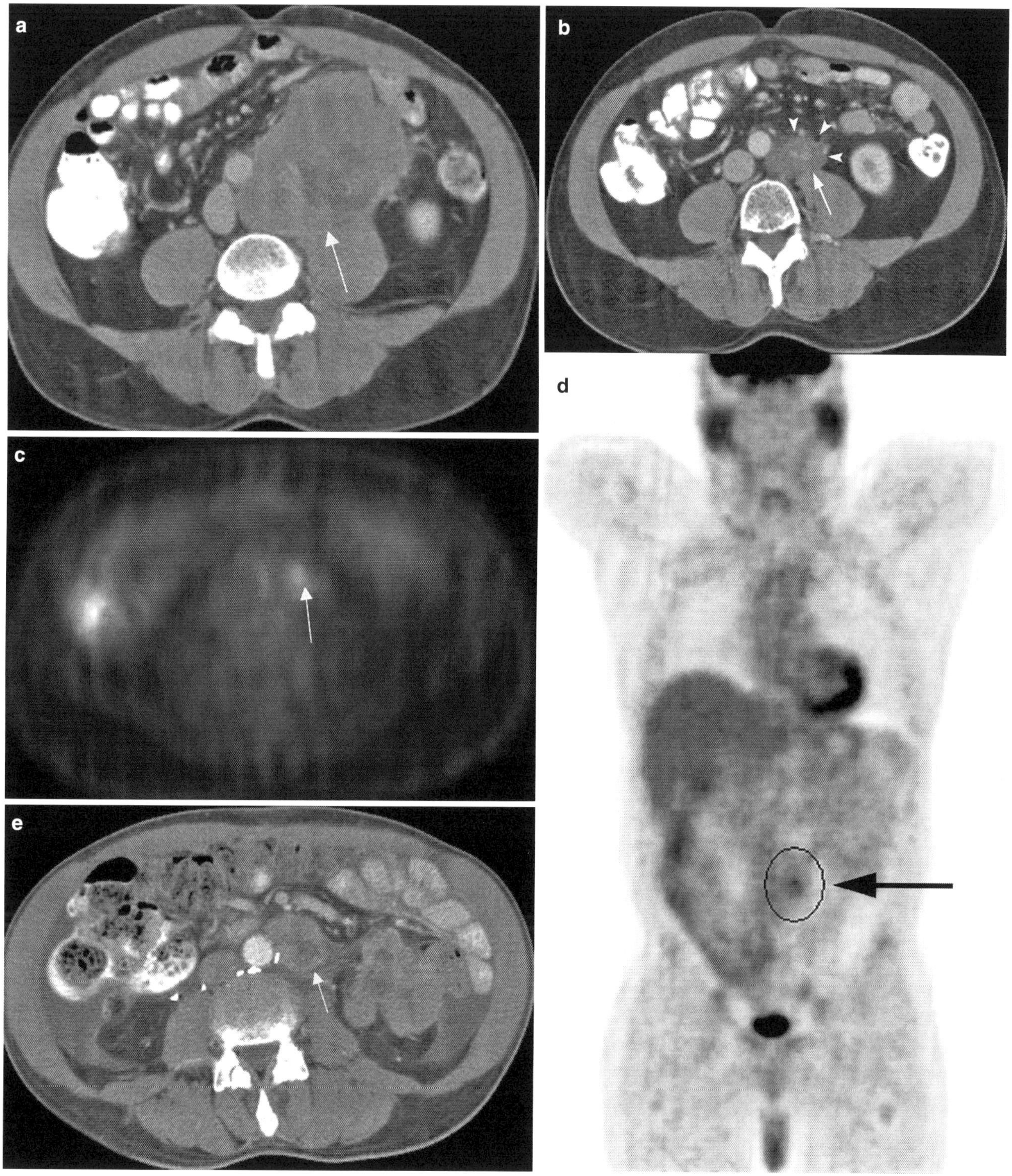

Fig. 6.53 Stage IIC seminoma with residual retroperitoneal metastasis after chemotherapy. Axial CT images of the abdomen with oral and intravenous contrast in a patient with a left testicular seminoma and retroperitoneal metastasis at presentation. (**a**) CT image at the time of diagnosis shows a large left para-aortic mass (*arrow*). Follow-up CT (**b**) and PET (**c**, **d**) scans after chemotherapy show the mass (*arrow*) has decreased in size but has increased FDG activity (*arrow*). This increased activity was suspicious for viable tumor so a retroperitoneal node dissection was performed. There is a surrounding ill-defined fibrotic reaction (*arrowheads*) around the mass on CT, which is typical in seminoma and makes complete resection difficult. At pathology there was a small 0.8 cm focus of metastatic seminoma, as well as extensive necrosis and histiocytic reaction. (**e**) Follow-up scan 4 months after surgery showed retroperitoneal recurrence of tumor (*arrow*), which responded to additional cycles of chemotherapy. For residual masses larger than 3 cm in patients with seminoma, tumor is found in up to 27 % of cases. FDG-PET can be helpful in assessing for viable tumor in these patients and triaging management [7]

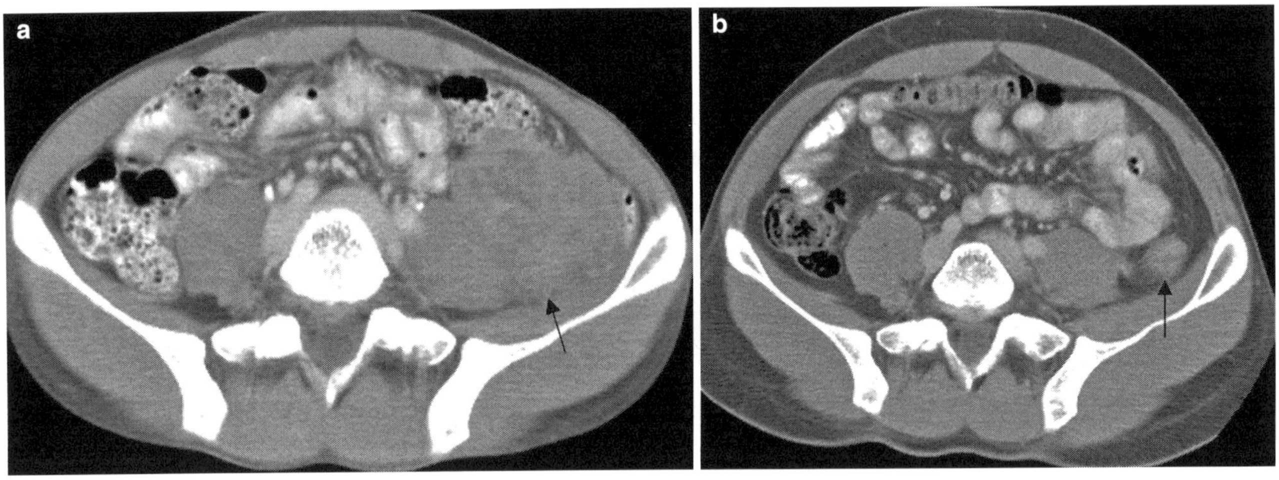

Fig. 6.54 Stage II seminoma with retroperitoneal recurrence after radiation therapy. Axial CT images of the abdomen with oral and intravenous contrast in a patient with a left testicular seminoma and retroperitoneal metastasis. CT at the time of diagnosis (*not shown*) showed small left paraaortic nodes and the patient was treated with radiation for probable stage IIA disease. On subsequent surveillance 2 years later, the patient's tumor markers were elevated and CT was performed. (**a**) CT shows a mass (*arrow*) lateral to the left psoas muscle due to recurrent tumor outside the radiation field. (**b**) Follow-up CT after chemotherapy shows the mass has decreased with a small amount of residual soft tissue (*arrow*) that remained stable on follow-up and was probably desmoplastic in nature without viable tumor

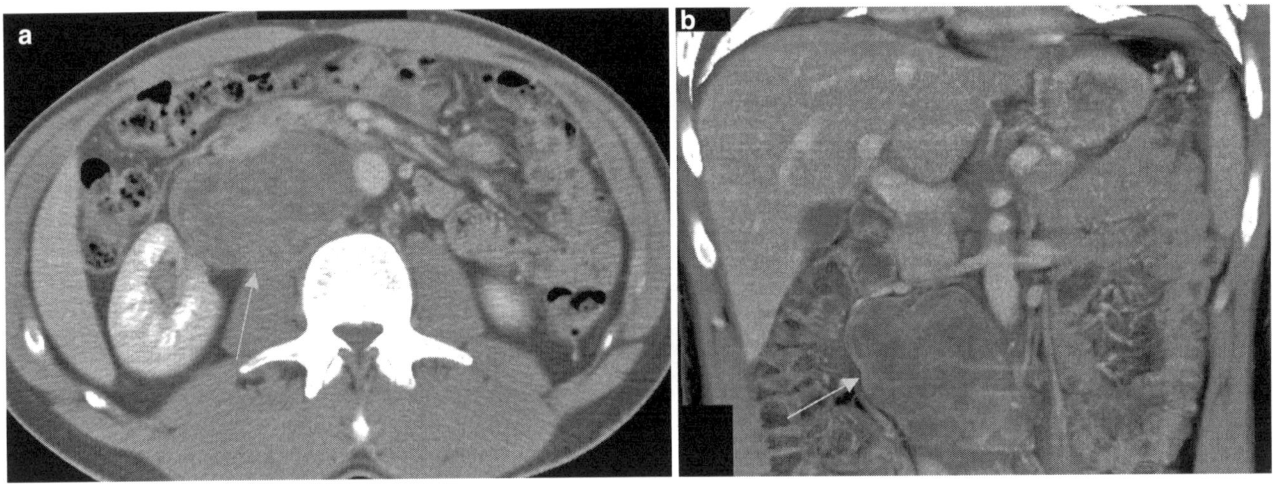

Fig. 6.55 Stage II seminoma with growing teratoma syndrome after chemotherapy. Axial CT images of the abdomen with oral and intravenous contrast in a patient with a left testicular seminoma and retroperitoneal metastasis at presentation. The patient had retroperitoneal adenopathy (*not shown*), which was treated with chemotherapy. Post-chemotherapy axial (**a**) and coronal (**b**) CT images show a large heterogeneous retrocaval mass (*arrows*) that had increased from the initial scan despite chemotherapy. The patient was asymptomatic and there was no FDG avidity in this mass on PET scan (*not shown*). Resection of the mass was performed and demonstrated metastatic mature teratoma. Teratomatous change after chemotherapy is typically seen in nonseminomatous germ cell metastases to the retroperitoneum. Teratoma is pathologically benign but tends to grow and compress local structures. It is also chemoresistant and there is a potential for malignant transformation into sarcoma or other tumors. Surgical resection is therefore performed for teratomas of the retroperitoneum [7]

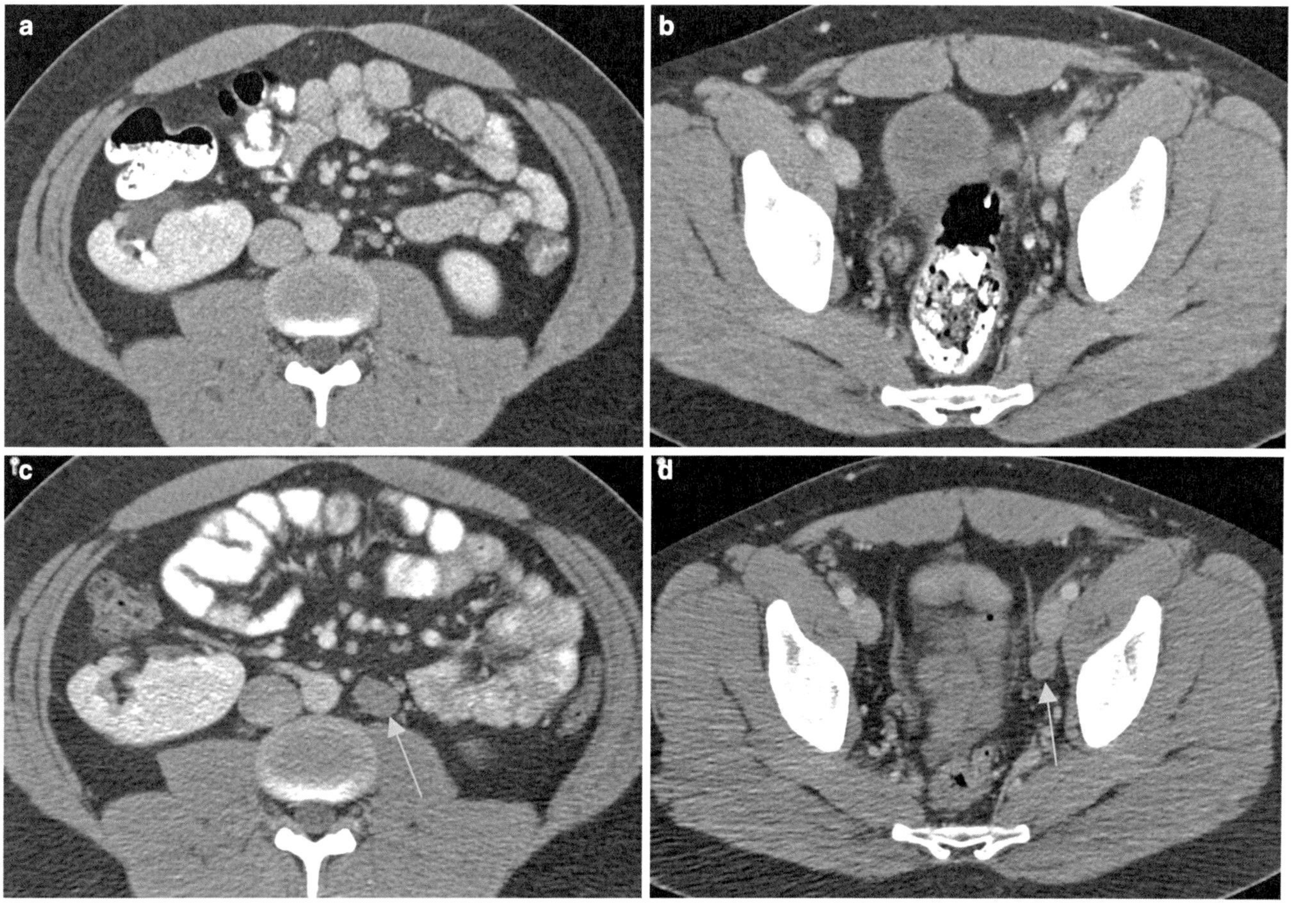

Fig. 6.56 Stage II NSGCT with enlarging nodes. Axial CT images of the abdomen with intravenous contrast in a patient with a left testicular embryonal carcinoma. CT images of the abdomen (**a**) and pelvis (**b**) at the time of the diagnosis of the testicular cancer show no adenopathy. Resection of the patient's primary tumor in the testis showed vascular invasion, which placed him at risk for metastatic disease, and a repeat CT was performed 6 weeks after the initial scan. Follow-up CT scans of the abdomen (**c**) and the pelvis (**d**) show increased left paraaortic and left external iliac nodes (*arrows*). These were suspicious for metastatic disease, given the patient's histology of embryonal carcinoma with vascular invasion, and chemotherapy was initiated

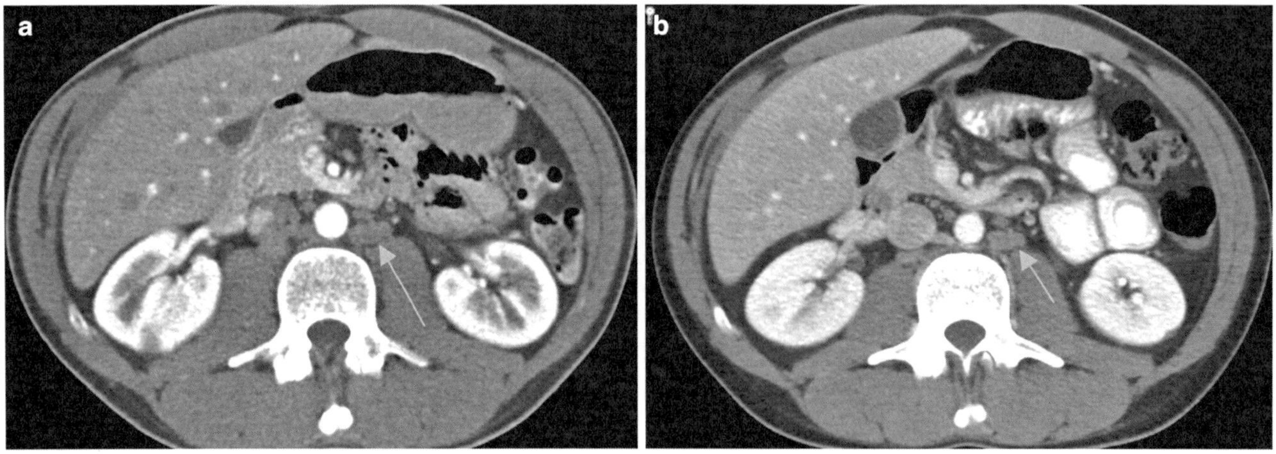

Fig. 6.57 Clinical stage II NSGCT with a benign retroperitoneal node. Axial CT images of the abdomen with intravenous contrast in a patient with a left testicular mixed germ cell tumor. The patient had an enlarged left para-aortic node that was in the nodal drainage pathway of a left testicular malignancy and was therefore considered suspicious for metastatic disease. (**a**) Initial CT shows a mildly enlarged left para-aortic node (*arrow*). The patient was given chemotherapy. Follow-up CT after 3 months (**b**) shows the node (*arrow*) is persistent and stable. The patient was at a high risk for recurrent tumor as he had a predominant embryonal carcinoma with vascular invasion in the testis. Retroperitoneal node dissection was therefore performed. The node was benign at pathology. It also did not demonstrate fibrosis to suggest treated tumor

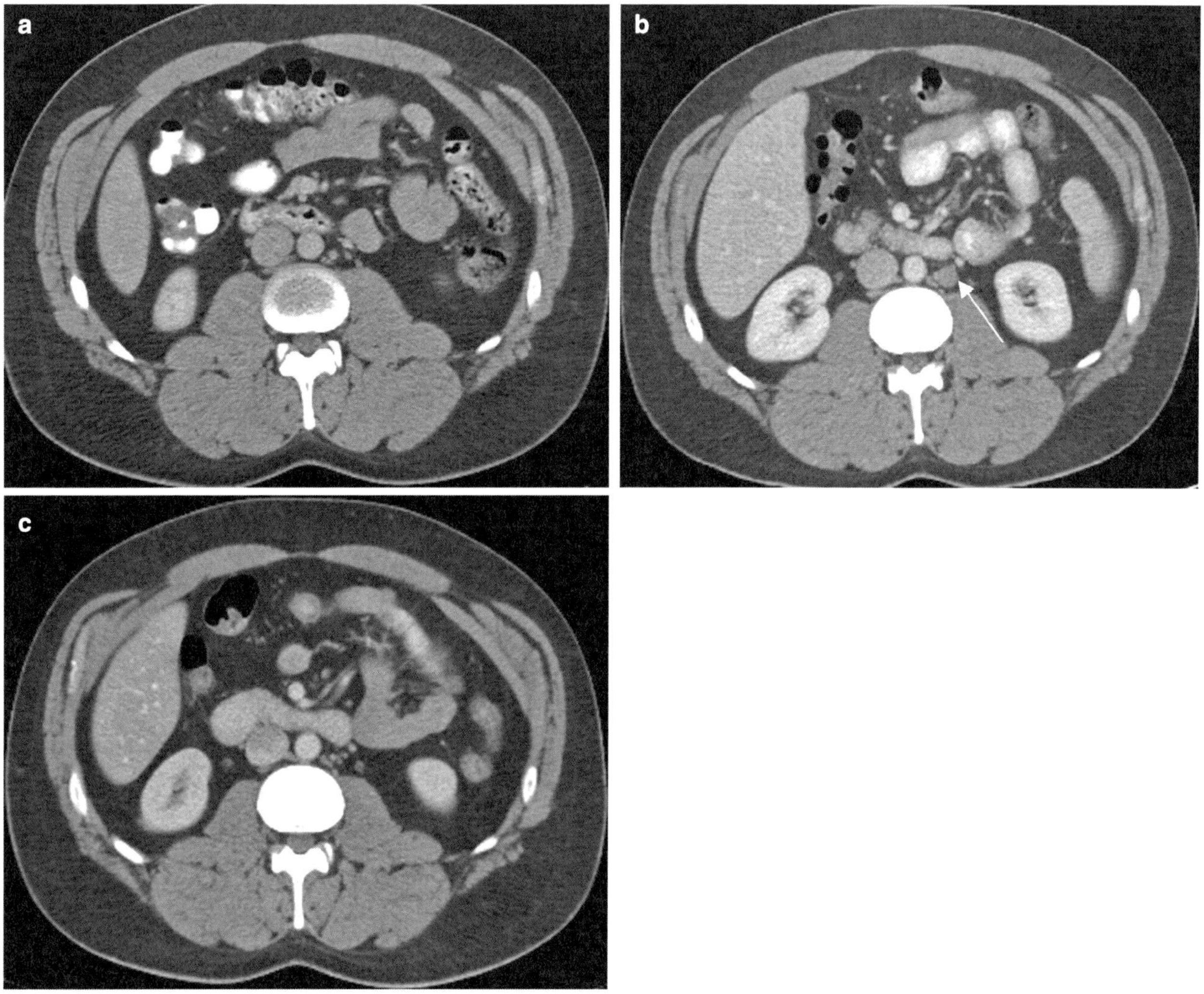

Fig. 6.58 Stage II NSGCT with resolution of a retroperitoneal node after chemotherapy. Axial CT images of the abdomen with oral and intravenous contrast in a patient with a left testicular mixed germ cell tumor, which was mainly embryonal carcinoma with vascular invasion. (**a**) CT at the time of diagnosis of a testicular mass shows no retroperitoneal adenopathy. (**b**) Follow-up CT 1 month later at the time of orchiectomy shows a new left para-aortic node (*arrow*). The patient was given chemotherapy and a subsequent CT 3 months later (**c**) showed resolution of the enlarged node. A retroperitoneal node dissection was performed and the resected nodes showed fibrosis and necrosis but no viable tumor. Retroperitoneal node dissection can also help cure 65 % of patients with stage II disease and normal serum tumor markers [7]

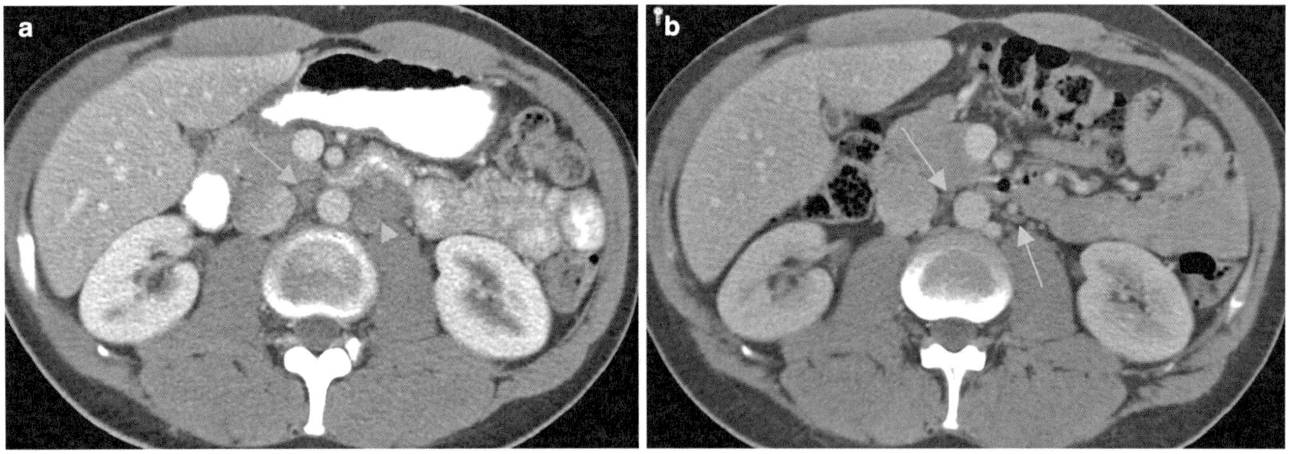

Fig. 6.59 Stage II mixed germ cell tumor with retroperitoneal node dissection for subcentimeter residual nodes after chemotherapy. Axial CT images of the abdomen with oral and intravenous contrast in a patient with a left testicular mixed germ cell tumor with a dominant embryonal carcinoma component and smaller seminomatous component. (**a**) CT at the time of diagnosis shows enlarged left para-aortic (*arrowhead*) and aortocaval nodes (*arrow*). The patient was given chemotherapy and follow-up CT (**b**) shows the nodes have decreased and are now subcentimeter (*arrows*). Due to the risk of residual or recurrent disease, the patient underwent a retroperitoneal node dissection, which revealed the nodes to have fibrosis with foamy macrophages but no viable tumor

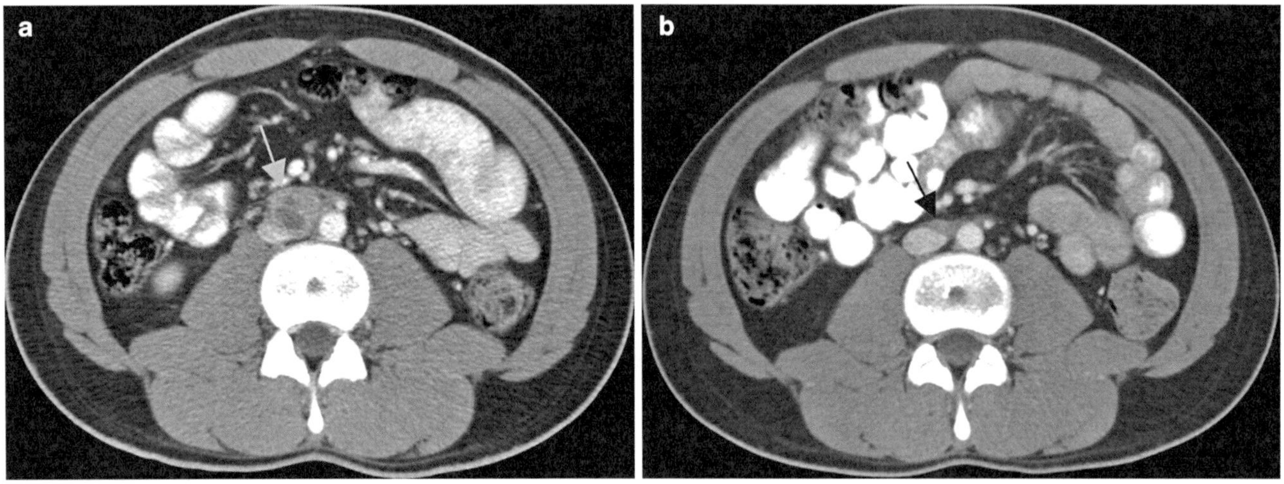

Fig. 6.60 Stage II NSGCT with residual nonmalignant mass after chemotherapy. Axial CT images of the abdomen with oral and intravenous contrast in a patient with a right testicular embryonal carcinoma and retroperitoneal metastasis with elevated tumor markers at presentation. (**a**) CT at the time of diagnosis shows a necrotic aortocaval node (*arrow*). The patient was given chemotherapy. Follow-up CT (**b**) after 6 weeks shows the node has decreased with residual soft tissue (*arrow*) in the aortocaval region. Subsequent retroperitoneal node dissection revealed necrotic tissue but no viable tumor or teratoma in the residual mass. The patient developed a 6 mm basal ganglia metastasis (*not shown*) successfully treated with radiation and has been free of disease for 5 years. Residual masses after chemotherapy are typically resected in patients with NSGCT due to a risk of remnant tumor or teratomatous elements

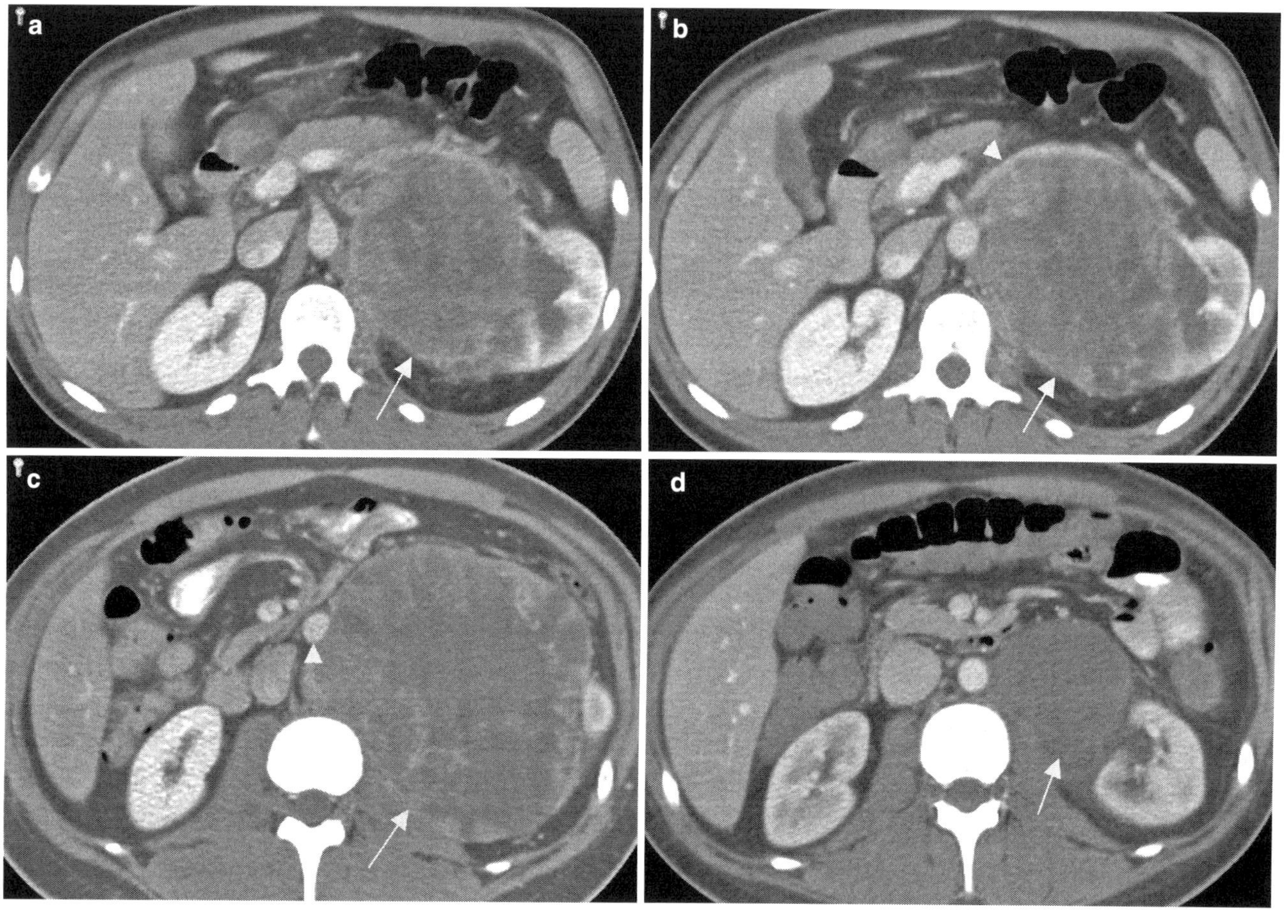

Fig. 6.61 Stage II NSGCT with a necrotic retroperitoneal mass after chemotherapy. Axial CT images of the abdomen with intravenous contrast in a patient with a left testicular mixed germ cell tumor, mainly yolk sac tumor without vascular invasion. (**a**–**c**) CT images at the time of diagnosis show a large necrotic left retroperitoneal mass (*arrows*) abutting the aorta (*arrowhead*) and splaying the left renal vessels (*arrowhead*). The mass is inseparable from the left psoas muscle. The patient was given chemotherapy and follow-up CT (**d**) shows the retroperitoneal mass (*arrow*) has decreased and is now hypodense. (**e**) A PET scan was performed to assess for viable disease and showed increased FDG uptake in the periphery of the mass (*arrow*), which was suspicious for viable tumor. A retroperitoneal node dissection was subsequently performed and demonstrated necrosis but no viable tumor in the residual mass

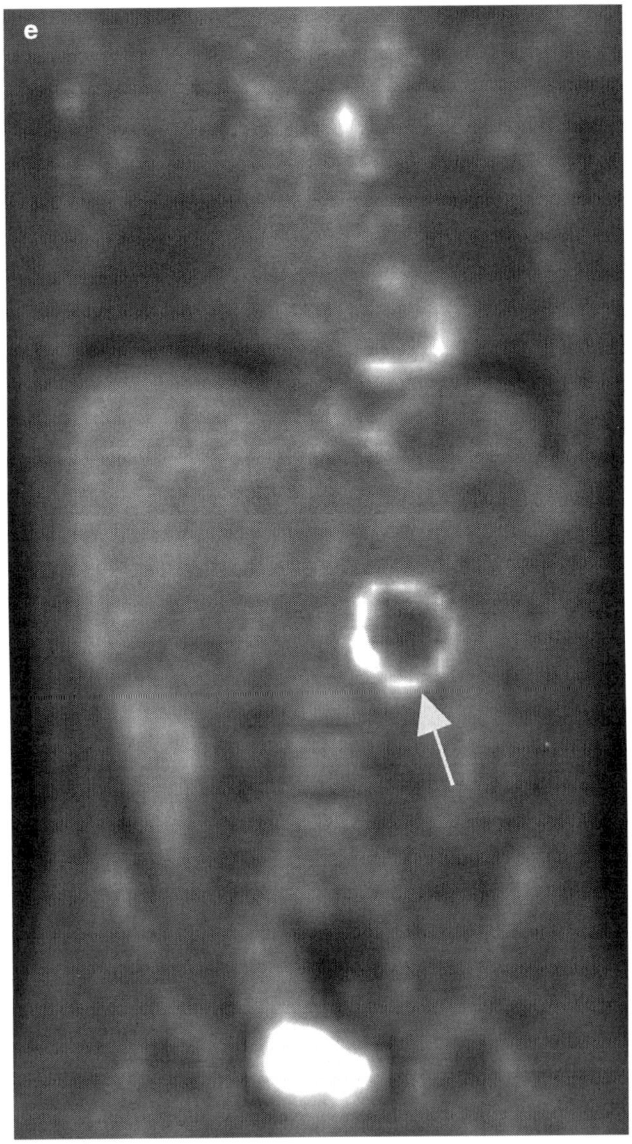

Fig. 6.61 (continued)

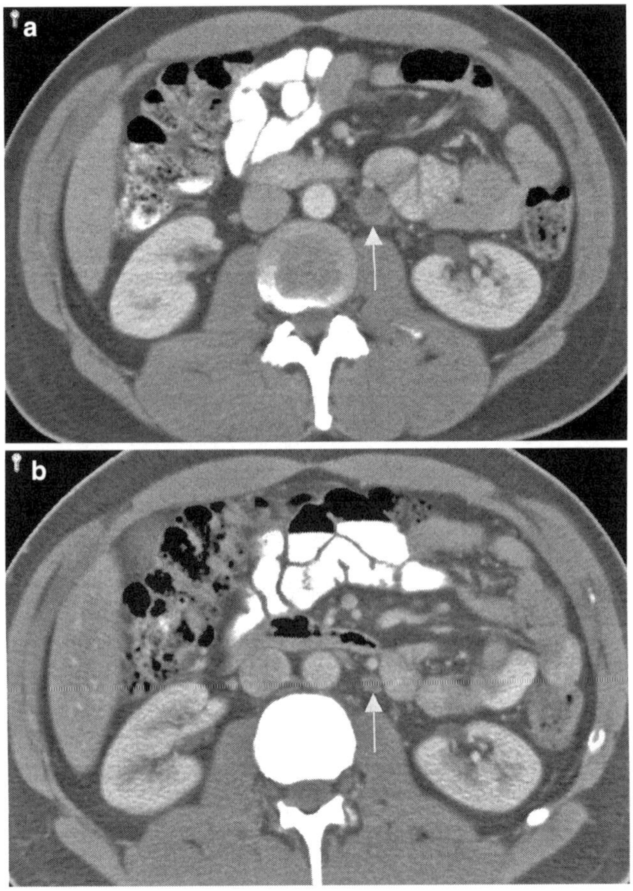

Fig. 6.62 Stage II NSGCT with residual tumor in retroperitoneal node after chemotherapy. Axial CT images of the abdomen with oral and intravenous contrast in a patient with a left testicular mixed germ cell tumor, which was primarily embryonal carcinoma. (**a**) CT at the time of diagnosis shows a heterogeneous left para-aortic node (*arrow*). (**b**) Follow-up CT 3 months later after chemotherapy shows the node (*arrow*) has decreased in size. A retroperitoneal node dissection was performed due to a high risk of recurrence and the node had a small 0.7 cm focus of viable embryonal carcinoma. Other resected nodes showed treatment-related changes such as necrosis and fibrosis

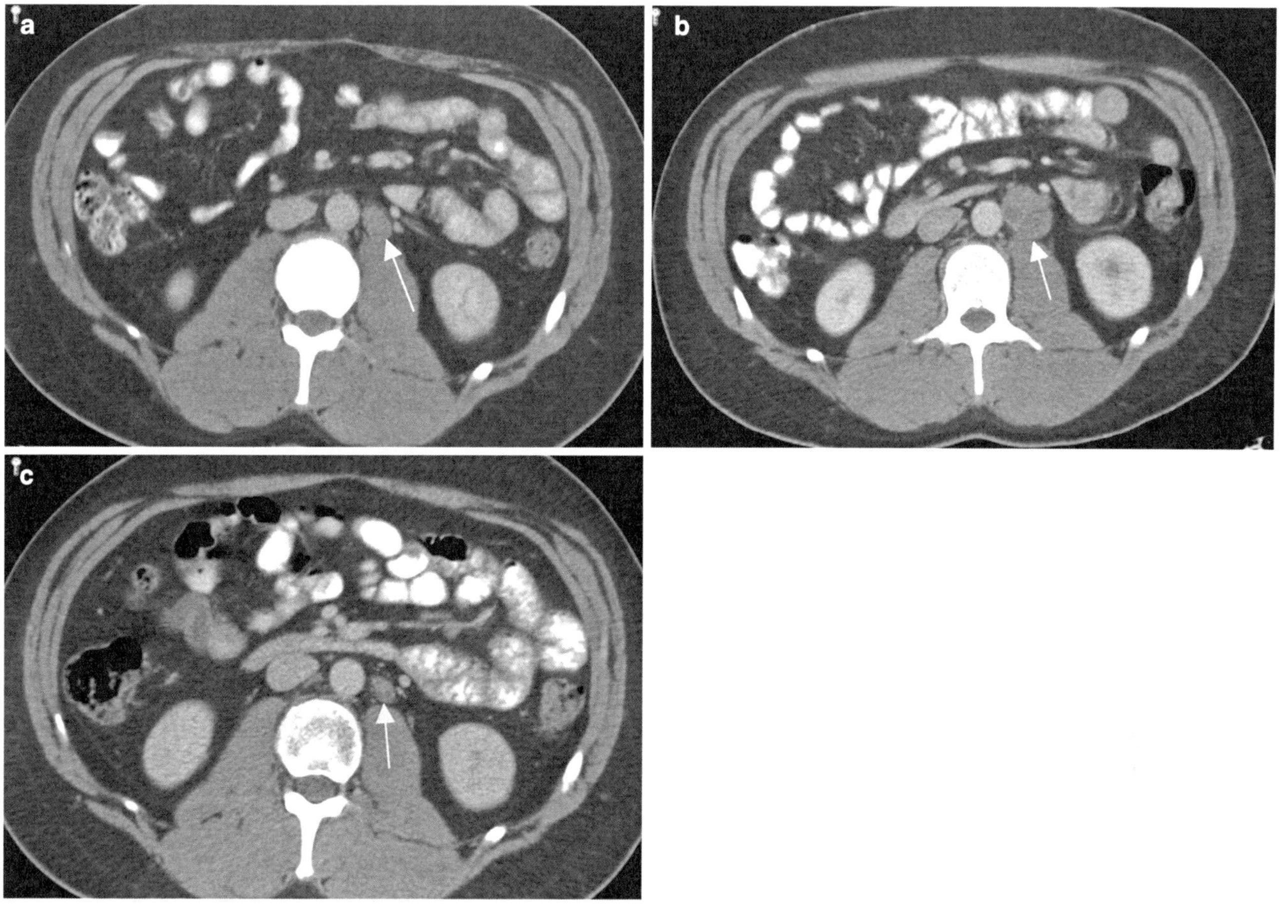

Fig. 6.63 Stage II NSGCT with teratoma in residual node after chemotherapy. Axial CT images of the abdomen with oral and intravenous contrast in a patient with a left testicular embryonal carcinoma. (**a**) CT at the time of diagnosis shows a small left para-aortic node (*arrow*). (**b**) CT performed 2 months later due to rising tumor markers showed interval enlargement of the node (*arrow*). The patient received chemotherapy. Follow-up CT (**c**) showed the node had decreased in size with a small amount of residual soft tissue (*arrow*). The node was resected to reveal mature teratoma with treatment effect

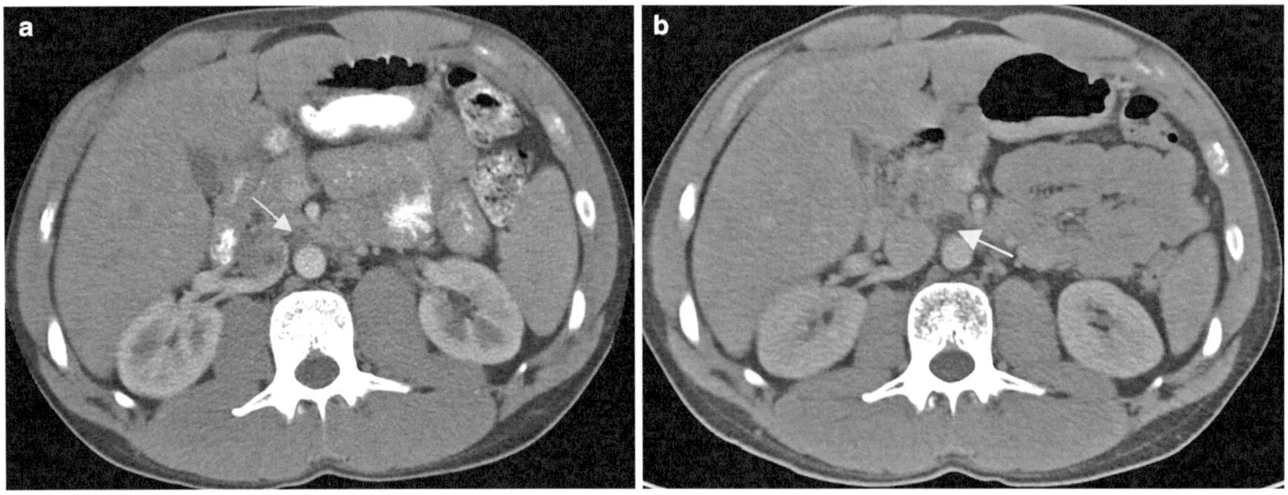

Fig. 6.64 Stage II NSGCT with teratoma in residual node after chemotherapy. Axial CT images of the abdomen with intravenous contrast in a patient with a left testicular mixed germ cell tumor. The patient had persistent elevation of tumor markers after orchiectomy and CT (**a**) revealed a prominent aortocaval node (*arrow*). The patient was given chemotherapy and follow-up CT (**b**) after 4 months shows the node has not significantly changed in size but is more hypodense (*arrow*). Due to the cystic change in the node, a teratoma was suspected and the node was resected. At pathology, the node had teratoma with fibrosis secondary to treatment effect. Patients with a residual mass post chemotherapy have teratoma in approximately half the cases and viable tumor in 10 %. Although approximately 45 % of patients have only necrosis in the residual mass, imaging cannot distinguish between necrosis, teratoma, and residual tumor. Therefore, a retroperitoneal node dissection is performed in NSGCT patients with a residual mass larger than 1 cm and normal serum tumor markers after chemotherapy. At pathology, if the residual mass is necrotic, the risk of relapse is less than 5 %. For patients with teratoma in the residual mass, the risk of relapse is also low, 7–14 %. However, for the 10 % of patients who have viable tumor in the residual mass, there is a 50–100 % risk of relapse and chemotherapy is typically given. FDG-PET is not helpful in NSGCT patients as teratoma in residual masses is not avid [7]

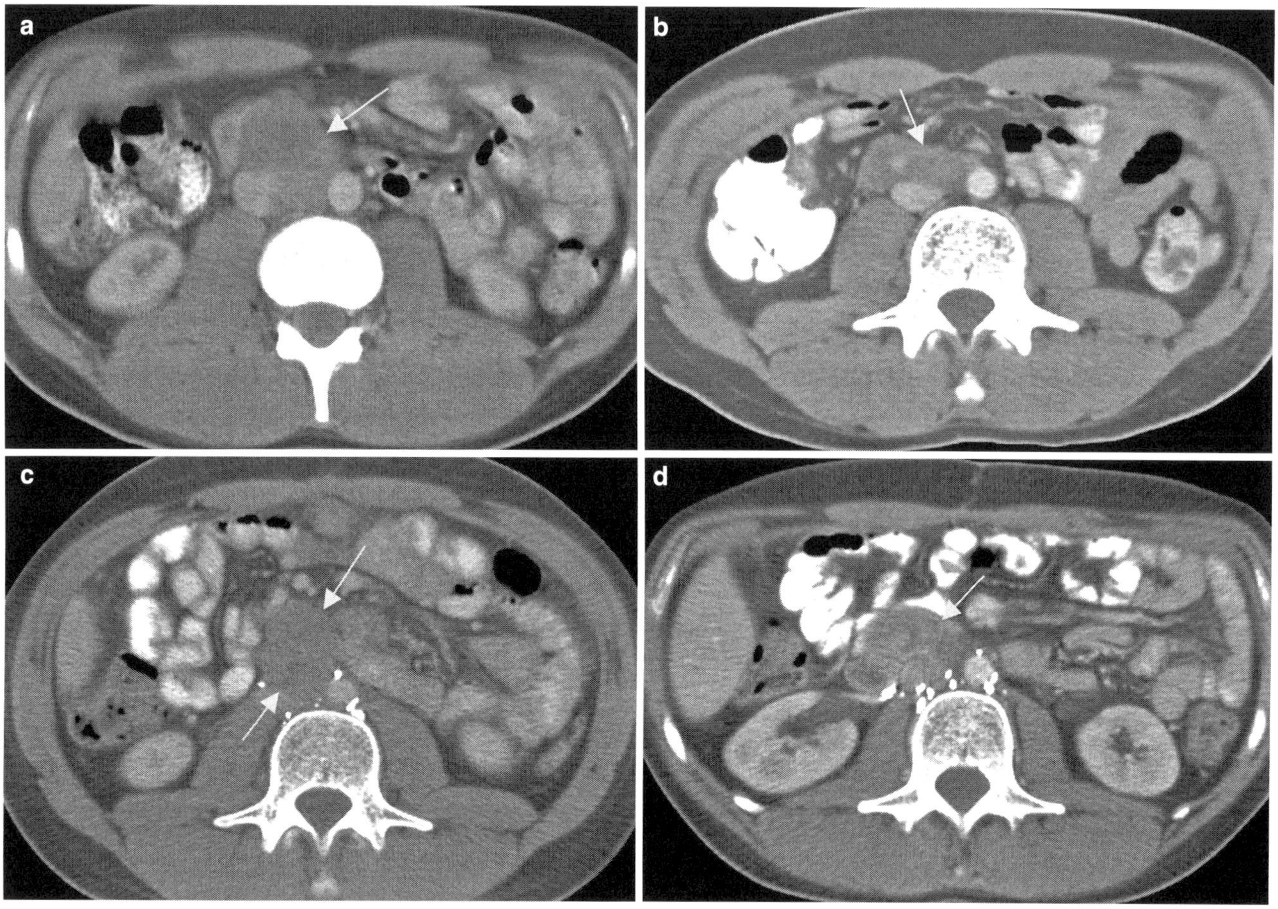

Fig. 6.65 Stage II NSGCT with recurrent teratoma in the retroperitoneum. Axial CT images of the abdomen with oral and intravenous contrast in a patient with a right testicular mixed germ cell tumor with a dominant teratoma component. (**a**) Initial CT shows an enlarged aortocaval node (*arrow*). The patient was given chemotherapy. Follow-up CT (**b**) shows decrease in the size of the mass with residual soft tissue (*arrow*). This was resected and pathology revealed metastatic teratoma with focal atypia, as well as necrosis, inflammation, and fibrosis consistent with treatment effect. 6 months after node dissection, the patient had an elevation in his serum tumor markers. (**c**) CT showed a recurrent retroperitoneal mass (*arrows*) adjacent to the surgical clips. An early relapse in the surgical field is unusual and the patient was given chemotherapy with a stem cell rescue. (**d**) Follow-up CT prior to a second retroperitoneal node dissection showed a heterogeneous residual mass (*arrow*). This proved to be metastatic mature teratoma at pathology

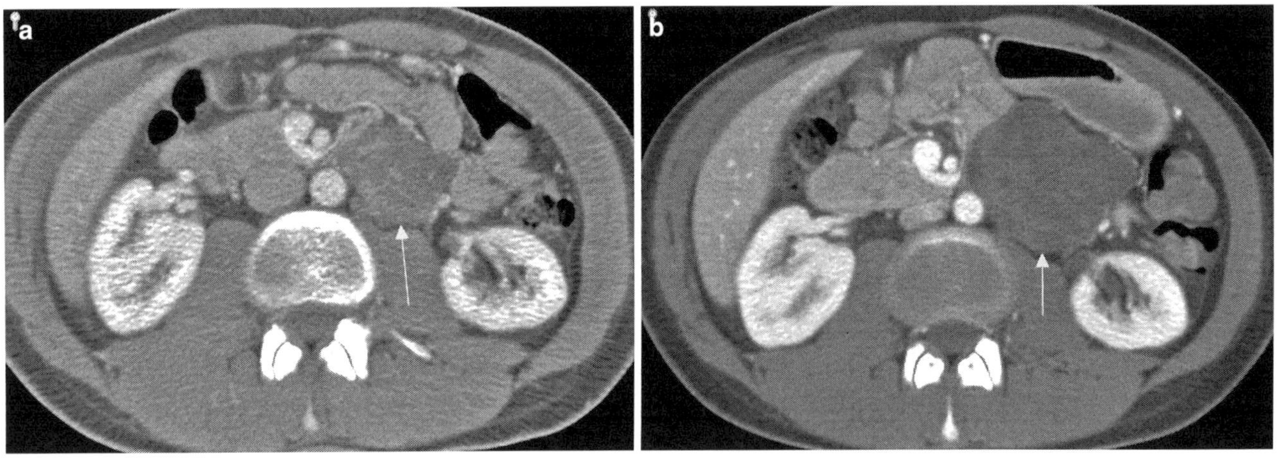

Fig. 6.66 Stage II NSGCT with growing teratoma syndrome on chemotherapy. Axial CT images with intravenous contrast in a patient with a left testicular mixed germ cell tumor, which consisted of seminoma, embryonal carcinoma, yolk sac tumor, and immature teratoma. (**a**) CT performed for back pain 2 weeks after orchiectomy showed a left para-aortic mass (*arrow*) that was consistent with adenopathy in an expected landing zone for a left testicular primary. Chemotherapy was administered but the patient presented 7 weeks later with worsening back pain. (**b**) Repeat CT demonstrated the left para-aortic mass (*arrow*) had increased in size and had a larger cystic component suspicious for growing teratoma syndrome. Pathology from a retroperitoneal node dissection showed metastatic mature teratoma and additional chemotherapy was given after surgery

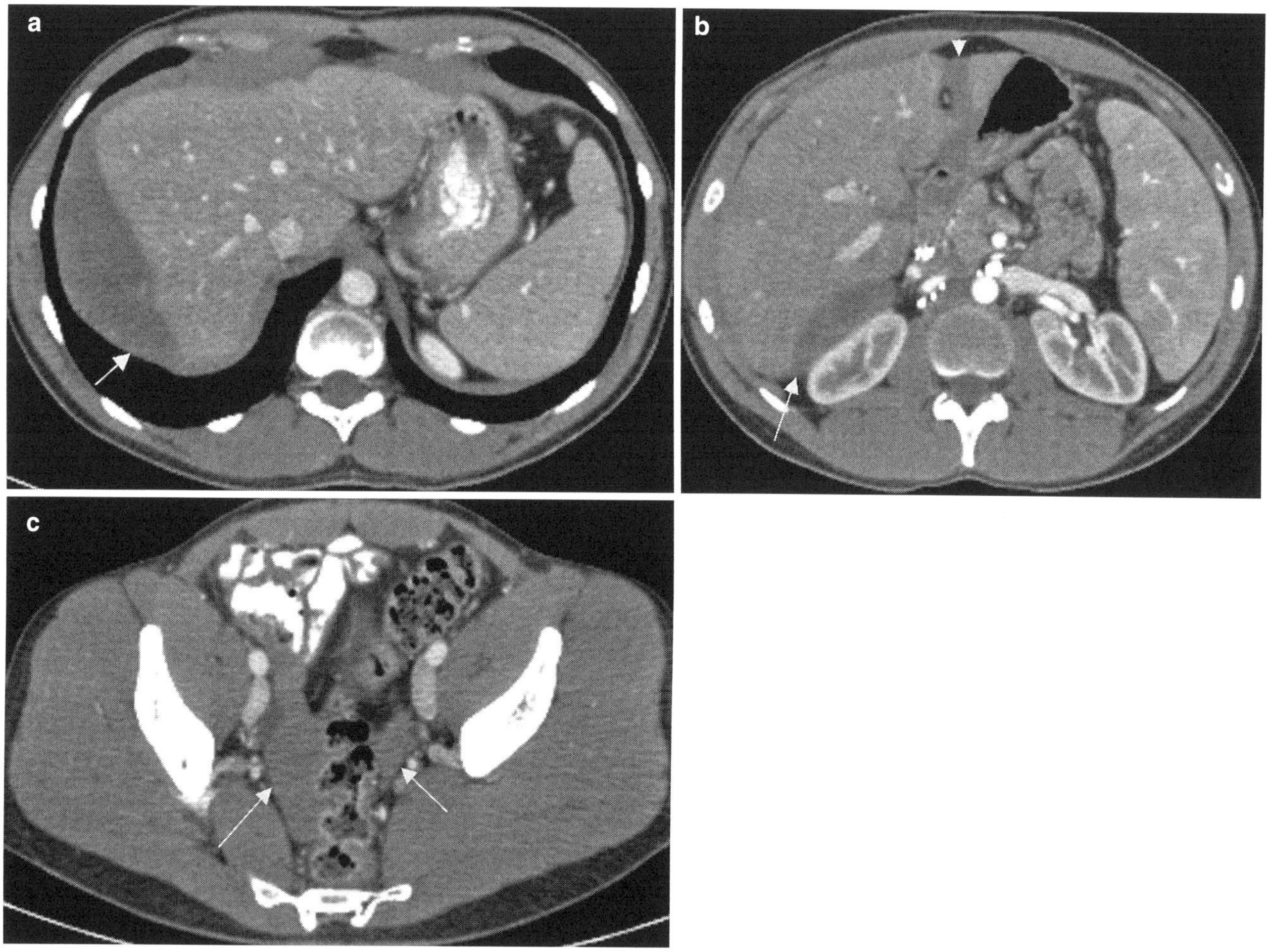

Fig. 6.67 Stage II NSGCT with teratoma in residual peritoneal masses after chemotherapy. Axial CT images of the abdomen with intravenous contrast in a patient with a right testicular mixed germ cell tumor with a dominant embryonal carcinoma. The patient was treated with orchiectomy and a laparoscopic retroperitoneal node dissection that revealed nodal metastases. 5 months later the patient had elevation of his serum tumor markers and imaging (*not shown*) revealed peritoneal metastases for which chemotherapy was given. Imaging 18 months later with CT showed multiple residual peritoneal masses that were not FDG avid at PET CT. (**a**) CT of the upper abdomen shows scalloping of the liver surface by implants (*arrow*). (**b**) CT at the mid abdomen level shows soft tissue in the falciform ligament (*arrowhead*) and an implant in Morrison's pouch (*arrow*). There are also retroperitoneal clips from previous nodal dissection. (**c**) Pelvic CT shows bilateral peritoneal masses (*arrows*). The patient underwent a debulking procedure similar to that performed in patients with metastatic ovarian cancer with removal of the peritoneal tumor deposits. Pathology showed the peritoneal deposits consisted of mature teratoma surrounded by a dense collagenized and inflamed fibroconnective tissue

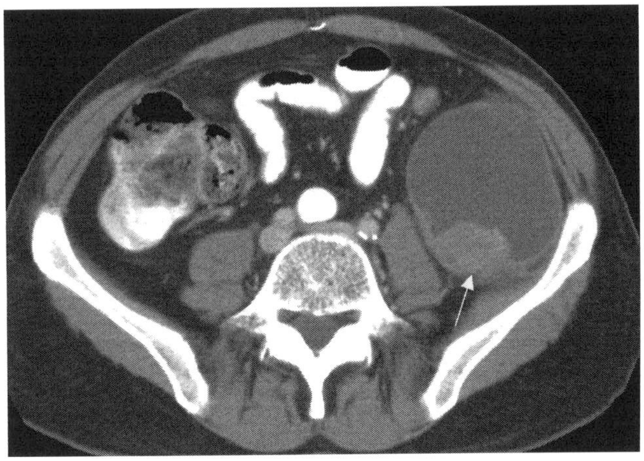

Fig. 6.68 Stage II NSGCT with late recurrence of teratoma. Axial CT image of the abdomen with oral and intravenous contrast in a patient with a previous orchiectomy as a teenager 26 years earlier for teratocarcinoma. A retroperitoneal node dissection performed at that time showed embryonal carcinoma and teratoma for which the patient was treated with radiation therapy to the retroperitoneum. The patient presented 26 years later with flank pain and CT showed a cystic and solid mass in the left iliac fossa (*arrow*). The mass was resected and pathology showed a mature teratoma composed of glandular and smooth muscle elements with focal necrosis. The patient has subsequently been followed for another 10 years without additional disease recurrence

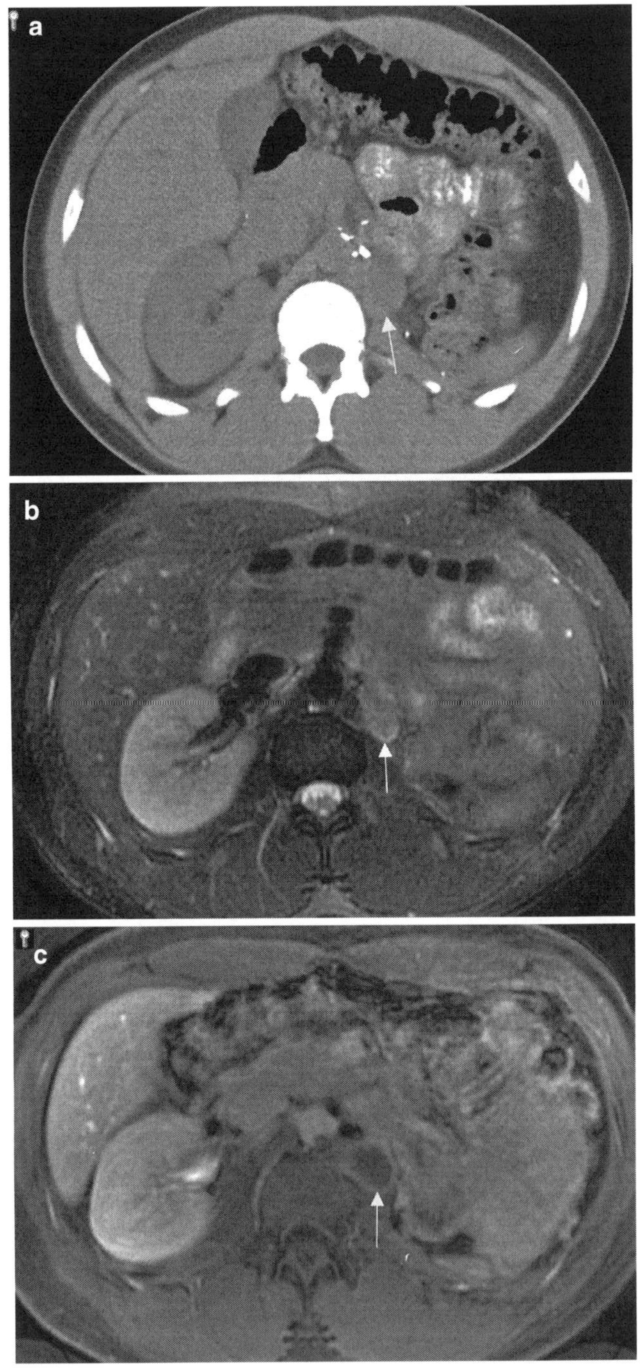

Fig. 6.69 Stage II NSGCT with late recurrence of malignant teratoma. Axial CT and MR images in a patient with previous left orchiectomy 4 years earlier for a mixed germ cell tumor. As part of the initial treatment, the patient had chemotherapy and a retroperitoneal node dissection for a residual retroperitoneal mass. (**a**) CT with oral contrast performed as part of routine imaging 4 years later showed a left para-aortic mass (*arrow*) adjacent to surgical clips. (**b**) Axial fat saturated T2-weighted MR image shows the mass (*arrow*) is intermediate in signal intensity. (**c**) Axial post contrast T1-weighted MR image shows peripheral enhancement of the mass (*arrow*) with central necrosis. The mass was suspicious for recurrent disease and was resected. Pathology demonstrated metastatic teratoma with necrosis, as well as a few foci of viable atypical glandular structures suspicious for adenocarcinomatous differentiation

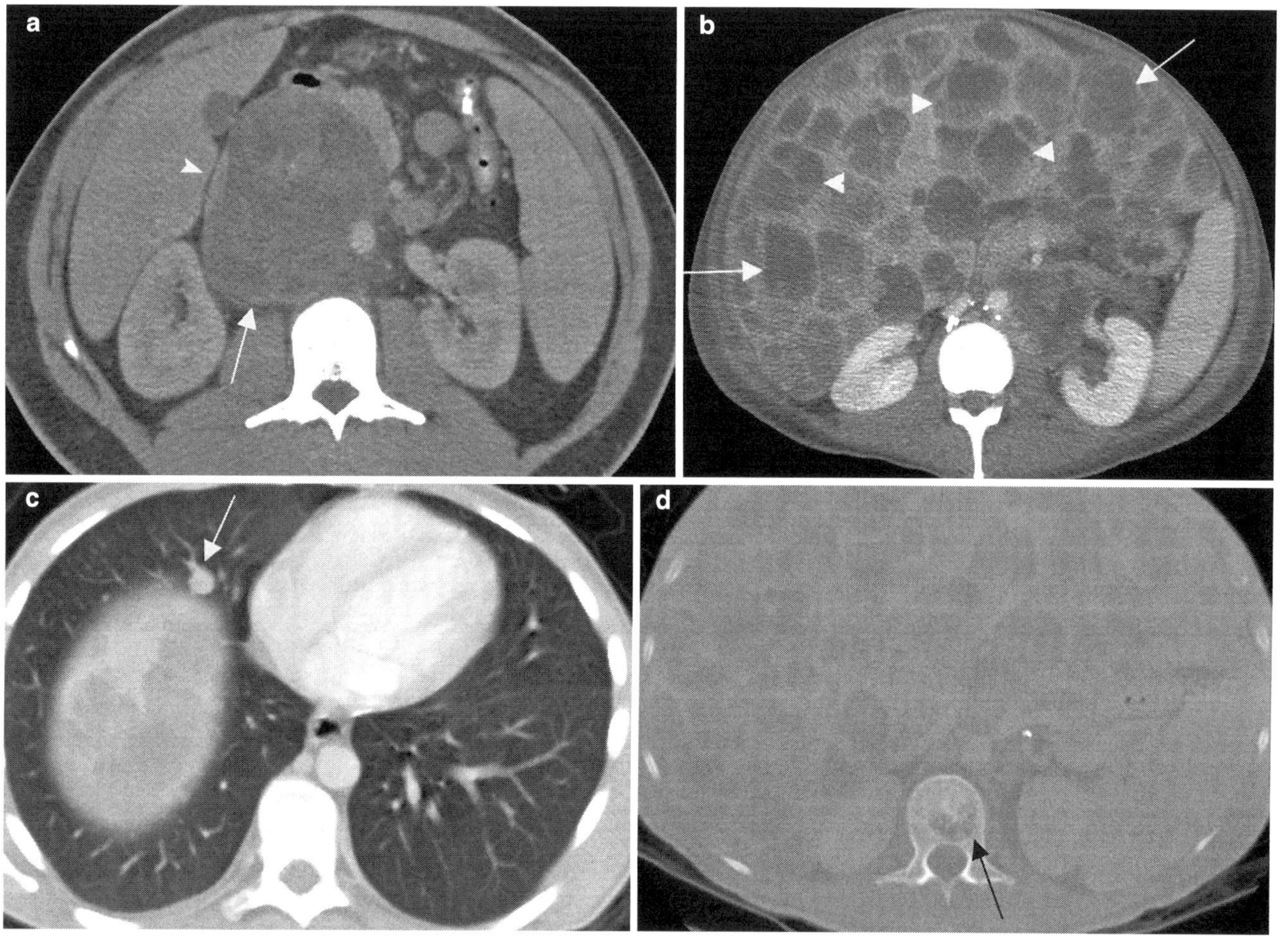

Fig. 6.70 Stage II NSGCT with cystic liver metastases. Axial CT images of the abdomen with intravenous contrast in a patient with a right testicular mixed germ cell tumor with a dominant yolk sac tumor and mature teratoma. (**a**) CT following orchiectomy showed a large paracaval metastatic node (*arrow*) displacing the IVC (*arrowhead*) and the patient was given chemotherapy. The patient had progressive disease despite chemotherapy and a CT scan obtained 2 years later showed liver, lung, and bone metastases. (**b**) CT shows numerous liver masses (*arrows*), many of which have a fluid–fluid level (*arrowheads*) with dependent high density fluid. Cystic liver metastases have been reported with teratoma and can also be seen following chemotherapy [16]. The fluid–fluid levels in the masses reflected intralesional hemorrhage and the patient had a low hemoglobin level that necessitated multiple transfusions. (**c**) CT with lung windows shows a right middle lobe metastasis (*arrow*). (**d**) CT with bone windows shows a lytic vertebral body lesion (*arrow*)

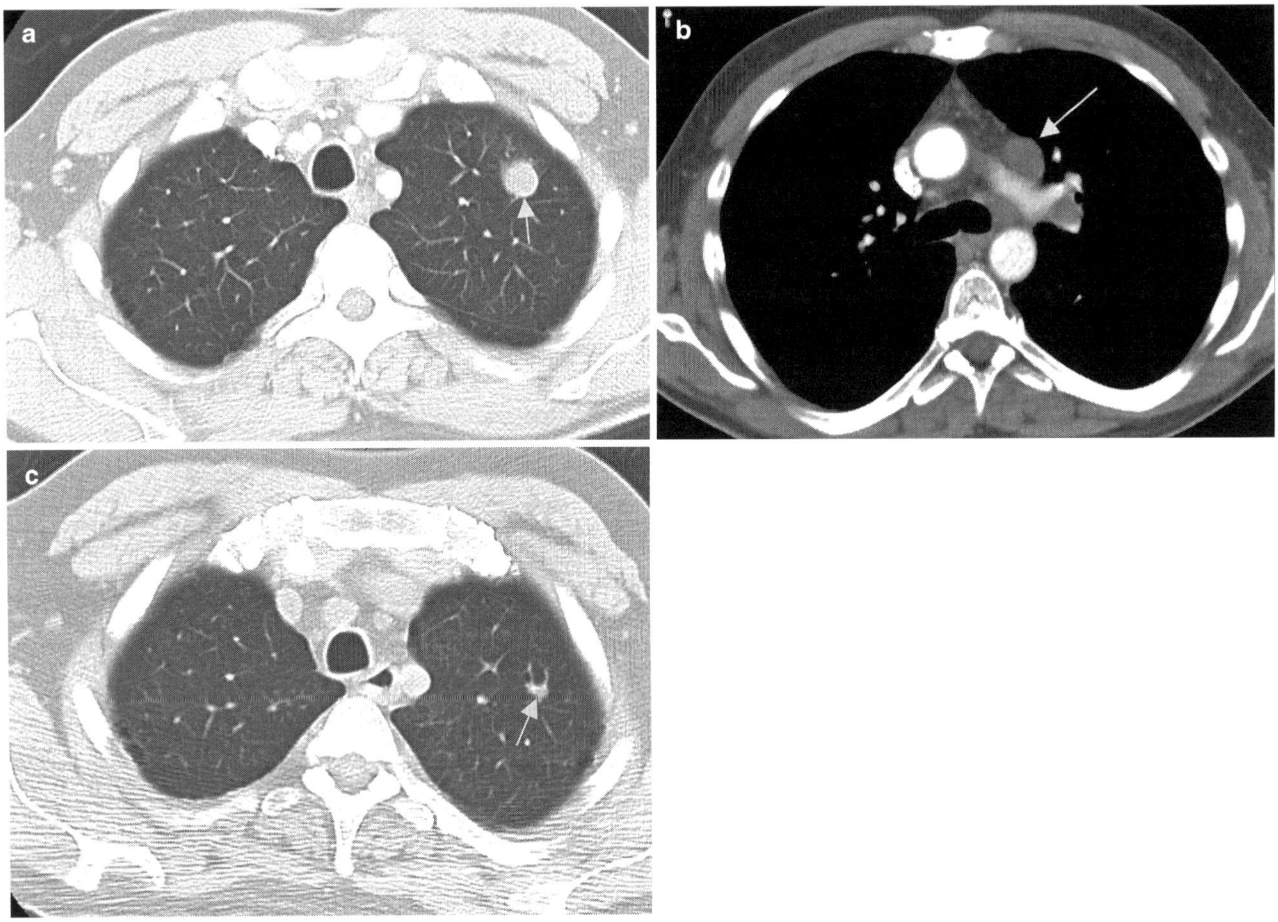

Fig. 6.71 Stage II NSGCT with lung metastases. Axial CT images of the chest with intravenous contrast in a patient with a testicular mixed germ cell tumor with a dominant embryonal carcinoma and a component of seminoma. The patient was treated with chemotherapy and then underwent retroperitoneal node dissection, which revealed mature teratoma and one 0.5 cm focus of embryonal carcinoma. (**a**, **b**) Images from a surveillance CT performed 1 year later showed an enlarging lung nodule (*arrow*), as well as mediastinal (*arrow*) and left hilar nodes. Biopsy of the lung nodule revealed a viable germ cell tumor, similar to the patient's primary testicular embryonal tumor. The patient received chemotherapy, with an interval decrease in size of the lung nodule (*arrow*) on follow-up CT (**c**)

Management of Stage III Disease

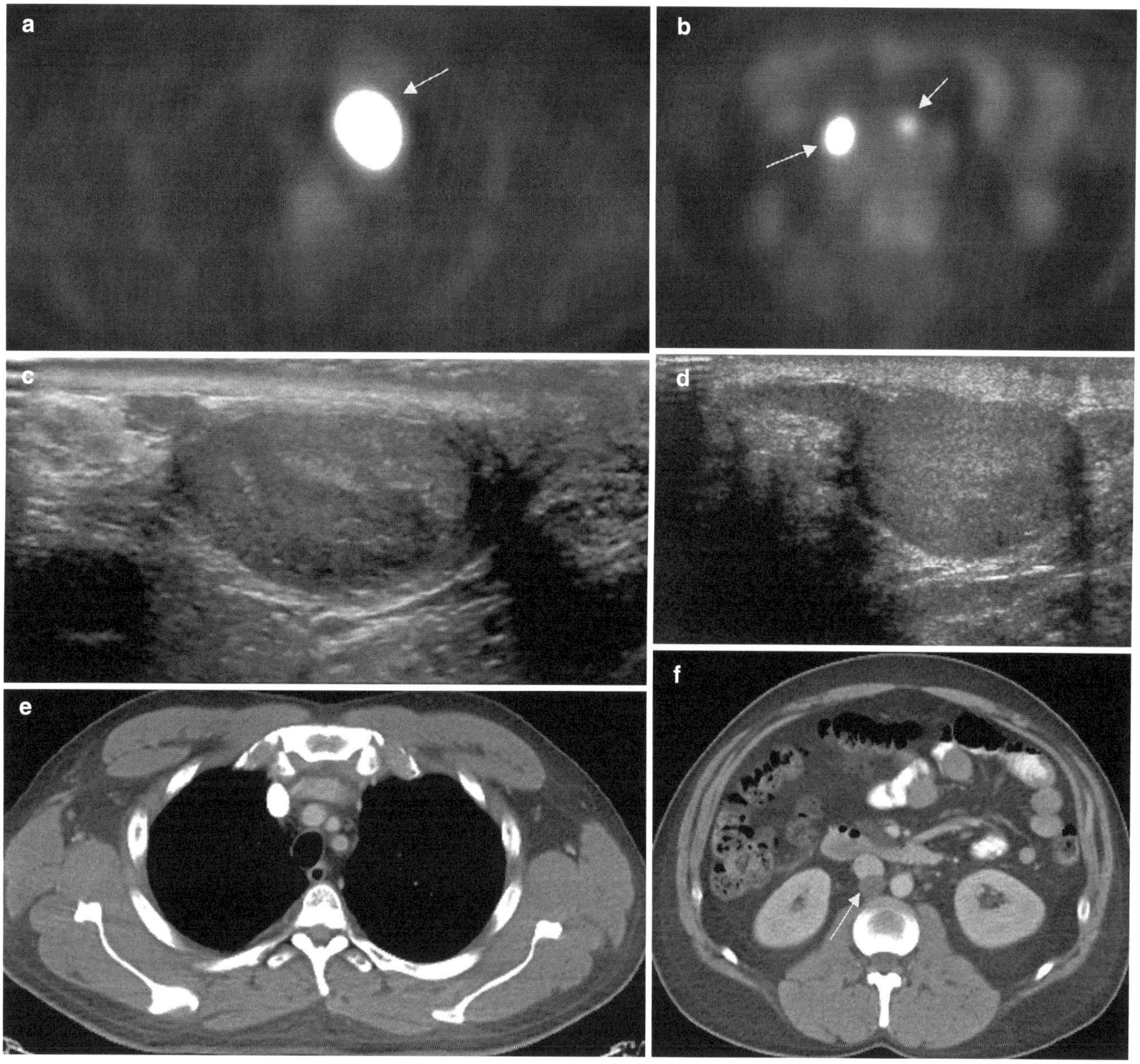

Fig. 6.72 Treatment of good risk stage IIIA seminoma. CT of the abdomen (*not shown*) in a patient with flank pain revealed retroperitoneal adenopathy in retrocaval, aortocaval, and left paraaortic regions. PET-CT performed for unknown primary showed a hypermetabolic mediastinal lesion and retroperitoneal adenopathy (*arrows* in **a**, **b**). Because of the patient's age and location of the adenopathy an ultrasound was performed, which demonstrated a hypoechoic right testicular mass (**c**). Mediastinoscopy and biopsy revealed seminoma and the patient was treated with chemotherapy with reduction in retroperitoneal nodal disease and resolution of mediastinal adenopathy. Post-chemotherapy ultrasound showed decrease in the hypoechoic testicular mass (**d**). Only fibrosis and scarring was identified at orchiectomy consistent with treatment effect. (**e**, **f**) Follow-up CT shows resolution of mediastinal node and decreased retroperitoneal adenopathy (*arrow* in **f**). This case also demonstrates the expected nodal drainage pathway from a right testicular primary with adenopathy in the interaortocaval and retrocaval sites, as well as contralateral left paraaortic node. Due to the cephalad extension along the thoracic duct to the retrocrural and prevascular regions the patient had stage III disease

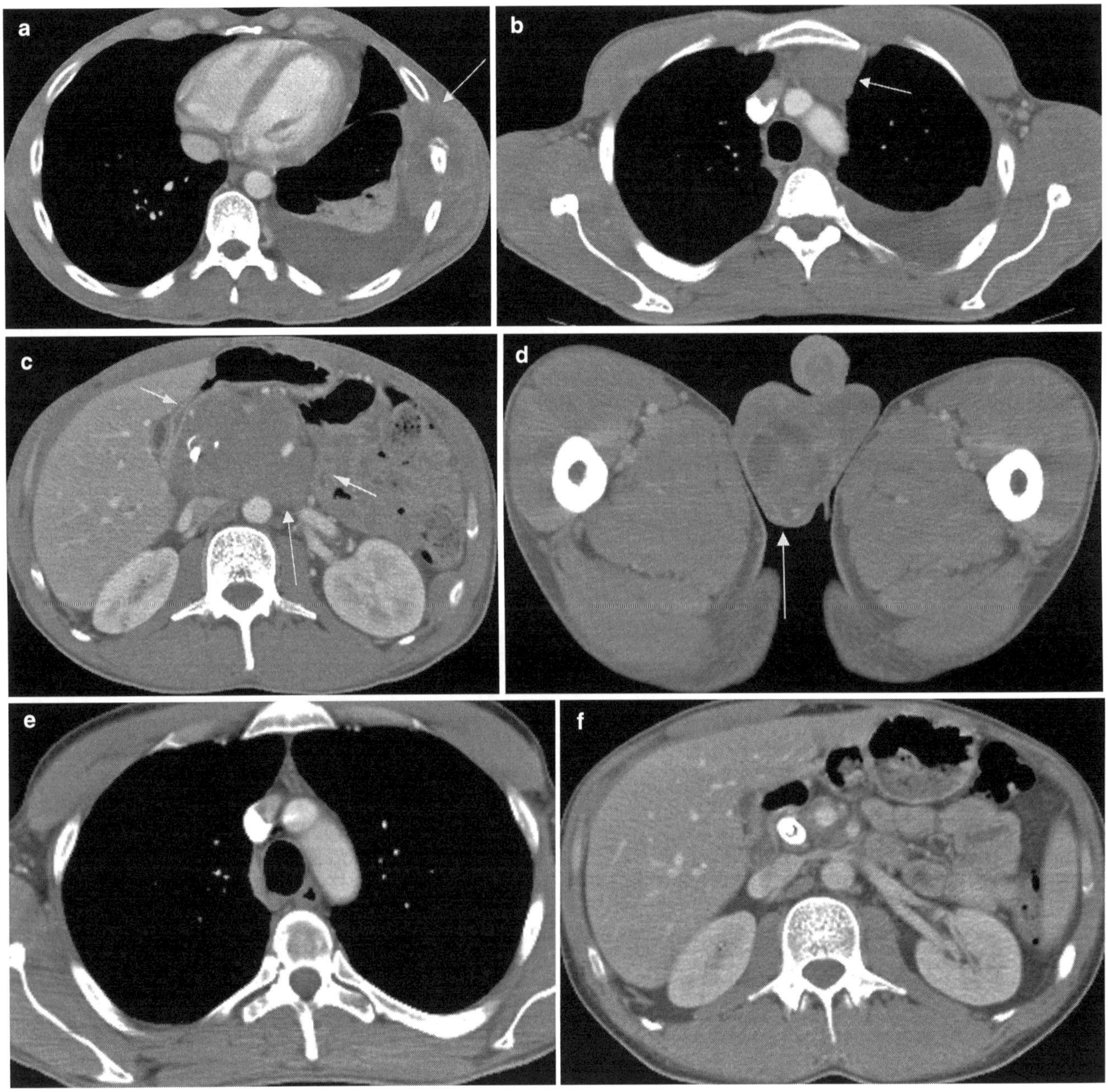

Fig. 6.73 Recurrent stage 3 seminoma. Axial CT images of the chest, abdomen, and pelvis with intravenous contrast performed for chest pain and history of weight loss revealed (**a**) a left rib metastasis with chest wall mass (*arrow*), moderate left effusion, (**b**) mediastinal adenopathy (*arrow*), (**c**) peripancreatic mass (*arrows*), and (**d**) a right scrotal mass (*arrow*). Rib biopsy was positive for seminoma and hCG was 2,000 mIU/mL. The patient also had jaundice and endoscopic retrograde cholangiopancreatography showed necrotic cells on brushings. An orchiectomy was performed to determine if the primary tumor had nonseminomatous elements that would classify the patient as poor risk versus intermediate risk for a pure seminoma. Right orchiectomy showed seminoma and radiation therapy was administered to the retroperitoneum followed by chemotherapy. The mediastinal adenopathy resolved (**e**). There was minimal residual soft tissue in the peripancreatic region (**f**) and at the left rib metastasis (**g**). PET-CT showed no avid disease. However, shortly thereafter there was regrowth of the left chest wall mass and a new lesion in the pancreatic head. Chest wall mass biopsy was positive for seminoma recurrence and the pancreatic biopsy was indeterminate. PET showed hypermetabolic activity in both sites. The decision was made to administer high-dose salvage chemotherapy with stem cell infusion and the recurrent disease decreased. After 11 months, Whipple procedure and rib resection confirmed that the tumor was eradicated. Pathology from both showed no tumor and extensive fibrosis. After chemotherapy, there is severe desmoplastic reaction in patients with seminoma at the site of disease. Post-chemotherapy surgery, especially in the retroperitoneum, is therefore very difficult. If residual mass is less than 3 cm, it is observed. If residual mass is larger than 3 cm, it is resected. We have begun doing PET-CT on these residual masses in patients with seminoma, as in this case. The PET-CT must be done after a certain amount of time (*see* chapter 10, "Nuclear Medicine") to avoid false-positive results. Any adenopathy or mass that has radiotracer uptake on PET is considered for resection

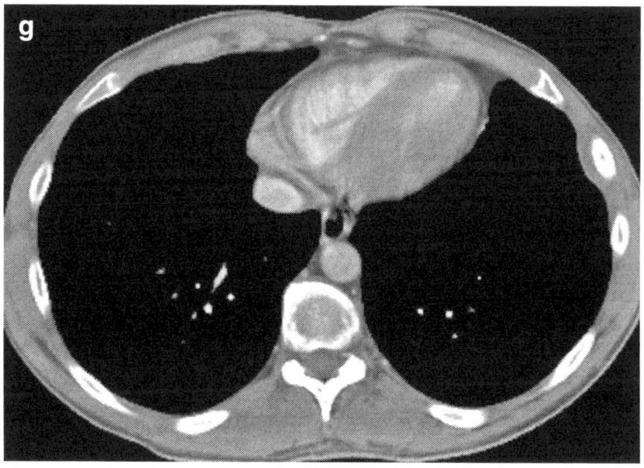

Fig. 6.73 (continued)

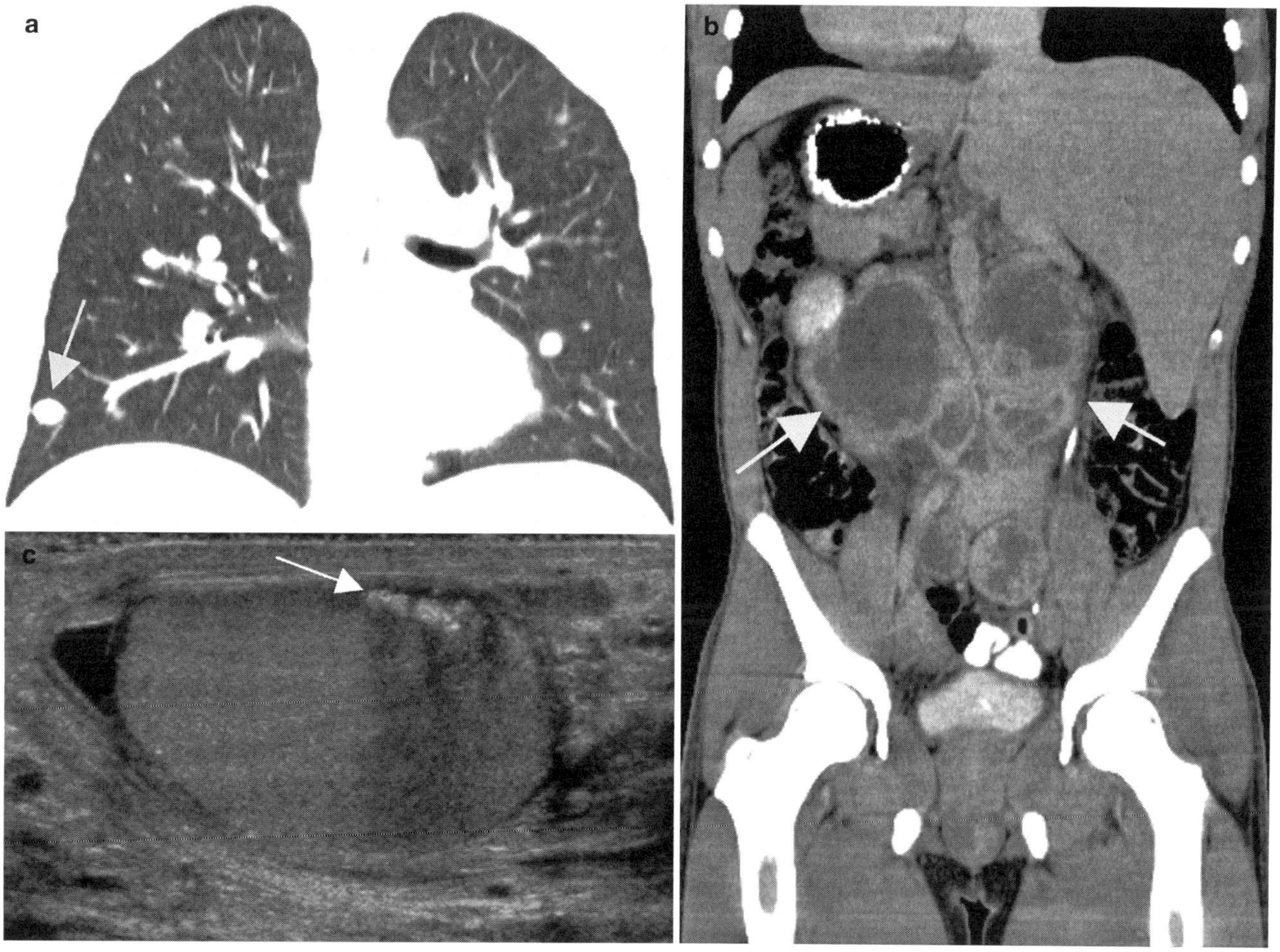

Fig. 6.74 Stage III NSGCT treated with primary chemotherapy and fibrosis in the residual mass. Coronal CT images of the chest, abdomen, and pelvis after intravenous contrast in a teenager with left flank pain, fatigue, and hematuria revealed lung metastases and retroperitoneal adenopathy (*arrows* in **a**, **b**). The hCG was more than 300,000 mIU/mL. Biopsy of retroperitoneal nodes revealed metastatic choriocarcinoma. He was considered poor-risk NSGCT. Chemotherapy was started after retroperitoneal node biopsy. Testicular ultrasound demonstrated coarse calcifications (*arrow* in **c**) and orchiectomy showed calcified scar with no viable tumor consistent with regressed or burnt-out tumor. This can be seen when the testicular tumor outgrows its blood supply and infarcts. After primary chemotherapy the residual mass or masses in patients with NSGCT, especially in the retroperitoneum are resected. Fibrosis is present in 45–50 %, teratoma in 40 % and viable germ cell tumor in 10–15 %. This is an example of a patient who had fibrosis in the resected masses. Those with fibrosis are considered free of disease

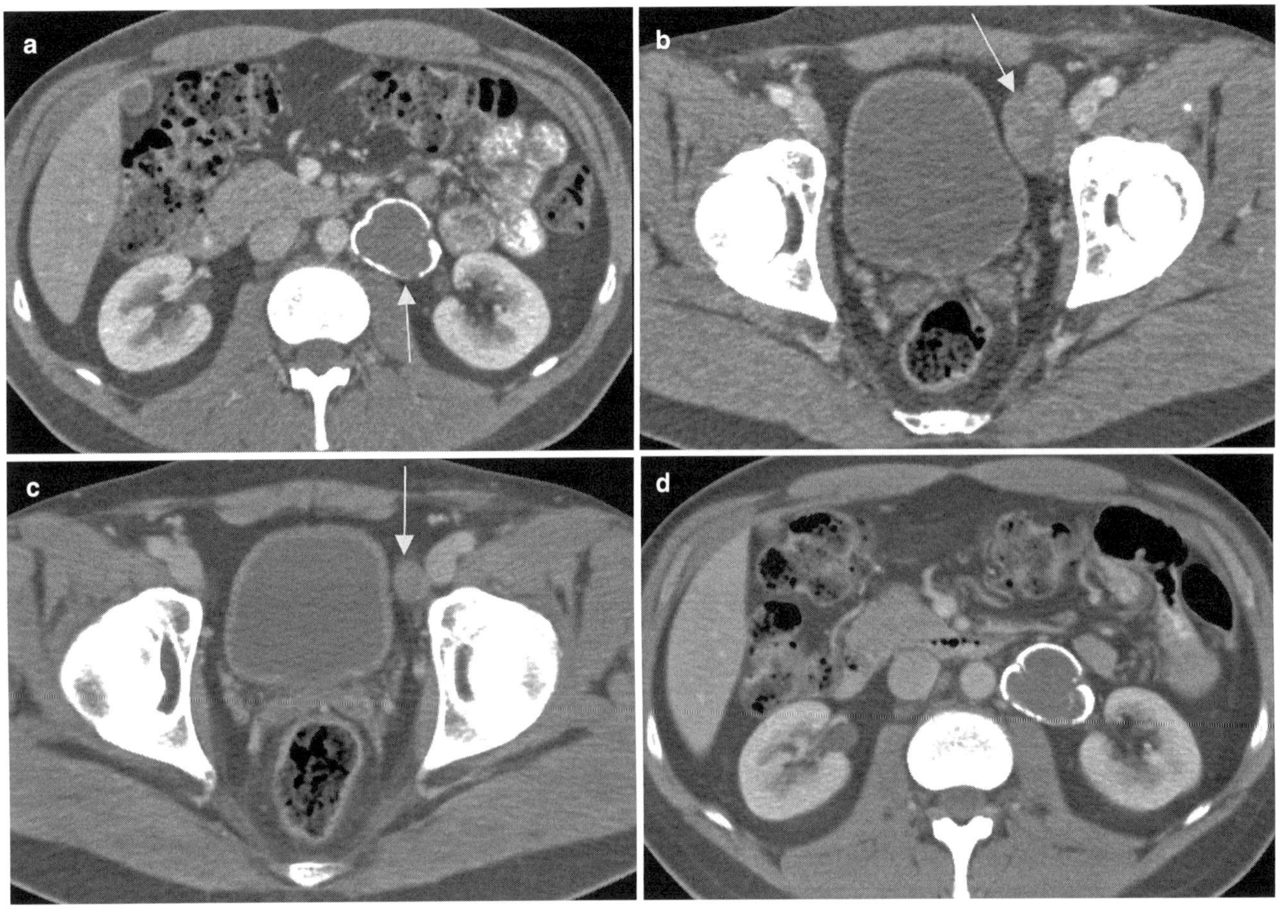

Fig. 6.75 Stage III NSGCT with teratoma in post-chemotherapy residual mass. Axial CT images of the abdomen and pelvis with oral and intravenous contrast in a 40-year-old with back pain showed a peripherally calcified left para-aortic mass (*arrow* in **a**) and an enlarged left external iliac node (*arrow* in **b**). Biopsy of the pelvic node showed poorly differentiated carcinoma. US examination of the testes documented a 1 cm calcified left testicular mass. Orchiectomy specimen showed intratubular germ cell neoplasia in a background of extensive sclerosis (partially burnt-out tumor). The patient was treated with chemotherapy, with a decrease in size of the pelvic node (*arrow* in **c**) but no change in the retroperitoneal mass (**d**). Retroperitoneal lymph node dissection showed metastatic teratoma in a background of necrosis, fibrosis, and histiocytic response. No viable germ cell component

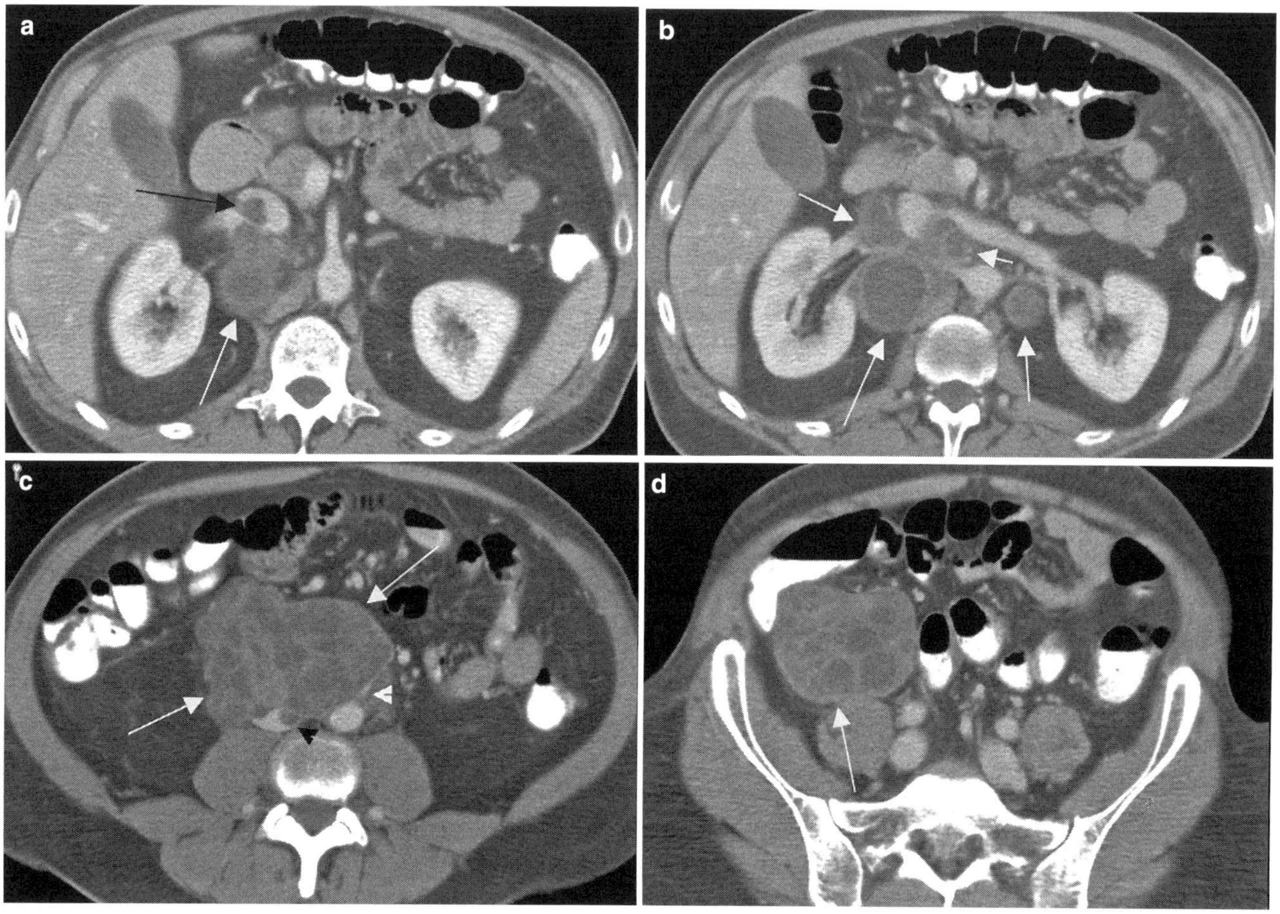

Fig. 6.76 Stage III NSGCT treated with primary chemotherapy and teratoma in bulky residual mass. Axial CT images of the abdomen and pelvis with oral and intravenous contrast in a patient with right mixed germ cell tumor; dominant teratoma, with embryonal carcinoma, yolk sac tumor, mature teratoma, immature teratoma. CT performed 5 months later demonstrated left supraclavicular and retroperitoneal disease. Images (**a**, **b**) show extensive bulky retroperitoneal adenopathy (*white arrow*) with thrombus in the IVC (*black arrow* in **a**; *black arrowhead* in **c**). (**c**) The inferior mesenteric artery (*white arrowhead*) is encased and stretched by adjacent tumor (*arrows*). (**d**) The right iliac fossa cystic mass (*arrow*) is along the expected course of the right gonadal vein. Primary chemotherapy was administered. Post-chemotherapy markers normalized but CT images revealed residual bulky mass with cystic change. Retroperitoneal node dissection showed mature teratoma in retroperitoneum and IVC thrombus; interaortocaval mass had extensive mature skeletal muscle component. Teratoma is present in 40 % of the residual post-chemotherapy masses in patients with NSGCT. It is benign but can grow, obstruct, invade adjacent structures, and become unresectable. There is a 3–6 % risk of malignant transformation. The teratomatous masses frequently contain cystic components. This patient has no evidence of disease 3 years later

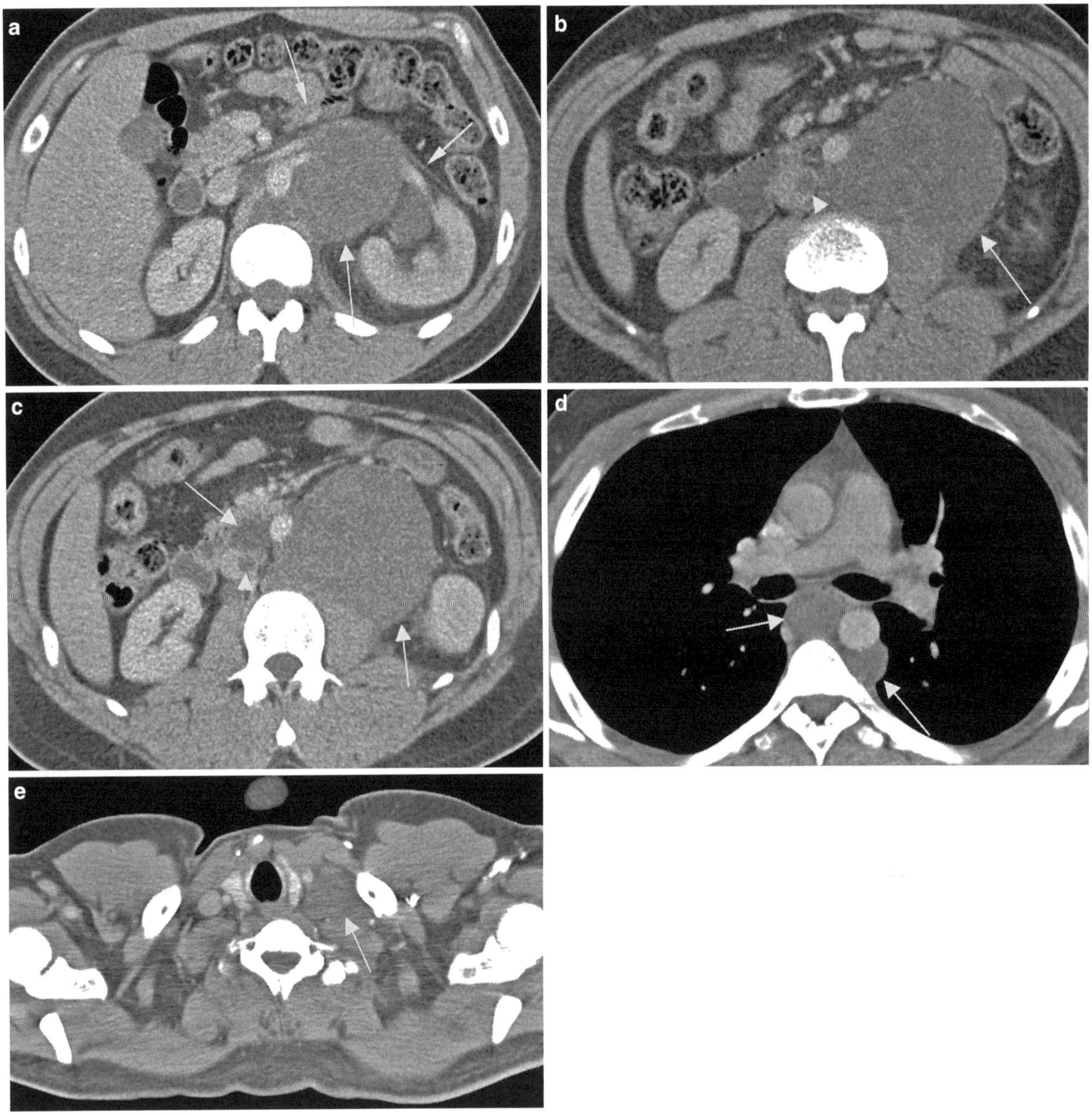

Fig. 6.77 Stage III NSGCT with growing testicular and nodal masses on chemotherapy consistent with growing teratoma. Axial CT images of the chest and abdomen with oral and intravenous contrast in a 25-year-old patient with left flank pain and elevated alpha fetoprotein. Patient was begun on chemotherapy for presumed diagnosis of testicular germ cell tumor. On chemotherapy, left testicle enlarged and became firm and patient developed left supraclavicular mass. (**a**) CT showed a large left paraaortic mass displacing the renal artery and vein anteriorly (*arrows*). Retrocrural extension is also noted. (**b**, **c**) Mass (*arrows*) extended into the interaortocaval and retrocaval region with invasion into the IVC (*arrowheads*). (**d**, **e**) Thoracic adenopathy (*arrows*) in posterior mediastinum and in the left supraclavicular chain. Orchiectomy and retroperitoneal node dissection showed mature teratoma in a background of fibrosis and focal necrosis. Mediastinal mass proved to be mature cystic teratoma. Intracaval mass was metastatic mature teratoma. In this case, the teratoma was growing. It is important to remember that increased size is not necessarily due to malignant tumor

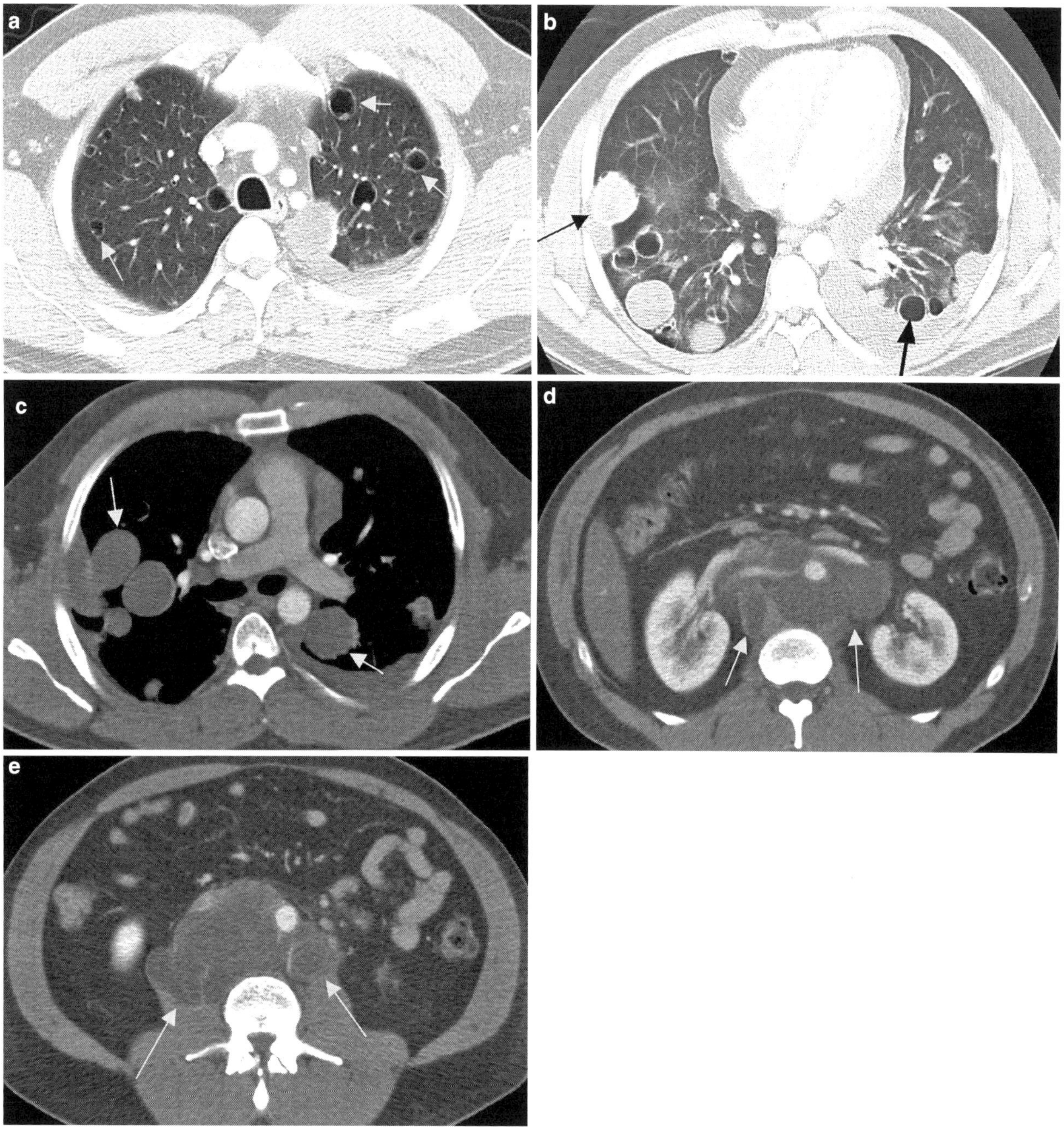

Fig. 6.78 Stage III NSGCT with increasing metastases during chemotherapy consistent with growing teratoma. Axial CT images of the chest and abdomen after oral and intravenous contrast in a patient diagnosed with right testicular mixed germ cell tumor cancer (70 % embryonal, yolk sac tumor, immature teratoma and choriocarcinoma with extensive necrosis) 2 years earlier. CT chest (**a**–**c**) demonstrated cystic and thin-walled cavitary pulmonary masses (*arrows*) on treatment with chemotherapy. Pulmonary function tests showed decreased residual volume, with an oxygen saturation in the lower 90 % range, which necessitated supplemental oxygen. Abdominal CT (**d**, **e**) shows bulky cystic mass (*arrows*) in the retroperitoneum displacing the aorta and IVC anteriorly. Because of the cystic appearance of these retroperitoneal masses and the increased size on treatment this was suggestive of teratoma and the decision was made to attempt to resect the retroperitoneal disease. RPLND showed metastatic teratoma with associated macrophage accumulation and foreign body giant cell reaction

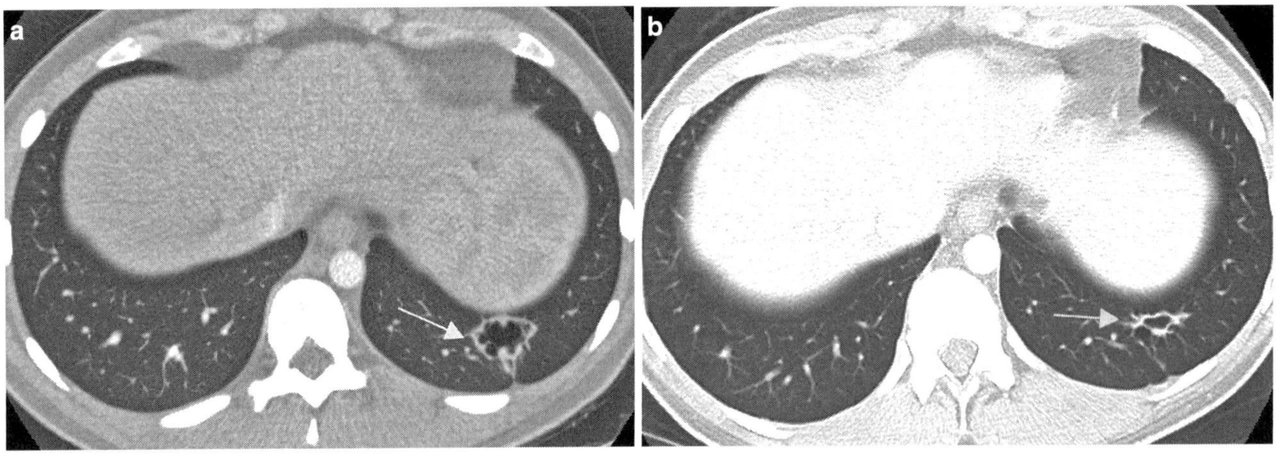

Fig. 6.79 Stage III NSGCT with cavitating pulmonary metastasis and minimal viable tumor after chemotherapy. Axial CT images of the chest with intravenous contrast in a patient with left mixed germ cell tumor (90 % embryonal carcinoma, yolk sac tumor, and immature teratoma). (**a**) 6 weeks after the orchiectomy, a left lower lobe lung mass (*arrow*) was identified on CT chest. (**b**) The metastasis decreased after chemotherapy to a residual cystic mass with a thick irregular wall (*arrow*). There was no retroperitoneal adenopathy. Wedge resection 6 months later showed metastatic germ cell tumor with more than 90 % treatment effect and less than 10 % viable tumor, consisting of predominantly mature teratoma with a minor component of immature teratoma. After primary chemotherapy, 10–15 % will have viable germ cell tumor in the resected specimen. An RPLND performed at the same time revealed no viable disease or teratoma

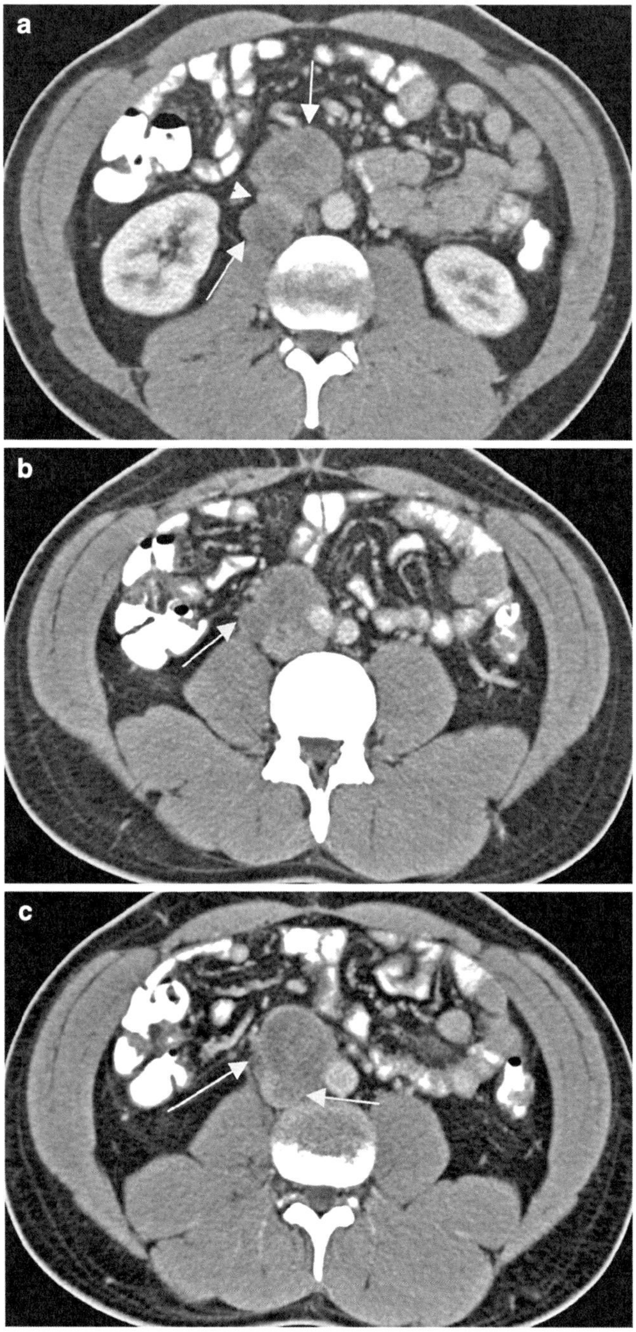

Fig. 6.80 Relapsed stage III, good-risk NSGCT. Axial CT images of the abdomen with oral and intravenous contrast in a patient with right testicular mixed germ cell tumor (dominant embryonal carcinoma, seminoma, and immature teratoma) shows (**a–c**) enlarged recurrent retroperitoneal nodes (*arrows*) in the interaortocaval and retrocaval region with IVC invasion (*arrowhead* in **a**). Note irregular margin of the anterior IVC and low attenuation tumor within the enhanced lumen of the IVC. The patient at presentation had lung metastases and retroperitoneal adenopathy. The lung metastases resolved with chemotherapy and the retroperitoneal disease decreased. The RPLND done elsewhere revealed mature teratoma. Patient came to our institution for follow-up 1 year later with rising tumor markers and recurrent disease in the retroperitoneum as described above with IVC invasion. Patient was treated with four cycles of salvage chemotherapy. Repeat RPLND revealed mature teratoma

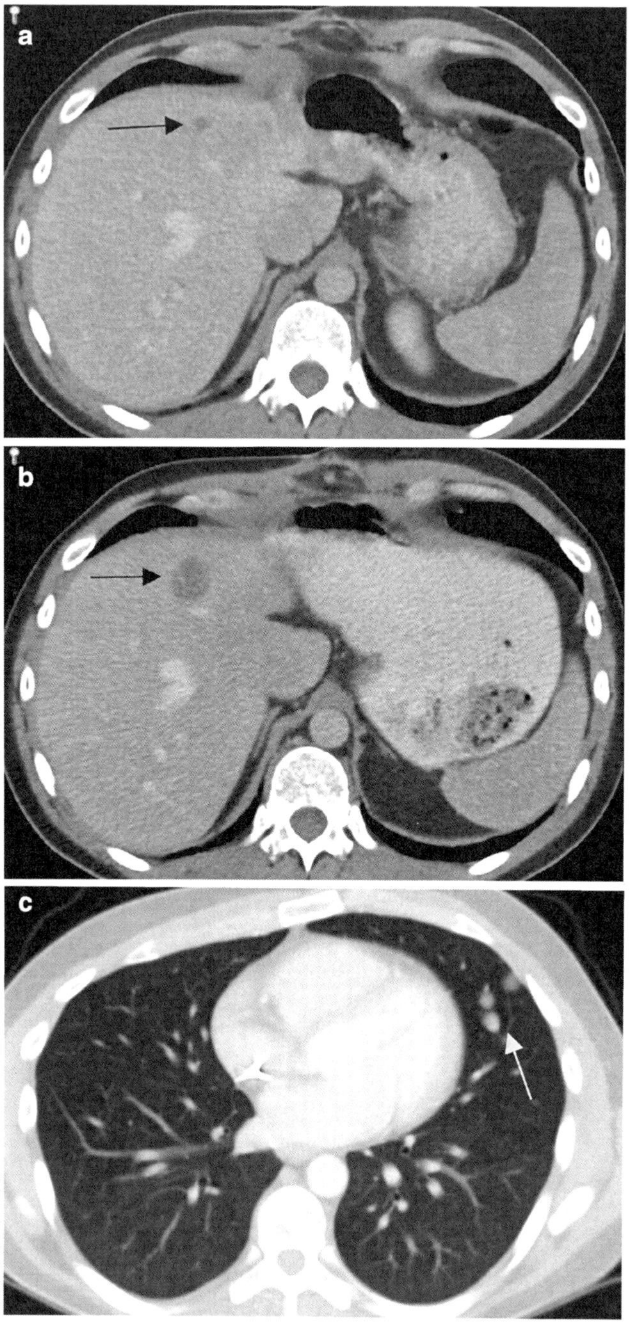

Fig. 6.81 Stage III mixed germ cell tumor with recurrence in lungs and liver. Surveillance axial CT images of the chest and abdomen with oral and intravenous contrast in a 30-year-old man demonstrated recurrence with (**a**, **b**) enlarging hepatic metastasis (*arrows*) and (**c**) lung metastases (*arrow*). He was treated with chemotherapy as he was considered to have a favorable prognosis because he had a complete response to chemotherapy previously. 2 years before, the patient had had a CT scan for back pain which revealed lung nodules consistent with metastases and retroperitoneal adenopathy. Because of the patient's age and tumor distribution, a testicular US was performed, which showed a right testis mass. Orchiectomy revealed pure seminoma, however, the AFP was elevated to more than 7,000 ng/mL, so the patient was treated in a similar fashion to NSGCT with chemotherapy followed by a retroperitoneal node dissection which showed necrosis with viable tumor—75 % teratoma (primitive neuroectodermal tumor) and 25 % yolk sac tumor

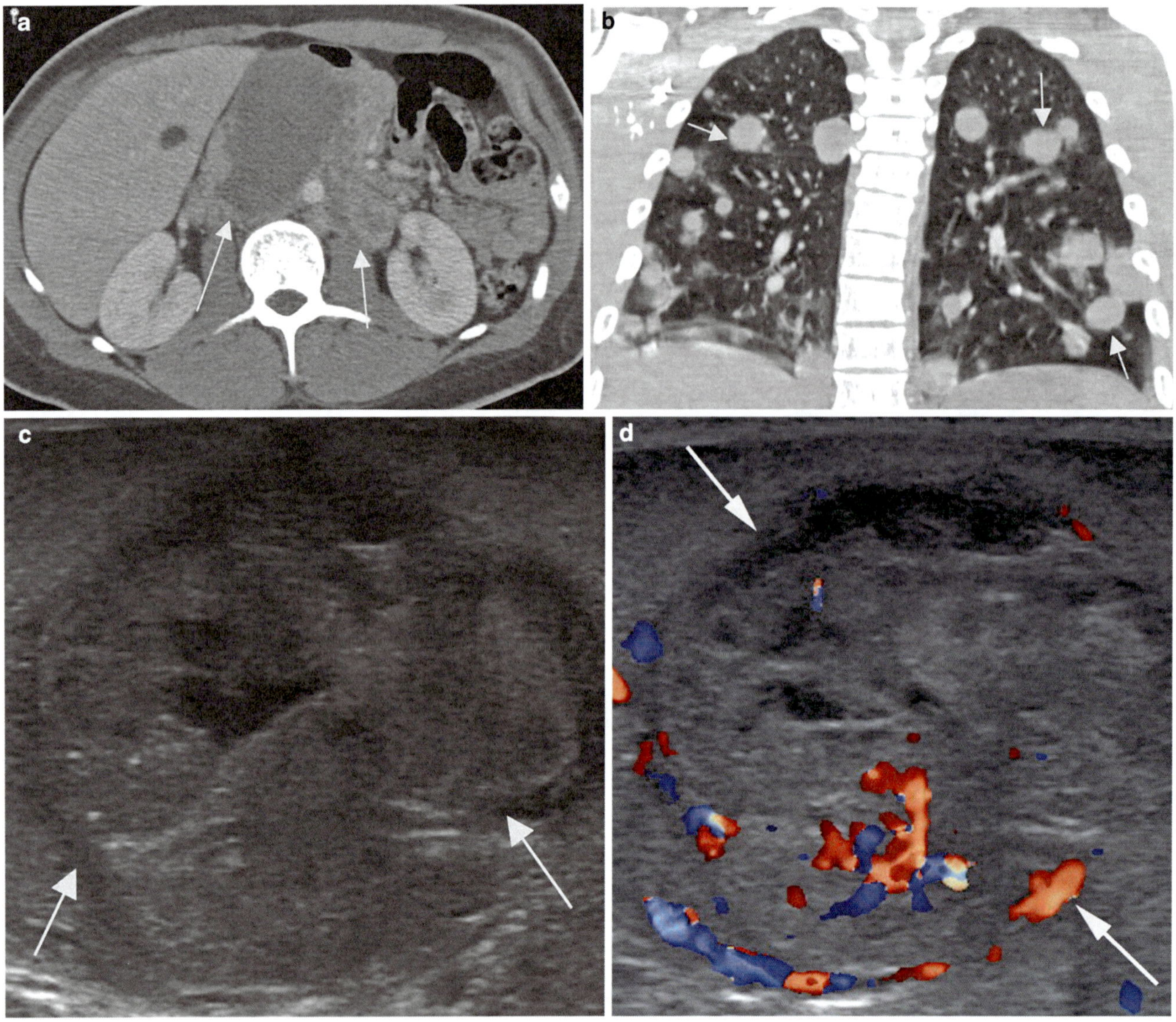

Fig. 6.82 Stage III NSGCT with recurrence in the brain despite response in the retroperitoneum and chest. CT images of the chest and abdomen with intravenous contrast in a 20-year-old male with progressive back pain and emesis. Abdominal CT showed (**a**) enlarged retroperitoneal nodes (*arrow*) and a very large interaortocaval mass (*arrow*) encasing the IVC. Chest radiograph (*not shown*) showed multiple lung nodules that were demonstrated on subsequent CT (*arrows* in **b**). (**c**, **d**) Scrotal US with color flow Doppler showed a hypervascular heterogeneous mass (*arrows*) with mixed echogenicity. Pathologic examination of the orchiectomy specimen revealed mixed germ cell tumor with dominant embryonal carcinoma and choriocarcinoma, yolk sac tumor, and mature teratoma. (**e**) Chemotherapy was administered and the lung metastases decreased in size. (**f**) The patient developed a new brain metastasis (*arrow*), which was resected. Pathology showed choriocarcinoma with hemorrhagic necrosis. Most patients relapse/recur within 2 years. Eighty percent of patients relapse in the retroperitoneum, with poor survival rates of 30–40 %. This patient is part of the 20 % that relapse outside the retroperitoneum

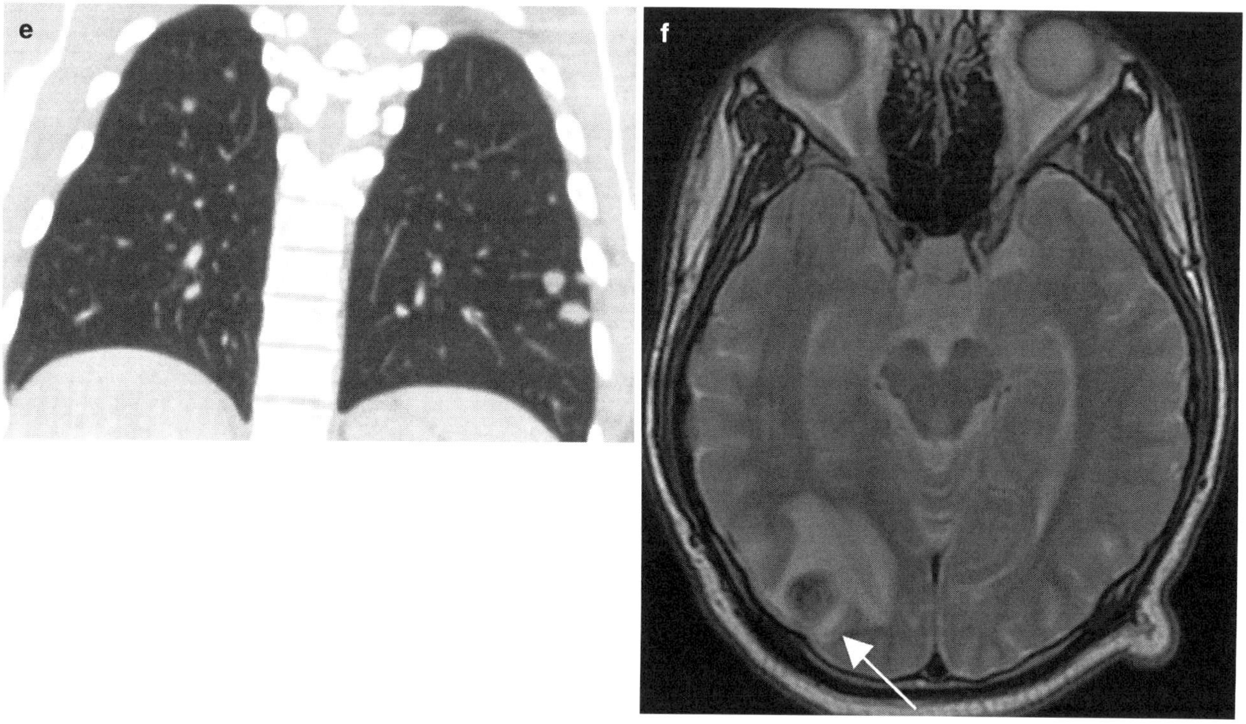

Fig. 6.82 (continued)

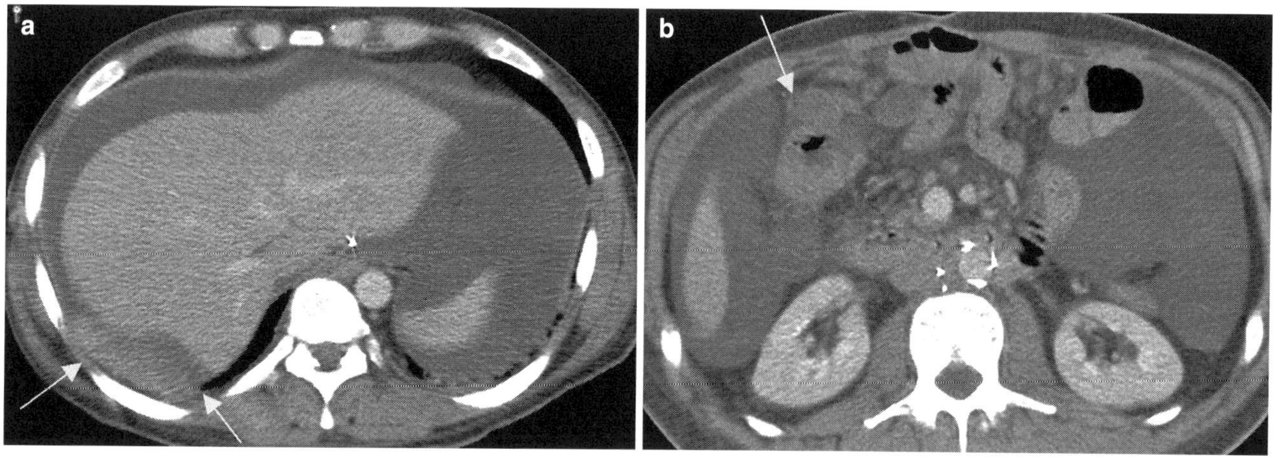

Fig. 6.83 Stage III NSGCT with late relapse in peritoneum in a patient with multiple prior recurrences. Axial CT images of the abdomen with oral and intravenous contrast in a patient with NSGCT who developed peritoneal disease on surveillance CT 10 years after initial presentation. The patient initially presented with retroperitoneal adenopathy and lung metastases and was treated with chemotherapy. Subsequent RPLND showed teratoma after which the patient had multiple relapses in the retroperitoneum and bone metastases showing teratoma at pathology. (**a**, **b**) CT demonstrates ascites and peritoneal nodular thickening (*arrows*). Surgery was performed on the peritoneal disease to improve the long-term survival and for histologic confirmation. Pathology revealed metastatic teratoma in background of fibrosis and macrophages, but no other viable tumor. Two to 4 % of patients relapse beyond 2 years after initial diagnosis. This is considered a late relapse as defined as a recurrence of disease 2 years or more following initial treatment. Treatment of late relapse is usually surgery because the recurrence is often chemoresistant. The pathology is viable germ cell tumor in 80 % cases and teratoma in 20 %. Relapse can occur at any time, reported up to 32 years later with a median of 6 years

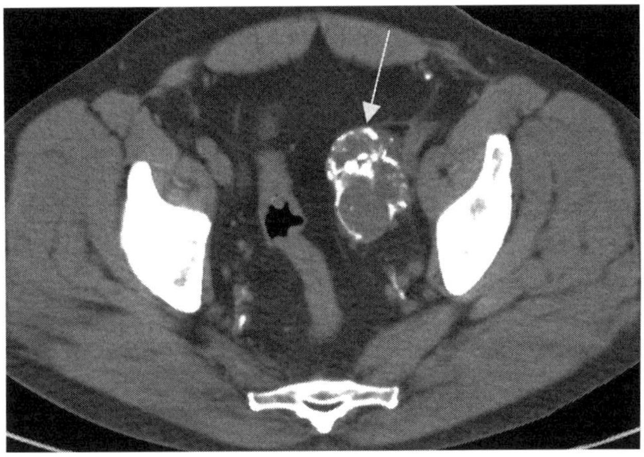

Fig. 6.84 Stage III NSGCT with late relapse 31 years after initial diagnosis. Axial CT image of the pelvis in a patient who had an orchiectomy 31 years earlier followed by chemotherapy for stage III NSGCT. RPLND performed 30 years earlier demonstrated mature teratoma and pulmonary nodules were resected without viable tumor. The patient had a relapse 1 year later (29 years earlier) for which he received chemotherapy. The patient presented now with elevated LDH and slowly increasing back pain. Axial CT image of the pelvis without oral or intravenous contrast demonstrated a peripherally calcified left pelvic mass (*arrow*). The patient also had a liver mass, which was excised and showed enteric type adenocarcinoma with 70 % necrosis. Biopsies of the pelvic mass showed necrosis, calcification, and fragments of adenocarcinoma of the colonic type. This was felt to be a somatic-type mutation or somatic-type malignant transformation of a prior mature teratoma. Radiation therapy was recommended for probable somatic transformation to enteric-type adenocarcinoma. The treatment of relapsing NSGCT depends on whether the patient is considered to have a favorable or unfavorable prognosis. Patients with favorable prognosis are those who have had a complete response to chemotherapy with testis primary. These patients are treated with more chemotherapy. The patient in this case had a favorable prognosis as there was no viable tumor after the initial chemotherapy at surgery in the retroperitoneum or chest and was considered to have had an initial complete response. Patients with unfavorable prognosis have had prior incomplete response to chemotherapy and testis primary. These patients receive high-dose chemotherapy and stem cell transplant

Mimics and Postoperative Complications

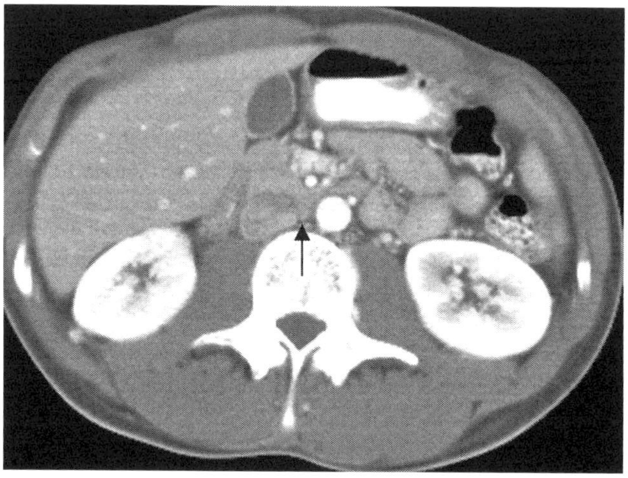

Fig. 6.85 Duodenum mimicking retroperitoneal node. Axial CT image of the abdomen with intravenous and oral contrast shows aortocaval soft tissue density (*arrow*), which can mimic a node. The soft tissue was contiguous with the duodenum and represented normal duodenum. Coronal reconstructions can be helpful to distinguish normal duodenum from lymphadenopathy

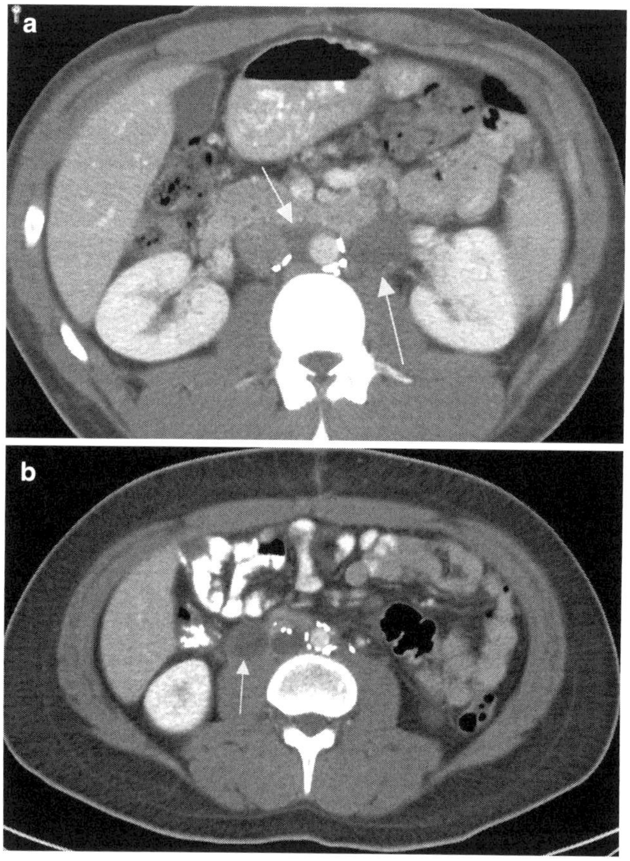

Fig. 6.86 Postoperative lymphocele following retroperitoneal lymph node dissection. Axial CT image with oral and intravenous contrast in a patient who had undergone a left orchiectomy 6 months earlier for embryonal carcinoma with vascular invasion. The patient preferred to undergo a retroperitoneal node dissection rather than surveillance due to a high risk of recurrence. At surgery, four left para-aortic and 21 interaortocaval nodes were resected and all were benign. (**a**) Follow-up CT obtained 3 months after node dissection shows characteristic low attenuation retroperitoneal fluid collections in the surgical bed (*arrows*) compatible with lymphoceles. These usually resolve completely with time. (**b**) Axial CT image with oral and intravenous contrast in a different patient who had undergone a retroperitoneal node dissection showing paracaval lymphoceles (*arrow*). There is a low rate of complications for primary retroperitoneal node dissection. In a series of more than 450 patients, superficial wound infections comprised the majority of complications, lymphoceles occurred in 0.4 % of patients and chylous ascites in one patient [7]

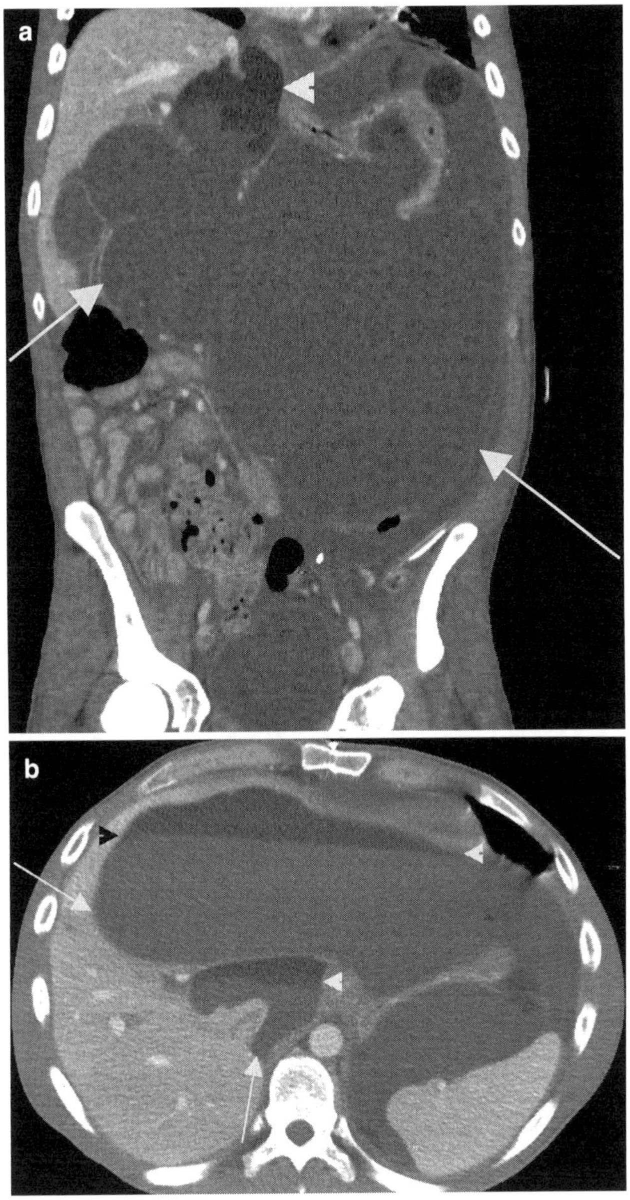

Fig. 6.87 Massive chylous ascites following retroperitoneal lymph node dissection. Axial and coronal CT images with intravenous contrast in a 20-year-old male patient who presented with back pain and dyspnea. CT (*not shown*) showed a mass in the superior vena cava extending through the heart to the pulmonary artery. This was resected and proved to be metastatic sarcomatous component of a germ cell neoplasm. Ultrasound examination of the right testis showed a small mass that was a scar at orchiectomy and felt to be a "burned-out" tumor. The patient was subsequently treated with chemotherapy and a retroperitoneal lymph node dissection, which showed metastatic sarcoma in a few nodes and teratoma. Postoperatively after the node dissection, the patient developed abdominal distention. (**a**) Coronal CT image shows moderate abdominal ascites (*arrows*) with some hypodense areas (*arrowhead*). (**b**) Axial CT image shows that the abdominal ascites (*arrows*) has fat–fluid levels (*arrowhead*) and is compatible with chylous ascites. The patient was placed on a low-fat diet without benefit. Due to persistent abdominal distention, a peritoneal drainage catheter was placed and had a daily output of 1 l of chylous ascites. The patient's diet was further restricted by placing him on total parenteral nutrition without dietary fat and the chylous ascites decreased

Acknowledgment The authors wish to thank Mr. Hans Michell for his extensive help with preparing the images for publication.

References

1. Carver BS, Sheinfeld J. Germ cell tumors of the testis. Ann Surg Oncol. 2005;12:871–80.
2. Husband JE, Koh DM. Multimodality imaging of testicular tumors. Cancer Imaging. 2004;4:S1–7.
3. Hahn N, Foster RS. Testis cancer. In: Markman M, editor. Atlas of cancer. 2nd ed. Philadelphia: Springer; 2008. p. 488–99.
4. Woodward PJ, Sohaey R, O'Donoghue MJ, Green DE. From the archives of the AFIP: tumors and tumorlike lesions of the testis: radiologic-pathologic correlation. Radiographics. 2002;22:189–216.
5. Hilton S, Herr HW, Teitcher JB, et al. CT detection of retroperitoneal lymph node metastases in patients with clinical stage I testicular nonseminomatous germ cell cancer: assessment of size and distribution criteria. AJR Am J Roentgenol. 1997;169:521–5.
6. Eggener SE, Carver BS, Sharp DS, et al. Incidence of disease outside modified retroperitoneal lymph node dissection templates in clinical stage I or IIa nonseminomatous germ cell testicular cancer. J Urol. 2007;177:937–42.
7. Jacobsen NE, Foster RS, Donohue JP. Retroperitoneal lymph node dissection in testicular cancer. Surg Oncol Clin N Am. 2007;16:199–220.
8. Sohaib SA, Koh DM, Husband JE. The role of imaging in the diagnosis, staging, and management of testicular cancer. Am J Roentgenol. 2008;191:387–95.
9. Sohaib SA, Koh DM, Barbachano Y, et al. Prospective assessment of MRI for imaging retroperitoneal metastases from testicular germ cell tumours. Clin Radiol. 2009;64:362–7.
10. Carver BS, Sheinfeld J. Management of post-chemotherapy extra-retroperitoneal residual masses. World J Urol. 2009;27:489–92.
11. Panicek DM, Toner GC, Heelan RT, Bosl GJ. Nonseminomatous germ cell tumors: enlarging masses despite chemotherapy. Radiology. 1990;175:499–502.
12. Kollmannsberger C, Oechsle K, Dohmen BM, et al. Prospective comparison of [^{18}F]fluorodeoxyglucose positron emission tomography with conventional assessment by computed tomography scans and serum tumor markers for the evaluation of residual masses in patients with nonseminomatous germ cell carcinoma. Cancer. 2002;94:2353–62.
13. De Santis M, Becherer A, Bokemeyer C, et al. 2-18fluoro-deoxy-D-glucose positron emission tomography is a reliable predictor for viable tumor in postchemotherapy seminoma: an update of the prospective multicentric SEMPET trial. J Clin Oncol. 2004;22:1034–9.
14. Feldman DR, Bosl GJ, Sheinfeld J, Motzer RJ. Medical treatment of advanced testicular cancer. JAMA. 2008;299:672–84.
15. Dogra VS, Gottlieb RH, Oka M, Rubens DJ. Sonography of the scrotum. Radiology. 2003;227:18–36.
16. Connor S, Guest P. Conversion of multiple solid testicular teratoma metastases to fatty and cystic liver masses following chemotherapy: CT evidence of "maturation". Br J Radiol. 1999;72:1114–6.

General Chemotherapy Imaging

7

Jean M. Torrisi, Tunc A. Iyriboz, and Han Xiao

Toxicity assessments on patients undergoing chemotherapy or targeted molecular therapy are performed regularly by the referring oncologist. Some toxicities have radiologic manifestations (*see* Table 7.1). Occasionally, the radiologist is asked by the oncologist to assess for a clinically suspected toxicity that has an associated radiologic presentation. An example of this is bleomycin-induced pulmonary toxicity encountered during the treatment of metastatic germ cell tumor of the testis. Some classic chemotherapy agents and particularly the newer targeted therapies have toxicities with radiologic manifestations that are asymptomatic [1]. Therefore the radiologist may be the first to detect these toxicities. A summary of the treatment options and radiographic presentations of the more common side effects encountered during treatment of genitourinary tumors is presented here.

Table 7.1 Radiographically evident toxicities associated with chemotherapy agents used in the treatment of genitourinary tumors by organ

Agent	Organ	Toxicity
Bevacizumab	GI	GI perforation, pneumatosis, bleeding
Bleomycin	Pulmonary	Interstitial infiltrates/fibrosis
Cisplatin	Vascular	Arterial and venous thrombosis
Etoposide	Secondary malignancy	Leukemia
Gemcitabine	Pulmonary	Capillary leak syndrome, diffuse alveolar damage, alveolar hemorrhage
	Vascular	Arterial and venous thrombosis
Interleukin–2	Pulmonary	Interstitial edema, capillary leak syndrome
Methotrexate	Pulmonary	Hypersensitivity pneumonitis, COP, noncardiogenic pulmonary edema
Sunitinib/ sorafenib	GI	Enteritis
Temsirolimus/ everolimus	Pulmonary	Ground glass infiltrates, COP

Renal Cell Cancer

Treatment Options for Metastatic Renal Cell Cancer

The treatment of advanced renal cell carcinoma (RCC) has undergone major advances in recent years as a result of the development of new targeted molecular agents [2–5]. These include the vascular endothelial growth factor receptor (VEGFR) tyrosine kinase inhibitors (TKI), the mTOR inhibitors, and the VEGFR monoclonal antibodies. The three orally administered VEGFR TKI agents that are U.S. Food and Drug Administration approved for the treatment of advanced RCC are sunitinib, sorafenib, and pazopanib. These agents inhibit multiple tyrosine kinases involved in cell proliferation, including VEGFR and platelet-derived growth factor receptors (PDGFR), which are activated in the majority of sporadic clear cell RCCs [5, 6]. The mTOR inhibitors, temsirolimus and everolimus, inhibit a key intracellular pathway represented by a protein kinase known as the mammalian target of rapamycin (mTOR) [6]. Inhibition of this key intracellular pathway results in interruption of cell proliferation, cell growth, and tumor angiogenesis. The anti-VEGF monoclonal antibody bevacizumab exerts its anti-angiogenic effects by binding to the circulating VEGF. Current evidence

J.M. Torrisi, M.D. (✉)
Department of Radiology, Memorial Sloan Kettering Cancer Center, 136 Mountain View Boulevard, Basking Ridge, NJ 07920, USA
e-mail: torrisij@mskcc.org

T.A. Iyriboz M.D.
Department of Radiology, Memorial Sloan-Kettering Cancer Center, 1275 York Avenue, New York, NY 10065, USA
e-mail: iyribozt@mskcc.org

H. Xiao, M.D.
Department of Medicine,
Memorial Sloan-Kettering Cancer Center at Basking Ridge, 136 Mountain View Boulevard, Basking Ridge, NJ 07920, USA
e-mail: xiaoh@mskcc.org

A.M. Bach, J. Zhang (eds.), *Atlas of Genitourinary Oncological Imaging*, Atlas of Oncology Imaging,
DOI 10.1007/978-1-4614-4872-3_7, © Springer Science+Business Media New York 2013

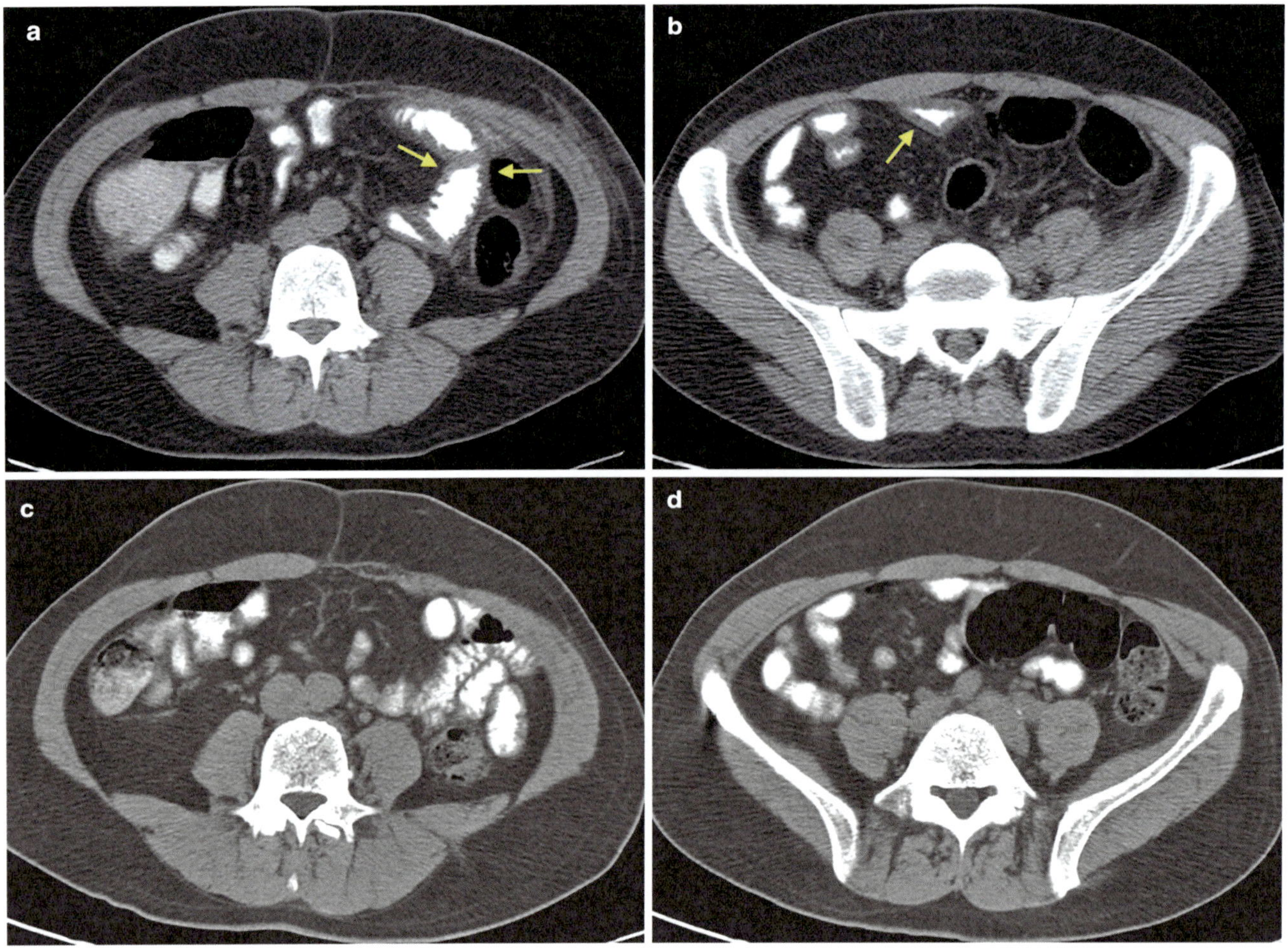

Fig. 7.1 Sunitinib-associated enteritis on CT in the treatment of metastatic RCC. A postnephrectomy patient presented with metastatic recurrence and was started on oral sunitinib at 50 mg daily, 4 weeks on and 2 weeks off. The patient developed grade I mucositis, neuropathy, skin changes, and epistaxis at the end of cycle 1. The patient continued to tolerate therapy with good treatment response. During the treatment break of cycle 7, the patient reported an episode of self-limiting abdominal pain and cramps. 2 weeks later, the routine follow-up CT demonstrated stable disease and a new finding of mild small bowel wall thickening. Representative axial CT images in the mid and lower abdomen demonstrated mild small bowel wall thickening, involving several loops of mid (**a**, *arrows*) and distal small bowel (**b**, *arrow*). During cycle 8, the patient had another episode of abdominal pain and diarrhea. The patient requested to continue treatment with no reduction in dose. At the end of cycle 9, clinical symptoms and radiographic findings resolved (**c**, **d**). He continued to tolerate therapy well with intermittent treatment breaks

supports the use of sunitinib, pazopanib, and the combination of bevacizumab plus α-interferon for treatment-naïve patients with good- and intermediate-risk advanced RCC and temsirolimus for treatment-naïve patients with poor-risk RCC. Standard second-line therapies include sorafenib and pazopanib for patients who are cytokine refractory, everolimus for patients who failed VEGFR TKI therapy, and axitinib, which is most recently approved for patients who have received one prior systemic therapy that contained sunitinib, temsirolimus, bevacizumab, or a cytokine [3, 4, 7–13].

Historical treatment with the immunotherapy cytokines interleukin (IL)-2 and interferon (INF)-α remains an option for selected cases of advanced RCC, but has increasingly less clinical implications [4]. These treatments are associated with significant toxicity, in particular IL-2–associated capillary leak syndrome [14, 15].

Radiographically Evident Toxicities Associated with Immunotherapy and Targeted Therapeutic Agents Used in the Treatment of Metastatic Renal Cell Cancer

Interleukin-2. The most frequent and severe complication of IL-2 therapy is the capillary leak syndrome characterized by hypotension, generalized edema, and renal insufficiency [16]. Patients receiving IL-2 therapy may develop pulmonary interstitial edema accompanied by pleural and pericardial effusions within 2–8 days following therapy. This may progress to diffuse air space disease similar to adult respiratory distress syndrome [17, 18]. These findings are detectable on chest radiograph or computed tomography (CT) imaging. This syndrome in most cases is reversible with discontinuation of therapy.

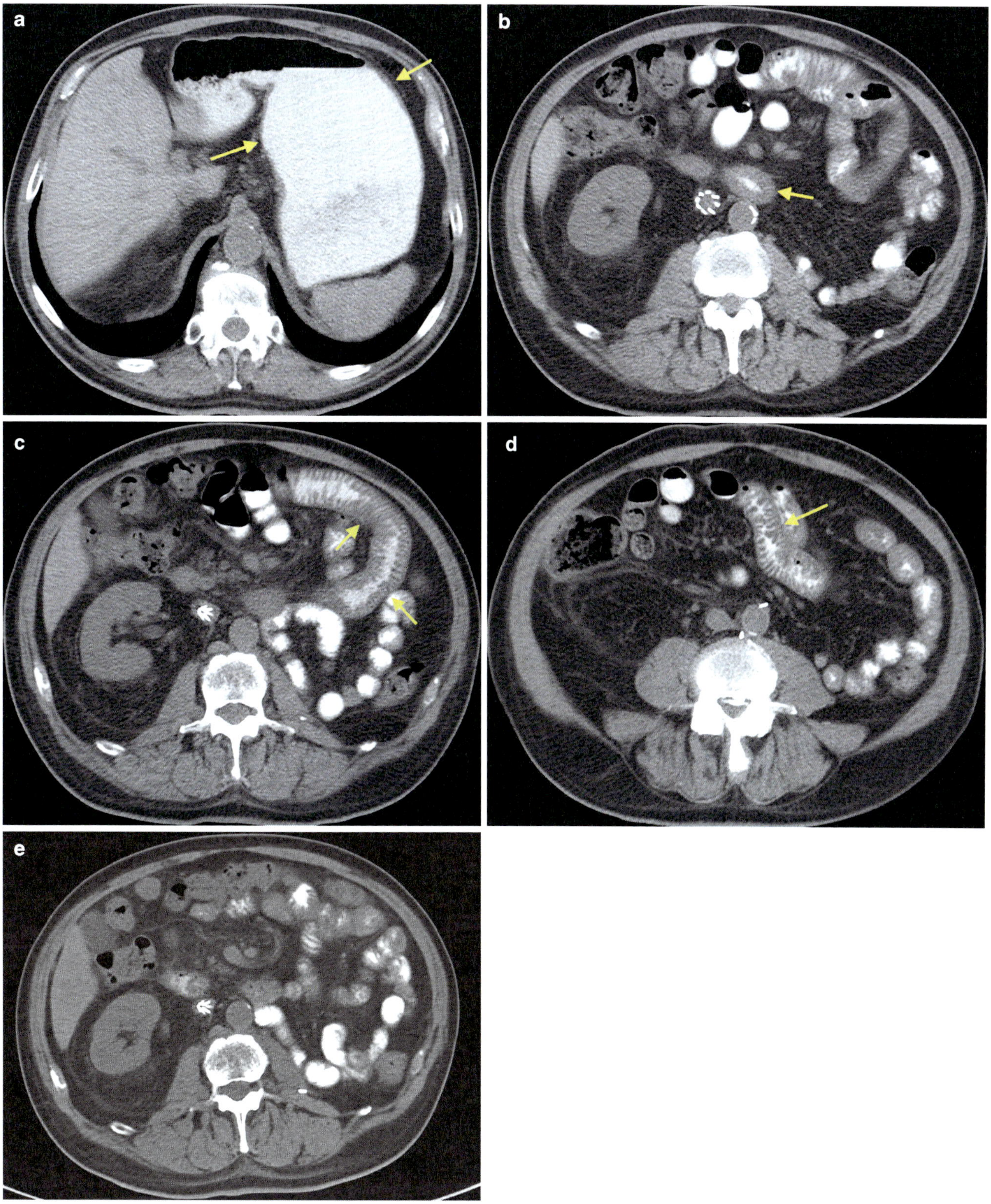

Fig. 7.2 Sunitinib-associated enteritis in the treatment of metastatic RCC. A patient with metastatic RCC was started on oral sunitinib 50 mg daily, 4 weeks on and 2 weeks off. The patient complained of grade I nausea during cycle 1 and grade III HFS during cycle 3. A follow-up CT after cycle 4 revealed good treatment response. A repeat CT after cycle 6 showed stable disease and incidental note of small bowel wall thickening. Axial CT images demonstrated mild gastric dilatation (**a**, *arrows*), bowel wall thickening of the crossing duodenum (**b**, *arrow*), mild bowel wall thickening of the proximal jejunum (**c**, *arrows*), and thickening of a distal loop of small bowel (**d**, *arrow*). The patient was asymptomatic at the time of imaging, however, during the following treatment cycle, the patient reported several episodes of nausea and vomiting. The patient continued to tolerate therapy at full dose but treatment was suspended for worsening hypertension. Radiographic manifestations of GI toxicity had resolved on follow-up CT (**e**). Sunitinib was ultimately discontinued due to progression of disease

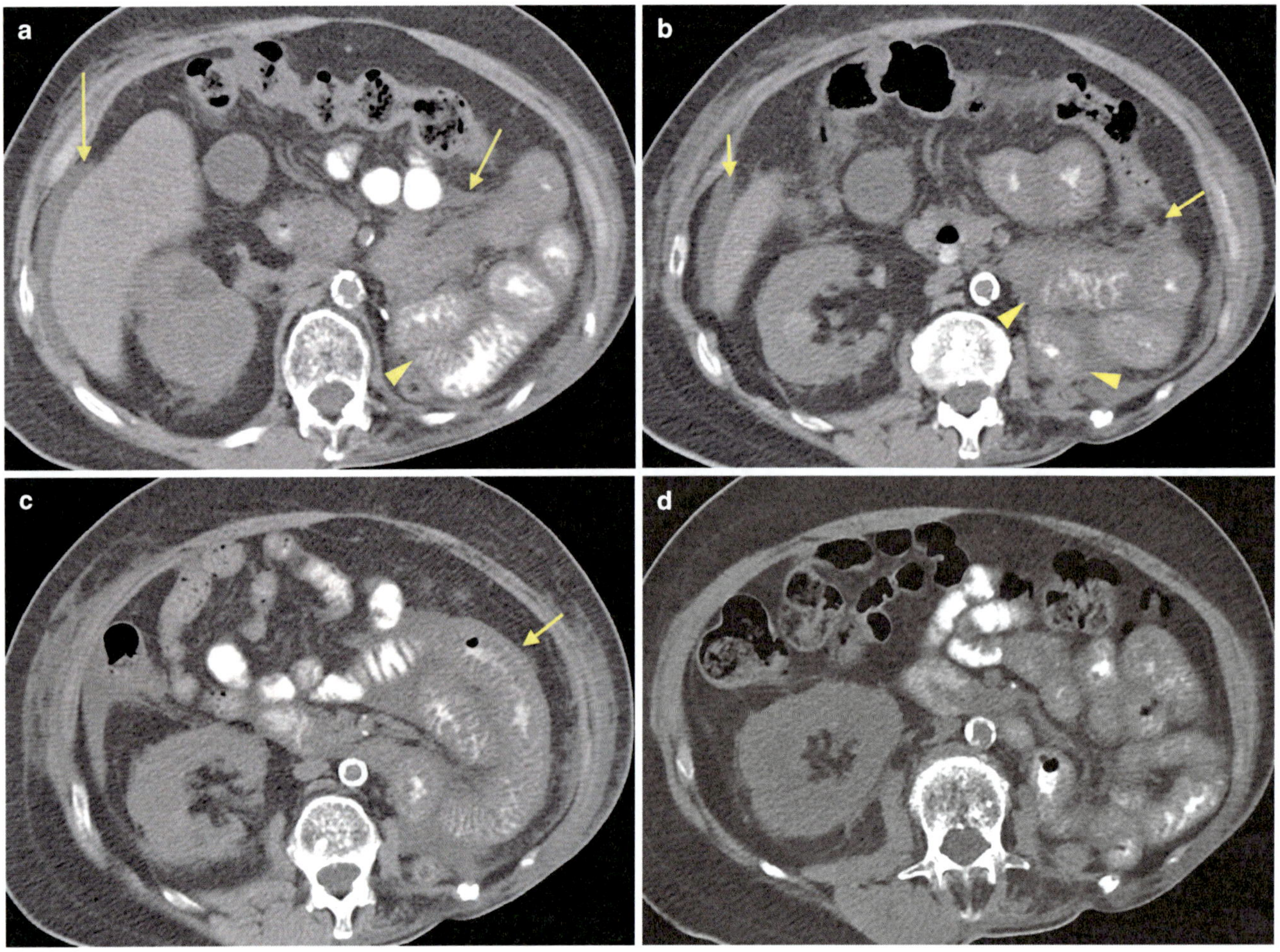

Fig. 7.3 Sunitinib-associated enteritis in the treatment of metastatic RCC. A patient with metastatic RCC was started on sunitinib with a dosing schedule of 4 weeks on and 2 weeks off. The patient complained of bloating within the first 4 weeks of therapy. Follow-up CT without intravenous contrast obtained at the end of cycle 1 revealed good treatment response, with new small volume ascites and stranding of the mesentery (**a**, *arrows*). Bowel wall thickening of the proximal jejunum was attributed to under distention at the time of the initial reading (**a**, *arrowhead*). The patient complained of general malaise, fatigue, and abdominal swelling during cycle 2. Repeat CT at the end of cycle 2 revealed stable disease, stable small-volume ascites, mesenteric stranding (**b**, *arrows*), and moderate to marked proximal small bowel wall thickening (**b**, *arrowhead*). Since bowel wall thickening was a persistent finding, a differential was offered, including edema, hemorrhage, or an infectious or inflammatory process. During the 4 weeks of treatment in cycle 3, the patient noted increasing abdominal girth that had dissipated during the 2 weeks off at the end of cycle 3. CT after cycle 3 revealed persistent small bowel wall thickening (**c**, *arrow*). The dose of sunitinib was reduced due to sores on the bottom of his feet. The follow-up CT after cycle 5 demonstrated resolution of ascites and marked improvement in mesenteric infiltration and small bowel wall thickening (**d**) with clinical improvement of abdominal swelling

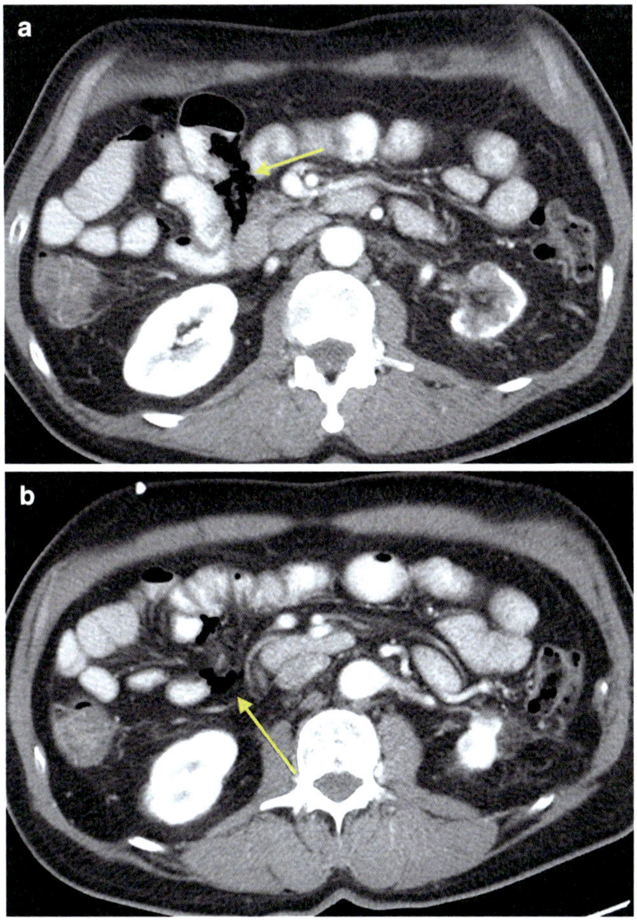

Fig. 7.4 Sunitinib-associated pneumatosis in treatment of metastatic RCC. A patient was randomized to pazopanib on a clinical trial for metastatic RCC. His treatment was changed to sunitinib due to progression of disease. At the end of cycle 1, the patient developed grade III neutropenia. Treatment was held temporarily and he was restarted at a lower dose. Follow-up CT at the end of cycle 3 revealed stable disease with incidental finding of small bowel pneumatosis. CT images reveal discrete and linear arrangement of gas bubbles within the wall of small bowel loops in the mid abdomen consistent with pneumatosis intestinalis (**a**, *arrow*). Air within the mesentery is also noted (**b**, *arrow*) with no portal venous gas. The patient was asymptomatic. Treatment was temporarily discontinued and restarted at a lower dose with no further problems

Anti-VEGF therapy: sunitinib, sorafenib, pazopanib, bevacizumab. The most common adverse events associated with the VEGFR TKIs sunitinib, sorafenib, pazopanib, and axitinib include hypertension (HTN), fatigue, hand-foot syndrome (HFS), anorexia, mucositis, diarrhea, hypothyroidism, elevated lipase, metabolic disturbances, and myelosuppression. The most frequent toxicities that occur during treatment with the monoclonal antibody bevacizumab include hypertension, proteinuria, bleeding, thrombosis, and gastrointestinal (GI) perforation [19–21]. Arterial thrombosis has been reported in 3 % of patients treated with pazopanib [8].

Diarrhea or abdominal pain during treatment with sunitinib may be accompanied radiographically by the finding of new bowel wall thickening. Sunitinib-associated enteritis may involve any part of the small bowel, with thickening of the proximal jejunum and mid and distal small bowel observed (Figs. 7.1–7.3).

Diarrhea occurs in 6–20 % of patients undergoing sunitinib treatment for RCC [19, 22]. The time to onset of this finding following the initiation of treatment is variable. The frequency of the radiographic manifestation of enteritis has not yet been reported but may be less common than the clinical correlate of abdominal pain, bloating, and diarrhea. In some cases, the radiographic manifestations are not accompanied by concurrent clinical symptoms and therefore deemed "asymptomatic"; in other cases, the CT manifestations of enteritis may precede the clinical symptoms (Fig. 7.2). Drug-induced diarrhea may be managed with dose reduction or interruption but does not typically require discontinuation of treatment [19]. In our experience, clinical and radiographic manifestations of sunitinib-associated enteritis can be self-limited (Fig. 7.1)

Other GI complications potentially encountered include pneumatosis (Fig. 7.4) and hemorrhage (Fig. 7.5). Pneumatosis intestinalis has been reported during certain types of chemotherapy, but of the molecular-targeted therapies it has been described with bevacizumab, an anti-VEGFR agent. Pneumatosis may be asymptomatic, detected first on routine

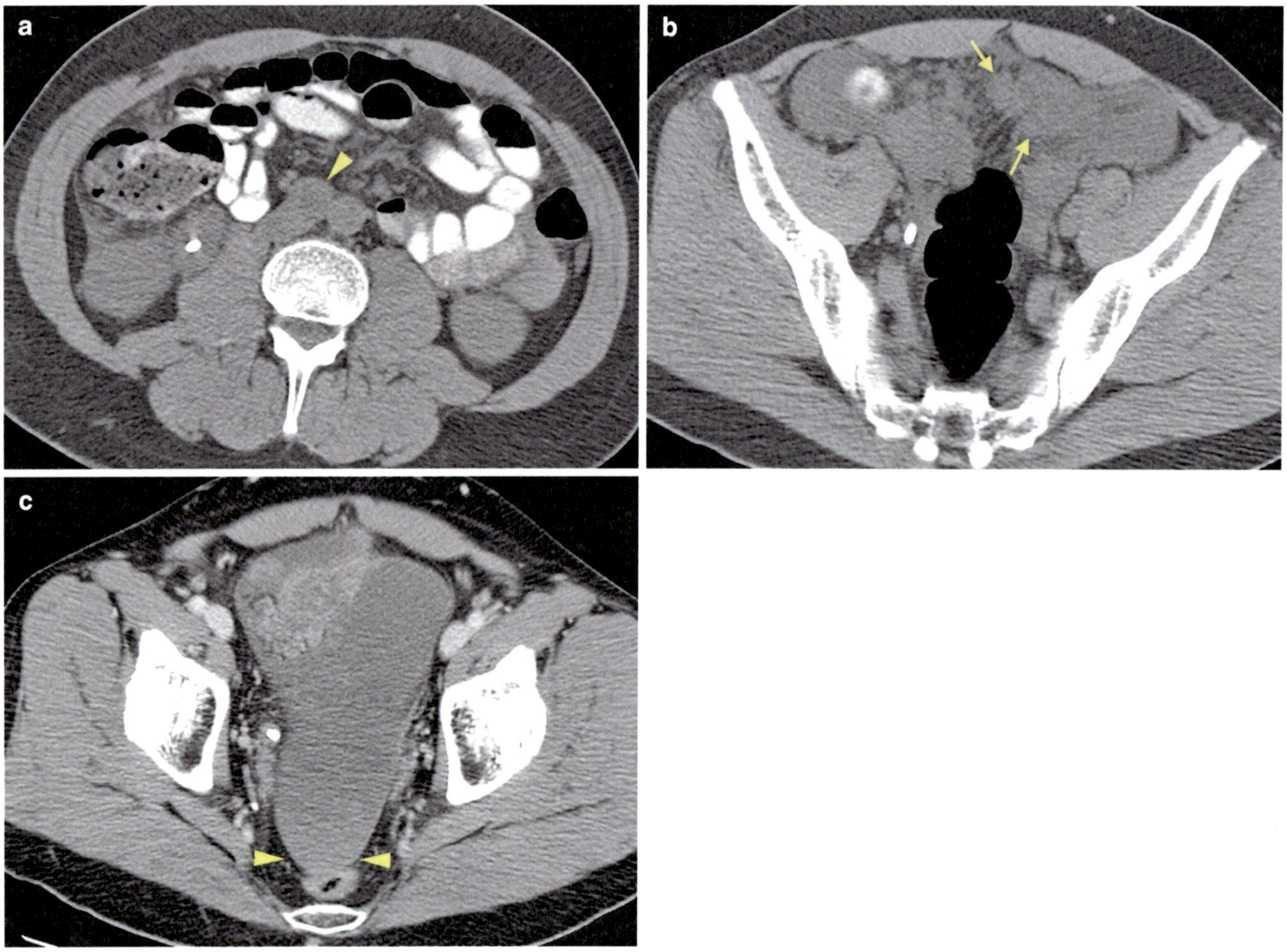

Fig. 7.5 Sunitinib-induced hemorrhage in treatment of metastatic RCC. A patient underwent partial nephrectomy for RCC and was followed with surveillance imaging studies. The patient developed retroperitoneal nodal metastases and was treated with IL-2. Due to subsequent progression of disease, he was enrolled in a clinical trial of sunitinib. A restaging CT scan prior to sunitinib revealed retroperitoneal adenopathy (**a**, *arrowhead*) and peritoneal carcinomatosis (**b**, *arrows*). At the end of cycle 1, the patient complained of abdominal distention and was found to have a drop in hemoglobin. CT examination revealed increased adenopathy, peritoneal carcinomatosis, and a large amount of high attenuation ascites (HU 40) consistent with hemoperitoneum, considered to be treatment related (**c**, *arrowheads*). The dose of sunitinib was reduced. The patient went on to have a mixed response on sunitinib, and was then offered further treatment options

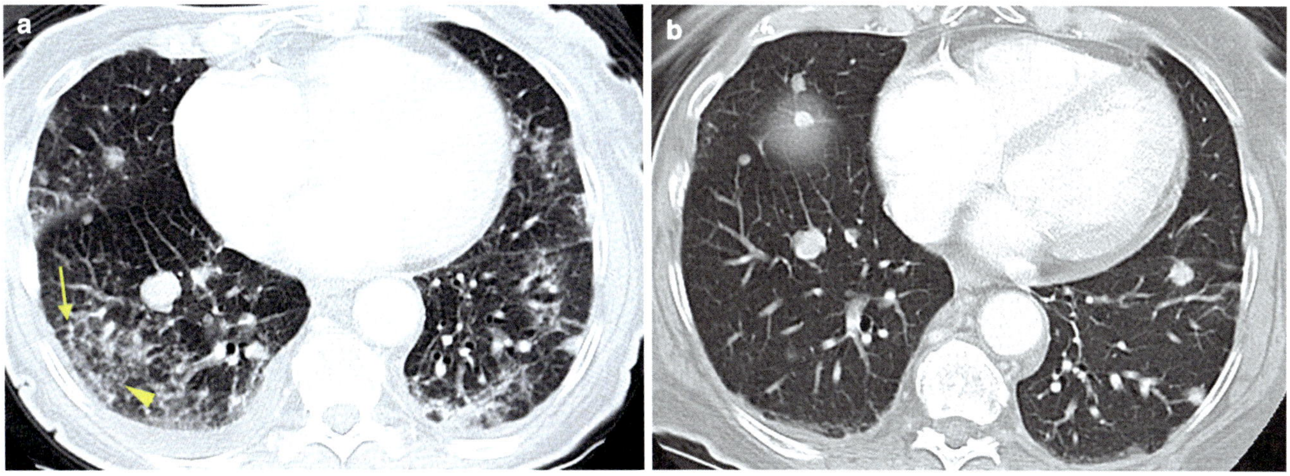

Fig. 7.6 Temsirolimus-associated pneumonitis in treatment of metastatic RCC. A patient presented with pulmonary metastases several years after initial nephrectomy. He was treated with sunitinib followed by sorafenib. Following progression of disease, his treatment was changed to temsirolimus, with the standard weekly dosing schedule. After 4 weeks of temsirolimus, asymptomatic interstitial infiltrates were incidentally noted on a CT performed for treatment evaluation. Axial images of the lower lungs demonstrate new coarse peripheral reticular interstitial thickening (**a**, *arrows*) and mild ground glass opacities (**a**, *arrowhead*) when compared to baseline CT images prior to initiation of therapy (**b**). Temsirolimus was eventually discontinued due to leukopenia and thrombocytopenia

surveillance imaging. Management is conservative in the absence of symptoms of peritonitis [23]

Temsirolimus/everolimus. Toxicities associated with mTOR inhibitors, such as temsirolimus and everolimus, include rash, mucositis, metabolic changes (elevated triglycerides, hyperglycemia, and hypophosphatemia), thrombocytopenia, and nonspecific pneumonitis [19].

Clinical pneumonitis occurs in approximately 15 % of patients treated with everolimus [24]. Patients may present with cough, dyspnea, or both. The incidence of asymptomatic pneumonitis encountered as a new radiographic finding detected during treatment ranges from 39 to 50 % with everolimus and temsirolimus [24, 25]. The high incidence of new pulmonary abnormalities reported during treatment with temsirolimus and everolimus may represent a low-grade drug toxicity that is not clinically detected [24]. The onset of pulmonary findings develops between approximately 3 and 37 weeks after starting treatment [24]. Imaging findings may include patchy ground glass infiltrates and multifocal areas of cryptogenic organizing pneumonitis (COP) with traction bronchiectasis (Figs. 7.6–7.8). The patterns are variable and may change over time. Management options include drug withdrawal, dose reduction, or treatment with steroids [24].

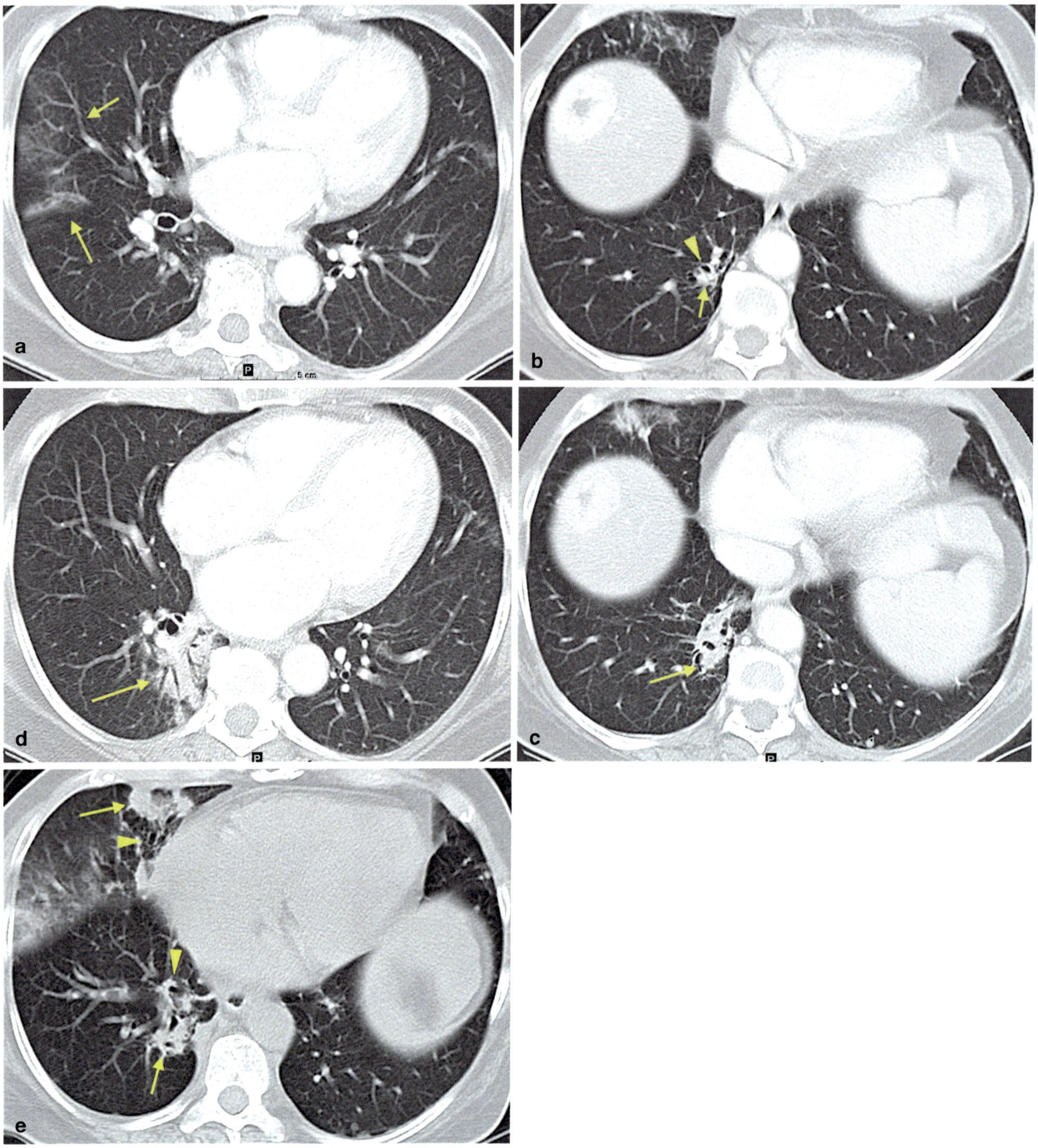

Fig. 7.7 Temsirolimus-associated pneumonitis in treatment of metastatic RCC. A patient was started on temsirolimus after progression of disease while on sunitinib and then on sorafenib. Early in the course of temsirolimus therapy, the patient developed a dry cough that gradually worsened with intermittent low-grade fevers. A chest radiograph revealed "atypical pneumonia." She continued to have intermittent low-grade fevers on antibiotics. The first CT scan obtained 3 weeks after initiation of treatment revealed multifocal infiltrates. Axial images from two different levels of the lower lungs reveals new ground glass peripheral infiltrate in the right middle lobe (**a**, *arrows*) and patchy consolidation (**b**, *arrow*) with bronchiectasis (**b**, *arrowhead*) in the right lower lobe. CT findings were reported with differential diagnosis of an infectious or inflammatory process. Respiratory symptoms were mild and therapy was continued. Follow-up CT during week 7 demonstrated areas of improvement and areas of worsening consolidation. Axial images from the same levels as in Fig. 7.7a,b revealed improvement in the ground glass infiltrates in the right middle lobe and worsening of COP infiltrates in the right lower lobe with persistent foci of bronchiectasis (**c** and **d**, *arrow*). Follow-up CT during week 13 later revealed increased air-space disease and peripheral COP opacities (**e**, *arrows*) with associated bronchiectasis (**e**, *arrowheads*) in the anterior right middle and right lower lobes. There was no change in clinical presentation of mild respiratory symptoms. A pulmonary consult determined that the slowly progressive infiltrates associated with mild respiratory symptoms temporally related to initiation of temsirolimus therapy were consistent with drug-induced pneumonitis. A bronchoscopy was performed due to the intermittent fevers and revealed a nonspecific interstitial inflammation and organizing pneumonia without infection. Therapy was held and steroid therapy was initiated with both clinical and radiographic improvement

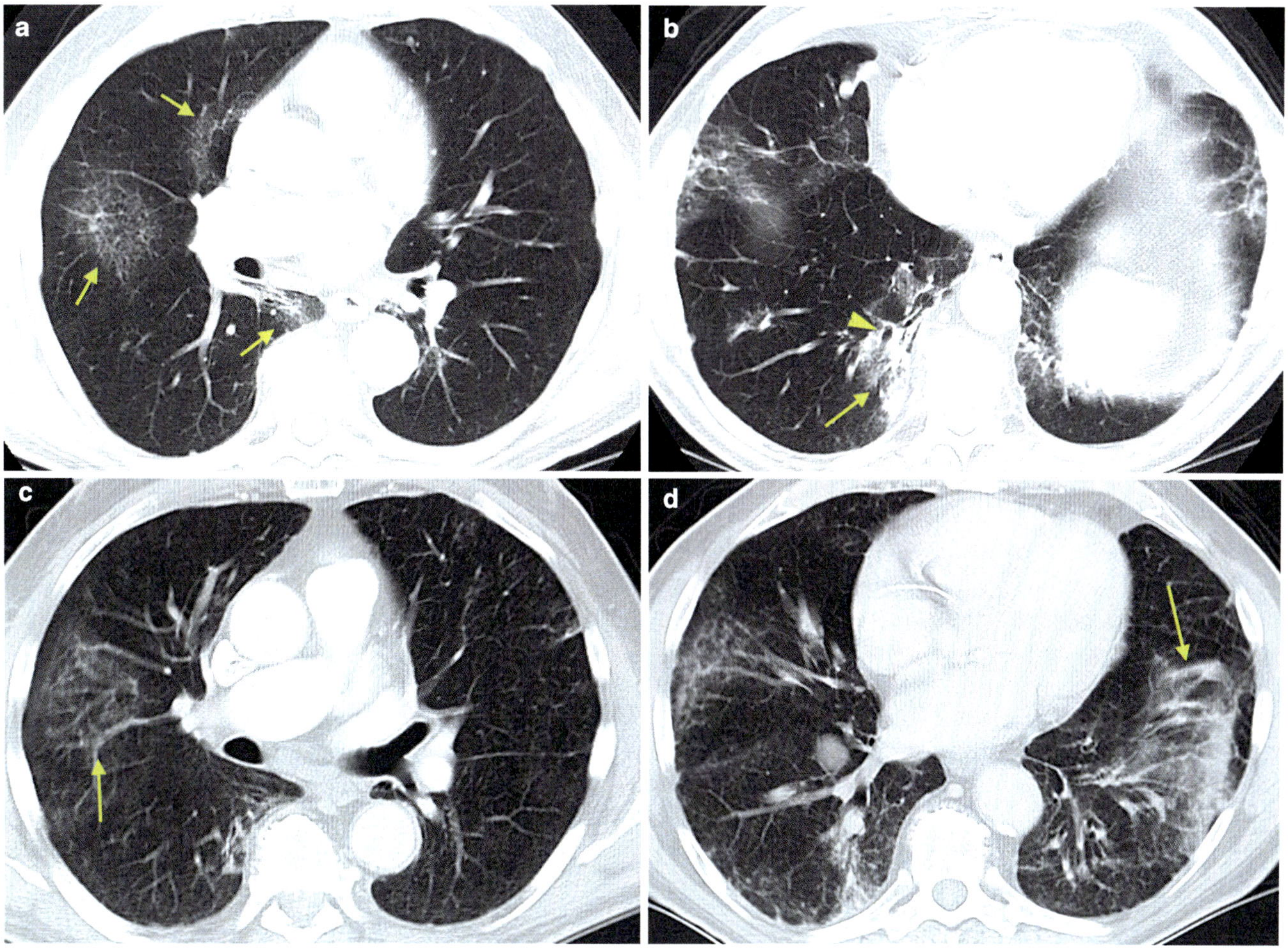

Fig. 7.8 Temsirolimus-associated pneumonitis in the treatment of metastatic RCC. A patient with metastatic RCC to lung was started on temsirolimus after progression on sunitinib. Follow- up CT on week 8 of temsirolimus revealed treatment response and new ground glass infiltrates predominantly in the right middle lobe (**a**, *arrows*) and COP infiltrates (**b**, *arrow*) with associated bronchiectasis in the lower lobes (**b**, *arrowhead*). Infiltrates were reported as new, consistent with infectious or inflammatory process, possibly treatment-related. The patient was treated with antibiotics for an upper respiratory infection with slight improvement of symptoms. 6 weeks later, the patient complained of a persistent dry cough. Repeat CT revealed improvement of right middle lobe ground glass infiltrate (**c**, *arrow*) and new peripheral ground glass infiltrate in the left lower lobe and lingua (**d**, *arrow*) reported as consistent with an infectious or inflammatory process. Temsirolimus was held with dramatic improvement in dyspnea on exertion and improved infiltrates on follow-up imaging

Bladder Cancer

Treatment Options for Urothelial Carcinoma of the Bladder

Treatment of non–muscle-invasive urothelial carcinoma (previously termed *superficial bladder cancer*) is transurethral resection with adjuvant intravesical chemotherapy or immunotherapy with BCG (bacillus Calmette–Guérin). The complications of intravesical BCG therapy are discussed elsewhere (*see* Chap. 3).

The standard of care for muscle-invasive urothelial carcinoma is radical cystoprostatectomy in men and anterior pelvic exenteration in women performed with bilateral pelvic lymphadenectomy and urinary diversion. About 30–50 % of patients are clinically understaged at the time of cystectomy [26]. The use of neoadjuvant chemotherapy before cystectomy in patients with locally advanced disease offers theoretical and real advantage to early treatment of microscopic metastases beyond the margins of local therapy already present at the time of diagnosis of invasive bladder cancer [27]. There is currently insufficient evidence to recommend adjuvant chemotherapy [28].

The treatment for advanced urothelial carcinoma presenting with metastatic disease is chemotherapy and is palliative in intent [29]. Historically, the standard regimen is MVAC (methotrexate, vinblastine, doxorubicin, cisplatin). The toxicities associated with the chemotherapy regimen of MVAC include mucositis, neutropenic fever, and drug-related deaths [29]. The combination of gemcitabine and cisplatin (GC) is associated with decreased toxicity and has become a favorable option in both the metastatic and neoadjuvant settings [30].

Radiographically Evident Toxicities Associated with Chemotherapy Agents Used in Treatment of Urothelial Carcinoma of the Bladder

Methotrexate. Methotrexate-induced pulmonary toxicity occurs in 2–8 % of patients and is typically a hypersensitivity pneumonitis [31]. Most patients present within the first year of therapy, usually within weeks to months of initiation of therapy. It is associated with high fever, nonproductive cough, severe dyspnea, hypoxemia, and peripheral eosinophilia with good response to cessation of therapy and steroids [31]. Radiographic findings may include bilateral interstitial opacities progressing to alveolar infiltrates and pleural effusions. Other pulmonary manifestations include COP and noncardiogenic pulmonary edema.

Gemcitabine. Gemcitabine pulmonary toxicity is a rare but serious complication [31]. Its pulmonary toxicity has been attributed to capillary leak syndrome, diffuse alveolar damage, or alveolar hemorrhage [32]. Toxicity can present as early as the first dose or several weeks after initiation of therapy. The clinical presentation is indolent with dry cough, dyspnea and fine rales on exertion, and low-grade temperature on physical examination. There is generally a good response to steroids but response is not universal, with reported fatalities [33, 34].

Vascular toxicities associated with gemcitabine include venous and arterial thrombosis, capillary leak syndrome (as described above), necrotizing vasculitis, acute coronary events, digital ischemia, and hematologic disorders such as thrombotic microangiopathy [35]. Necrotizing vasculitis may affect a variety of organs such as myalgia with swelling of extremities and GI tract with enterocolitis. Arterial events such as renal and splenic infarctions have been reported.

Cisplatin. Cisplatin-associated vascular toxicity also includes venous and arterial events (see discussion on testicular cancer below). Vascular toxicities have been described in cisplatin-based combination chemotherapy regimens for the treatment of head and neck cancer, genitourinary tumors, lymphoma, and breast cancer [36]. Vascular complications described in patients with urothelial carcinoma of the bladder treated with cisplatin-based therapy include deep vein thrombosis, pulmonary emboli, arterial thrombotic, cerebrovascular events, and angina pectoris [37]. Most events occur early in treatment within the first two cycles.

Testicular Cancer (Germ Cell Tumor)

Treatment Options for Germ Cell Tumor

Management of germ cell tumor (GCT) depends on origin of the tumor, pathology, risk stratification, and stage at the time of diagnosis. Treatment modalities include surgery, radiation, and chemotherapy. Patients with stage I of either testicular seminoma or nonseminomatous germ cell tumor (NSGCT) without lymphovascular invasion and rete testis involvement can be managed with orchiectomy followed by surveillance, whereas radiation and retroperitoneal lymph node dissection may be indicated for other stage I and early stage II testicular seminoma and nonseminoma, respectively. However, for patients with advanced GCT, including mediastinal primary GCT, systemic chemotherapy plays an important role in providing a long-term cure for these patients. Four cycles of etoposide and cisplatin (EP) has been accepted as the preferred treatment for patients with good-risk GCT, whereas three cycles of bleomycin, etoposide, and cisplatin (BEP) remain an acceptable alternative. Patients with intermediate- and poor-risk GCT are treated with four cycles of BEP. Acute toxicities associated with BEP include bone marrow suppression (with risk of neutropenic sepsis, thrombocytopenia, and bleeding), nausea and vomiting, alopecia, rashes, pneumonitis, neuropathy, nephrotoxicity, ototoxicity, infertility, and Raynaud phenomenon.

Radiation therapy for seminomatous tumors is accompanied with risk of secondary malignancy, cardiovascular toxicity, and infertility [38, 39]. Retroperitoneal lymph node dissection (RPLND) in the treatment of NSGCTs is associated with risk of retrograde ejaculation. Modified templates of dissections and nerve-sparing techniques have reduced this morbidity [40].

Radiographically Evident Toxicities Associated with Chemotherapy Agents Used in Treatment of Testicular Cancer

Bleomycin. The onset of symptoms of bleomycin-induced toxicity can occur weeks to months after initiation of therapy with clinical presentation of a fever, dry cough, and progressive dyspnea. Pulmonary syndromes such as cryptogenic organizing pneumonia (COP) and hypersensitivity pneumonitis with eosinophilia can occur, but most patients develop subacute to chronic interstitial pneumonitis [39, 41]. The most common abnormalities encountered are bilateral reticular or nodular infiltrates, typically bibasilar, which can progress to alveolar infiltrates and eventually fibrosis (Fig. 7.9) [42].

Well-established risk factors include dose of bleomycin, age of the patient, and impaired renal function [42]. Other probable risk factors are oxygen therapy, radiation exposure, cigarette smoking, and lung metastases.

Cisplatin. Venous thrombosis and pulmonary embolism have been associated with cisplatin treatment but can occur in the hypercoagulable state of malignancy (Fig. 7.10).

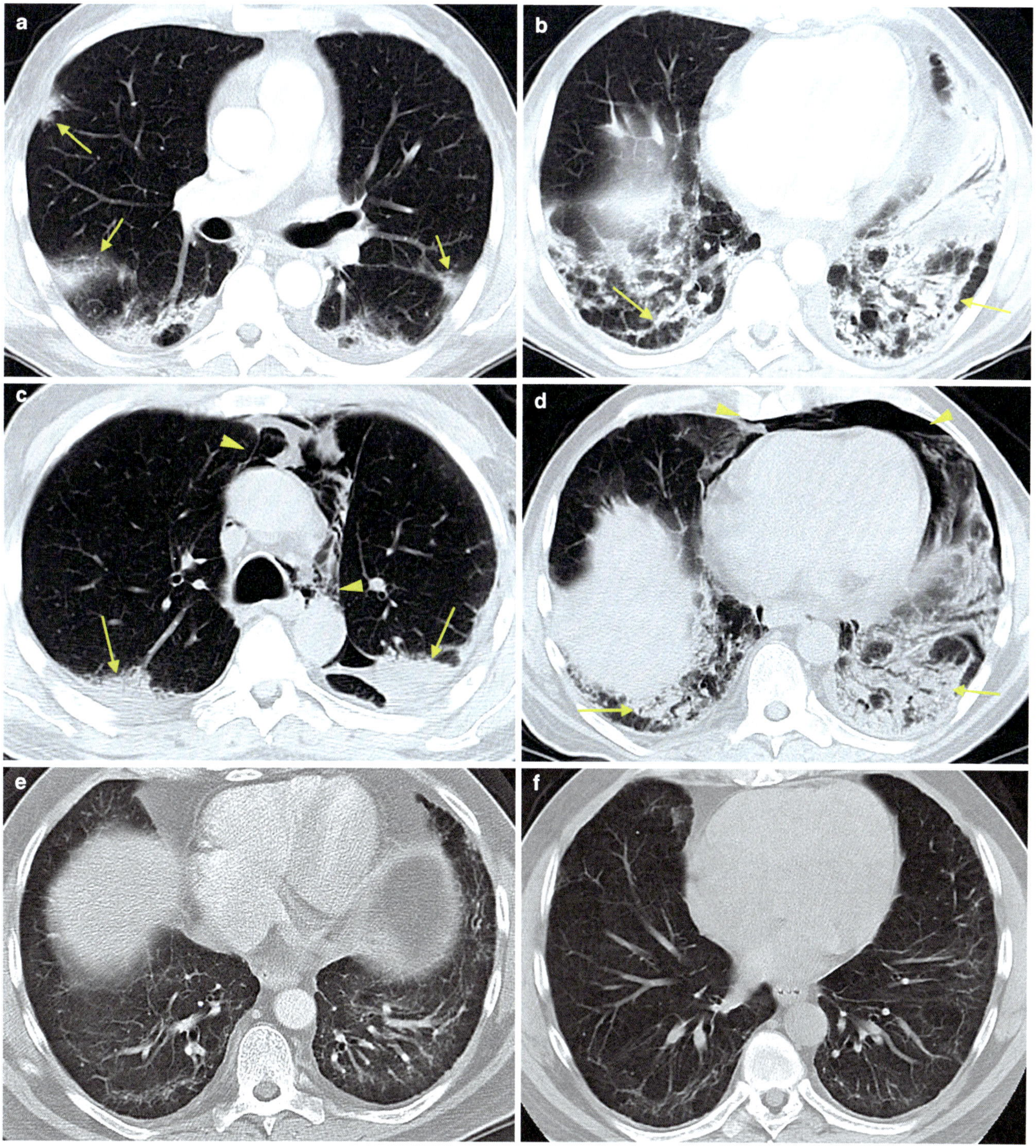

Fig. 7.9 Bleomycin-induced pneumonitis during treatment of testicular cancer. A patient with nonseminomatous germ cell tumor presented with bulky retroperitoneal lymphadenopathy and pulmonary metastases at the time of diagnosis. He was treated with BEP. At completion of therapy, he complained of dyspnea. CT chest scan revealed bilateral peripheral areas of consolidation suggestive of COP (**a**, *arrows*) and bibasilar coarse reticular interstitial thickening (**b**, *arrows*). Findings were consistent with infectious or inflammatory process, including drug toxicity. The patient was treated for pneumonia and a follow-up CT scan 2 weeks later revealed new and worsening consolidation and a pneumomediastinum. CT demonstrates worsening lower lobe infiltrates with new peripheral areas of consolidation in the upper lobes (**c**, *arrows*) and worsening consolidation in the lower lobes (**d**, *arrows*; compared to **b**) with a new left pneumothorax and pneumomediastinum (**c** and **d**, *arrowheads*). The patient slowly improved on steroid therapy and underwent a delayed retroperitoneal dissection following recovery from bleomycin pulmonary toxicity. CT scans obtained at 1 year (**e**) and 4 years after completion of BEP (**f**) revealed mild residual interstitial fibrosis with bronchiectasis

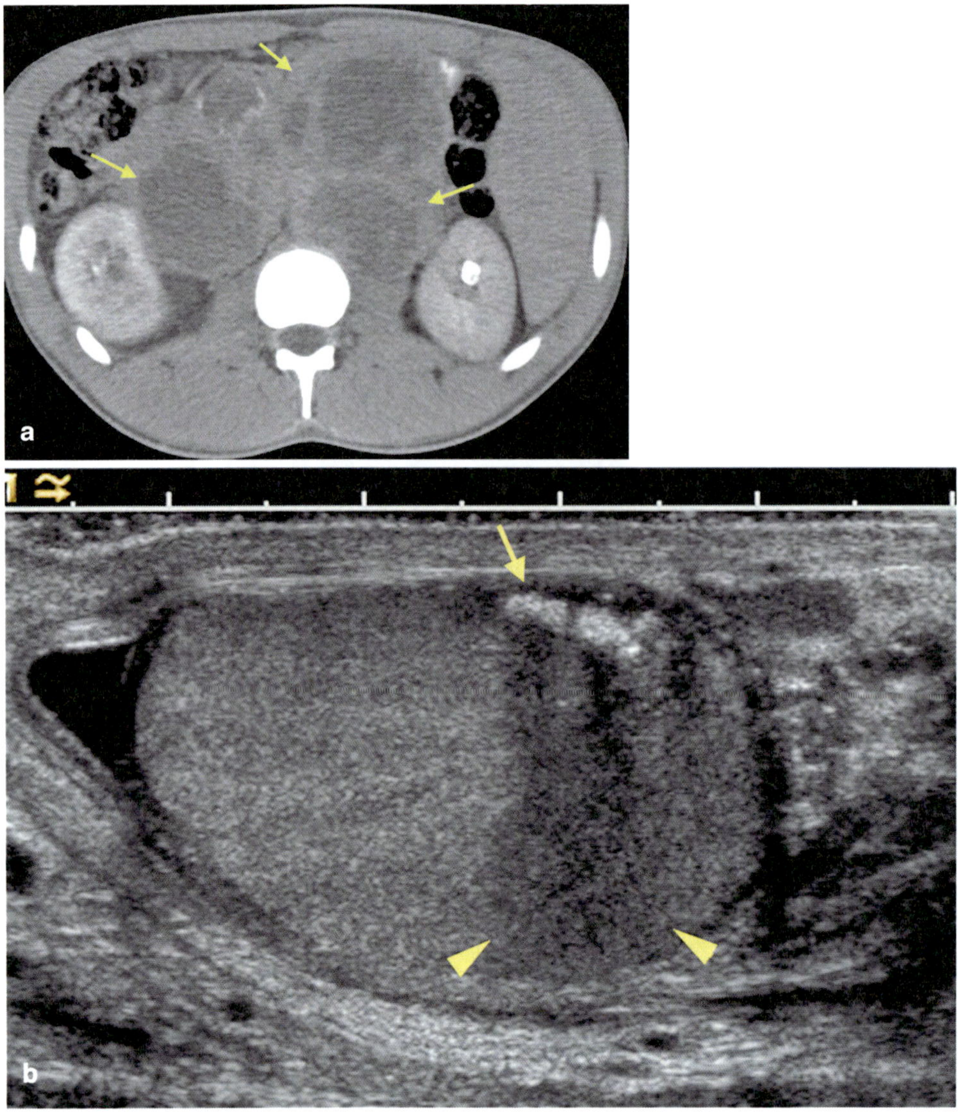

Fig. 7.10 Cisplatin-induced arterial thrombosis during treatment of testicular cancer. A patient with metastatic GCT presented with bulky retroperitoneal nodes (**a**, *arrows*) and visceral metastases (*not shown*). A biopsy of the retroperitoneal mass was consistent with metastatic choriocarcinoma with extensive necrosis. A scrotal ultrasound revealed a coarse calcification (**b**, *arrow*) with shadowing (**b**, *arrowheads*) without associated mass consistent with a burned-out GCT. Tumor markers revealed marked elevation of human chorionic gonadotropin and lactate dehydrogenase. The patient was started on a cisplatin-based chemotherapy regimen consisting of paclitaxel, ifosfamide, and cisplatin (TIP) with good clinical response (drop in serum tumor markers) and evidence of treatment response on subsequent imaging. CT obtained at completion of chemotherapy revealed marked improvement in retroperitoneal and pelvic adenopathy (**c**, *arrows*) and incidental bilateral lower lobe pulmonary emboli (**d**, *arrows*). A follow-up CT showed continued regression of the retroperitoneal nodes with a residual mass (**e**, *arrow*). Resection of residual disease was delayed for a course of anticoagulation

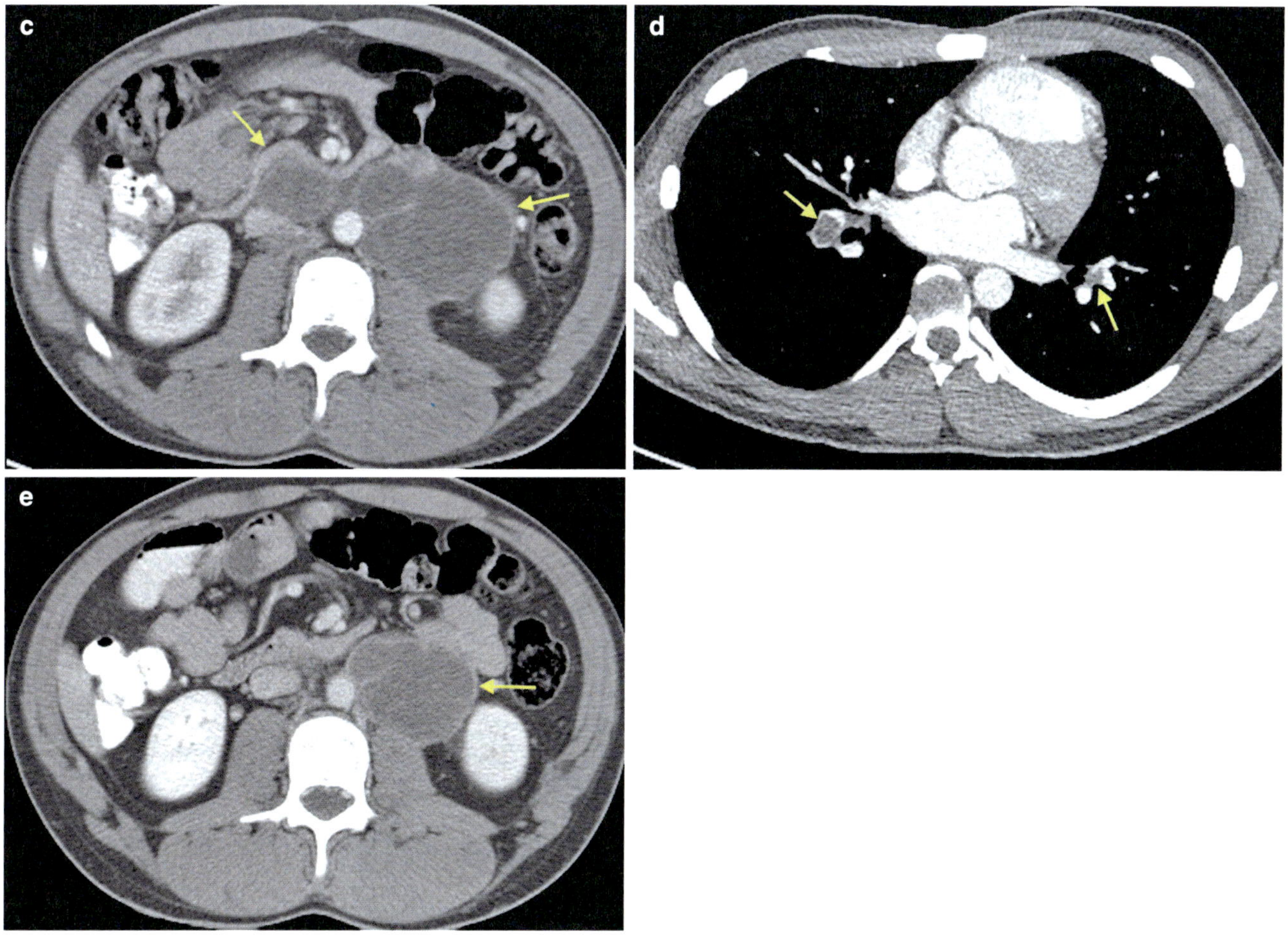

Fig. 7.10 (continued)

Of interest are arterial events such as cerebrovascular accidents and arterial occlusions that have been reported during cisplatin-based therapy for GCTs [38, 43–45]. Case reports described thromboembolic events such as splenic infarcts and peripheral arterial occlusions involving the external iliac artery, popliteal artery, and lower extremity (Fig. 7.11) [45, 46].

Long-term complications of BEP. Testicular cancer survivors treated with BEP are also at risk of second malignancies and cardiovascular disease [38, 39]. Up to 10 % of GCT patients develop either angina pectoris or myocardial infarction within 20 years after receiving chemotherapy treatment. The combination of chemotherapy and radiation predicts the greatest risk, especially with radiation to the mediastinum. Secondary malignancies have been described in the pleura, stomach, pancreas, urinary bladder, retroperitoneum, and connective tissue. Increased risk of hematologic malignancies, such as myelodysplastic syndrome and secondary leukemia, are due to chemotherapy and are predominantly linked to etoposide [38]. Other chronic toxicities include GI disorders (intestinal vascular lesions, hepatobiliary disease, and ulcers), cardiovascular disease, infections, respiratory illnesses, infertility, anxiety, Raynaud phenomenon, ototoxicity, and persistent neuropathy [38].

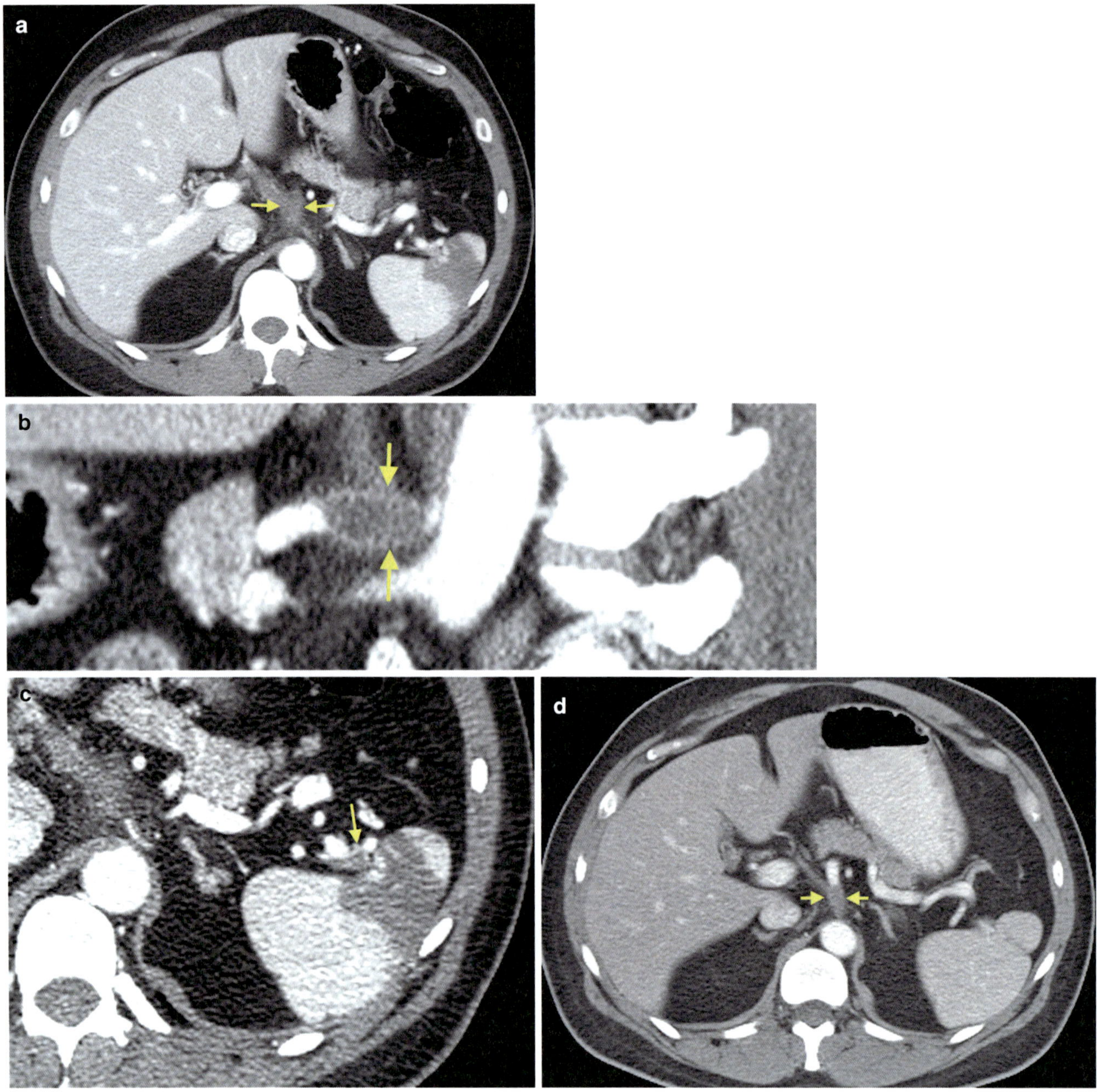

Fig. 7.11 Cisplatin-induced arterial thrombosis during treatment of testicular cancer. A patient with nonseminomatous GCT underwent a radical orchiectomy that revealed embryonal carcinoma. A staging CT scan revealed enlarged retroperitoneal lymph nodes and he was started on systemic therapy including EP. Following one cycle of EP, the patient developed mild nausea and left upper quadrant pain. Unscheduled CT examination revealed a thrombus in the celiac artery shown in axial (**a**, *arrows*) and sagittal (**b**, *arrows*) images, right hepatic artery thrombosis and a new peripheral wedge shaped defect in the spleen compatible with an infarct (**a**). High resolution images of the hilar splenic vessels revealed a small splenic artery thrombus in a distal branch (**c**, *arrow*). He was treated with anticoagulation. Follow-up CT images revealed improvement of the celiac and hepatic artery thrombosis and the splenic infarct (**d**, *arrows*). The patient's treatment was changed to carboplatin and etoposide with the consideration that the risk of another potential catastrophic arterial thrombosis was higher than the risk of relapse on the substitute therapy. The patient completed therapy without further incident

References

1. Torrisi JM, Schwartz LH, Gollub MJ, et al. CT findings of chemotherapy-induced toxicity: what radiologists need to know about the clinical and radiologic manifestations of chemotherapy toxicity. Radiology. 2011;258:41–56.
2. Agarwala SS, Case S. Everolimus (RAD001) in the treatment of advanced renal cell carcinoma: a review. Oncologist. 2010;15:236–45.
3. Motzer RJ, Hutson TE, Tomczak P, et al. Sunitinib versus interferon α in metastatic renal-cell carcinoma. N Engl J Med. 2007;356:115–24.
4. Summers J, Cohen MH, Keegan P, Pazdur R. FDA drug approval summary: bevacizumab plus interferon for advanced renal cell carcinoma. Oncologist. 2010;15:104–11.
5. Bukowski RM. Pazopanib: a multikinase inhibitor with activity in advanced renal cell carcinoma. Expert Rev Anticancer Ther. 2010;10:635–45.
6. Mulders P. Vascular endothelial growth factor and mTOR pathways in renal cell carcinoma: differences and synergies of two targeted mechanisms. BJU Int. 2009;104:1585–9.
7. RECORD-1 Study Group, Motzer RJ, Escudier B, Oudard S, et al. Phase 3 trial of everolimus for metastatic renal cell carcinoma: final results and analysis of prognostic factors. Cancer. 2010;116:4256–65.
8. Sternberg CN, Davis ID, Mardiak J, et al. Pazopanib in locally advanced or metastatic renal cell carcinoma: results of a randomized phase III trial. J Clin Oncol. 2010;28:1061–8.
9. Escudier B, Eisen T, Stadler WM, et al. Sorafenib in advanced clear-cell renal-cell carcinoma. N Engl J Med. 2007;356:125–34.
10. Escudier B, Eisen T, Stadler WM, et al. TARGET Study Group. Temsirolimus, interferon α, or both for advanced renal-cell carcinoma. N Engl J Med. 2007;356:2271–81.
11. Escudier B, Pluzanska A, Koralewski P, et al. for the AVOREN Trial investigators. Bevacizumab plus interferon α-2a for treatment of metastatic renal cell carcinoma: a randomised, double-blind phase III trial. Lancet. 2007;370:2103–11.
12. Rini BI, Halabi S, Rosenberg JE, et al. Bevacizumab plus interferon α compared with interferon α monotherapy in patients with metastatic renal cell carcinoma: CALGB 90206. J Clin Oncol. 2008;26:5422–8.
13. Rini BI, Escudier B, Tomczak P, et al. Comparative effectiveness of axitinib versus sorafenib in advanced renal cell carcinoma (AXIS): a randomised phase 3 trial. Lancet. 2011;378:1931–9.
14. Rock EP, Goodman V, Jiang JX, et al. Food and drug administration drug approval summary: sunitinib malate for the treatment of gastrointestinal stromal tumor and advanced renal cell carcinoma. Oncologist. 2007;12:107–13.
15. Eklund JW, Kuzel TM. Interleukin-2 in the treatment of renal cell carcinoma and malignant melanoma. Cancer Treat Res. 2005;126:263–87.
16. Vial T, Descotes J. Clinical toxicity of interleukin-2. Drug Saf. 1992;7:417–33.
17. Davis SD, Berkmen YM, Wang JC. Interleukin-2 therapy for advanced renal cell carcinoma: radiographic evaluation of response and complications. Radiology. 1990;177:127–31.
18. Saxon RR, Klein JS, Bar MH, et al. Pathogenesis of pulmonary edema during interleukin-2 therapy: correlation of chest radiographic and clinical findings in 54 patients. AJR Am J Roentgenol. 1991;156:281–5.
19. Hutson TE, Figlin RA, Kuhn JG, Motzer RJ. Targeted therapies for metastatic renal cell carcinoma: an overview of toxicity and dosing strategies. Oncologist. 2008;13:1084–96.
20. Boehm S, Rothermundt C, Hess D, Joerger M. Antiangiogenic drugs in oncology: a focus on drug safety and the elderly—a mini-review. Gerontology. 2010;56:303–9.
21. Di Lorenzo G, Porta C, Bellmunt J, et al. Toxicities of targeted therapy and their management in kidney cancer. Eur Urol. 2011;59:526–40.
22. Motzer RJ, Rini BI, Bukowski RM, et al. Sunitinib in patients with metastatic renal cell carcinoma. JAMA. 2006;295:2516–24.
23. St Peter SD, Abbas MA, Kelly KA. The spectrum of pneumatosis intestinalis. Arch Surg. 2003;138:68–75.
24. White DA, Camus P, Endo M, et al. Noninfectious pneumonitis after everolimus therapy for advanced renal cell carcinoma. Am J Respir Crit Care Med. 2010;182:396–403.
25. Duran I, Siu LL, Oza AM, et al. Characterisation of the lung toxicity of the cell cycle inhibitor temsirolimus. Eur J Cancer. 2006;42:1875–80.
26. Jacobs BL, Lee CT, Montie JE. Bladder cancer in 2010: how far have we come? CA Cancer J Clin. 2010;60:244–72.
27. Babjuk M. Current value of neoadjuvant chemotherapy prior to cystectomy. Eur Urol. 2010;9(Suppl):424–7.
28. Sternberg CN, Calabro F. Adjuvant chemotherapy for bladder cancer. Expert Rev Anticancer Ther. 2005;5:987–92.
29. Flechon A, Droz JP. Chemotherapy practices and perspectives in invasive bladder cancer. Expert Rev Anticancer Ther. 2006;6:1473–82.
30. Morgan TM, Clark PE. Bladder cancer. Curr Opin Oncol. 2010;22:242–9.
31. Meadors M, Floyd J, Perry MC. Pulmonary toxicity of chemotherapy. Semin Oncol. 2006;33:98–105.
32. Vahid B, Marik PE. Pulmonary complications of novel antineoplastic agents for solid tumors. Chest. 2008;133:528–38.
33. Vander Els NJ, Stover DE. Chemotherapy-induced lung disease. Clin Pulm Med. 2004;11:84–91.
34. Pavlakis N, Bell DR, Millward MJ, Levi JA. Fatal pulmonary toxicity resulting from treatment with gemcitabine. Cancer. 1997;80:286–91.
35. Dasanu CA. Gemcitabine: vascular toxicity and prothrombotic potential. Expert Opin Drug Saf. 2008;7:703–16.
36. Shahab N, Haider S, Doll DC. Vascular toxicity of antineoplastic agents. Semin Oncol. 2006;33:121–38.
37. Czaykowski PM, Moore MJ, Tannock IF. High risk of vascular events in patients with urothelial transitional cell carcinoma treated with cisplatin based chemotherapy. J Urol. 1998;160(6 Pt 1):2021–4.
38. Feldman DR, Bosl GJ, Sheinfeld J, Motzer RJ. Medical treatment of advanced testicular cancer. JAMA. 2008;299:672–84.
39. van den Belt-Dusebout AW, de Wit R, et al. Treatment-specific risks of second malignancies and cardiovascular disease in 5-year survivors of testicular cancer. J Clin Oncol. 2007;25:4370–8.
40. Yoon GH, Stein JP, Skinner DG. Retroperitoneal lymph node dissection in the treatment of low-stage nonseminomatous germ cell tumors of the testicle. Expert Rev Anticancer Ther. 2005;5:75–85.
41. Cordier JF. Cryptogenic organising pneumonia. Eur Respir J. 2006;28:422–6.
42. Kawai K, Akaza H. Bleomycin-induced pulmonary toxicity in chemotherapy for testicular cancer. Expert Opin Drug Saf. 2003;2:587–96.
43. Weijl NI, Rutten MF, Zwinderman AH, et al. Thromboembolic events during chemotherapy for germ cell cancer: a cohort study and review of the literature. J Clin Oncol. 2000;18:2169–78.
44. Cantwell BM, Mannix KA, Roberts JT, et al. Thromboembolic events during combination chemotherapy for germ cell-malignancy. Lancet. 1988;2:1086–7.
45. Vos AH, Splinter TA, van der Heul C. Arterial occlusive events during chemotherapy for germ cell cancer. Neth J Med. 2001;59:295–9.
46. Cheng E, Berthold DR, Moore MJ, Duran I. Arterial thrombosis after cisplatin-based chemotherapy for metastatic germ cell tumors. Acta Oncol. 2009;48:475–7.

Genitourinary Interventions

8

Bradley B. Pua and Stephen B. Solomon

Interventional radiology plays an important role in the management of patients with genitourinary neoplasms. This role ranges from imaging diagnosis to biopsy, to palliation of symptoms, to definitive treatment of both primary and metastatic lesions. Biopsy of solid renal masses and metastatic foci for staging is commonplace. Furthermore, relief of obstruction of the collecting system has evolved from simply placing a tube in the renal pelvis to more advanced techniques to optimize patient comfort. For treatment of primary or metastatic lesions in the kidney, procedures such as arterial embolization may play an important definitive or adjunctive role to surgery. In addition to treatment of symptomatic osseous metastasis, symptomatic osseous metastasis are now playing a larger role in primary therapy of solid renal tumors and prostate cancers. This chapter provides a pictorial review of common procedures performed in oncologic patients, including urologic biopsies; ablation of renal tumors; arterial embolization; radiologic therapies in ureteral obstruction; prostate biopsy and focal therapies; and management of pelvic lymphoceles.

Urologic Biopsies

Nontargeted Medical Renal Biopsy

Nontargeted renal parenchymal biopsy remains an important tool in the diagnosis of certain parenchymal renal diseases to determine prognosis and guide treatment strategies [1]. The goal of these biopsies is to sample multiple glomeruli to provide a confident diagnosis. Multiple strategies exist in obtaining renal tissue, the most common being image-guided percutaneous renal biopsy. Some authors have demonstrated feasibility of transvenous biopsy in patients with high risk associated with a percutaneous approach [2]. A large body of literature exists pertaining to the determination of the best type and size of needle for core biopsies, the common goal being to obtain the greatest number of intact glomeruli with the lowest risk [3, 4]. More recently, Patel et al. [5] described a cortical tangential approach in obtaining core specimens in renal transplants, which appears to be associated with a 95 % sample adequacy rate according to Banff 97 assessment criteria. Perinephric hemorrhage can be seen in some patients after biopsy. Fortunately, only rarely is this hemorrhage clinically significant, with even a smaller percentage requiring further therapy for either pseudoaneurysm or arteriovenous fistula [6].

Indeterminate Masses and Renal Cell Carcinoma

Since surgical excision is the standard treatment plan for renal cell carcinoma (RCC), biopsy of renal masses was traditionally limited to those who, on imaging and history, did not fit classic criteria for RCC [7]. More recently, advances in adjuvant and medical therapy have made delineation of renal tumor histopathologic subtype by core biopsy important, as it directly impacts treatment [8]. Results from a presurgical biopsy may redirect treatment from total nephrectomy, to nephron sparing, or to ablative techniques. In fact, as more lesions are ablated rather than resected, the role of biopsy will expand, as no resected specimen will be available for histopathologic correlation. Recent literature confirms that for the diagnosis of renal masses, core needle biopsy is superior to fine needle aspiration (FNA), with some authors citing 97.7 % sensitivity and 100 % specificity for core biopsy and FNA sensitivities as low as 50 % [9]. Improvements in fluorescence in situ hybridization (FISH) techniques have also resulted in improved accuracy of renal tumor biopsies and may play an increasing role, providing important information regarding tumor subtypes that can guide management [10].

B.B. Pua, M.D. (✉)
Department of Interventional Radiology, New York—Presbyterian Hospital /Weill Cornell Medical Center,
525 East 68th Street, Payson Pavilion, 5, New York, NY 10065, USA
e-mail: brp9018@med.cornell.edu

S.B. Solomon, M.D.
Department of Radiology, Memorial Sloan-Kettering Cancer Center,
1275 York Avenue, H-118, New York, NY 10021, USA
e-mail: solomons@mskcc.org

A.M. Bach, J. Zhang (eds.), *Atlas of Genitourinary Oncological Imaging*, Atlas of Oncology Imaging,
DOI 10.1007/978-1-4614-4872-3_8, © Springer Science+Business Media New York 2013

Biopsy of Metastasis

As with any biopsies, biopsy of a potential metastatic focus requires thorough discussion with the primary treating physician, patient, and pathologist. Knowledge of the goal of biopsy, such as staging, or necessity of histologic type, can guide biopsy of certain lesions over others, as well as dictate needle gauge and number of samples taken. Furthermore, as each type of tumor tends to metastasize to different tissues and lymph node chains, a firm grasp of these common sites is important. Often, it is left to the physician performing the biopsy to identify the metastatic focus to biopsy.

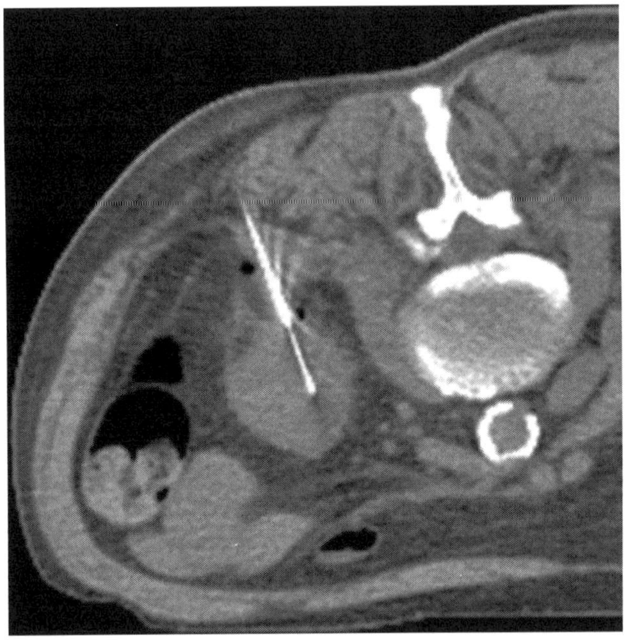

Fig. 8.1 Computed tomography (CT)–guided renal biopsy (nontargeted). A noncontrast axial CT image demonstrates a biopsy needle within the right kidney. Note the tangential course of the needle with respect to the renal cortex

Ablation of Renal Tumors

Although surgical resection remains the standard of care for localized renal cell carcinoma, ablative techniques such as cryoablation and radiofrequency ablation are rapidly becoming viable alternatives for treatment of small renal lesions in patients who may not be able to tolerate surgical resection. Ablative techniques can be applied either through an open, laparoscopic, or percutaneous approach.

Cryoablation uses a rapid freeze–thaw cycle to both mechanically disrupt cell membranes and draw out intracellular fluid resulting in alterations in intracellular pH. Radiofrequency ablation uses frictional energy to heat surrounding tissues, resulting in cell death. A recent meta-analysis suggests that, based on short-term oncologic outcomes, ablative treatments are reasonable options in the treatment of small renal masses [11]. Levinson et al. [12] published early long-term outcomes following patients treated with radiofrequency ablation to a mean of 61.6 months, citing an overall recurrence-free survival of 90.3 %. Such results lead these authors to suggest that radiofrequency ablation can play a role in the management of small renal lesions in patients who are high-risk surgical candidates or have a limited life expectancy [12].

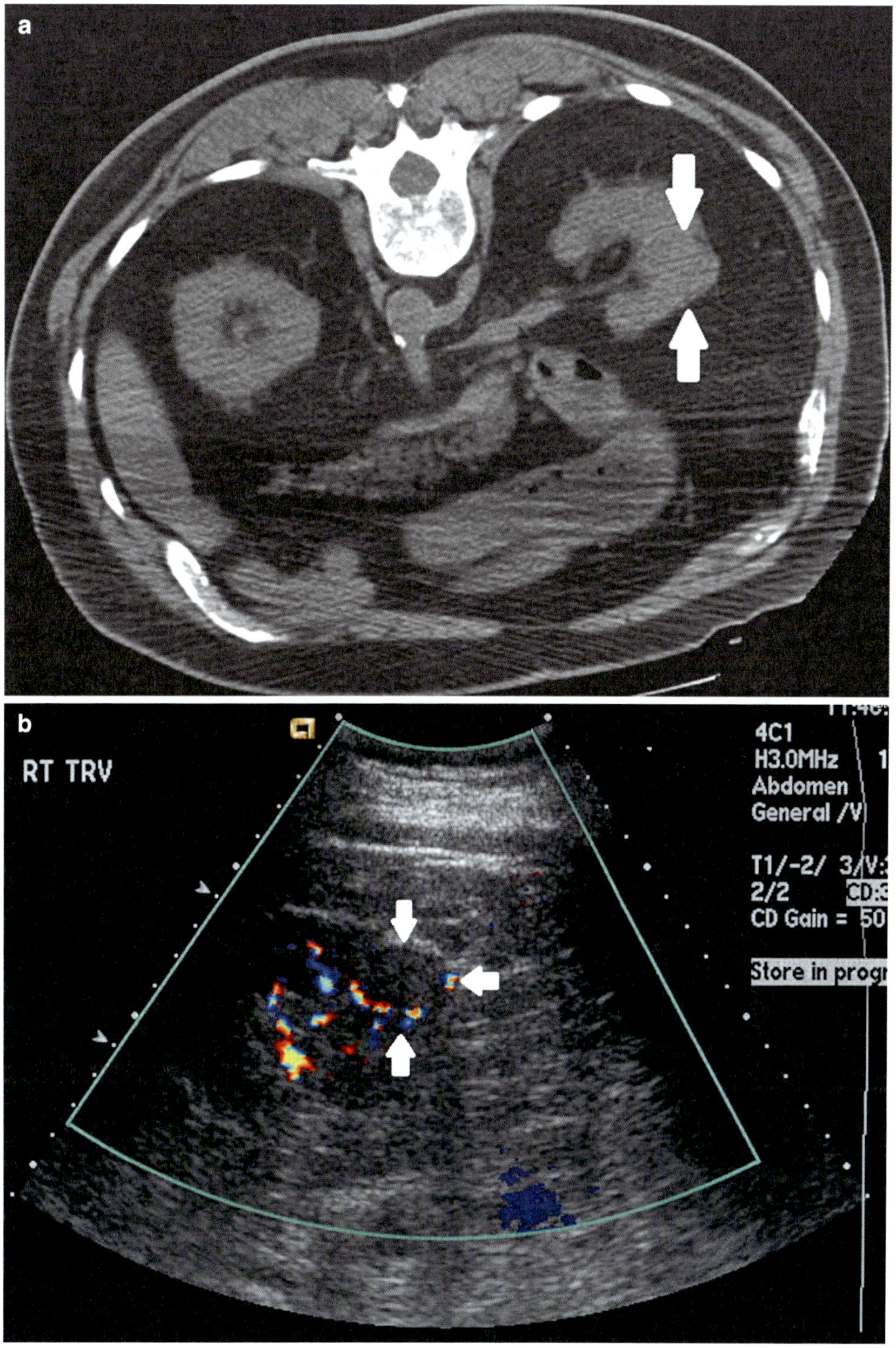

Fig. 8.2 Renal mass. (**a**) Noncontrast images demonstrate contour irregularity of the right kidney at the level of the known renal mass (*arrows*), better appreciated on a preprocedural contrast-enhanced CT (*not shown*). (**b**) Due to the inconspicuous nature of this lesion, initial targeting was done by ultrasound. Ultrasound through the same region clearly demonstrates a mass with peripheral vascularity (*arrows*). Targeting needles or the ablation probe can be placed in the renal mass under ultrasound guidance while the patient is on the CT gantry

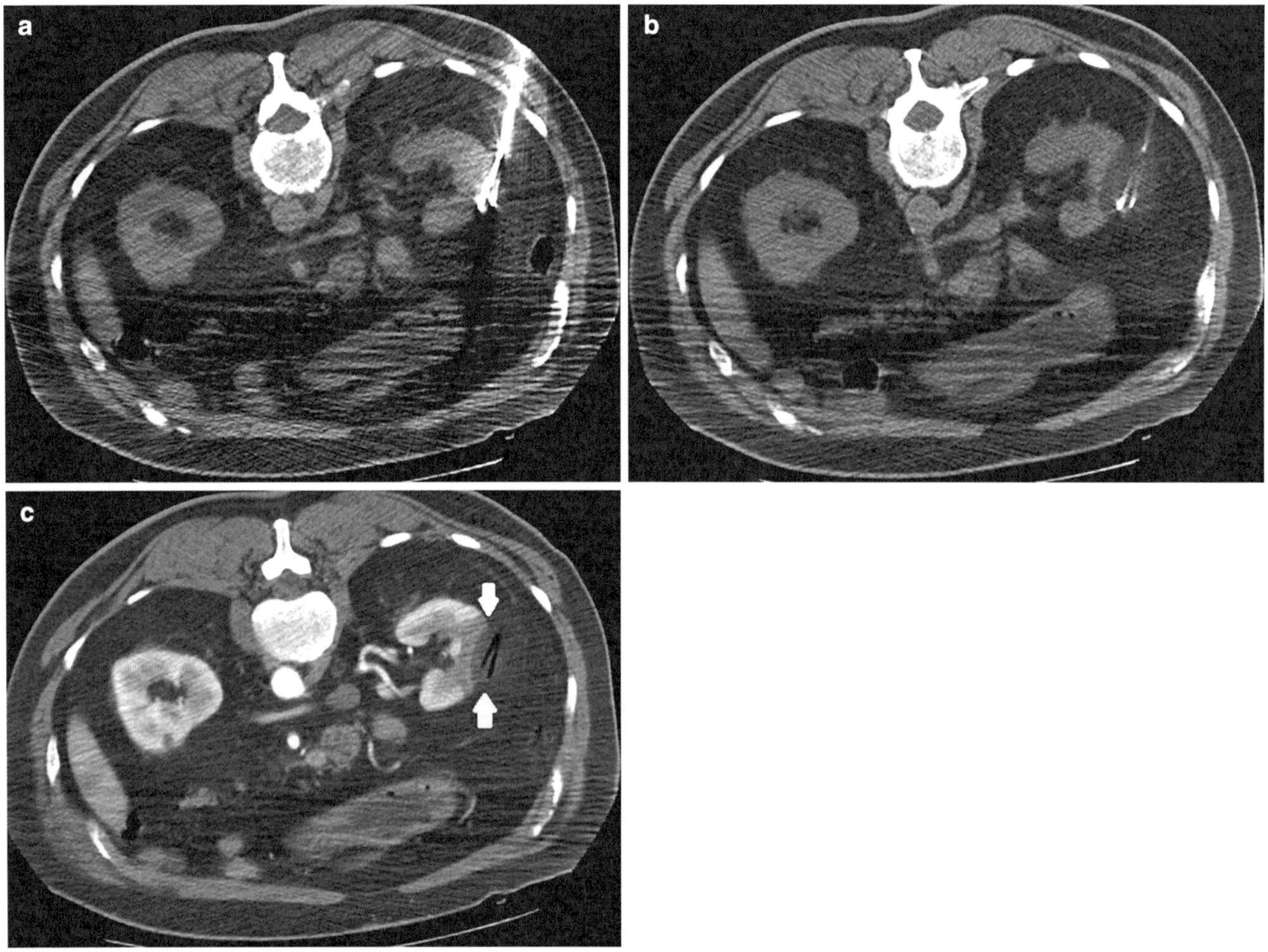

Fig. 8.3 Cryoablation. Axial images demonstrating the cryoprobes in place (**a**) with low density surrounding the probes (**b**) representing ice ball formation. In solid organs such as the kidney, ice ball formation can be well visualized and allows for better approximation of ablation margins. (**c**) Post-contrast CT after ablation demonstrates a low-density defect (*arrows*) representing the ablated area with air density in the probe tract

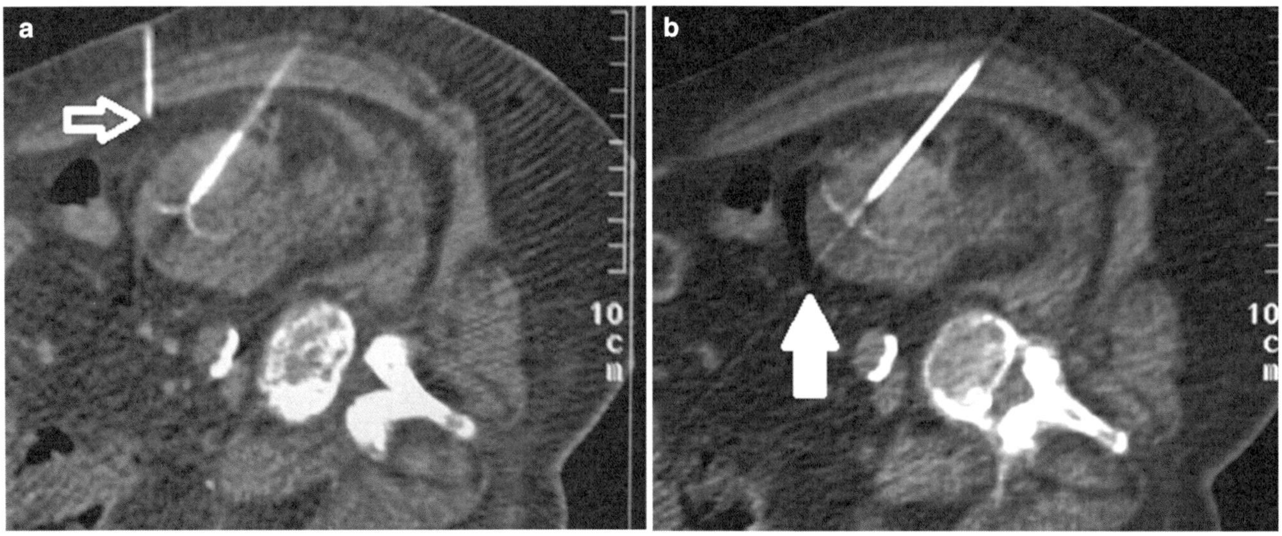

Fig. 8.4 Advanced separation techniques. On occasion, vital structures such as hollow viscera (bowel) or vasculature may be too close to the target lesion for that lesion to be safely ablated. (**a, b**) An ablation probe is fully deployed in the target renal lesion; however, the edge of the tumor is too close to the adjacent bowel. Air or fluid can be used as an insulator to the ablation energy. A small needle (*open arrow* in **a**) was in the space between the target lesion and bowel. Air was subsequently injected to separate the organs (*solid arrow* in **b**)

Role of Arterial Embolization

Embolization of Renal Angiomyolipomas

Renal angiomyolipoma (AML) is the most common benign renal neoplasm. Treatment of an AML is generally reserved for patients presenting with hemorrhage or pain, or with the goal to preempt possible spontaneous bleeding from a large lesion. Transcatheter arterial embolization is an important adjunct before complete or partial nephrectomy, and in many cases can serve as the primary therapy [13]. Although there is little argument for the emergent treatment of a hemorrhagic AML, controversy exists regarding treatment of minimally symptomatic and asymptomatic AML. Most centers use a size cutoff of 4 cm for elective treatment. The vast majority of tumors larger than 4 cm are symptomatic and more than half are associated with a risk of spontaneous hemorrhage [14, 15].

Transcatheter arterial embolization can be performed with various agents: absolute ethanol, with or without ethiodized oil, polyvinyl alcohol particles, absorbable gelatin powder, spherical particles, coils, or a combination. There remains no consensus as to the embolic material of choice. Technical success rates have been reported in the range of 90–100 %. Recurrence rates (same site), especially in those patients with associated tuberous sclerosis complex, can be up to 30 % [16]. For patients treated for symptoms secondary to mass effect or for primary size reduction, long-term mean size reduction can be seen ranging from 43 to 70.2 % [17, 18].

Angiographically, the vessels of an AML are tortuous, as is the case for tumor vasculature. Active contrast extravasation in the setting of acute hemorrhage may not always be seen on angiography as the surrounding hematoma may partially obscure the bleeding. Authors have described the use of a "light bulb" sign to direct embolization. Similar to a light bulb, a bleeding nidus/aneurysm resembles a filament of an incandescent and the surrounding hematoma resembles the bulb [19].

Postembolization follow-up imaging generally demonstrates cessation of bleeding (if treatment was for hemorrhage) and decreased tumor size. Since the fatty component of the AML is relatively insensitive to embolization, there is much variability in size reduction, and thus size itself cannot be used to determine treatment success [18]. There is currently no consensus on the follow-up of patients after embolization for AML. Some authors suggest that short-term imaging is predictive of long-term outcome [17]. Kothary et al. [16] have suggested lifelong follow-up for patients with associated tuberous sclerosis complex, secondary to high tumor-recurrence rates.

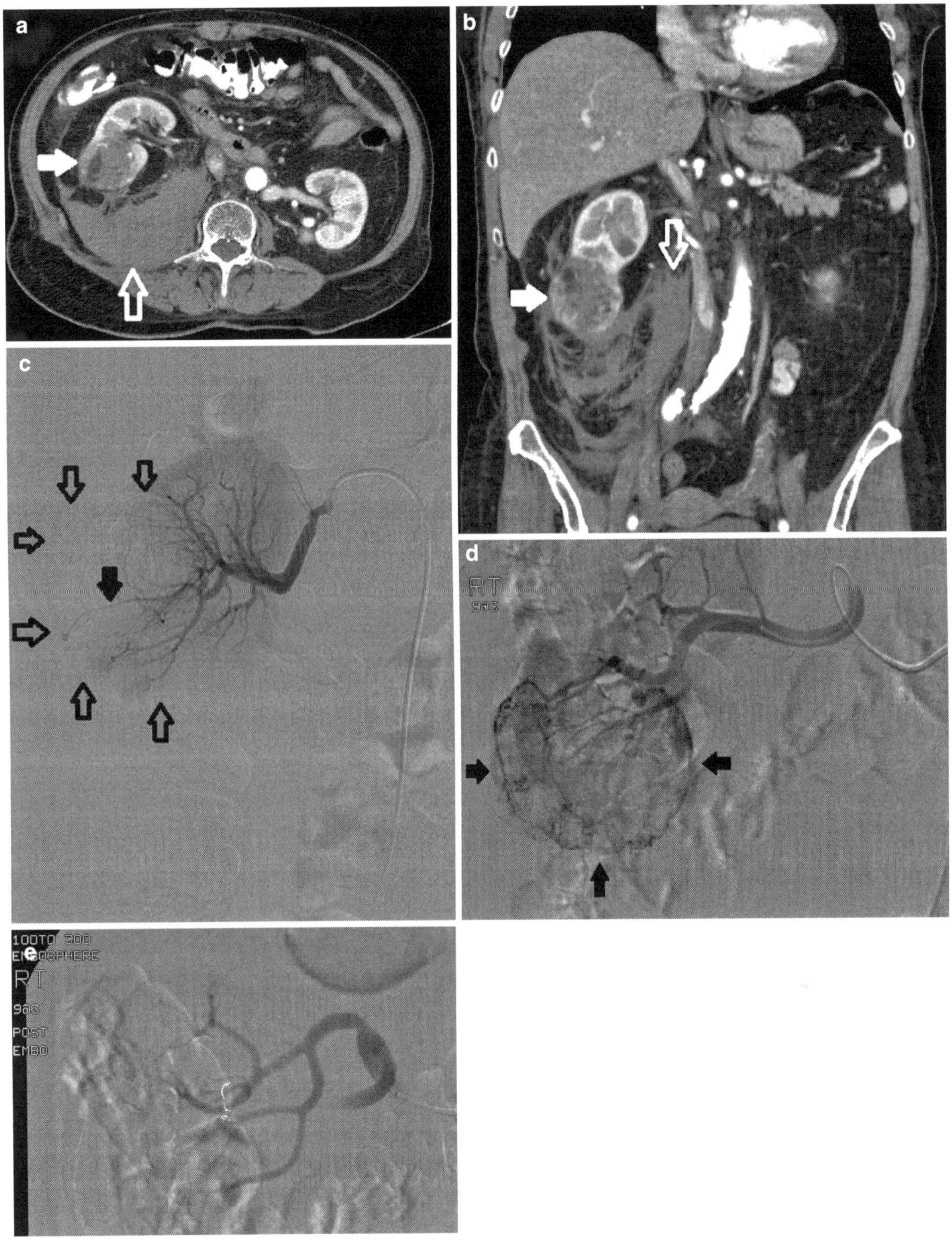

Fig. 8.5 Ruptured AML. Post-contrast axial (**a**) and reformatted coronal CT images (**b**) demonstrate an exophytic mass (*solid arrows*) arising from the right kidney containing macroscopic fat. There is a large amount of perirenal and retroperitoneal hemorrhage (*open arrows*), consistent with a ruptured AML. (**c**) Selective renal arteriogram demonstrating an irregular renal parenchymal contour secondary to surrounding hematoma. Additionally, a single tortuous vessel (*solid arrow*) with a nidus and surrounding lack of parenchymal blush (*open arrows*) is seen, compatible with the region of hemorrhage, the "light bulb sign." (**d**) Superselective renal arteriogram with microcatheter demonstrates filling of the tumor (*solid arrows*) with associated tortuous tumor vasculature. (**e**) Postembolization arteriogram demonstrates stasis of contrast in the renal artery with no filling of the tumor

Preoperative Embolization for Renal Neoplasms

A relatively controversial indication for renal artery embolization is that of preoperative embolization of tumor prior to partial or complete nephrectomy [20, 21]. Proponents of this procedure cite decreased operative time and blood loss, and ease of tissue dissection created by edema in dissection planes after embolization [22]. One retrospective analysis suggests decreased perioperative blood loss in patients undergoing preoperative embolization of tumors larger than 10 cm [23]. However, prospective randomized trials are lacking and thus are required to identify the role of embolization in the preoperative setting.

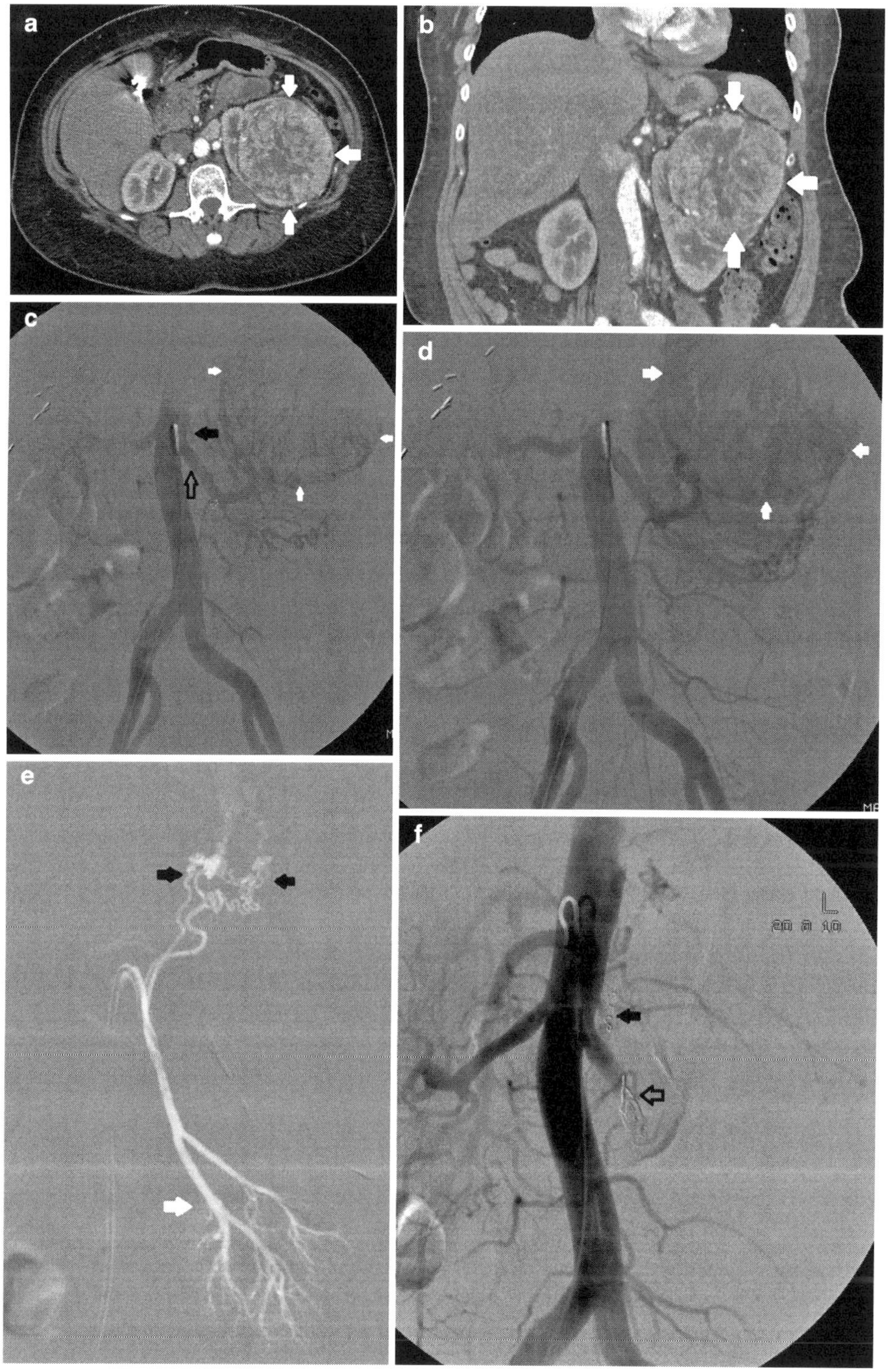

Fig. 8.6 Renal mass. Axial (**a**) and reformatted coronal (**b**) CT images demonstrate a large heterogeneously enhancing renal mass (*arrows*) replacing a large portion of left renal parenchyma. Due to its size, preoperative arterial embolization was performed with the goal of decreasing intraoperative blood loss. (**c**) Aortogram demonstrates multiple tumor vessels supplying the mass (*solid white arrows*) as noted on CT. Of note, an accessory renal artery (*solid black arrow*) in addition to the main renal artery (*open black arrow*) is seen. (**d**) Aortogram mid-embolization demonstrates contrast within the mass (*arrows*). (**e**) Accessory renal artery. Selective arteriogram demonstrates that the accessory renal artery feeds both tumor (*white arrows*) and normal residual renal parenchyma (*black arrow*). Because this patient would be undergoing total nephrectomy, coil embolization after particle embolization was performed. (**f**) Completion angiogram demonstrates no filling distal to the coils within the left main (*open arrow*) or accessory renal artery (*solid arrow*)

Embolization of Pseudoaneurysm After Partial Nephrectomy

A recent 5-year outcomes analysis suggests that laparoscopic and open partial nephrectomy are comparable in overall and cancer-specific survival in the treatment of small tumors [24]. Hemorrhage after both open and laparoscopic partial nephrectomy is a known complication, with one study citing a 9.5 % hemorrhage rate after laparoscopic partial nephrectomy [25, 26]. Rarely do patients require therapy beyond conservative management; however, a small subset of patients may develop pseudoaneurysms, resulting in gross hematuria and decreased hematocrit, some of which are potentially life threatening. Catheter-directed embolization of these pseudoaneurysms can be performed with excellent technical and clinical success [27]. Pseudoaneurysms may also be seen rarely after renal biopsy, placement of percutaneous nephrostomies or tumor ablations, and are treated in a similar fashion.

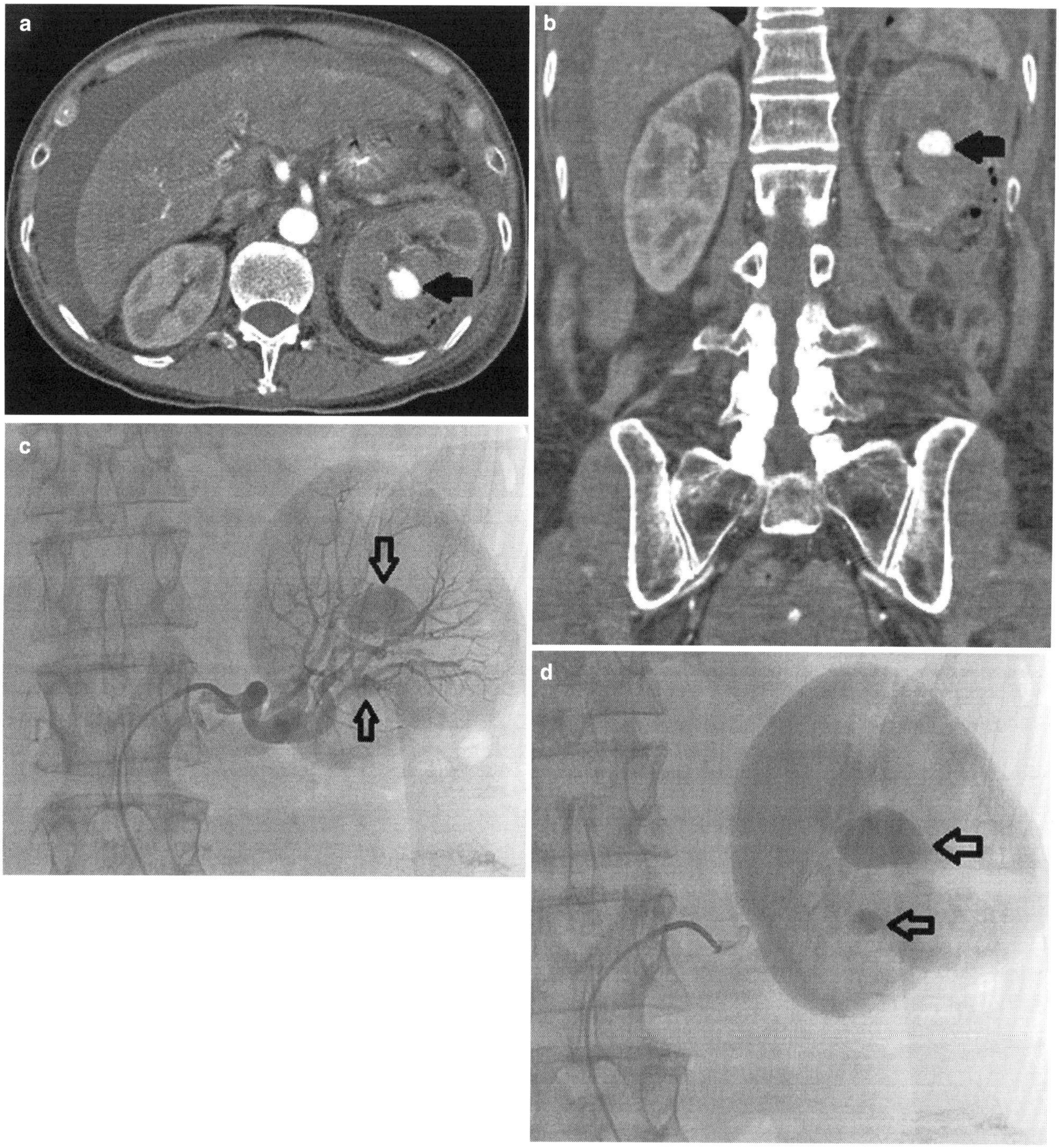

Fig. 8.7 CT. Post-contrast axial (**a**) and reformatted coronal CT images (**b**) demonstrate a large pseudoaneurysm (*arrows*) abutting the left partial nephrectomy bed. This patient has had persistent hematuria and decreased hematocrit for several days postoperatively. One of the most common causes of postnephrectomy-delayed hemorrhage is pseudoaneurysm [28]. (**c**) A selective left renal arteriogram demonstrates two pseudoaneurysms (*open arrows*) abutting the surgical bed (early arterial), which become more apparent as focal pools of contrast on parenchymal phase (**d**). (**e**) Superselective injection. Superselective angiogram demonstrates that both pseudoaneurysms arise from the same subsegmental artery. Careful diagnostic arteriogram technique should always be followed as it will often guide therapy and, in this case, allow for minimal sacrifice of normal residual renal parenchyma. (**f, g**) Postembolization. After coil embolization, repeat arteriogram, both subselective (**f**) and from the main renal artery (**g**), demonstrates complete exclusion of the pseudoaneurysms

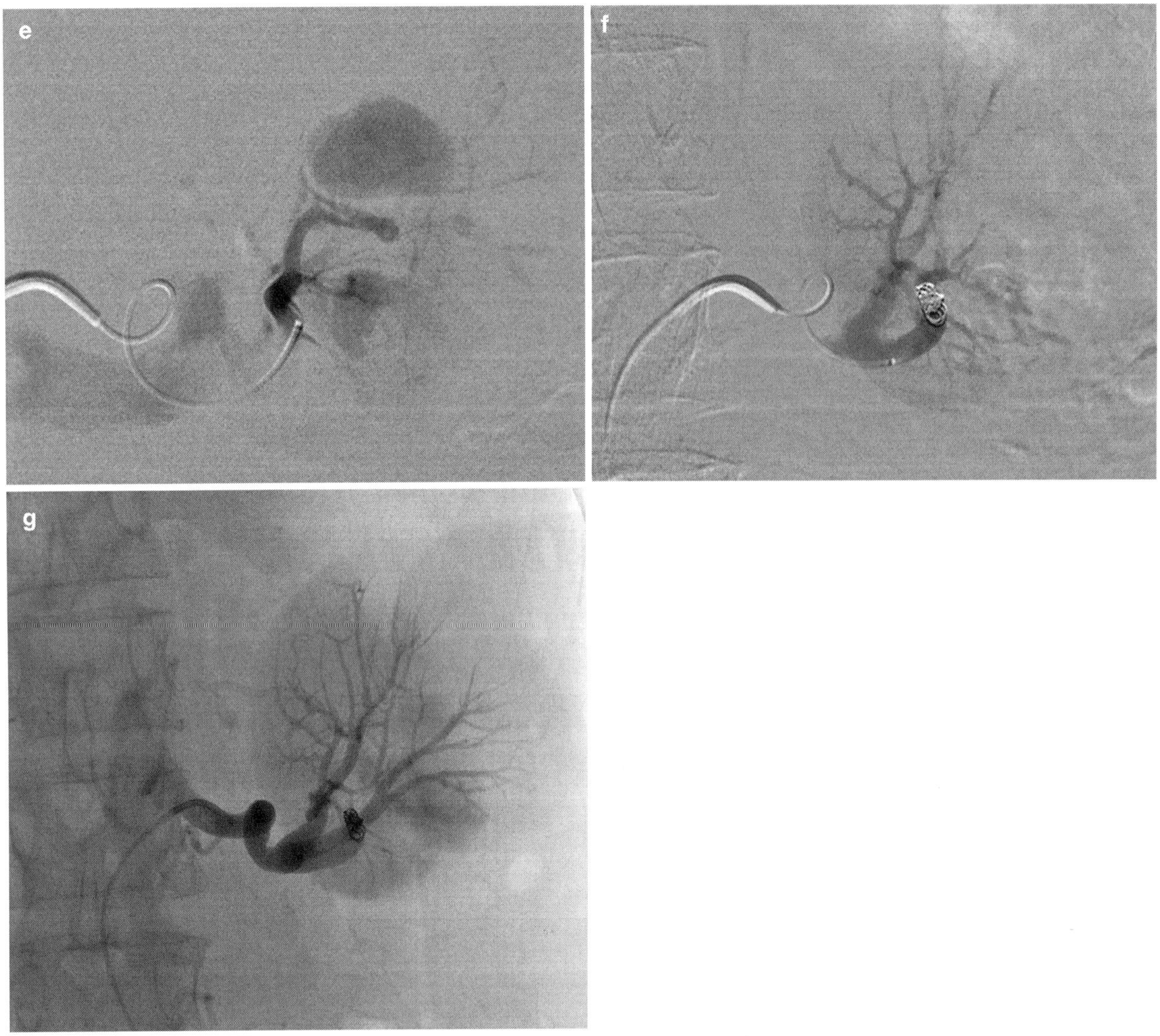

Fig. 8.7 (continued)

Radiologic Therapies in Ureteral Obstruction

Percutaneous access and tube placement within an obstructed renal collecting system was first described in 1955 by Goodwin et al. [29]. Since then, indications for nephrostomy tube placement have evolved to include obstructive uropathy, urinary diversion, treatment of nephrolithiasis, and treatment of obstructive urosepsis. Furthermore, technological advances have yielded multiple different types of percutaneously placed catheters, such as the nephrostomy tube, nephroureterostomy tube, and the ureteral stent (JJ stent).

In the oncologic patient, the choice of these different catheters is based on the etiology of the obstruction, disease prognosis, and patient comfort. For instance, a completely internalized ureteral stent, would be the most comfortable as patients would not be required to have a catheter with or without an attached bag extending from the flank. However, a completely internalized catheter would ideally need to be placed and replaced in a retrograde fashion and would initially require visualization and access to the ureteral orifice. Thus, patients with bladder tumors that distort underlying anatomy may not be ideal candidates. Generally, if the urinary bladder is normal, placement of internal stents is suggested as the first choice for patients. For those immediately involved in placement and management of these catheters, it is important to be aware of the advantages and disadvantages of each, which is beyond the scope of this chapter. Dyer et al. [30], however, provide an excellent review of these catheters.

It is important for those reviewing these films to be aware of the different types of catheters, as well as situations where these catheters may be placed in nonstandard positions, as demonstrated in the following images.

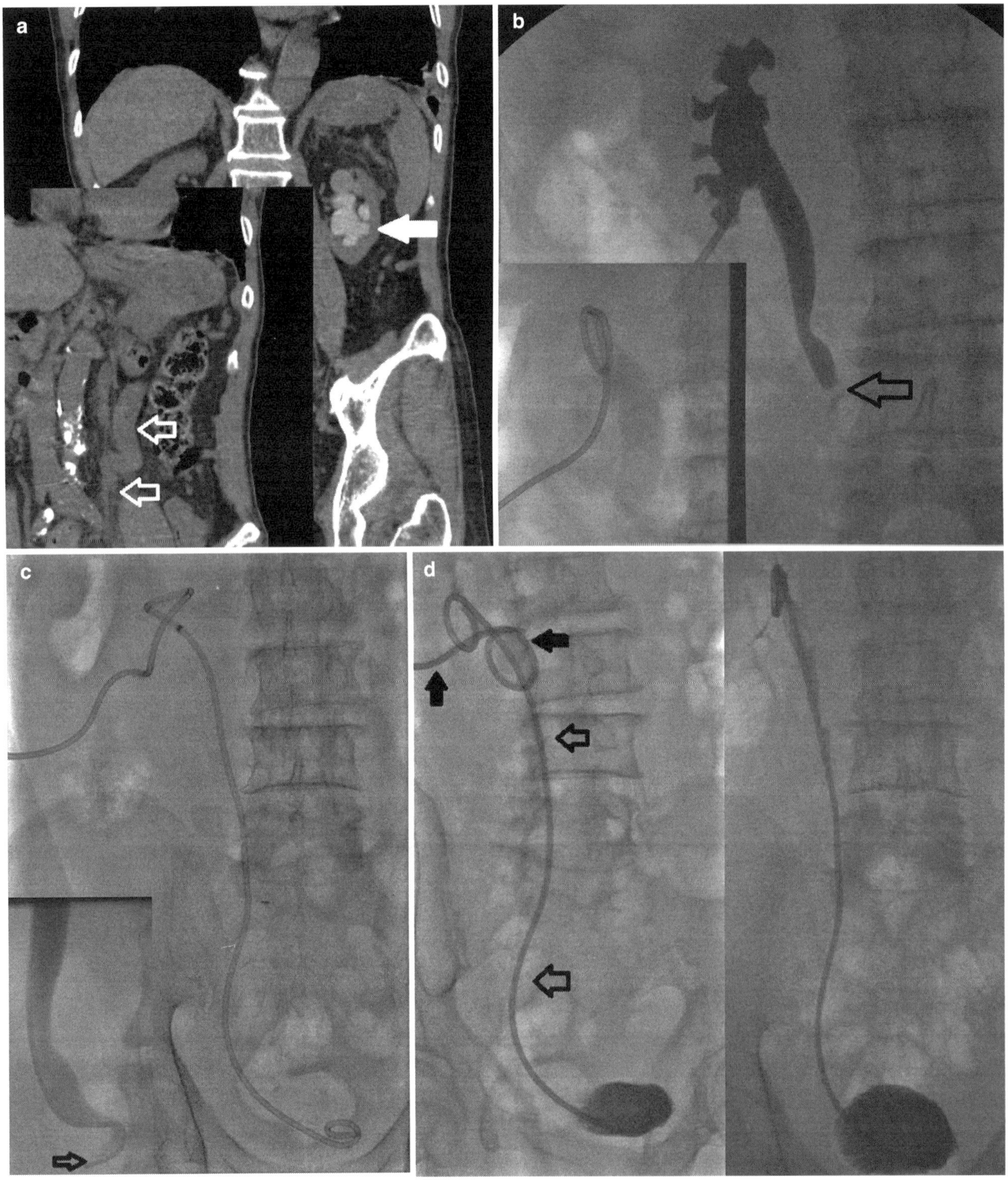
a
b
c
d

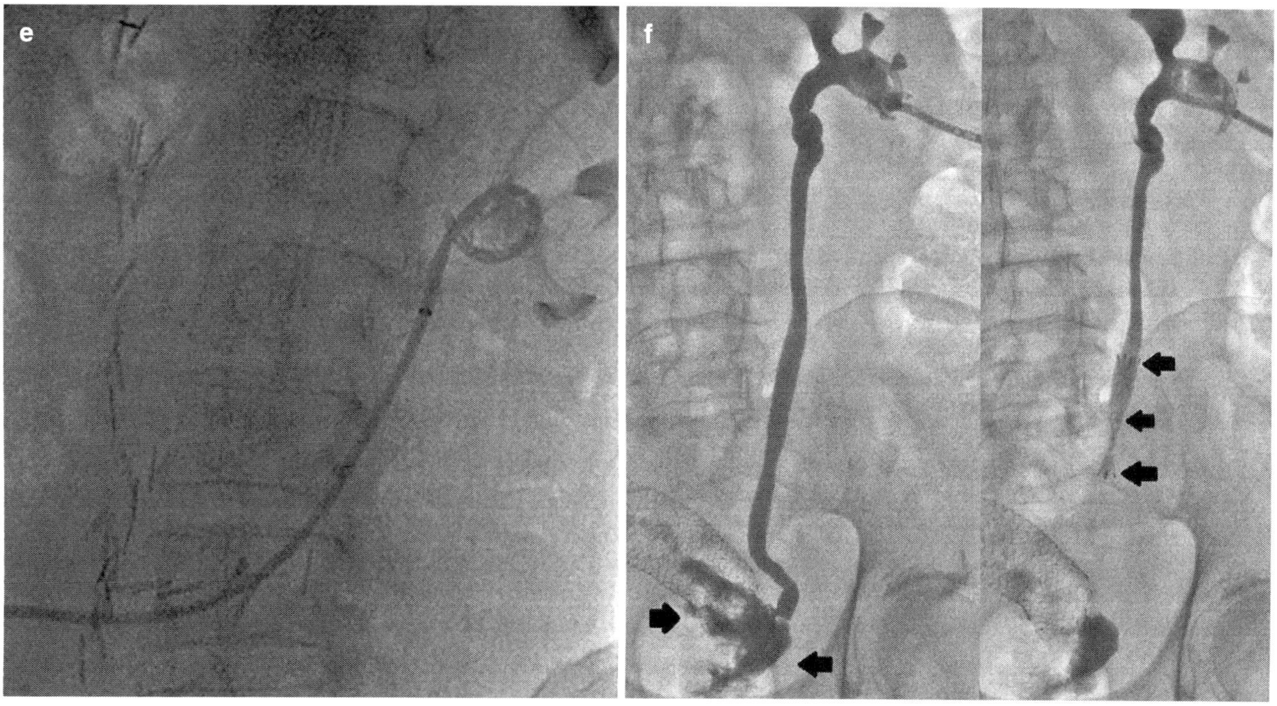

Fig. 8.8 (continued)

Fig. 8.8 Hydronephrosis. (**a**) Reformatted coronal CT images through the left kidney and ureter demonstrating left hydroureteronephrosis to the level of the mid ureter (*open arrows; inset*). This patient was found on further work-up to have metastatic gastric cancer with a small implant resulting in obstruction. Contrast is noted in the renal collecting system secondary to failed attempt at placing a stent under cystoscopy (*solid arrow*). (**b**) Nephrostomy. Nephrostomy tube was placed in the target kidney to divert urine in the immediate obstructive setting to preserve renal function (*inset*). Nephrostogram through the tube demonstrates high-grade obstruction at the level of the mid ureter (*arrow*), as noted on CT (**a**). (**c**) Nephroureterostomy. A wire was placed crossing the high-grade obstruction (*arrow, inset*) that allowed subsequent placement of a nephroureterostomy tube, which offers better stability (decreased risk of dislodgement) and the ability to cap the external portion of the tube. *Capping* refers to the ability to place a cap on the external tubing to allow for the tube to drain internally. With capping, a patient no longer needs a urine bag attached to the tube. (**d**) Ureteral stent (JJ tube). For comfort, patients may also have a completely internalized stent placed (*right panel*). On the date of placement, a covering catheter is often left (*solid arrows*) with the patient overnight (*left panel*) to make sure the internal stent (*open arrows*) works before removing the external catheter. (**e**) Retrograde nephroureterostomy tube (also known as *an upside-down NUT*). For patients who have had an ileal conduit creation or Indiana pouch creation requiring external drainage, a retrograde ureteral stent may be utilized to optimize comfort. The stent is open and drains directly into the ostomy bag associated with the ileal conduit, obviating the need for an additional bag. (**f**) Ureteral embolization for urinary diversion. Occasionally, postsurgical urinary leaks or continued bleeding from a tumor may require urinary diversion. For cases in which simple diversion with percutaneous nephrostomy is not adequate, embolization of the distal ureter utilizing a partially deployed covered stent, may be used [31]. A nephrostogram (*left panel*) demonstrates contrast freely flowing into an irregular urinary bladder (*arrows*). After stent deployment in the mid-ureter (*arrows; right panel*), contrast injection demonstrates occlusion of the ureter at the level of the stent

Prostate Biopsy and Focal Therapies

Biopsy

Transrectal ultrasonographic (TRUS)–guided prostate biopsy is the most widely accepted method to confirm and diagnose prostate cancer. Unfortunately, grayscale ultrasound has limited specificity and sensitivity in detecting tumor [32]. Recent advances in sonographic technology have allowed for utilization of color and power Doppler, as well as elastography to improve detection and therefore guidance [33]. At the same time, MRI has been found to be superior in delineating prostate cancer foci [34]. This has resulted in a tremendous interest in utilizing fusion imaging of real-time TRUS fused with pre-biopsy MRI to guide biopsy. Early clinical experience has demonstrated both feasibility and safety [35]. MRI-guided biopsy of the prostate has also been shown to be feasible, however this technique may be limited by high cost associated with the technology [36]. It remains to be seen what modality or combination of modalities will be the most efficacious and cost-effective while maintaining a low-risk profile.

Focal Therapies

Traditional management of localized prostate cancer involves either surveillance or more radical therapy such as total prostatectomy or radiotherapy. A growing number of focal therapies are being developed that could potentially offer the advantage of preserving normal prostate tissue and diminish morbidity of radical treatments such as incontinence, impotence, and hemorrhage [37]. Current focal therapeutic options include cryotherapy, high-intensity focused ultrasound (HIFU), photodynamic therapy, and laser ablation.

Cryotherapy utilizes image guidance to place multiple probes that act to destroy tumor cells by ice-crystal formation and induce cellular responses resulting in apoptosis. HIFU, generally performed under MR guidance, utilizes sonographic vibrational energy originating from multiple sources outside the body, triangulated in a way to focus the energy on the target tumor, thus destroying it. Photodynamic therapy utilizes an intravenously administered medication activated by a certain wavelength of light. Optical fibers are placed, via image guidance, into the target tumor, allowing for administration of the laser light that activates the drug. Finally, laser ablation utilizes multiple introducers, usually placed under MR guidance, that direct laser heat energy, destroying the target lesion.

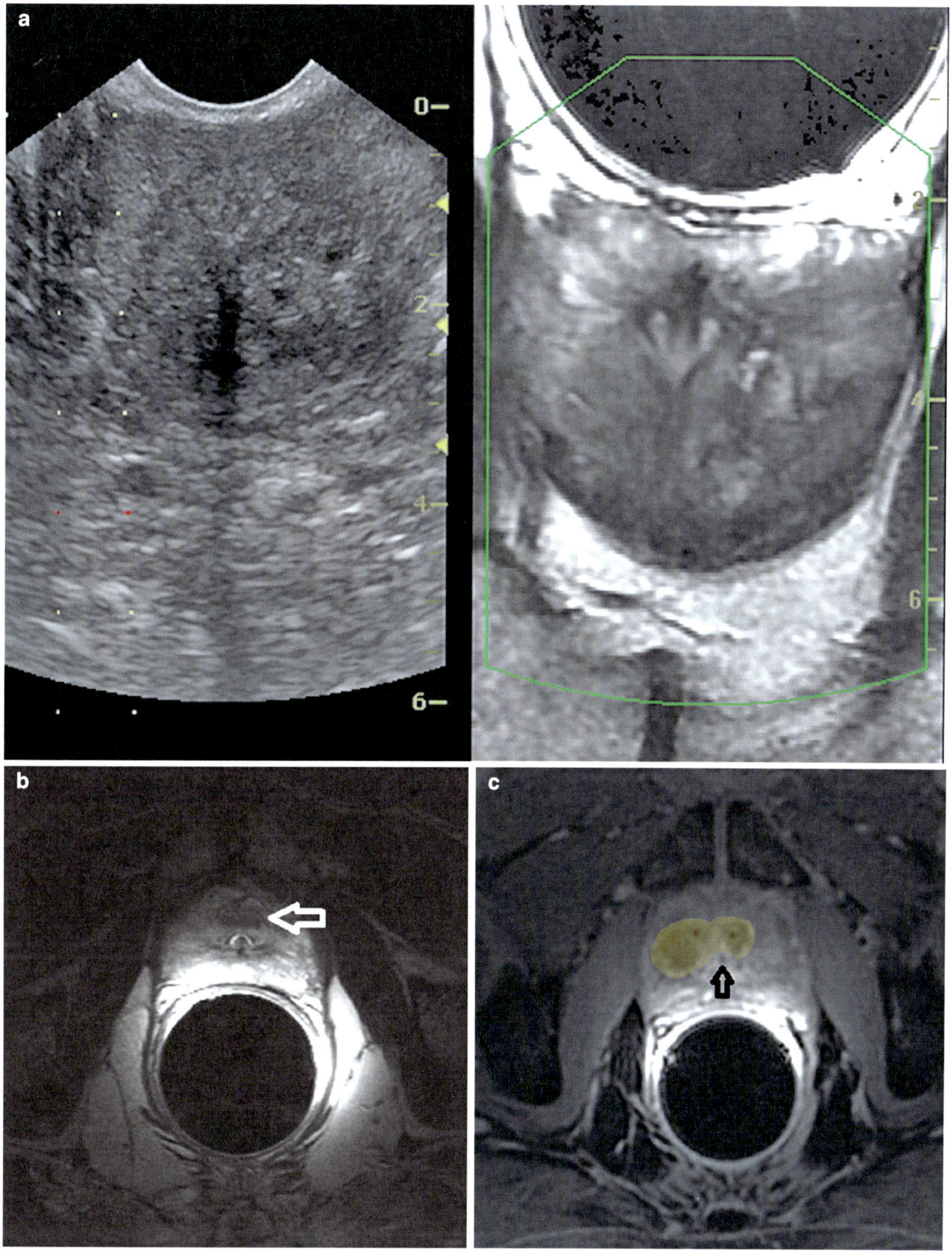

Fig. 8.9 (**a**) Fusion imaging. Real-time sonographic images during prostate biopsy (*left panel*) are registered with preoperative MRI images of the prostate (*right panel*). Image registration to guide biopsy takes advantage of the increased delineation of the tumor focus within the prostate on MRI with the advantages of real-time imaging and low cost of sonography. (**b, c**) MR-guided laser ablation. Pre-ablation T2-weighted MR image (**b**) demonstrates a low-intensity focus corresponding to a central prostate tumor (*open arrow*). Post-ablation contrast-enhanced images (**c**) demonstrates post-ablation foci (*shaded region*), abutting the urethra (*open arrow*). The utilization of MR allows for a temperature map to be created, which can potentially increase ablation efficacy. (**d**) Treatment temperature maps are created (*open arrow*; *left panel*) with estimates of irreversible damage made (*open arrow*; *right panel*)

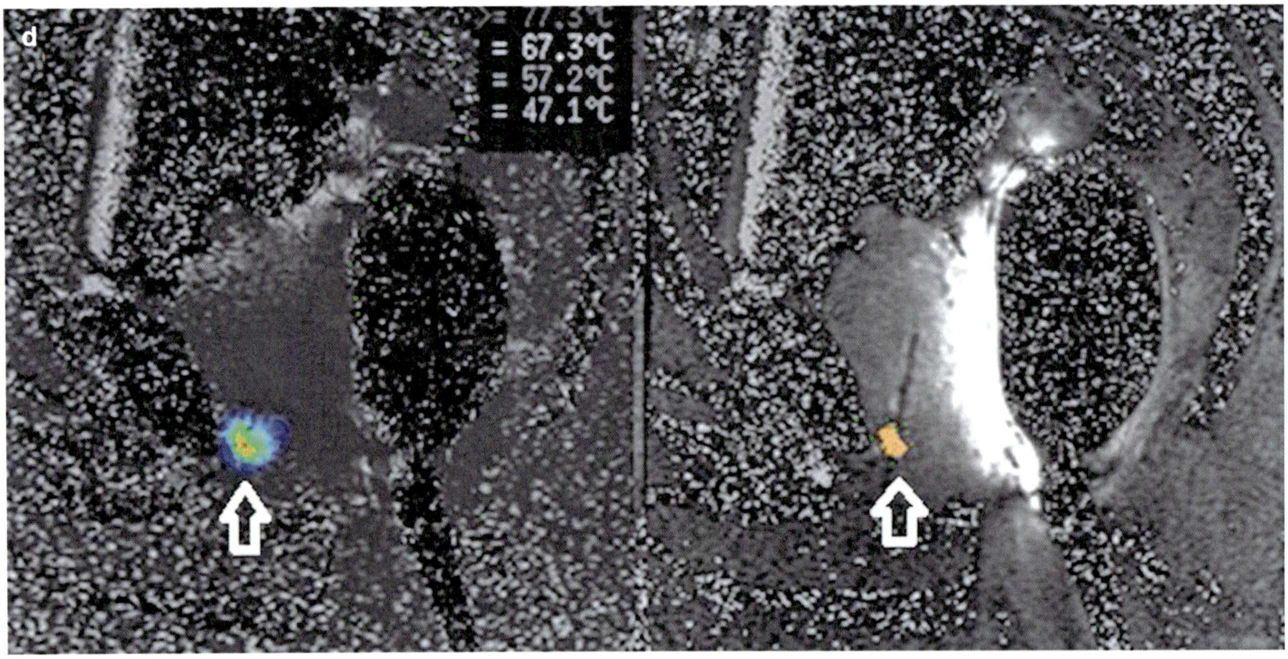

Fig. 8.9 (continued)

Management of Pelvic Lymphoceles

Pelvic or retroperitoneal lymphoceles are common complications after pelvic lymphadenectomy. These entities are cystic structures that arise from lymphatic injury during tissue dissection. Generally, lymphoceles cause symptoms secondary to mass effect and, occasionally, can become secondarily infected [38]. Various treatment options are available ranging from surgical marsupialization to transcatheter drainage with or without sclerotherapy [39]. The use of a sclerosant appears to be associated with higher success and lower recurrence rates, especially in patients with persistently increasing catheter drainage outputs.

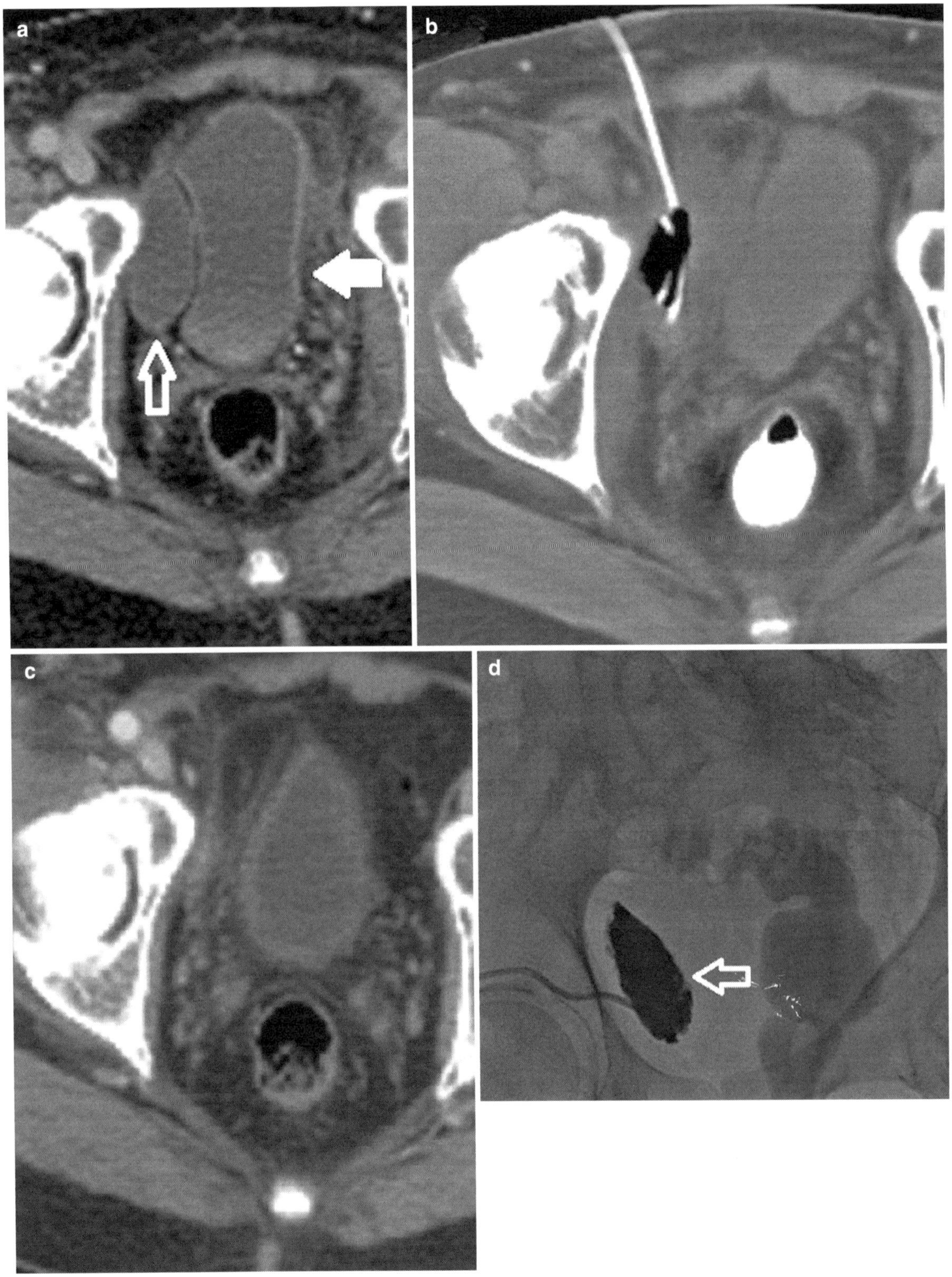

Fig. 8.10 CT-guided lymphocele drainage. A lymphocele (*open arrow*) is noted adjacent to the urinary bladder (*solid arrow*) after prostatectomy (**a**). CT-guided drainage was performed, with drainage catheter in place (**b**). After treatment with a sclerosant [40] for persistently increasing outputs, the catheter was eventually removed 1 month later. Repeat CT demonstrates resolution of the lymphocele (**c**). Patients can be followed with injection of the catheter under fluoroscopy. The initial image demonstrates filling of a large lymphocele cavity (*open arrow* in **d**). Interval follow-up demonstrates that the cavity had decreased in size (*open arrow* in **e**)

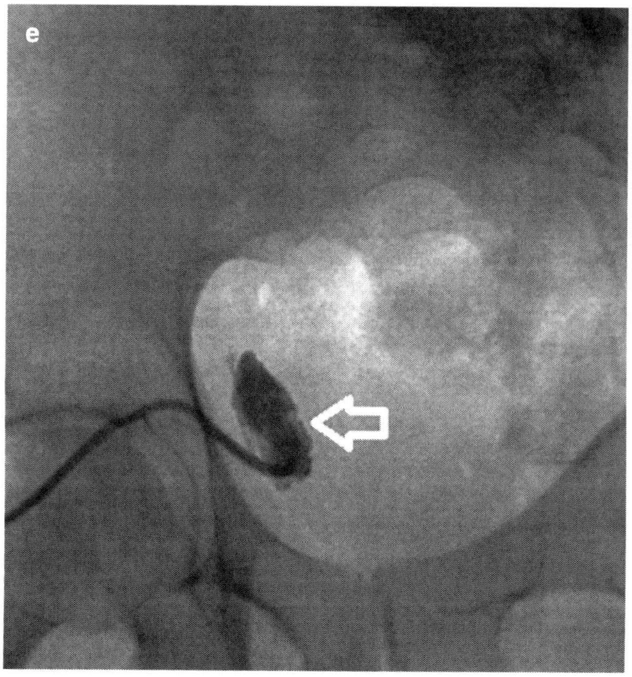

Fig. 8.10 (continued)

References

1. Whittier WL, Korbet SM. Renal biopsy: update. Curr Opin Nephrol Hypertens. 2004;13:661–55.
2. Misra S, Gyamlani G, Swaminathan S, et al. Safety and diagnostic yield of transjugular renal biopsy. J Vasc Interv Radiol. 2008;19:546–51.
3. Constantin A, Brisson ML, Kwan J, et al. Percutaneous US-guided renal biopsy: a retrospective study comparing the 16-gauge end-cut and 14-gauge side-notch needles. J Vasc Interv Radiol. 2010;21:357–61.
4. Song JH, Cronan JJ. Percutaneous biopsy in diffuse renal disease: comparison of 18- and 14-gauge automated biopsy devices. J Vasc Interv Radiol. 1998;9:651–5.
5. Patel MD, Phillips CJ, Young SW, et al. US-guided renal transplant biopsy: efficacy of a cortical tangential approach. Radiology. 2010;256:290–6.
6. Ralls PW, Barakos JA, Kaptein EM, et al. Renal biopsy-related hemorrhage: frequency and comparison of CT and sonography. J Comput Assist Tomogr. 1987;11:1031–4.
7. Singh JC, Kekre NS. Role of needle biopsy in solid renal masses: when does the pudding require a proof? Indian J Urol. 2006;22:61–3.
8. Ficarra V, Brunelli M, Cheng L, et al. Prognostic and therapeutic impact of the histopathologic definition of parenchymal epithelial renal tumors. Eur Urol. 2010;58:655–68.
9. Maturen KE, Nghiem HV, Caolli EM, et al. Renal mass core biopsy: accuracy and impact on clinical management. AJR Am J Roentgenol. 2007;18:563–70.
10. Barocas DA, Mathew S, DelPizzo JJ, et al. Renal cell carcinoma sub-typing by histopathology and fluorescence in situ hybridization on a needle-biopsy specimen. BJU Int. 2007;99:290–5.
11. Kunkle DA, Uzzo RG. Cryoablation or radiofrequency ablation of the small renal mass. A meta-analysis. Cancer. 2008;113:2671–80.
12. Levinson AW, Su LM, Agarwal D, et al. Long-term oncological and overall outcomes of percutaneous radiofrequency ablation in high risk surgical patients with a solitary small renal mass. J Urol. 2008;180:499–504.
13. Halpenny D, Snow A, McNeill G, Torreggiani WC. The radiological diagnosis and treatment of renal angiomyolipoma—current status. Clin Radiol. 2010;65:99–108.
14. Steiner MS, Goldman SM, Fishman EK, et al. The natural history of renal angiomyolipoma. J Urol. 1993;150:1782–6.
15. Oesterling JE, Fishman EK, Goldman SM, et al. The management of renal angiomyolipoma. J Urol. 1986;135:1121–4.
16. Kothary N, Soulen MC, Clark TW, et al. Renal angiomyolipoma: long-term results after arterial embolization. J Vasc Interv Radiol. 2005;16:45–50.
17. Lee SY, Hsu HH, Chen YC, et al. Embolization of renal angiomyolipomas: short-term and long term outcomes, complications, and tumor shrinkage. Cardiovasc Interv Radiol. 2009;32:1171–8.
18. Han YM, Kim JK, Roh BS, et al. Renal angiomyolipoma: selective arterial embolization—effectiveness and changes in angiomyogenic components in long term follow-up. Radiology. 1997;204:65–70.
19. Lenton J, Kessel D, Watkinson AF. Embolization of renal angiomyolipoma: immediate complications and long term outcomes. Clin Radiol. 2008;63:864–70.
20. Loffroy R, Rao P, Ota S, et al. Correspondence: renal artery embolization prior to radical nephrectomy for renal cell carcinoma: when, how and why? Br J Radiol. 2010;83:630.
21. May M, Brookman-Amissah S, Pflanz S, et al. Preoperative renal arterial embolization does not provide survival benefit in patients with radical nephrectomy for renal cell carcinoma. Br J Radiol. 2009;82:724–31.
22. Bakal CW, Cynamon J, Lakritz PS, et al. Value f preoperative renal artery embolization in reducing blood transfusion requirements during nephrectomy for renal cell carcinoma. J Vasc Interv Radiol. 1993;4:727–31.
23. Schwartz MJ, Smith EB, Trost DW, et al. Renal artery embolization: clinical indications and experience from over 100 cases. BJU Int. 2006;99:881–6.
24. Lane BR, Gill IS. 5-Year outcomes of laparoscopic partial nephrectomy. J Urol. 2007;177:70–4.
25. Huber J, Pahernik S, Hallscheidt P, et al. Risk factors and clinical management of haemorrhage after open nephron-sparing surgery. BJU Int. 2010;106:1488–93.
26. Ramani AP, Desai MM, Steinberg AP, et al. Complications of laparoscopic partial nephrectomy in 200 cases. J Urol. 2005;173:42–7.
27. Shapiro EY, Hakimi AA, Hyams ES, et al. Renal artery pseudoaneurysm following laparoscopic partial nephrectomy. J Urol. 2009;74:819–23.
28. Sing D, Gill IS. Renal artery pseudoaneurysm following laparoscopic partial nephrectomy. J Urol. 2005;174:2256–9.
29. Goodwin WE, Casey WC, Woolf W. Percutaneous trocar (needle) nephrostomy in hydronephrosis. J Am Med Assoc. 1955;157:891–4.
30. Dyer RB, Regan JD, Kavanagh PV, et al. Percutaneous nephrostomy with extensions of the technique: step by step. Radiographics. 2002;22:503–25.
31. Lynch FC. Use of a covered stent for percutaneous transrenal occlusion of the ureter. J Vasc Interv Radiol. 2007;18:1456–8.
32. Punnen S, Nam RK. Indications and timing for prostate biopsy, diagnosis of early prostate cancer and its definitive treatment: a clinical conundrum in the PSA era. Surg Oncol. 2009;18:192–9.
33. Loch T. Urologic imaging for localized prostate cancer. World J Urol. 2007;25:121–9.
34. Futterer JJ, Heijmink SW, Scheenen TW, et al. Prostate cancer: local staging at 3-T endorectal MR imaging—early experience. Radiology. 2006;238:184–91.

35. Singh AK, Kruecker J, Xu S, et al. Initial clinical experience with real-time transrectal ultrasonography-magnetic resonance imaging fusion-guided prostate biopsy. BJU Int. 2008;101:841–5.
36. Yakar D, Hambrock T, Hoeks C, et al. Magnetic resonance-guided biopsy of the prostate: feasibility, technique and clinical applications. Top Magn Reson Imaging. 2008;19:291–5.
37. Ahmen HU, Moore C, Emerton M. Minimally-invasive technologies in uro-oncology: the role of cryotherapy, HIFU and photodynamic therapy in whole gland and focal therapy of localized prostate cancer. Surg Oncol. 2009;18:219–32.
38. Karcaaltincaba M, Akhan O. Radiologic imaging and percutaneous treatment of pelvic lymphocele. Euro J Radiol. 2005;55:340–54.
39. Kim JK, Jeong YY, Kim YH, et al. Postoperative pelvic lymphocele: treatment with simple percutaneous catheter drainage. Radiology. 1999;212:390–4.
40. Gilliland JD, Spies JB, Brown SB, et al. Lymphoceles: percutaneous treatment with povidone-iodine sclerosis. Radiology. 1989; 171:227–9.

9 Nuclear Medicine Imaging in Genitourinary Oncology

Mark Dunphy

Noninvasive diagnostic imaging with radioactive pharmaceuticals is often referred to as *nuclear imaging* or *scintigraphy*. General nuclear medicine texts offer technical details of nuclear imaging technology and the large pharmacopoeia of radiopharmaceuticals in clinical use and research. This chapter focuses on radiolabeled agents given intravenously in small, nontherapeutic trace amounts for scintigraphic tumor detection as part of disease staging and response evaluation in genitourinary (GU) oncology, including preeminent radiotracers in current use and selected new tracers now in trials, which likely will be more widely available in clinical practice to GU oncologists in the next 10 years. Sentinel lymph node scintigraphy is also discussed as a promising diagnostic adjunct for nodal staging being explored in certain GU malignancies.

Nuclear imaging technology includes positron emission tomography (PET) and single-photon detection scintigraphy, the latter including single-photon emission computed tomography (SPECT) and traditional two-dimensional (2D) or planar imaging. PET imaging can only be performed with positron-emitting tracers, such as the now-common agent fluorodeoxyglucose (FDG), which carries the PET isotope fluorine-18 (^{18}F). To date, PET is the best noninvasive imaging modality available for *in vivo* quantification of labeled compounds, with picomolar sensitivity. State-of-the-art PET scanners offer a spatial resolution of approximately 4–5 mm (full-width half-maximum [FWHM]), whereas SPECT scanners offer approximately 12–15 mm FWHM. PET imaging spatial resolution is inferior to other standard clinical modalities, including MRI, CT, and ultrasound (US).

The superior signal-sensitivity of PET has been combined with the superior spatial resolution of CT in integrated PET-CT scanners. Numerous clinical studies have fairly consistently demonstrated that fusion imaging has a synergistic effect in improving the diagnostic accuracy of both PET and CT image analyses. The clinical PET-CT experience spurred development of SPECT-CT hybrid scanners, now in routine clinical use, and integrated PET-MRI and SPECT-MRI scanners now in clinical testing.

All US Food and Drug Administration (FDA)-approved radiotracers used to date for tumor detection are known to potentially yield false-positive and false-negative results scintigraphically due to a variety of conditions, generally including the limited sensitivity and/or specificity of a particular radiotracer for cancerous tissues (*e.g.*, other noncancerous pathologies might also accumulate tracer); normal variations in tracer biodistribution that may mimic tumor or obscure tumor detection; and tracer interactions with endogenous or exogenous substances. Like other pharmaceuticals, each radiotracer has a characteristic pharmacological profile, sometimes including potential interactions with over-the-counter or prescription drugs or other substances. The oncologist unfamiliar with a particular diagnostic nuclear imaging study should contact an imaging specialist for information on patient preparation.

FDG-PET Versus FDG-PET-CT

FDG is a glucose analog labeled with the positron-emitting isotope ^{18}F. FDG-PET is frequently mentioned in disease management guidelines issues by genitourinary cancer societies. GU oncologists should be aware of recommendations that focus on FDG-PET studies (particularly citations before 2000) rather than fusion FDG-PET-CT literature—the latter representing the current state-of-the-art, which in addition to advances in PET data processing and analyses is fundamentally superior in diagnostic accuracy versus PET alone.

M. Dunphy, DO
Department of Radiology, Memorial Sloan-Kettering Cancer Center, 1275 York Avenue, New York, NY 10065, USA
e-mail: dunphym@mskcc.org

A.M. Bach, J. Zhang (eds.), *Atlas of Genitourinary Oncological Imaging*, Atlas of Oncology Imaging, DOI 10.1007/978-1-4614-4872-3_9, © Springer Science+Business Media New York 2013

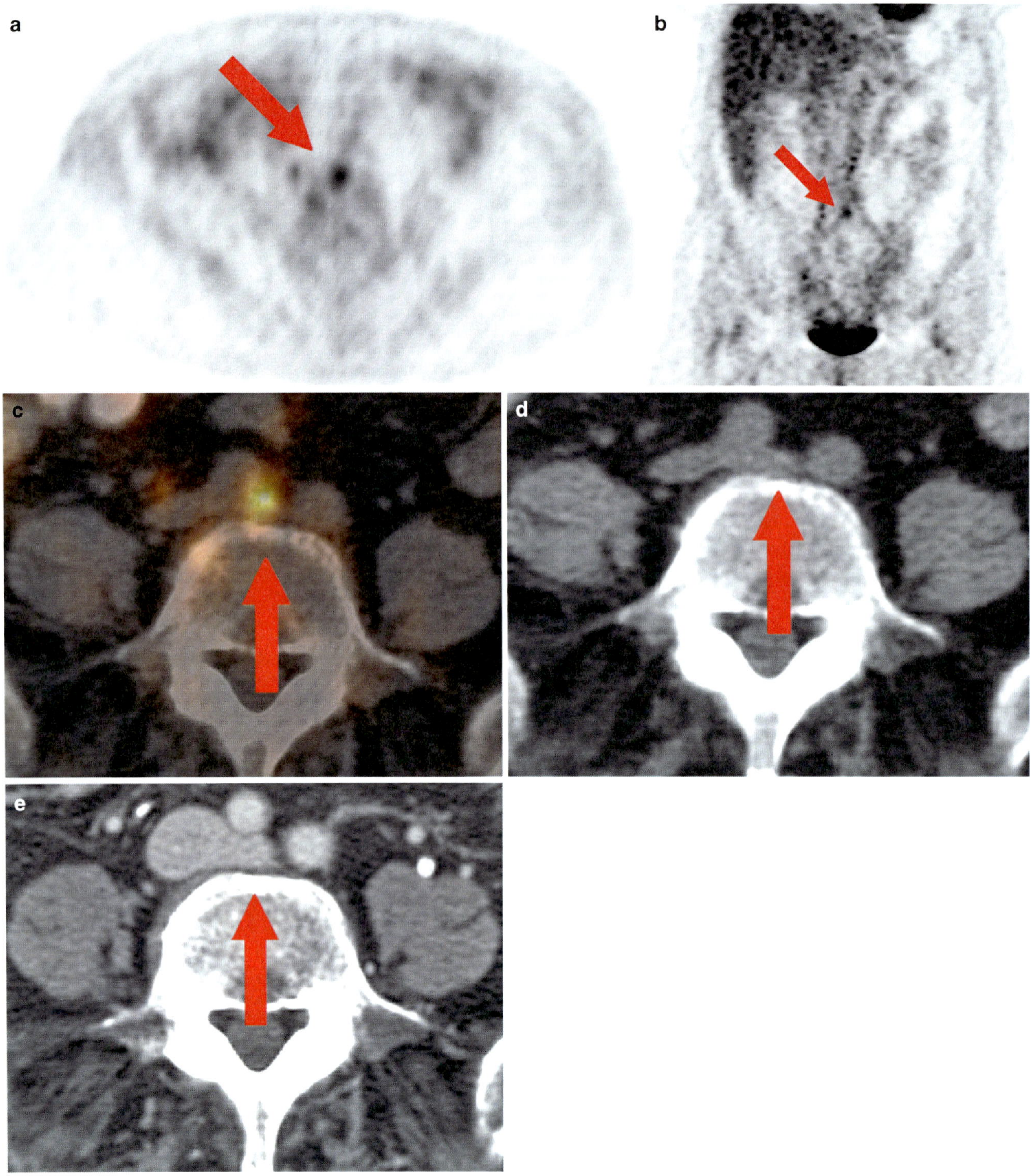

Fig. 9.1 A 66-year-old female with bladder cancer referred for staging. PET imagery (transaxial slice, **a**; coronal slice, **b**) visualizes a focus of FDG activity at the bifurcation of the iliac vessels (*arrow*). Without CT fusion, such a focus is concerning for hypermetabolic metastatic adenopathy. With fusion imaging (**c**), the PET focus localized to the iliac vein (as artifact) on CT without IV contrast (**d**); further identified by a same-day CT with IV contrast (**e**). PET-CT fusion yields significantly higher diagnostic accuracy than PET alone, both in sensitivity and specificity. Moreover, fusion imagery has been shown to have a synergistic impact on PET and CT analyses: analysis of PET-CT fusion imagery has a higher diagnostic yield than the sum of independent PET and CT readings

Bone Scintigraphy and Osteoblastic Versus Osteolytic Lesions

Single photon-emitter technetium 99 m (^{99m}Tc)-labeled bisphosphonate scintigraphy, often referred to as *the bone scan*, visualizes the skeleton by a bisphosphonate, commonly methylene diphosphonate (MDP) or hydroxymethyl diphosphonate (HDP) labeled with ^{99m}Tc. Bone scintigraphy is for the detection of osseous lesions, usually by planar body imaging, with or without SPECT or SPECT-CT of selected body regions. The radiotracer localizes by chemical adsorption to the inorganic hydroxyapatite matrix of bone. Genitourinary cancer cells in bone metastases do not accumulate bisphosphonate tracer. Bisphosphonate scintigraphy detects osseous metastases indirectly by detecting the local response of a bone to a metastasis. Some GU cancers, notably prostate metastases, classically cause osteoblastic reactions that evoke a relatively high local exposure of hydroxyapatite matrix, which tracer can absorb. This manifests on scintigraphy as a bony hotspot. Osteolytic-type metastases, typical of renal and bladder cancer, disintegrate compact bone, sometimes without any osteoblastic-type bone reaction. Nonosteoblastic disease may be invisible to the bone scan. CT can detect osteolytic metastases of clinically relevant, macroscopic size, as well as radiodense-appearing osteoblastic-type metastases.

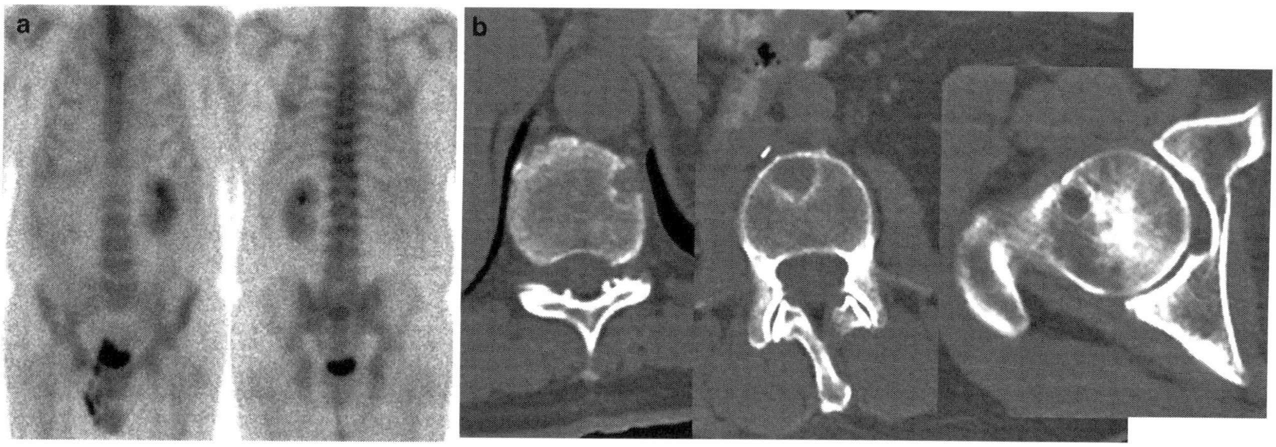

Fig. 9.2 Renal cancer patient with known metastatic disease referred for bone evaluation. Bone scintigraphy showed no osseous lesions of clear concern for a metastatic etiology (anterior planar torso projection, **a**; posterior projection, **b**). However, same-day CT study visualized multiple osteolytic metastases invisible to scintigraphy, for example, in several vertebrae (*left* and *middle* transaxial CT images in **b**) and right femoral neck (*right* transaxial CT image in **b**)

Radiographically Occult Osseous Metastasis

Other macroscopic intraosseous metastases may cause neither an osteoblastic-type reaction nor osteolytic damage detectable by CT. However, a radiographically occult bony reaction may be detected by bone scintigraphy. This is usually followed by changes on CT within several weeks.

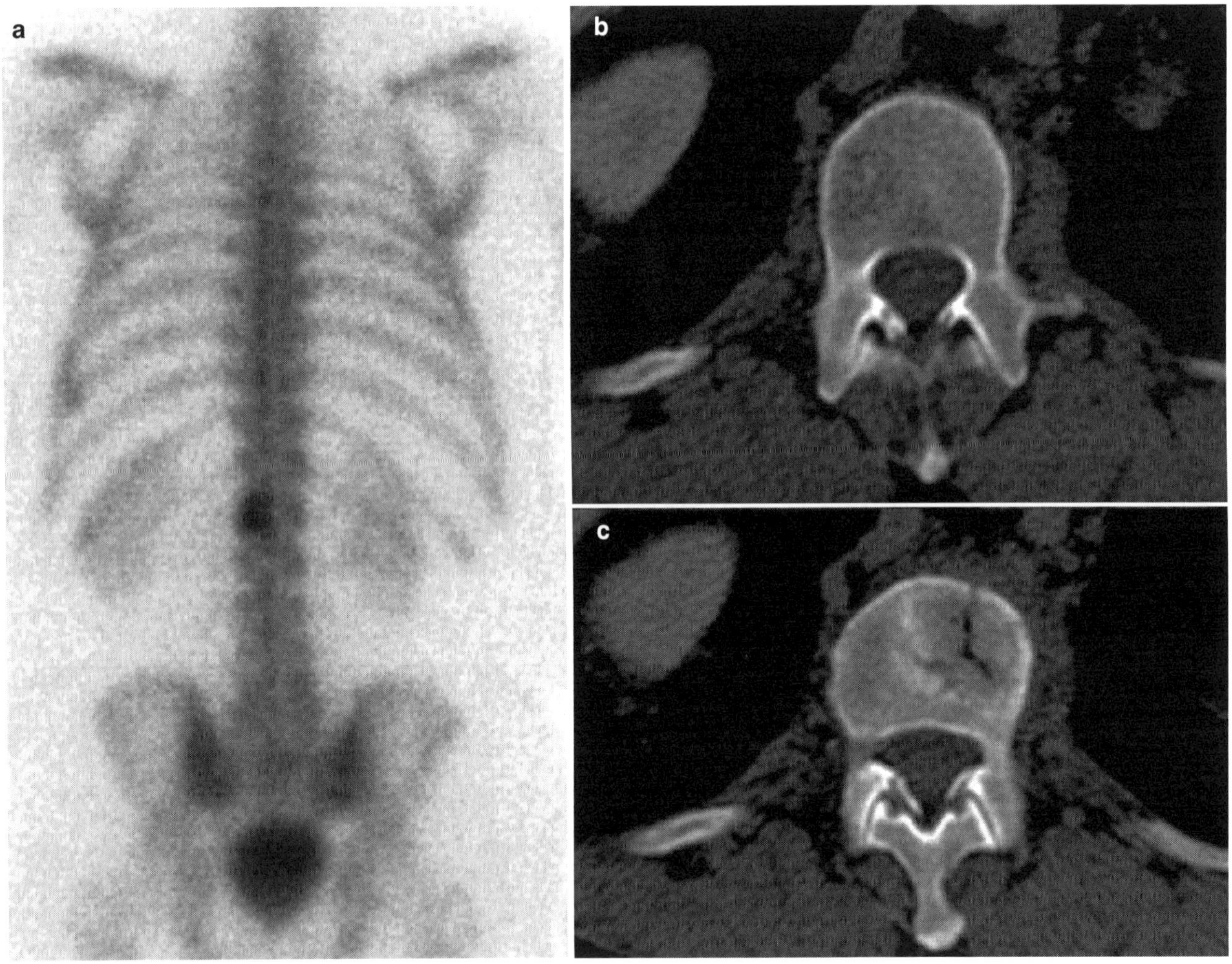

Fig. 9.3 Prostate cancer patient having follow-up bone scintigraphy during disease surveillance. Suspicious lesion of the L1 vertebra was newly visualized, scintigraphically (**a**), but same-day CT (transaxial slice through L1, **b**) showed no clear radiographic correlate of concern. Three months later, the lesion persisted on bone scintigraphy (*not shown*), and same-day follow-up CT (**c**) showed a corresponding L1 radiodense changes, with a pathological fracture. Osseous lesions may manifest on bone scintigraphy before CT changes become apparent

Flare Response Phenomenon

Other macroscopic intraosseous metastases may be present but invisible on both CT imagery and bone scintigraphy but can often be visualized by PET and/or MRI imaging. Such invisible osseous marrow metastases have an added complication: the scan flare-response phenomenon. The scan flare-response, also called *pseudoprogression*, is a well-documented (but probably underrecognized) biological-imaging phenomenon observed in serial imaging studies of cancer patients receiving anticancer therapy. In the scan flare-response, the effect of interim anticancer therapy induces the new visualization of osseous lesions (of metastatic etiology) that were preexistent but previously invisible in the prior study. Newly visualized osseous findings can easily be (mis-)attributed to interim development of a new osteoblastic-type osseous metastasis, when in fact metastatic cells might no longer be present in the osseous lesion (remembering that *lesion* is synonymous with *wound* and not synonymous with *metastasis*), possibly having been eradicated by interim therapy. Newly visualized osteoblastic-type changes may represent bony healing at the site. The 2008 guidelines of the Prostate Cancer Clinical Trials Working Group (PCCTWG) make the important recommendation that therapy ought not be discontinued, if bone scintigraphy shows new foci of osseous activity at the first (12 week) post-therapy assessment time-point but no other clear indications of disease progression are evident to avoid potentially being misled by flare response phenomenon, or pseudoprogression [1, 2]. Rather, bone scintigraphy should be repeated at least 6 weeks later. If this second post-therapy bone scan documents >2 additional, suspicious, new scintigraphic foci, then the findings are accepted as confirming disease progression [3].

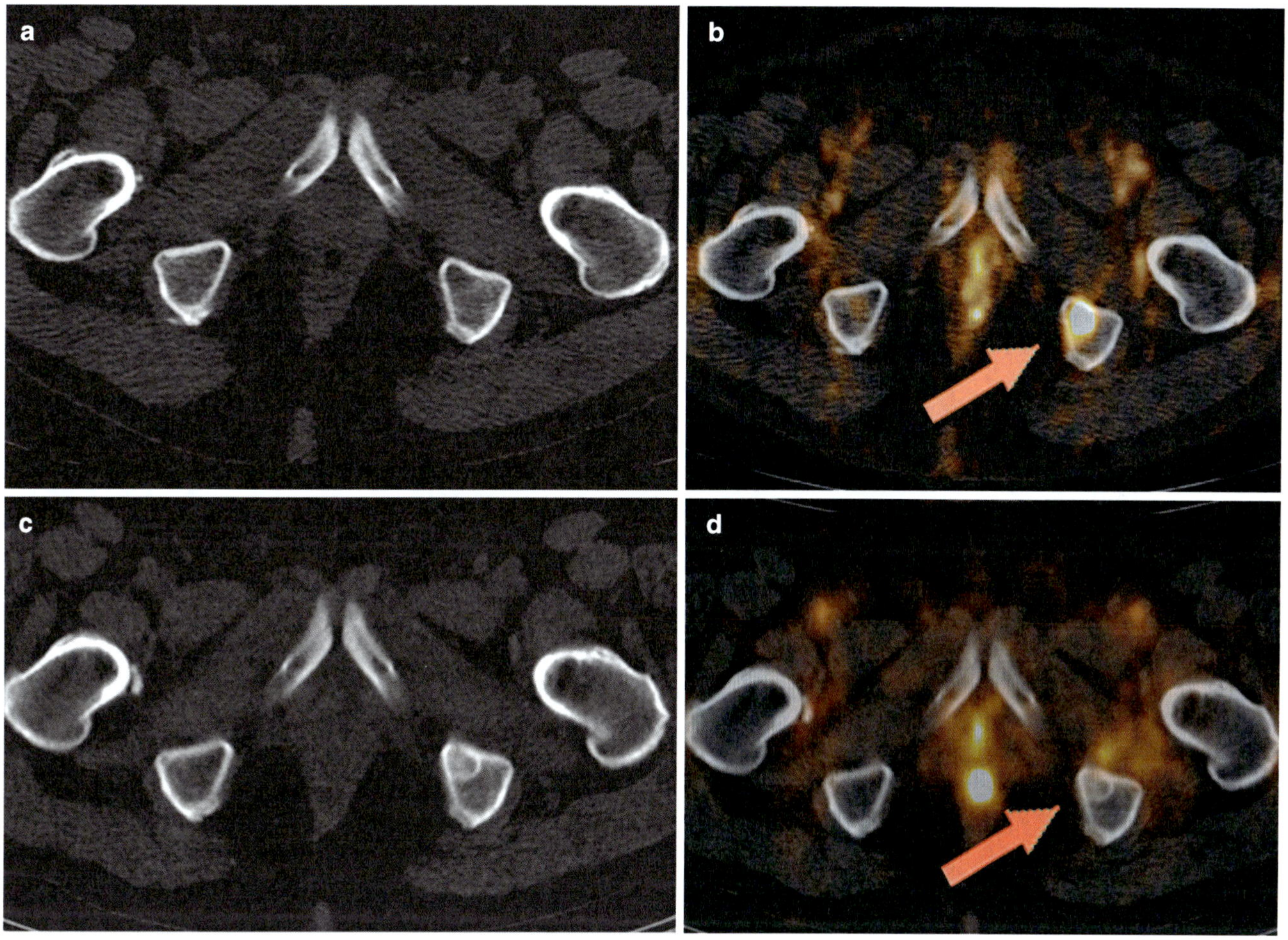

Fig. 9.4 Prostate cancer patient, with postsurgical rise in PSA, referred for imaging for restaging. (**a**,**b**) show a transaxial fusion FDG-PET-CT image (**b**) that visualized a previously unidentified lesion of the left ischium (*red arrow*) suspicious for metastatic disease. Same-day standard CT (**a**) showed no ischial lesion. Next-day biopsy confirmed metastatic prostate cancer in left ischium. Patient received salvage radiotherapy. (**c**,**d**) show restaging imaging, 20 months later. Standard CT (**c**) newly visualized a radiodense lesion of the left ischium, reported as a new osseous metastasis (though previously identified by prior PET, **b**). Same-day follow-up PET-CT (**d**) shows no residual FDG uptake in the previously identified metastatic ischial lesion, consistent with a favorable response to treatment, the newly visualized radiodense changes being consistent with bony healing (CT flare response)

Slow Healing of Osseous Lesions

During follow-up of patients with a history of osseous metastases, many imaging specialists will describe persistent lesions, on bone scintigraphy, as "metastases" in their reports, whereas others prefer phrasing such as "osseous lesions of metastatic etiology," recognizing that bone scintigraphy does not visualize osseous metastases directly, only the osseous wounds that metastases cause. More than mere semantics, the latter phrase recognizes a fundamental limitation of bone scintigraphy: the bone scan and CT are both often unable to identify in a timely fashion bony metastasis response, in osteoblastic lesions, to anticancer therapy. At best, usually, osteoblastic lesions appear stable in the short term, generally lingering for months or years after an osseous metastasis has been essentially eradicated at that site [2]. Hence, in prostate cancer, for example, Prostate Cancer Clinical Trials Working Group guidelines consider a favorable therapeutic response of osseous disease as the absence of new bony lesions and the stable scintigraphic appearance of previously identified bony lesions [1].

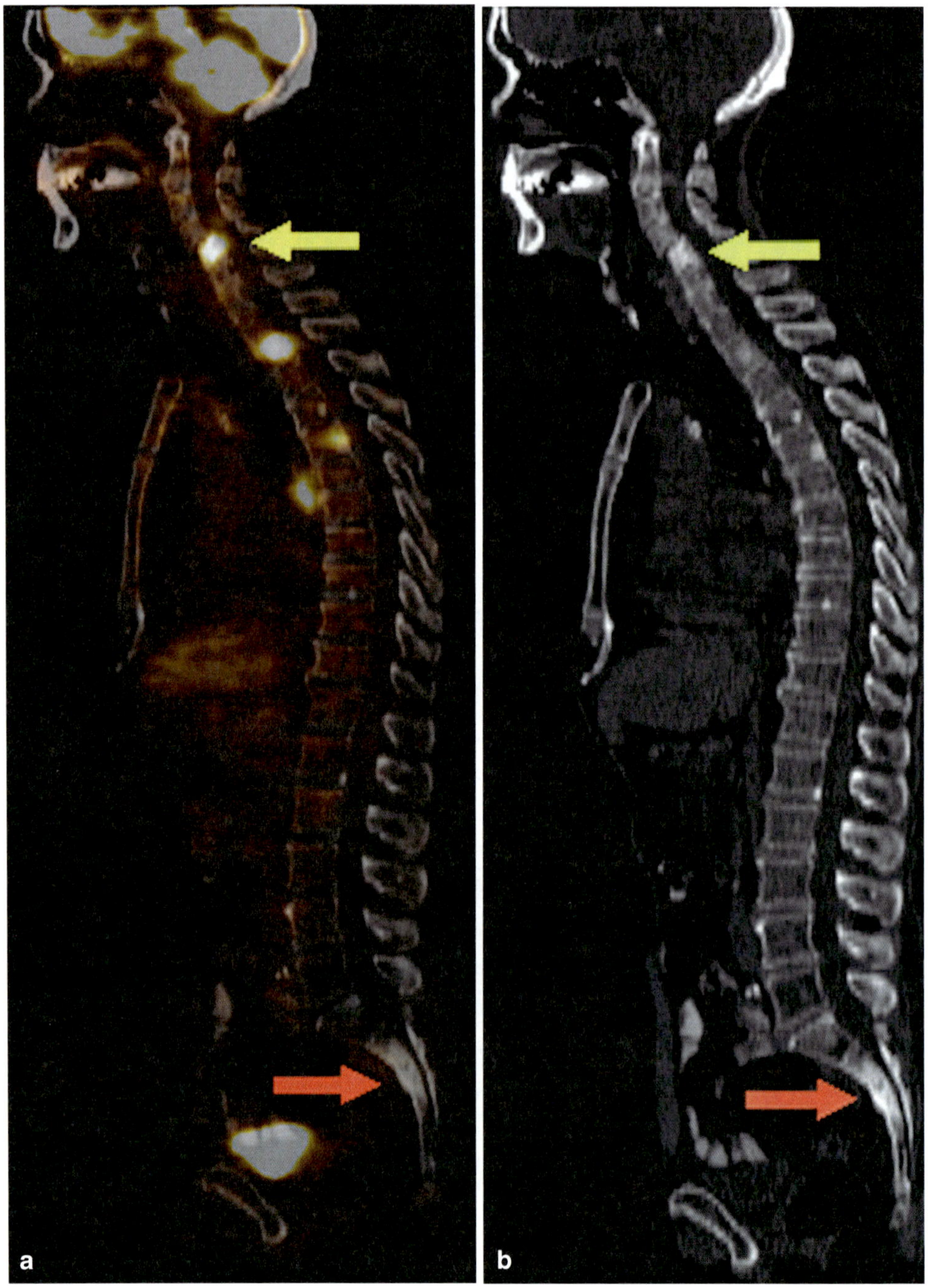

Fig. 9.5 Prostate cancer patient with bony metastases. (**a**), Fusion FDG-PET-CT, sagittal tomograph. (**b**), Companion CT, bone window setting. Note that multiple radiodense vertebral lesions are FDG avid (*e.g., yellow arrow*), consistent with viable osteoblastic-type metastases. However, the radiodense sacral lesion (*red arrow*), a site of biopsy-proven metastatic disease in the past, is not FDG avid, consistent with treated-disease (*i.e.*, a lesion of metastatic etiology lacking viable tumor)

Lymphoscintigraphy in GU Oncology

The sentinel lymph node paradigm involves injecting a lymphatic tracer around the tumor region and then using imaging and intraoperative radioprobes to find the node or lymph nodes that drain the tumor region, indicated by nodal radioactivity due to uptake of the lymphatic tracer. Initial histological sampling is restricted to these sentinel nodes, followed by more extensive lymphadenectomy if intraoperative histology identifies sentinel nodal metastasis. If sentinel nodes reveal no metastatic involvement, this is taken to be sufficient for pathological staging (as pN0, in American Joint Committee on Cancer parlance), and the patient is spared extensive nodal dissections and the morbidity it too frequently entails [4–7]

Lymphoscintigraphy has long been [8, 9] and continues to be an active area of clinical research in prostate cancer [10] and penile cancer for guiding nodal sampling for pathological staging. No noninvasive imaging technique currently available offers a reliable substitute for histopathology in prostate and penile cancer nodal staging, fundamentally because micrometastatic disease is undetectable by currently available imaging methods [4]. The technique shows promising accuracy [4, 10, 11]. Exceptions [12, 13] point to a need for technical improvements and application of the sentinel node approach to appropriate patient populations. Presurgical SPECT-CT will likely improve lymphoscintigraphy imagery as an intraoperative reference aid to the surgeon [14]. Penile cancer research suggests lymphoscintigraphy is probably best-applied to patients with no palpable inguinal adenopathy (cN0), in which the technique is highly accurate [15, 16].

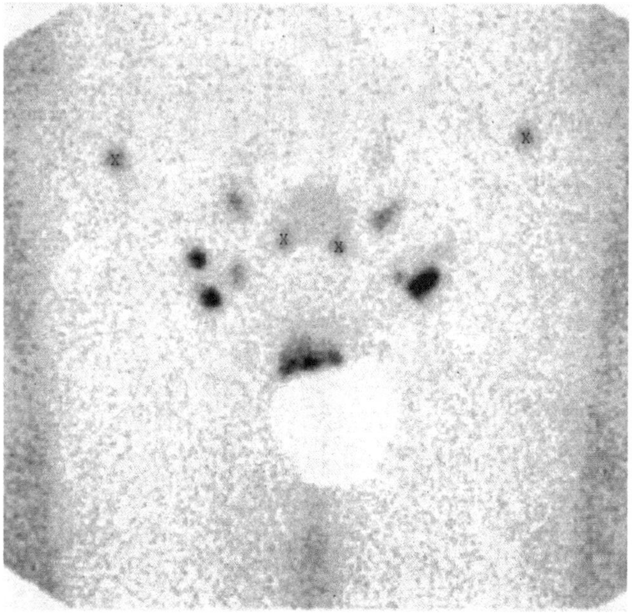

Fig. 9.6 Planar pelvic lymphoscintigraphy 3 h after injection of ^{99m}Tc tracer adjacent to a cancer of glans penis. Bilateral scintigraphic hotspots indicate draining sentinel lymph nodes draining the penile region. An external lead shield covers the penis and manifests as a "cold" region. The shield improves image clarity because residual radioactivity at the injection site can potentially obscure adjacent nodal uptake, scintigraphically. (*Images courtesy of* Jørgen Bjerggaard Jensen, MD, Department of Urology, Aarhus University Hospital, Skejby, Denmark)

Cancer cells in enlarged metastatic lymph nodes might have thoroughly displaced the phagocytic cells responsible for nodal tracer uptake, resulting in false negatives.

FDG-PET Value in Prostate Cancer Staging

Older clinical trials predating PET-CT suggested FDG-PET had poor diagnostic sensitivity for prostate cancer [17, 18], possibly explaining why current prostate cancer guidelines do not include FDG-PET, even as an optional imaging study [1, 19]. However, in clinical practice, as of 2008, the US National Oncologic PET Registry (NOPR) found that prostate cancer patients were most frequently studied by FDG-PET and that FDG-PET results changed therapeutic management in a third of prostate cancer patients studied, with prognostic implications [20, 21]. Though metastatic prostate cancer can indeed manifest with mild or no FDG avidity, recent clinical data using state-of-the-art technology suggest that FDG-PET, particularly PET-CT [22], is an effective modality for disease (re)staging in high-yield prostate patient populations defined by threshold values of serum prostate-specific antigen (PSA) level or velocity [23, 24] and progressive, castration-resistant disease [17, 25–27]. In such patients, FDG-PET offers a means for evaluating bony tumor response in a timely fashion [26], potentially avoiding the pitfalls and limitations of bone scintigraphy [28]. CT and MRI also have difficulty distinguishing viable versus treated osseous metastases and even misleading increases in serum PSA levels (a tumor biomarker commonly used as a surrogate index of systemic prostatic tumor burden) can occur, preceding a favorable tumor response to treatment, not uncommonly—a so-called PSA flare response [29]. PET visualization of skeletal foci of FDG uptake, consistent with metastases, however, reliably indicates the presence of viable metastases at those sites [23, 28]. FDG-PET may be useful when conventional biochemical and imaging assays are discordant or suspected to be false-negative [25] (*e.g.*, PSA-negative prostate cancer [30]).

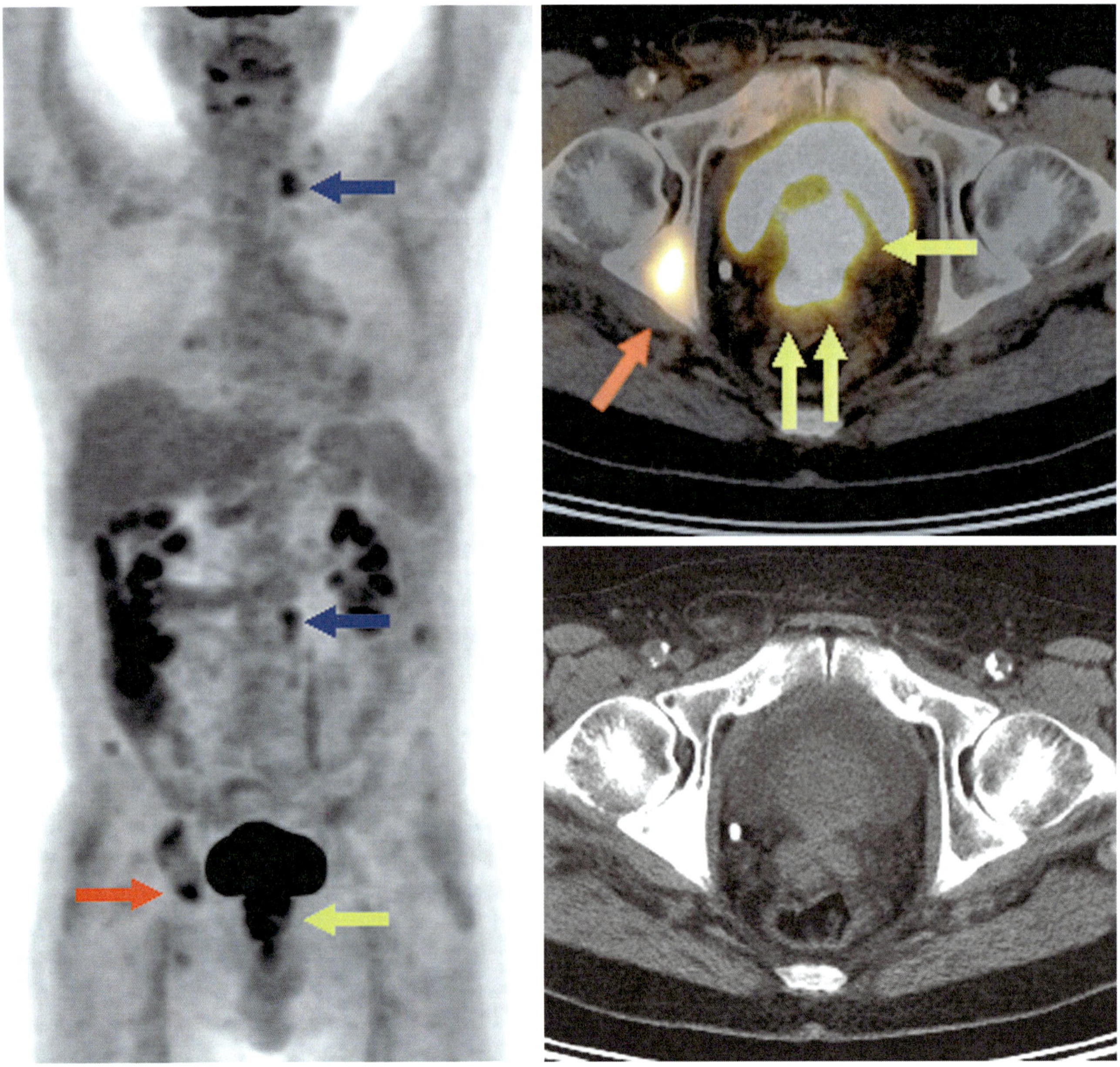

FDG-PET and the Primary Prostate Lesion

For evaluation of a known or suspected primary prostate tumor, MRI is the modality of choice [31], providing excellent detection of extracapsular extension and involvement of the seminal vesicles or other neighboring tissues [23]. If an FDG-avid lesion of the prostate lesion is discovered incidentally in a patient without known prostate cancer (*i.e.*, having a PET scan for another indication), the finding must receive further appropriate evaluation to exclude a neoplasm [30]. Most untreated primary prostate tumors are FDG avid [20]. The differential diagnosis also includes other FDG-avid diseases, such as benign prostatic hyperplasia and focal prostatitis [18, 32], which may require further clinical management. In the prostate cancer patient, after radical prostatectomy, FDG-PET appears unable to distinguish local recurrence from scarring [33].

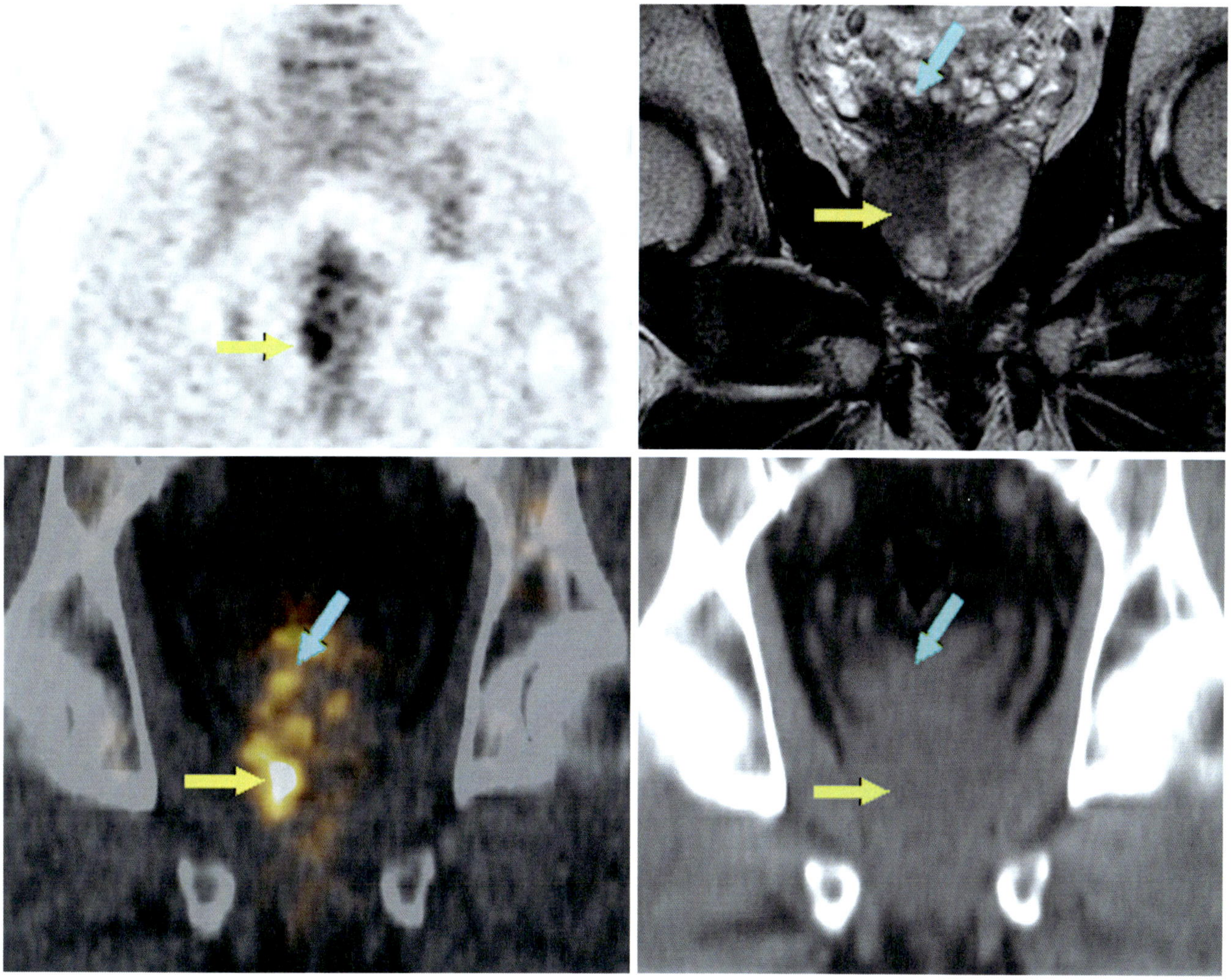

Fig. 9.8 FDG PET-CT imagery of a 50-year-old man with a history of synovial sarcoma. PET visualized an incidental hypermetabolic lesion in the rightward region of the prostate gland (*yellow arrow*). Prostatic MRI evaluation confirmed a large prostatic tumor, also showing gross right seminal vesical invasion not evident on PET (*blue arrow*). Coronal PET image of pelvis (*top left*). Coronal T2W MRI prostate image (*top right*). Coronal CT image of prostate region (*bottom right*). Coronal PET-CT fusion image of prostate region (*bottom left*)

Fig. 9.7 PET-CT imagery shows FDG-avid primary prostate cancer invading seminal vesicles bilaterally (*yellow arrows*), metastatic adenopathy in the neck and abdomen (*blue arrows*), and multiple osseous metastases, including, for example, in the right acetabulum (*red arrow*)

New PET Tracers Selective for Prostate Histology

A commonly noted fundamental limitation of FDG, as a tumor tracer, is that a wide variety of nonneoplastic diseases are also FDG avid. New tracers selective for prostate histology are in development as imaging agents for tumor detection. 16β-[^{18}F]fluoro-5α -dihydrotestosterone (FDHT) is an analog of the main prostatic form of testosterone, radiolabeled for PET. FDHT-PET has already undergone initial testing, in prostate cancer patients, demonstrating the feasibility of its use, in tumor detection [34–36].

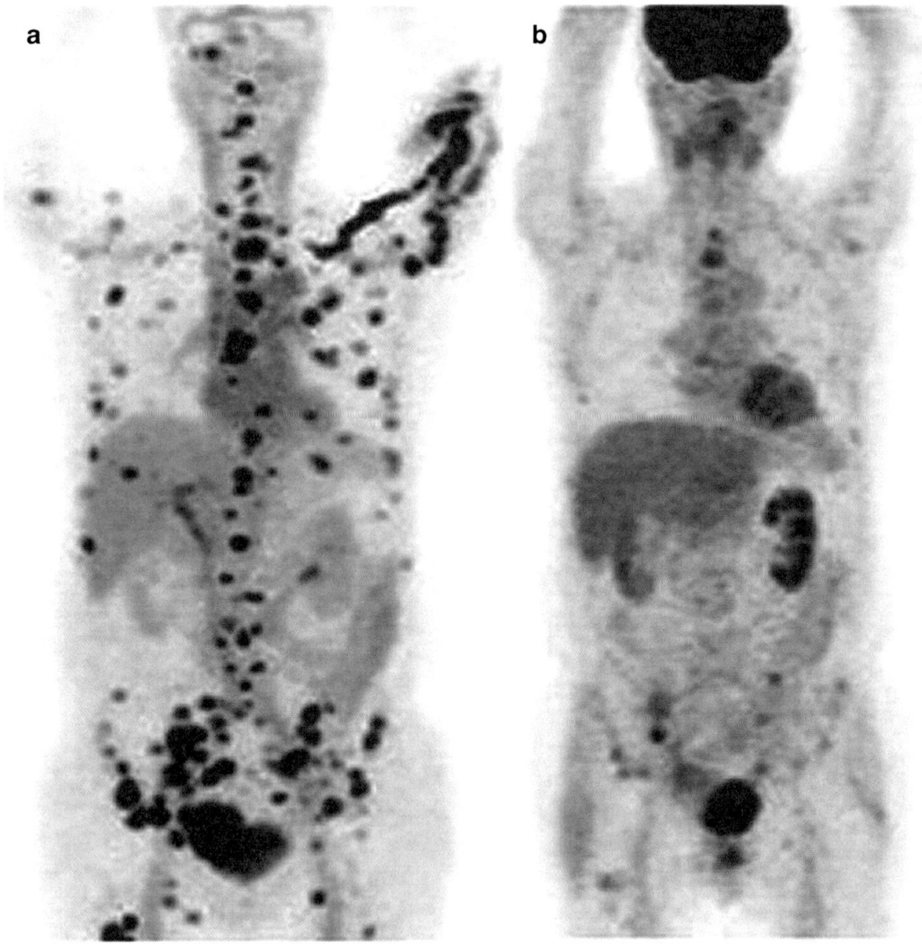

Fig. 9.9 A 69-year-old male with metastatic prostate cancer. FDHT-PET image (**a**) reveals far more scattered widespread metastases than evident on FDG-PET (**b**). The two PET studies were obtained 24 h apart (Images courtesy of Dr. Josef Fox, Memorial Sloan Kettering Cancer Center, NY)

Capromab Pendetide Scintigraphy and Prostate Cancer

Early clinical trial data showed the feasibility of detecting metastatic prostate cancer in patients, scintigraphically, by use of a radiolabeled antibody, capromab pendetide (ProstaScint; EUSA Pharma, Langhorne, PA), which targets glutamate carboxypeptidase II, also known as prostate-specific membrane antigen (PSMA) [37, 38]. National Comprehensive Cancer Network (NCCN) prostate cancer guidelines support capromab pendetide radioimmunoscintigraphy as an optional diagnostic tool in salvage setting evaluation. FDA approved in 1996 with promising early trials [39, 40], postmarketing clinical experience with capromab pendetide radioimmunoscintigraphy has been criticized by some as being of low diagnostic yield, both in the diagnostic clarity of the imagery it provides and in terms of its incremental diagnostic value beyond standard imaging assays (CT and MRI) [41, 42]. Recent technological advances in scintigraphic imaging hardware and software have spurred a reevaluation of the clinical diagnostic performance of radiolabeled capromab pendetide. Notably, SPECT-CT fusion imaging appears to increase the diagnostic sensitivity and specificity of capromab pendetide radioimmunoscintigraphy [43]. Increasing the diagnostic yield of capromab pendetide radioimmunoscintigraphy, in routine clinical practice, may also require better patient selection: identifying clinical variables that provide a higher pretest likelihood that capromab pendetide radioimmunoscintigraphy results will be positive (similar to the aforementioned discussion of FDG-PET in prostate cancer) [44]. Capromab pendetide radioimmunoscintigraphy is utilized predominantly for detection of metastatic disease, with no clear evidence that it can supplant MRI for evaluation of local tissue invasion at the primary site [45]. Recent research has explored a novel application of capromab pendetide radioimmunoscintigraphy in defining a biological target volume in planning conformal prostate brachytherapy [46].

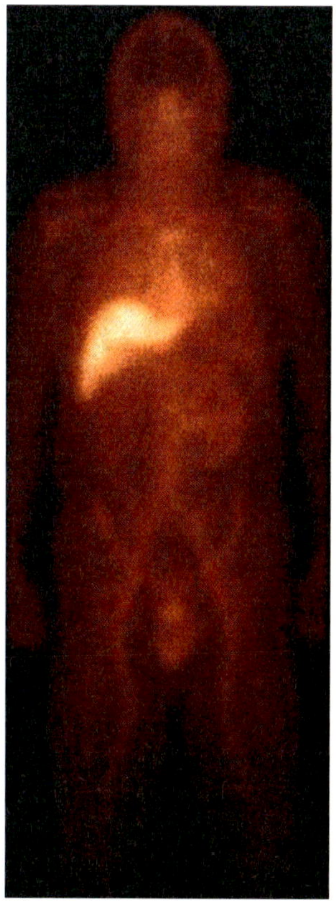

Fig. 9.10 An anterior planar scintigraphic image of the head, neck, and torso, showing the normal biodistribution of radiolabeled capromab pendetide (ProstaScint). (Image courtesy of Gary Ulaner, MD, Memorial Sloan-Kettering Cancer Center, New York, NY)

FDG-PET Value in Bladder Cancer Staging

For detection and evaluation of primary tumors and local recurrence, nonradiological approaches remain the standard [47, 48]; CT urography offers no clear advantages over cystoscopy, histopathology, and urinalysis [49, 50]. Hence, recommendations regarding the use of FDG-PET in urinary bladder cancer should focus on its potential role in detecting synchronous upper urinary tract neoplasms, which are of significant incidence, in urinary bladder cancer patient populations [49] and detecting nodal or distant metastatic disease [48–50]. Pretreatment imaging guides tissue biopsy and helps determine what course of treatment is appropriate in bladder cancer [47].

Neither NCCN [47], European Association of Urology [51], nor American College of Radiology guidelines [49, 50] currently recommend a role for FDG-PET in the management of bladder cancer. Yet FDG-PET imaging results change bladder cancer management in 38 % of patients [20]. FDG-PET/CT is sensitive and specific for detecting metastatic bladder cancer. When added to standard imaging, PET/CT information changed clinical management in 68 % of cases [52]. State-of-the-art fusion PET/CT and iterative PET image reconstruction algorithms improve diagnostic accuracy [22], as these were unavailable for FDG-PET in the 1990s.

As is typical for FDG-PET (and all current imaging modalities), patients with microscopic lymph node metastases were the most common false-negatives [53, 54]. Yet FDG-PET/CT can identify occult nodal metastases in patients with prior negative conventional abdominopelvic CT [53].

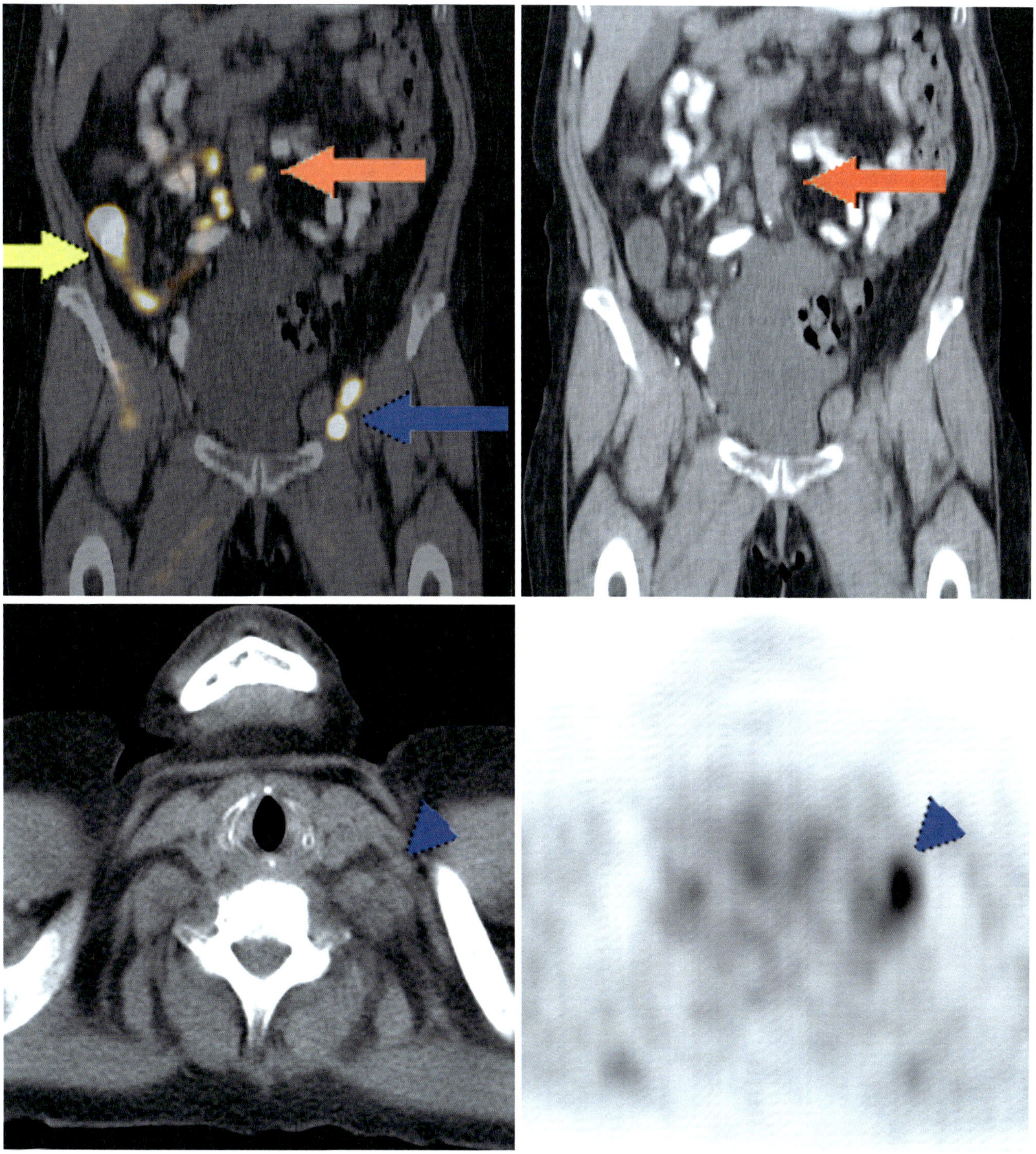

Fig. 9.11 A 58-year-old female with bladder cancer, status postcystectomy with ileal conduit (*yellow arrow*) filled with excreted FDG. Hypermetabolic adenopathy in the left external iliac region (*blue arrows*) was also evident on CT by its enlarged size. Markedly hypermetabolic para-aortic adenopathy (*red arrow*), suspicious for metastatic disease, was subcentimeter in transaxial short axis, reported as equivocal on same-day dedicated CT. Not identified by CT was adenopathy in the left supraclavicular region (*blue arrowhead*), hypermetabolic on PET, suspicious for a Virchow nodal metastasis

FDG Excretion Is a Problem in Urinary Tract/ Renal PET Imaging

FDG is excreted via the urinary tract and the radioactive signal from excreted FDG can obscure PET evaluation of the urinary tracts, as well as renal parenchyma and adjacent nodal groups [55–57]. Yet multiple studies have shown that FDG-PET has excellent diagnostic accuracy for detection of urothelial neoplasms in the bladder and upper tracts when imaging is performed after clearance of excreted FDG, with urinary clearance facilitated by delayed imaging [56, 57] (*e.g.*, imaging at 2 h after tracer injection instead of the more conventional 1-h time-point); oral or intravenous hydration [53, 56, 57]; diuretics [53, 56, 57]; urinary bladder drainage and irrigation [55, 58]; and/or combined use of excreted radiographic contrast [59]. However, because such practices to facilitate urinary clearance for FDG-PET are probably not in widespread use, referring clinicians may wish to approach their local imaging specialists to discuss the matter.

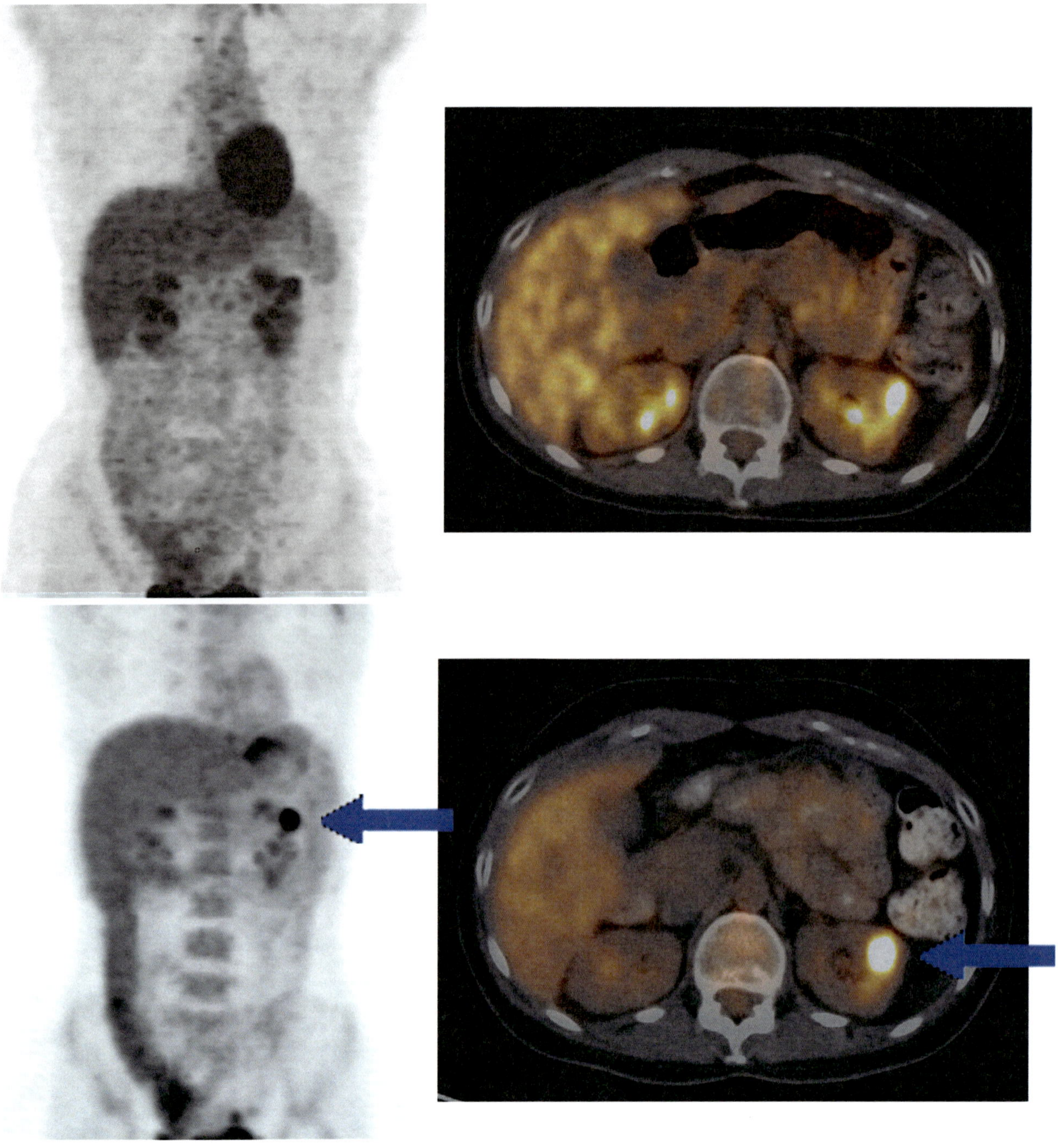

Fig. 9.12 PET scan was performed standard 60 min after FDG injection and was negative. Follow-up PET scan obtained 120 min after FDG injection. A hypermetabolic upper-pole parenchymal lesion of left kidney (*blue arrow*) is more conspicuous because the 2-h imaging delay allowed for clearance of excreted FDG from the renal calyceal system. Biopsy revealed renal oncocytoma

Renal PET Imaging: FDG-PET and Beyond

For evaluation of the patient with a suspicious renal mass prior to histological evaluation, data from multiple small studies suggest FDG-PET sensitivity is 85–90 % for malignancy [60–64]. Note that these reports were older studies using PET, not PET-CT, and usually did not employ diuretic administration or other procedural techniques that subsequently have been shown to clear excreted FDG that can obscure evaluation of the upper urinary tracts and renal parenchyma. The sensitivity of FDG-PET is probably lower for lesions that are predominantly cystic, whereas solid malignant renal masses have a high density of cells to produce a detectable signal on PET, malignant cells lining the periphery of a cystic renal lesion will produce a less-concentrated uptake signal less easily detected on PET imagery.

Focal accumulations of excreted tracer in the renal pelvicaliceal system can mimic hypermetabolic renal parenchymal tumors. Renal oncocytomas in multiple cases have demonstrated high FDG avidity on PET imagery, presenting another false-positive (for malignancy). (*See* Fig. 9.12)

A PET tracer highly selective for clear cell carcinoma has been studied, in clinical trials: the iodine124-labelled antibody chimeric G250 (124I-cG250) [65]. Interestingly, in a pilot study of 25 renal cancer patients, this PET radioantibody did not accumulate in nine non–clear cell carcinomas (including two papillary cell carcinomas), but accumulated in 15 of 16 clear cell carcinomas. A larger clinical study, using iodine131-labeled cG250 in renal cancer patients, supports the concept that the radioantibody is histology specific [66].

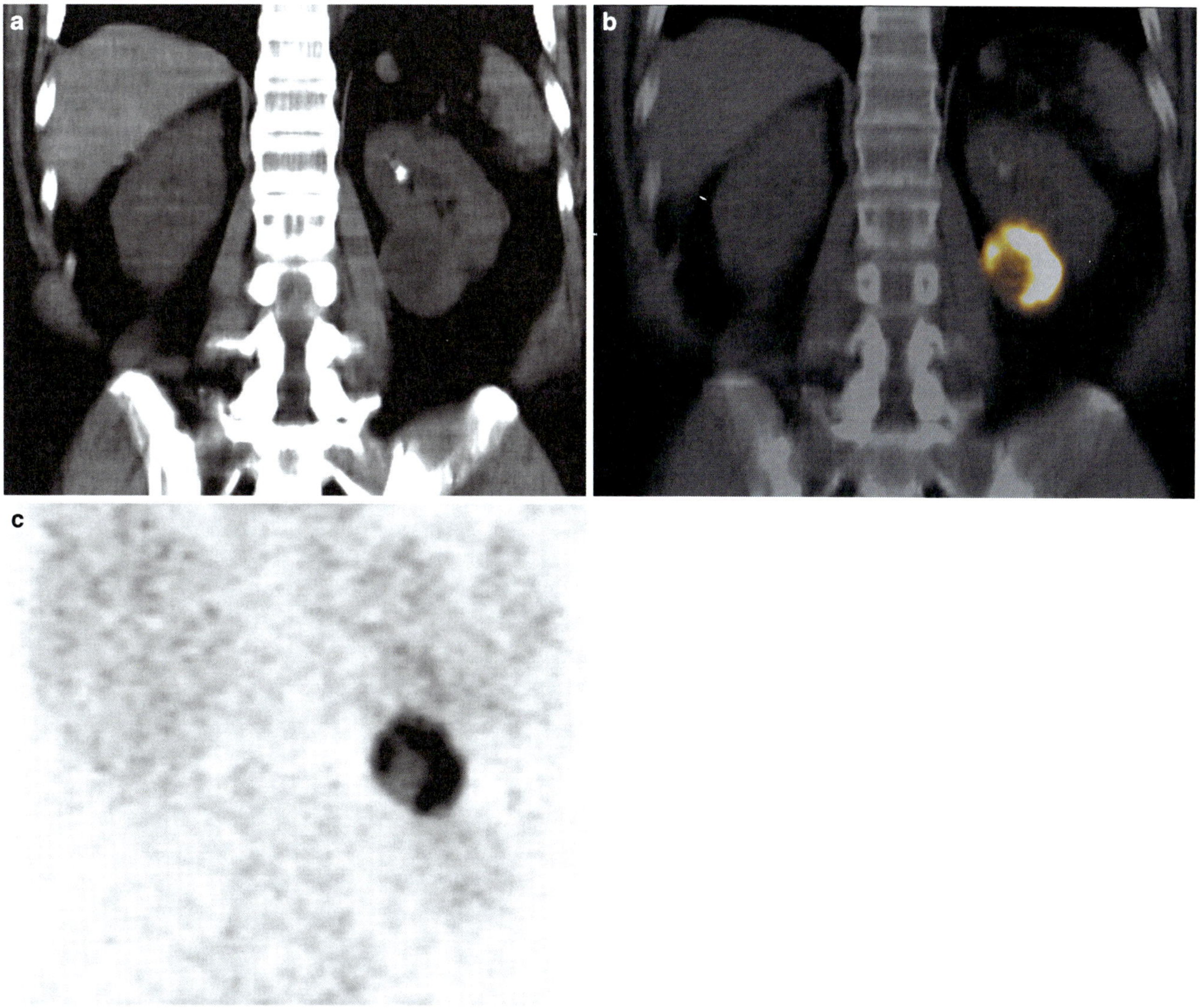

Fig. 9.13 124I-cG250 PET-CT of a 63-year-old man with a clear cell carcinoma of left kidney, shown on a coronal abdominal tomograph by CT (**a**), fusion (**b**), and PET (**c**). Note the utter lack of background PET activity and the intense tumor uptake, illustrating the potential of diagnostic PET imaging with radiolabeled antibodies

The Value of FDG-PET in Testicular Cancer

FDG-PET has been found sensitive both for seminoma [67] and nonseminomatous germ cell tumors (NSGCT) in general [68], with some researchers suggesting histology-specific variations in tumor FDG avidity [69–72]. FDG is the preeminent radiopharmaceutical for imaging of seminoma in current practice [73, 74]. For stage IIC-III seminoma patients with normal serum markers, current NCCN guidelines recommend FDG-PET as the preferred test for evaluating a residual mass when present following primary chemotherapy and for identifying whether viable cancer is present within the mass. The use of FDG-PET is also recommended, when no residual mass is present, during follow-up "as clinically indicated" [73]. Additionally, the NCCN suggests FDG-PET can be considered for stage IIB-III seminoma patients with elevated but stable β-human chorionic gonadotropin levels. FDG-PET is not suggested for the evaluation of nonseminomatous germ cell tumors (NSGCT) patients nor for initial staging of seminoma patients, per guidelines of the NCCN and the European Germ Cell Cancer Consensus group (EGCCC) [73, 74].

Guidelines suggest that FDG-PET can be used "as clinically indicated" for follow-up of stage IIC-III seminoma patients [73]. Yet FDG-PET is not considered of proven clinical benefit in the follow-up of NSGCT patients [73, 74]. For example, in one study, a negative FDG-PET/CT did not have a statistical impact upon relapse risk in stage I NSGCT patients at high-risk for recurrence [75], even though FDG-PET/CT identifies metastatic disease in up to 21 % of stage I NSGCT patients with serum tumor markers and CT showing no evidence of disease [75, 76].

Guidelines suggest that FDG-PET cannot be recommended for initial staging of GCT patients [73, 74]. The EGCCC suggested that available FDG-PET research in GCT staging was not conclusive as of 2008. None of the research articles cited offered the same conclusion. In fact, the EGCCC statements cite multiple articles which reported that FDG-PET was more sensitive for tumor detection than CT [70, 75, 76], offering improved staging of GCT patients compared to CT alone [70, 76, 77]. These guidelines did not clearly distinguish between FDG-PET and FDG-PET/CT technology and sometimes cited certain older research that used outmoded PET methodology [78, 79].

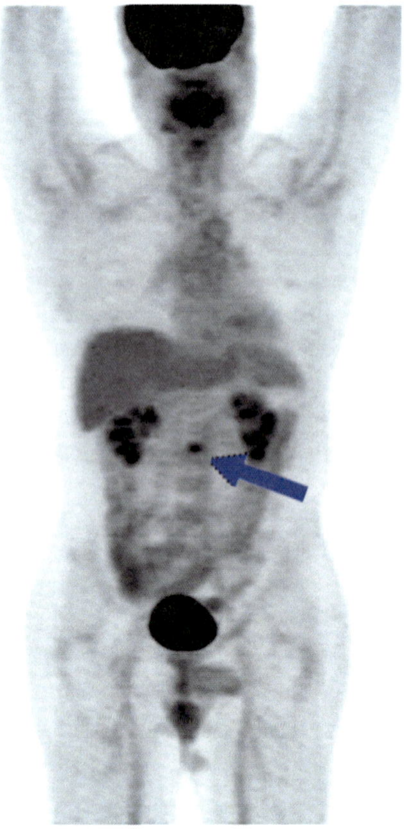

Fig. 9.14 A 44-year-old male with seminoma postorchiectomy referred for FDG-PET to rule out relapse during surveillance. Hypermetabolic aortocaval lymph node is visualized (*blue arrow*), consistent with metastatic disease

Adenopathy Detected by FDG-PET

In the seminoma patient with a residual mass, postchemotherapy, FDG-PET is efficacious for noninvasively identifying the presence of viable tumor cells [67, 68, 71, 80, 81]. FDG-PET should be performed 6 weeks after the end of chemotherapy, as false-positive PET findings are more frequent in the early postchemotherapy period—probably due to a greater presence of FDG-avid inflammatory/phagocytic cells within the mass during that time [82–84]. If the residual mass is unremarkable on FDG-PET imagery, surveillance is appropriate, whereas FDG-PET visualization of suspicious metabolic activity within the mass provides an indication for biopsy of the mass and further therapeutic management [73]. FDG-PET does not perform as well for the NSGCT patient with a residual mass, postchemotherapy, in which the residual mass may contain carcinoma, teratoma, or infiltrating inflammatory cells clearing debris. FDG-PET frequently fails to detect mature teratoma within such masses [68, 69, 83, 84]. Resection of mature teratoma is important, as such teratomas can grow and dedifferentiate into carcinomatous disease.

Peripheral lymph nodes (in the neck, axillae, and inguinofemoral regions) sometimes appear mildly FDG avid and either mildly prominent in size or nonenlarged. Often, this a mild reactive adenopathy (*e.g.*, systemic viral illness). Similar reactive pulmonary perihilar adenopathy is not too uncommon on the PET scans of smokers and elderly patients, usually sparing the hilar and mediastinal regions. Retroperitoneal or mesenteric regions are not typical sites for reactive adenopathy, without a local abdominal/pelvic infection/inflammation being present (*e.g.*, appendicitis).

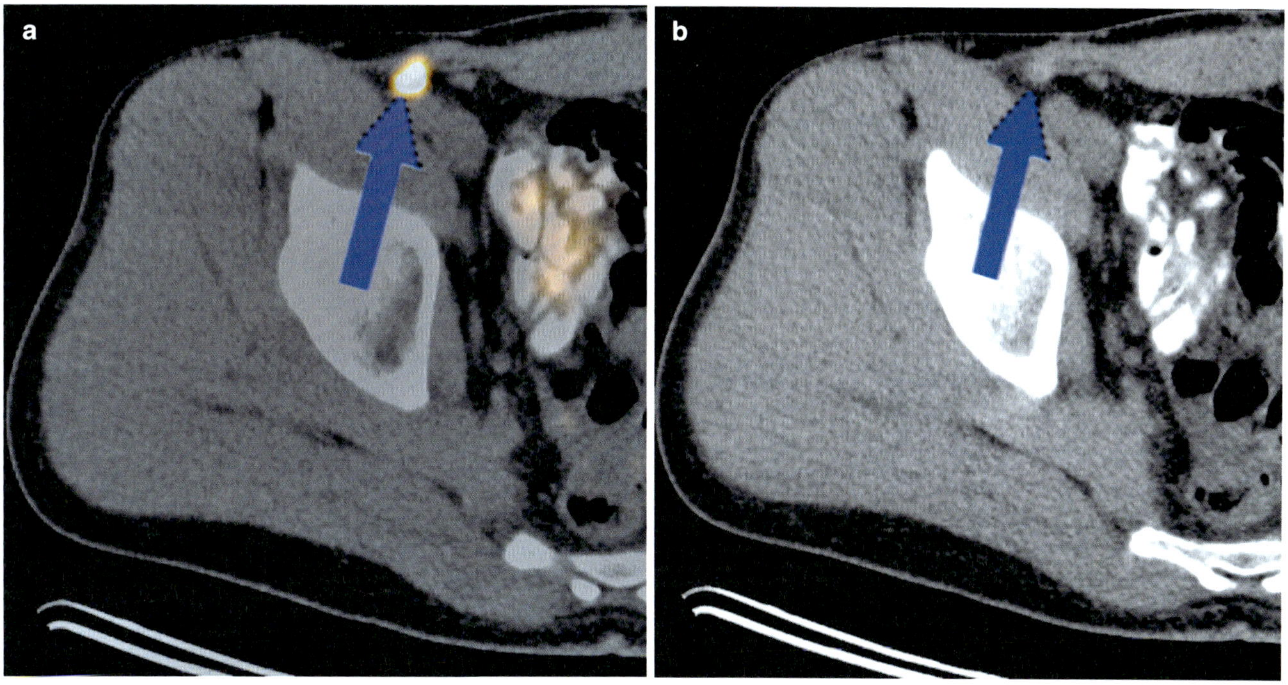

Fig. 9.15 A 31-year-old male with metastatic NSGCT status after prior orchiectomy and prior retroperitoneal lymph node dissection. FDG-PET-CT during disease surveillance showed a subcentimeter markedly hypermetabolic nodularity (*blue arrow* in **a**), slightly radiodense (**b**) in the deep right inguinal region, with standard contemporaneous CT (*not shown*) showing nodular contrast enhancement. Patient underwent salvage chemotherapy but follow-up PET-CT was unchanged 3 months later in hypermetabolic activity and nodule size. A right hemi-pelvic nodal dissection was performed, complicated by some postoperative internal bleeding requiring laparoscopic intervention. Pathology from the nodal dissection revealed an exuberant giant cell reaction to a small suture foreign body at the right internal inguinal ring (the suture being from the original abdominopelvic surgery). No metastatic adenopathy was found in nodes resected

PET and Adrenal Tumors

An adrenal tumor may be discovered during an FDG-PET or PET-CT study obtained for initial staging of a cancer patient. In that setting, FDG-PET-CT in trials at multiple medical centers has consistently demonstrated near-perfect sensitivity for detection of malignant adrenal tumors >1 cm in diameter [85–88]. FDG-PET appears to have lesser diagnostic sensitivity for malignant adrenal tumors smaller than 1 cm in diameter, presumably because of partial volume averaging effects that reduce apparent FDG-uptake inside subcentimeter cancers [88]. When an adrenal tumor >1 cm in diameter lacks distinct FDG avidity, on pretherapy PET imaging, such patients probably do not need further evaluation by adrenal CT or MRI, to exclude malignancy. In a patient who has received anticancer therapy, a malignant adrenal tumor (primary or metastatic) may undergo cytoreduction, reducing the apparent FDG avidity of the adrenal tumor [89].

However, benign adrenal neoplasms also can demonstrate FDG avidity. Further evaluation of an FDG avid adrenal by correlation with biochemical assays and/or adrenal CT or MRI may be helpful for further characterization, if clinically indicated.

Pheochromocytoma constitute an important fraction of adrenal incidentaloma. ^{18}F-fluorodihydroxyphenylalanine (FDOPA) PET imaging appears highly sensitive for detection of pheochromocytoma, both adrenal and extraadrenal, with a sensitivity of 98 % in a study of 30 patients. The specificity was 100 % but only 5 of the 30 patients had non-pheochromocytomas. Although more clinical data regarding tracer specificity are needed, these preliminary data are encouraging [90].

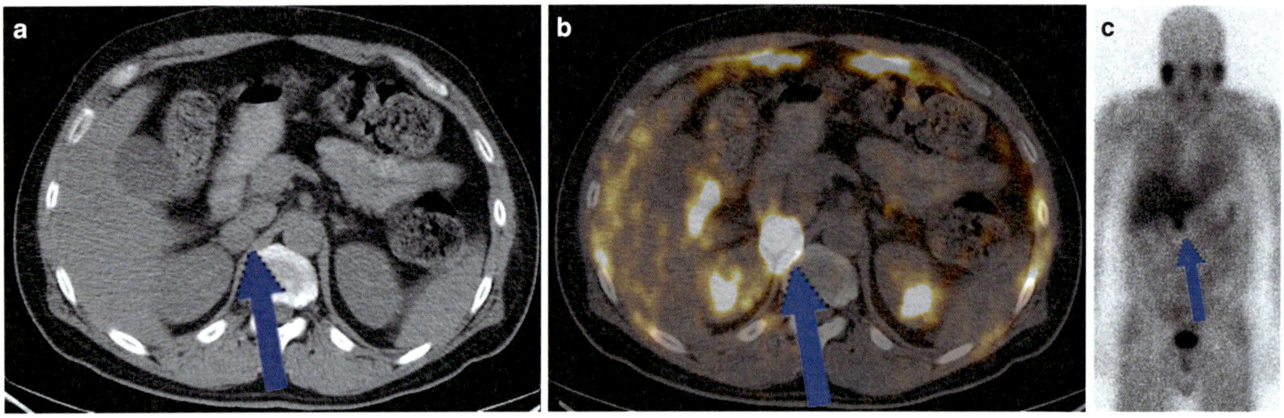

Fig. 9.16 A 50-year-old male with non–small cell lung carcinoma (large cell). FDG-PET staging. The malignant primary lung tumor and thoracic metastases are evident. An intensely hypermetabolic right adrenal nodule was also visualized (*blue arrow*; transaxial CT, **a**; PET-CT, **b**), with maximized standardized uptake volume (SUVmax) of 80.1, one of the highest SUVmax in the author's experience. Adrenal MRI findings (*not shown*) were not consistent with a benign adenoma. Metaiodobenzylguanidine (MIBG) scintigraphy (**c**) demonstrated scintigraphically intense right adrenal uptake (*blue arrow*) beyond normal variant adrenal MIBG uptake. Biopsy revealed a pheochromocytoma

Neuroblastoma, 123I-MIBG, and Fusion Imaging

Neuroblastoma is the most common extracranial solid malignancy of childhood. The majority of tumors arise in the abdomen and the majority of abdominal neuroblastomas arise from the adrenal medulla. MIBG, radiolabeled with either iodine-123 or -131, for single-photon scintigraphy, has a well-established role in the clinical staging or restaging of neuroblastoma [91, 92]. For surveillance of high-risk neuroblastoma patients, one group reported MIBG scintigraphy as being the most sensitive clinical assay for detection of relapse, compared to CT, bone marrow histology, and urinary catecholamines [93]. The advent of three-dimensional SPECT and, more recently, SPECT-CT fusion imaging has improved the diagnostic accuracy of MIBG scintigraphy to more than 90 % in most clinical studies.

MIBG has catecholamine-selective cellular uptake and retention mechanisms. Single-photon scintigraphy can detect metastatic foci as ectopic foci of neuroadrenergic tissues, with high diagnostic specificity. Other neurogenic/neuroendocrine tumors are known to be MIBG avid, but coincidental presentations with neuroblastoma are rare. False-positive MIBG uptake usually involves artifacts—biological or technical causes of focal MIBG accumulation that mimic tumor foci, yielding diagnostic misinterpretation or uncertainty. Uptake of MIBG occurs in normal adrenal glands, scintigraphically distinct uptake in the adrenal glands usually representing a "physiological variant," even when it appears asymmetrical [94]. Hence, MIBG scintigraphy has not been found useful for characterizing the nature of an incidental adrenal tumor per se. Rather, MIBG scintigraphy is useful for detecting metastatic neuroblastoma or recurrent neuroblastoma in an adrenalectomy bed.

The diagnostic sensitivity of MIBG scintigraphy can suffer from a variety of factors: lesions can be too small to detect scintigraphically or a recently treated tumor mass may contain only microscopic residual disease, internally; normal organ uptake and/or the presence of excreted tracer in the biliary fecal or urinary routes can obscure detection of tumor uptake in those regions; and certain neuroblastomas may lack scintigraphically distinct MIBG avidity, possibly because of tumor histological dedifferentiation. Patient preparation is vital for sensitive MIBG scintigraphy, requiring avoidance of various drugs known to interfere with MIBG uptake, including both prescription drugs and common over-the-counter medications that contain pseudoephedrine or phenylpropanolamine (often ingredients in nonprescription remedies for cough or flu-type symptoms). Such substances can have a significant, detrimental impact on the sensitivity of MIBG tumor imaging. The oncologist ordering MIBG scintigraphy should contact the imaging specialist for a list of prescribed substances.

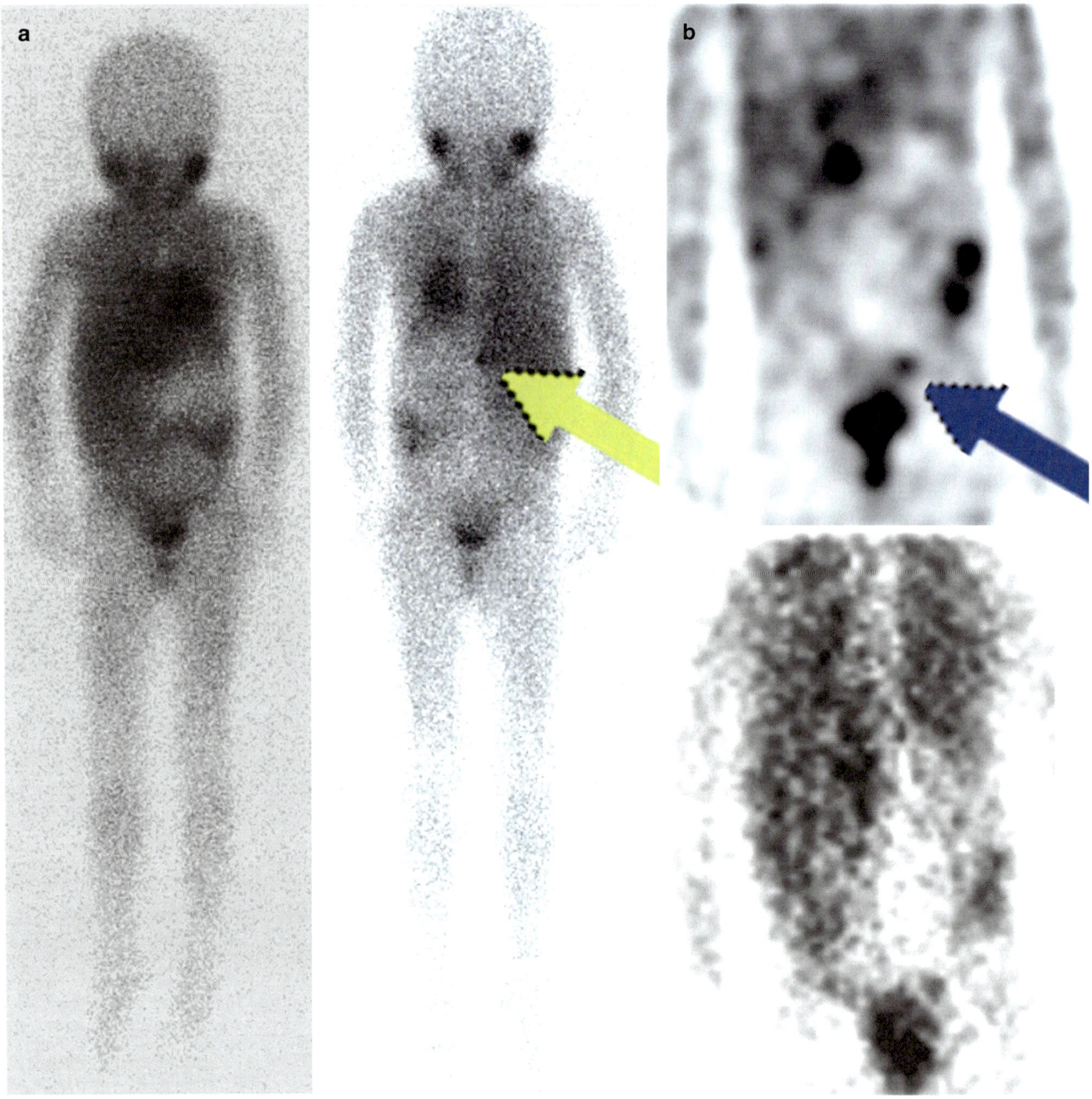

Fig. 9.17 MIBG scintigraphy of a 3-year-old female with previously treated neuroblastoma, clinically no evidence of disease, referred for tumor surveillance. Prior CT with IV contrast reported only an equivocal 1 cm left common iliac region soft tissue nodule. Planar scintigraphy (**a**, *lateral*, anterior planar; *medial image*, posterior) showed a possible lesion of the lumbar spine (*yellow arrow*) and no common iliac focus. SPECT imaging showed no foci of concern (**b**, *bottom image*: coronal MIBG SPECT tomograph, from lung apex to bladder region). Patient 2-h later had SPECT-CT (scanner previously occupied) that showed the concerning lumbar region focus to be physiological adrenal uptake (*not shown*) and showed the common iliac nodule (*blue arrow* in **c**, transaxial CT) to be MIBG avid (**d**, fusion SPECT-CT) consistent with metastatic disease, and revealed a 1 cm nodularity posterior to the descending colon (*blue arrowhead* in **e**, medial: sagittal SPECT-CT fusion; lateral: sagittal CT), which had been initially missed on the day-before standard CT. These MIBG findings were stable on a confirmatory repeat SPECT-CT 1 month later and then confirmed as metastatic disease histopathologically. Planar MIBG scintigraphy is often helpful in detecting osseous metastatic disease. SPECT (alone) improves evaluation of the soft tissues somewhat, but the case illustrates that such images are often noisy and lacking in anatomic reference points. As for PET-CT, fusion SPECT-CT provides the advantage of anatomic localization and SPECT quality improved by CT-based attenuation correction (and by state-of-the-art data-processing algorithms). However, in the author's experience, some currently marketed SPECT-CT hybrid scanner models provide companion CT data of extremely poor quality compared to other commercially available models, and anatomic localization on SPECT-CT is not as precise as for PET-CT (*e.g.*, see transaxial SPECT-CT fusion in **d**)

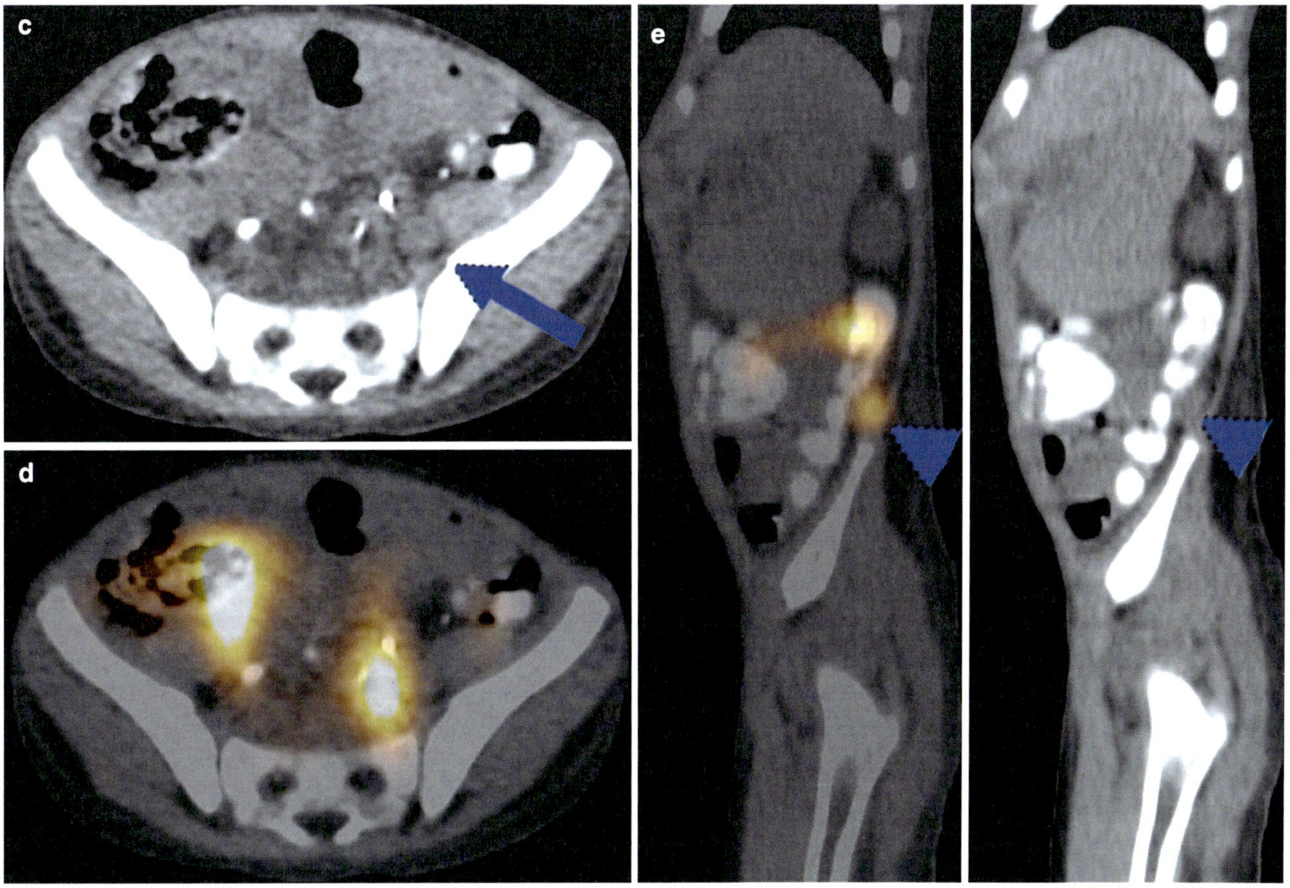

Fig. 9.17 (continued)

The Value of FDG-PET in Penile Carcinoma

Penile cancer is a rare disease. Medical literature describing the diagnostic value of FDG-PET for penile cancer management is also rare. Available clinical data are encouraging, however. FDG-PET/CT seems a sensitive, specific imaging tool for lymph node staging in the untreated penile cancer patient [95, 96] due to the scintigraphically distinct FDG avidity of penile cancer. However, as is typical even for FDG-avid diseases, FDG-PET/CT has difficulty detecting micrometastatic disease and cannot replace surgical staging as standard of care [97] but still may be useful in the staging of selected patients [98]. The utility of FDG-PET/CT in penile cancer management perhaps may be found in detection of unexpected distant metastases at initial staging [96], or other applications of FDG-PET/CT used in other cancer populations, such as surveillance for tumor recurrence, and/or evaluation of tumor response to therapy.

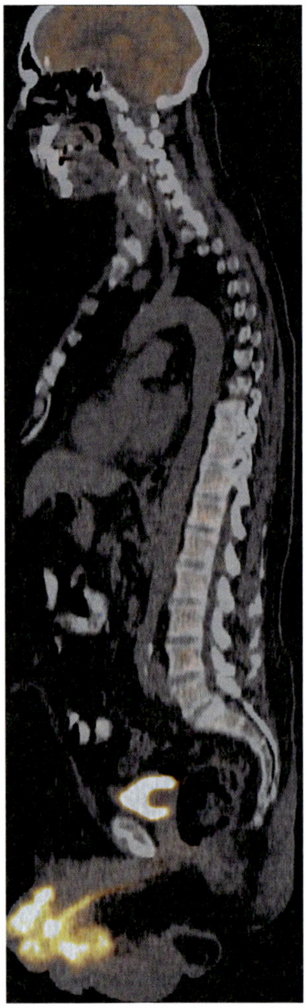

Fig. 9.18 FDG-PET-CT fusion image, sagittal tomograph, shows an intensely hypermetabolic infiltrative soft tissue mass occupying the penile region

References

1. Scher HI, Halabi S, Tannock I, et al. Design and end points of clinical trials for patients with progressive prostate cancer and castrate levels of testosterone: recommendations of the prostate cancer clinical trials working group. J Clin Oncol. 2008;26:1148–59.
2. Scher HI, Morris MJ, Kelly WK, et al. Prostate cancer clinical trial end points: "RECIST"ing a step backwards. Clin Cancer Res. 2005;11:5223–32.
3. Coleman RE, Mashiter G, Whitaker KB, et al. Bone scan flare predicts successful systemic therapy for bone metastases. J Nucl Med. 1988;29:1354–9.
4. Wawroschek F, Vogt H, Wengenmair H, et al. Prostate lymphoscintigraphy and radio-guided surgery for sentinel lymph node identification in prostate cancer. Technique and results of the first 350 cases. Urol Int. 2003;70:303–10.
5. Leijte JA, Hughes B, Graafland NM, et al. Two-center evaluation of dynamic sentinel node biopsy for squamous cell carcinoma of the penis. J Clin Oncol. 2009;27:3325–9.
6. Hadway P, Smith Y, Corbishley C, et al. Evaluation of dynamic lymphoscintigraphy and sentinel lymph-node biopsy for detecting occult metastases in patients with penile squamous cell carcinoma. BJU Int. 2007;100:561–5.
7. Hadway P, Smith Y, Corbishley C, et al. Sentinel lymph-node biopsy in patients with squamous cell carcinoma of the penis. BJU Int. 2009;103:1199–203.
8. Gardiner RA, Fitzpatrick JM, Constable AR, et al. Human prostatic lymphoscintigraphy. A preliminary report. Br J Urol. 1979; 51:300–3.
9. Zuckier LS, Finkelstein M, Kreutzer ER, et al. Technetium-99 m antimony sulphide colloid lymphoscintigraphy of the prostate by direct transrectal injection. Nucl Med Commun. 1990;11:589–96.
10. Silva Jr N, Anselmi CE, Anselmi OE, et al. Use of the gamma probe in sentinel lymph node biopsy in patients with prostate cancer. Nucl Med Commun. 2005;26:1081–6.
11. Hinev A, Klissarova A, Ghenev P, et al. Radioisotopic detection of sentinel lymph nodes in clinically localized high-risk prostate cancer. J BUON. 2009;14:661–7.
12. Spiess PE, Izawa JI, Bassett R, et al. Preoperative lymphoscintigraphy and dynamic sentinel node biopsy for staging penile cancer: results with pathological correlation. J Urol. 2007;177:2157–61.
13. Spiess PE, Izawa JI, Bassett R, et al. Role of dynamic sentinel node biopsy in penile cancer: our experience. J Surg Oncol. 2006; 93:181–5.
14. Vermeeren L, Valdés Olmos RA, Meinhardt W, et al. Value of SPECT/CT for detection and anatomic localization of sentinel lymph nodes before laparoscopic sentinel node lymphadenectomy in prostate carcinoma. J Nucl Med. 2009;50:865–70.
15. Hungerhuber E, Schlenker B, Frimberger D, et al. Lymphoscintigraphy in penile cancer: limited value of sentinel node biopsy in patients with clinically suspicious lymph nodes. World J Urol. 2006;24:319–24.
16. Heyns CF, Theron PD. Evaluation of dynamic sentinel lymph node biopsy in patients with squamous cell carcinoma of the penis and palpable inguinal nodes. BJU Int. 2008;102:305–9.
17. Shreve PD, Grossman HB, Gross MD, Wahl RL. Metastatic prostate cancer: initial findings of PET with 2-deoxy-2-[F-18]fluoro-D-glucose. Radiology. 1996;199:751–6.
18. Effert PJ, Bares R, Handt S, et al. Metabolic imaging of untreated prostate cancer by positron emission tomography with sup 18 fluorine-labeled deoxyglucose. J Urol. 1996;155:994–8.
19. National Comprehensive Cancer Network: NCCN clinical practice guidelines in oncology. *Prostate Cancer* v.2.2010. 2010.
20. Oyama N, Akino H, Suzuki Y, et al. Prognostic value of 2-deoxy-2-[F-18]fluoro-D-glucose positron emission tomography imaging for patients with prostate cancer. Mol Imaging Biol. 2002;4:99–104.
21. Hillner BE, Siegel BA, Shields AF, et al. Relationship between cancer type and impact of PET and PET/CT on intended management: findings of the national oncologic PET registry. J Nucl Med. 2008; 49:1928–35.
22. Wahl RL. Why nearly all PET of abdominal and pelvic cancers will be performed as PET/CT. J Nucl Med. 2004;45 Suppl 1:82S–95.
23. Schöder H, Herrmann K, Gönen M, et al. 2-[^{18}F] Fluoro-2-deoxyglucose positron emission tomography for the detection of disease in patients with prostate-specific antigen relapse after radical prostatectomy. Clin Cancer Res. 2005;11:4761–9.
24. Seltzer MA, Barbaric Z, Belldegrun A, et al. Comparison of helical computerized tomography, positron emission tomography and monoclonal antibody scans for evaluation of lymph node metastases in patients with prostate specific antigen relapse after treatment for localized prostate cancer. J Urol. 1999;162:1322–8.
25. Morris MJ, Akhurst T, Larson SM, et al. Fluorodeoxyglucose positron emission tomography as an outcome measure for castrate metastatic prostate cancer treated with antimicrotubule chemotherapy. Clin Cancer Res. 2005;11:3210–6.
26. Agus DB, Golde DW, Sgouros G, et al. Positron emission tomography of a human prostate cancer xenograft: association of changes in deoxyglucose accumulation with other measures of outcome following androgen withdrawal. Cancer Res. 1998;58:3009–14.

27. Oyama N, Kim J, Jones LA, et al. MicroPET assessment of androgenic control of glucose and acetate uptake in the rat prostate and a prostate cancer tumor model. Nucl Med Biol. 2002;29:783–90.
28. Morris MJ, Akhurst T, Osman I, et al. Fluorinated deoxyglucose positron emission tomography imaging in progressive metastatic prostate cancer. Urology. 2002;59:913–8.
29. Nelius T, Klatte T, de Riese W, Filleur S. Impact of PSA flare-up in patients with hormone-refractory prostate cancer undergoing chemotherapy. Int Urol Nephrol. 2008;40:97–104.
30. Bucerius J, Ahmadzadehfar H, Hortling N, et al. Incidental diagnosis of a PSA-negative prostate cancer by 18FDG-PET/CT in a patient with hypopharyngeal cancer. Prostate Cancer Prostatic Dis. 2007;10:307–10.
31. Watanabe H, Kanematsu M, Kondo H, et al. Preoperative detection of prostate cancer: a comparison with 11C-choline PET, ^{18}F-fluorodeoxyglucose PET and MR imaging. J Magn Reson Imaging. 2010;31:1151–6.
32. Liu IJ, Zafar MB, Lai YH, et al. Fluorodeoxyglucose positron emission tomography studies in diagnosis and staging of clinically organ-confined prostate cancer. Urology. 2001;57:108–11.
33. Hofer C, Laubenbacher C, Block T, et al. Fluorine-18-fluorodeoxyglucose positron emission tomography is useless for the detection of local recurrence after radical prostatectomy. Eur Urol. 1999;36:31–5.
34. Beattie BJ, Smith-Jones PM, Jhanwar YS, et al. Pharmacokinetic assessment of the uptake of 16beta-^{18}F-fluoro-5alpha-dihydrotestosterone (FDHT) in prostate tumors as measured by PET. J Nucl Med. 2010;51:183–92.
35. Dehdashti F, Picus J, Michalski JM, et al. Positron tomographic assessment of androgen receptors in prostatic carcinoma. Eur J Nucl Med Mol Imaging. 2005;32:344–50.
36. Larson SM, Morris M, Gunther I, et al. Tumor localization of 16beta-18F-fluoro-5alpha-dihydrotestosterone versus ^{18}F-FDG in patients with progressive, metastatic prostate cancer. J Nucl Med. 2004;45:366–73.
37. Elgamal AA, Troychak MJ, Murphy GP. ProstaScint scan may enhance identification of prostate cancer recurrences after prostatectomy, radiation, or hormone therapy: analysis of 136 scans of 100 patients. Prostate. 1998;37:261–9.
38. Polascik TJ, Manyak MJ, Haseman MK, et al. Comparison of clinical staging algorithms and 111indium-capromab pendetide immunoscintigraphy in the prediction of lymph node involvement in high risk prostate carcinoma patients. Cancer. 1999;85: 1586–92.
39. Manyak MJ, Hinkle GH, Olsen JO, et al. Immunoscintigraphy with indium-111-capromab pendetide: evaluation before definitive therapy in patients with prostate cancer. Urology. 1999;54:1058–63.
40. Manyak MJ, Hinkle GH, Olsen JO, et al. Multicenter radioimmunoscintigraphic evaluation of patients with prostate carcinoma using indium-111 capromab pendetide. Cancer. 1998;83:739–47.
41. Pucar D, Sella T, Schoder H. The role of imaging in the detection of prostate cancer local recurrence after radiation therapy and surgery. Curr Opin Urol. 2008;18:87–97.
42. Nagda SN, Mohideen N, Lo SS, et al. Long-term follow-up of 111In-capromab pendetide (ProstaScint) scan as pretreatment assessment in patients who undergo salvage radiotherapy for rising prostate-specific antigen after radical prostatectomy for prostate cancer. Int J Radiat Oncol Biol Phys. 2007;67:834–40.
43. Sodee DB, Sodee AE, Bakale G. Synergistic value of single-photon emission computed tomography/computed tomography fusion to radioimmunoscintigraphic imaging of prostate cancer. Semin Nucl Med. 2007;37:17–28.
44. Kahn D, Williams RD, Manyak MJ, et al. 111Indium-Capromab pendetide in the evaluation of patients with residual or recurrent prostate cancer after radical prostatectomy. The ProstaScint study group. J Urol. 1998;159:2041–6;discussion 2046–47.
45. Tsivian M, Wright T, Price M, Tsivian M, Wright T, Price M, et al. 111-In-capromab pendetide imaging using hybrid-gamma camera-computer tomography technology is not reliable in detecting seminal vesicle invasion in patients with prostate cancer. Urol Oncol. 2012;30:150–4.
46. Ellis RJ, Zhou H, Kim EY, et al. Biochemical disease-free survival rates following definitive low-dose-rate prostate brachytherapy with dose escalation to biologic target volumes identified with SPECT/CT capromab pendetide. Brachytherapy. 2007;6:16–25.
47. National Comprehensive Cancer Network: NCCN clinical practice guidelines in oncology. *Bladder Cancer*. v.2.2010. 2010.
48. Kaufman DS, Shipley WU, Feldman AS. Bladder cancer. Lancet. 2009;374:239–49.
49. American College of Radiology: ACR appropriateness criteria: pretreatment staging of invasive bladder cancer. Available at http://www.acr.org/SecondaryMainMenuCategories/quality_safety/app_criteria/pdf/ExpertPanelonUrologicImaging/PretreatmentStagingofInvasivebladdercancerDoc11.aspx. Accessed 17 Dec 2010.
50. American College of Radiology. ACR appropriateness criteria: follow-up imaging of bladder carcinoma. Available at http://www.acr.org/SecondaryMainMenuCategories/quality_safety/app_criteria/pdf/ExpertPanelonUrologicImaging/FollowUpImagingofBladderCarcinomaDoc4.aspx. Accessed 17 Dec 2010.
51. Stenzl A, Cowan NC, De Santis M, et al. The updated EAU guidelines on muscle-invasive and metastatic bladder cancer. Eur Urol. 2009;55:815–25.
52. Apolo AB, Riches J, Schöder H, et al. Clinical value of fluorine-18 2-fluoro-2-deoxy-D-glucose positron emission tomography/computed tomography in bladder cancer. J Clin Oncol. 2010; 28:3973–8.
53. Kibel AS, Dehdashti F, Katz MD, et al. Prospective study of [^{18}F]fluorodeoxyglucose positron emission tomography/computed tomography for staging of muscle-invasive bladder carcinoma. J Clin Oncol. 2009;27:4314–20.
54. Heicappell R, Müller-Mattheis V, Reinhardt M, et al. Staging of pelvic lymph nodes in neoplasms of the bladder and prostate by positron emission tomography with 2-[(18)F]-2-deoxy-D-glucose. Eur Urol. 1999;36:582–7.
55. Koyama K, Okamura T, Kawabe J, et al. Evaluation of ^{18}F-FDG-PET with bladder irrigation in patients with uterine and ovarian tumors. J Nucl Med. 2003;44:353–8.
56. Anjos DA, Etchebehere EC, Ramos CD, et al. ^{18}F-FDG-PET/CT delayed images after diuretic for restaging invasive bladder cancer. J Nucl Med. 2007;48:764–70.
57. Kamel EM, Jichlinski P, Prior JO, et al. Forced diuresis improves the diagnostic accuracy of ^{18}F-FDG-PET in abdominopelvic malignancies. J Nucl Med. 2006;47:1803–7.
58. Kosuda S, et al. Preliminary assessment of fluorine-18 fluorodeoxyglucose positron emission tomography in patients with bladder cancer. Eur J Nucl Med. 1997;24:615–20.
59. Kosuda S, Kison PV, Greenough R, et al. Anterior layering of excreted ^{18}F-FDG in the bladder on PET/CT: frequency and cause. Am J Roentgenol. 2007;189:W96–9.
60. Ak I, Can C. F-18 FDG-PET in detecting renal cell carcinoma. Acta Radiol. 2005;46:895–9.
61. Kumar R, Chauhan A, Lakhani P, et al. 2-Deoxy-2-[F-18]fluoro-D-glucose-positron emission tomography in characterization of solid renal masses. Mol Imaging Biol. 2005;7:431–9.
62. Kang DE, White Jr RL, Zuger JH, et al. Clinical use of fluorodeoxyglucose F 18 positron emission tomography for detection of renal cell carcinoma. J Urol. 2004;171:1806–9.
63. Jadvar H, Kherbache HM, Pinski JK, Conti PS. Diagnostic role of [F-18]-FDG positron emission tomography in restaging renal cell carcinoma. Clin Nephrol. 2003;60:395–400.

64. Goldberg MA, Mayo-Smith WW, Papanicolaou N, et al. FDG-PET characterization of renal masses: preliminary experience. Clin Radiol. 1997;52:510–5.
65. Divgi CR, Pandit-Taskar N, Jungbluth AA, et al. Preoperative characterisation of clear-cell renal carcinoma using iodine-124-labelled antibody chimeric G250 (124I-cG250) and PET in patients with renal masses: a phase I trial. Lancet Oncol. 2007;8:304–10.
66. Brouwers AH, Dorr U, Lang O, et al. 131 I-cG250 monoclonal antibody immunoscintigraphy versus [^{18}F]FDG-PET imaging in patients with metastatic renal cell carcinoma: a comparative study. Nucl Med Commun. 2002;23:229–36.
67. De Santis M, Bokemeyer C, Becherer A, et al. Predictive impact of 2-18fluoro-2-deoxy-D-glucose positron emission tomography for residual postchemotherapy masses in patients with bulky seminoma. J Clin Oncol. 2001;19:3740–4.
68. Kollmannsberger C, Oechsle K, Dohmen BM, et al. Prospective comparison of [^{18}F]fluorodeoxyglucose positron emission tomography with conventional assessment by computed tomography scans and serum tumor markers for the evaluation of residual masses in patients with nonseminomatous germ cell carcinoma. Cancer. 2002;94:2353–62.
69. Cremerius U, Effert PJ, Adam G, et al. FDG-PET for detection and therapy control of metastatic germ cell tumor. J Nucl Med. 1998; 39:815–22.
70. Cremerius U, Wildberger JE, Borchers H, et al. Does positron emission tomography using 18 fluoro-2-deoxyglucose improve clinical staging of testicular cancer? Results of a study in 50 patients. Urology. 1999;54:900–4.
71. Hain SF, O'Doherty MJ, Timothy AR, et al. Fluorodeoxyglucose PET in the initial staging of germ cell tumours. Eur J Nucl Med. 2000;27:590–4.
72. Nuutinen JM, Leskinen S, Elomaa I, et al. Detection of residual tumours in postchemotherapy testicular cancer by FDG-PET. Eur J Cancer. 1997;33:1234–41.
73. National Comprehensive Cancer Network: NCCN clinical practice guidelines in oncology. *Testicular Cancer*. v.2.2010. April 1, 2010.
74. Krege S, Beyer J, Souchon R, et al. European consensus conference on diagnosis and treatment of germ cell cancer: a report of the second meeting of the European germ cell cancer consensus group (EGCCCG): part I. Eur Urol. 2008;53:478–96.
75. Huddart RA, O'Doherty MJ, Padhani A, et al. 18fluorodeoxyglucose Positron emission tomography in the prediction of relapse in patients with high-risk, clinical stage I nonseminomatous germ cell tumors: preliminary report of MRC trial TE22—the NCRI testis tumour clinical study group. J Clin Oncol. 2007;25:3090–5.
76. Lassen U, Daugaard G, Eigtved A, et al. Whole-body FDG-PET in patients with stage I non-seminomatous germ cell tumours. Eur J Nucl Med Mol Imaging. 2003;30:396–402.
77. de Wit M, Hartmann M, Kotzerke J, et al. [^{18}F]-FDG-PET in clinical stage I and II non-seminomatous germ cell tumors: first results of the German multicenter trial (abstract). J Clin Oncol. 2005; 23:4504.
78. Albers P, Bender H, Yilmaz H, et al. Positron emission tomography in the clinical staging of patients with stage I and II testicular germ cell tumors. Urology. 1999;53:808–11.
79. Tsatalpas P, Beuthien-Baumann B, Kropp J, et al. Diagnostic value of ^{18}F-FDG positron emission tomography for detection and treatment control of malignant germ cell tumors. Urol Int. 2002; 68:157–63.
80. Becherer A, De Santis M, Karanikas G, et al. FDG-PET is superior to CT in the prediction of viable tumour in post-chemotherapy seminoma residuals. Eur J Radiol. 2005;54:284–8.
81. Lewis DA, Tann M, Kesler K, et al. Positron emission tomography scans in postchemotherapy seminoma patients with residual masses: a retrospective review from Indiana university hospital. J Clin Oncol. 2006;24:e54–5.
82. Haba Y, Williams MV, Neal DE, et al. Stage migration and pilot studies of reduced chemotherapy supported by positron-emission tomography findings suggest new combined strategies for stage 2 nonseminoma germ cell tumour. BJU Int. 2008;101:570–4.
83. Sugawara Y, Zasadny KR, Grossman HB, et al. Germ cell tumor: differentiation of viable tumor, mature teratoma, and necrotic tissue with FDG-PET and kinetic modeling. Radiology. 1999;211:249–56.
84. Stephens AW, Gonin R, Hutchins GD, Einhorn LH. Positron emission tomography evaluation of residual radiographic abnormalities in postchemotherapy germ cell tumor patients. J Clin Oncol. 1996;14:1637–41.
85. Stephens AW, Gonin R, Hutchins GD, Einhorn LH. Adrenal lesions: characterization with fused PET/CT image in patients with proved or suspected malignancy—initial experience 1. Radiology. 2006;238:970–7.
86. Erasmus JJ, Patz EF, McAdams HP, et al. Evaluation of adrenal masses in patients with bronchogenic carcinoma using ^{18}F-fluorodeoxyglucose positron emission tomography. Am J Roentgenol. 1997;168:1357–60.
87. Groussin L, Bonardel G, Silvéra S, et al. ^{18}F-Fluorodeoxyglucose positron emission tomography for the diagnosis of adrenocortical tumors: a prospective study in 77 operated patients. J Clin Endocrinol Metab. 2009;94:1713–22.
88. Metser U, Miller E, Lerman H, et al. ^{18}F-FDG-PET/CT in the evaluation of adrenal masses. J Nucl Med. 2006;47:32–7.
89. Metser U, Miller E, Lerman H, et al. Utility of PET/CT in differentiating benign from malignant adrenal nodules in patients with cancer. Am J Roentgenol. 2008;191:1545–51.
90. Fottner C, Helisch A, Anlauf M, et al. 6-^{18}F-Fluoro-L-dihydroxyphenylalanine positron emission tomography is superior to 123I-metaiodobenzyl-guanidine scintigraphy in the detection of extraadrenal and hereditary pheochromocytomas and paragangliomas: correlation with vesicular monoamine transporter expression. J Clin Endocrinol Metab. 2010;95:2800–10.
91. Cohn SL, Pearson AD, London WB, et al. The international neuroblastoma risk group (INRG) classification system: an INRG task force report. J Clin Oncol. 2009;27:289–97.
92. Monclair T, Brodeur GM, Ambros PF, et al. The international neuroblastoma risk group (INRG) staging system: an INRG task force report. J Clin Oncol. 2009;27:298–303.
93. Kushner BH, Kramer K, Modak S, Cheung NK. Sensitivity of surveillance studies for detecting asymptomatic and unsuspected relapse of high-risk neuroblastoma. J Clin Oncol. 2009;27:1041–6.
94. Jacobsson H, Bremmer S, Larsson SA. Visualisation of the normal adrenals at SPET examination with 111In-pentetreotide. Eur J Nucl Med Mol Imaging. 2003;30:1169–72.
95. Scher B, Seitz M, Reiser M, et al. ^{18}F-FDG-PET/CT for staging of penile cancer. J Nucl Med. 2005;46:1460–5.
96. Graafland NM, Leijte JA, Valdés Olmos RA, et al. Scanning with ^{18}F-FDG-PET/CT for detection of pelvic nodal involvement in inguinal node-positive penile carcinoma. Eur Urol. 2009;56:339–45.
97. Leijte JA, Graafland NM, Valdés Olmos RA, et al. Prospective evaluation of hybrid ^{18}F-fluorodeoxyglucose positron emission tomography/computed tomography in staging clinically node-negative patients with penile carcinoma. BJU Int. 2009;104:640–4.
98. Schlenker B, Scher B, Tiling R, et al. Detection of inguinal lymph node involvement in penile squamous cell carcinoma by ^{18}F-fluorodeoxyglucose PET/CT: a prospective single-center study. Urol Oncol. 2012;30:50–9.

Pediatric Genitourinary Tumor Imaging

10

Sara J. Abramson, Anita P. Price, and Michael J. Sohn

Wilms tumor (4 %) and neuroblastoma (8 %) make up the largest group of extracranial solid tumors of childhood. Most of these patients present before 5 years of age. Mesoblastic nephroma and stage IVS neuroblastoma are seen in children less than 1 year of age. Several other primary renal tumors may be seen in children. Adrenocortical carcinoma and pheochromocytoma are rare. The imaging features of these tumors will be shown. Rhabdomyosarcoma of the bladder will also be discussed

Renal Tumors

Renal tumors account for approximately 4 % of all malignancies in children [1]. Historically, many pediatric renal tumors were grouped together and categorized as Wilms tumor. However, the tumors are now separated into unique pathologic entities (*e.g.*, mesoblastic nephroma, clear cell sarcoma, rhabdoid tumor). Age at presentation, clinical history, and underlying genetic factors, as well as imaging characteristics, are useful in arriving at a diagnosis prior to biopsy. Nearly 90 % of pediatric renal masses are Wilms tumor [2]. Congenital anomalies and syndromes such as Beckwith-Wiedemann, isolated hemihypertrophy, WAGR (aniridia, genitourinary anomaly, and mental retardation), isolated aniridia, and Bloom syndrome are present in 10 % of patients with Wilms tumor [3]. Histopathology of the tumor is useful for prognosis and separate from staging. Patients are categorized according to stage and histopathology. Wilms tumor is divided into three groups: favorable histology, anaplastic histology, and nephrogenic rests. Anaplasia is found in 10 % of Wilms tumors. Focal anaplasia, unlike diffuse anaplasia, is not associated with a poor prognosis [3].

Table 10.1 Staging of Wilms tumor

Stage	Patients (%)	Characteristics
I	43	Limited to kidney
II	20	Extends beyond kidney but completely resected
III	21	Residual tumor confined to abdomen; nonhematogenous; abdominal/pelvic lymph nodes
		Tumor rupture, spillage confined to flank
IV	11	Hematogenous (lung, liver, brain); extra-abdominal lymph nodes
V	5	Bilateral disease at diagnosis

Congenital Mesoblastic Nephroma

CMN, also known as mesoblastic nephroma or fetal renal hamartoma, is the most common solid renal mass in infants under the age of 6 months [4]. The peak age of presentation is 1–3 months and 90 % of cases occur within the first year [5]. CMN is considered a low-risk renal tumor [2]. Although a palpable abdominal mass is the most common presentation in infants, some cases are detected on routine prenatal ultrasound examinations [2]. CMN is divided into classic and a more aggressive cellular subtype. Imaging in cases of the classic subtype demonstrates a large solid mass that may have peripheral enhancement. Necrosis/cystic changes, hemorrhage, focal enhancement, and infiltration of perinephric tissue can be seen in the cellular subtype [6]. Nephrectomy with wide margins may be the only treatment necessary. Although the tumor is generally considered as benign, local recurrence can occur in cases of incomplete resection. Metastases to lungs, brain, and bone are rare [2].

S.J. Abramson, M.D., FACR (✉) • A.P. Price, M.D.
Department of Radiology,
Memorial Sloan-Kettering Cancer Center,
1275 York Avenue, New York,
NY 10065, USA
e-mail: abramsos@mskcc.org; pricea@mskcc.org

M.J. Sohn
Department of Radiology, Breast and Imaging Center,
Memorial Sloan-Kettering Cancer Center,
1275 York Avenue, New York,
NY 10065, USA
e-mail: sohnm@mskcc.org

A.M. Bach, J. Zhang (eds.), *Atlas of Genitourinary Oncological Imaging*, Atlas of Oncology Imaging,
DOI 10.1007/978-1-4614-4872-3_10, © Springer Science+Business Media New York 2013

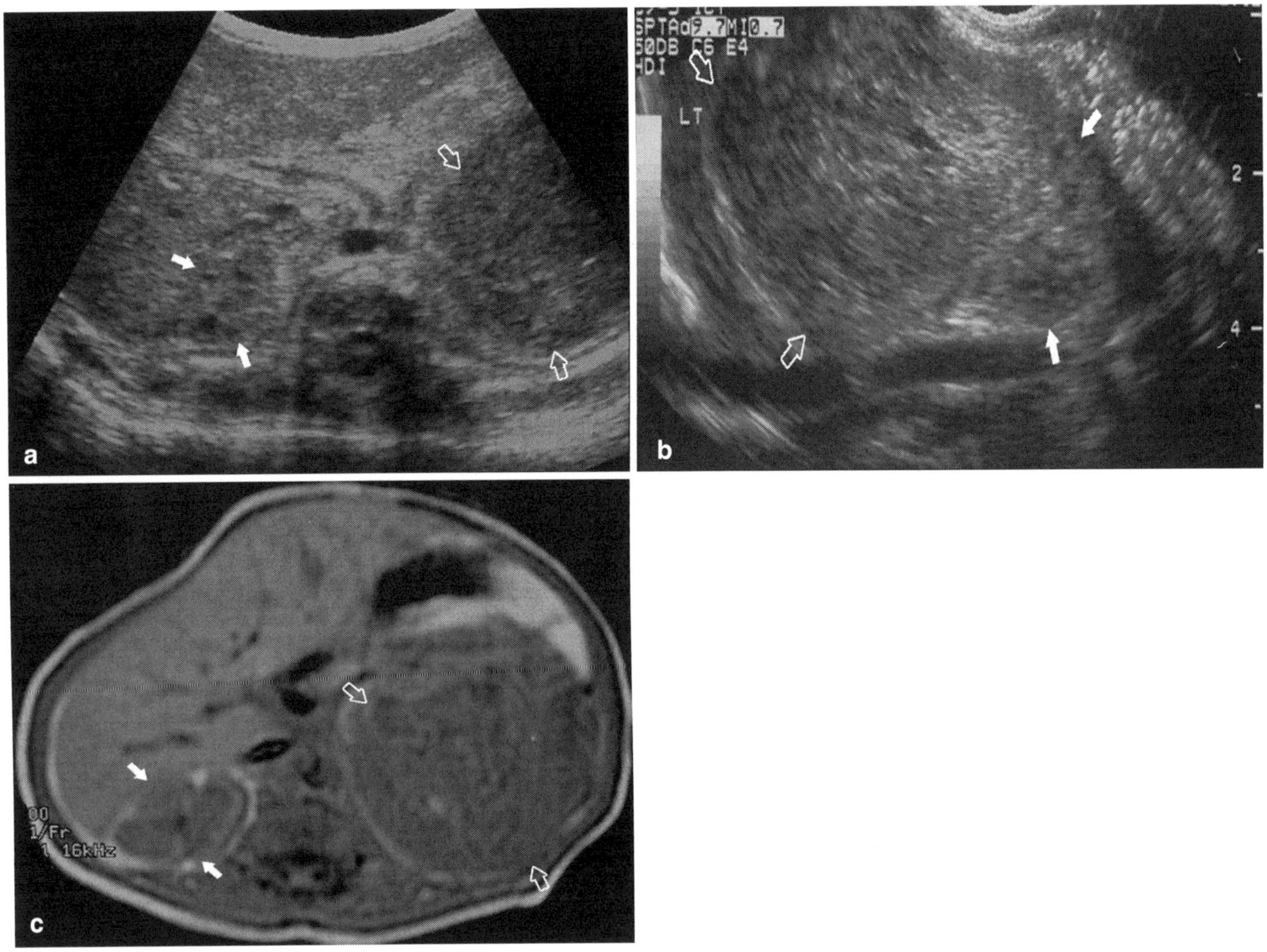

Fig. 10.1 An abdominal mass was palpated on 4-week-old male during a routine physical examination. Transverse abdominal ultrasound (**a**) demonstrates normal right kidney (*closed arrows*) and large left renal mass (*open arrows*). On sagittal ultrasound images (**b**) the heterogeneous left upper pole mass (*open arrows*) and normal lower pole renal parenchyma (*closed arrows*) are seen. Axial post-gadolinium T1-weighted MR (**c**) shows a large vascular left renal mass (*open arrows*) and a normal right kidney (*closed arrows*). Surgical resection confirmed the suspected diagnosis of congenital mesoblastic nephroma (CMN)

Nephroblastomatosis

Nephroblastomatosis refers to multifocal or diffuse distribution of nephrogenic rests [8]. Nephrogenic rests may be solitary or diffuse. Two subtypes exist: perilobar and intralobar. Perilobar nephrogenic rests occur in the peripheral renal cortex and are multiple whereas intralobar nephrogenic rests are usually solitary or few in number and occur anywhere within the renal lobe [9]. Wilms tumor is commonly associated with intralobar nephrogenic rests, although they occur less frequently than perilobar rests. Nephrogenic rests are associated with unilateral Wilms tumor in 41 % of cases and with bilateral Wilms tumor in 99 % of cases. Intralobar nephrogenic rests are associated with such Wilms tumor risk factors as Drash (ambiguous genitalia and progressive renal failure), sporadic aniridia, and WAGR [2, 9]. Perilobar rests are associated with Beckwith-Wiedemann syndrome and hemihypertrophy [9]. Nephrogenic rests exhibit homogenous appearance on ultrasound (US), and pre- and post-contrast computed tomography (CT) and magnetic resonance imaging (MRI) [7]. A heterogeneous or enlarging mass in a patient with nephroblastomatosis is concern for transformation to Wilms tumor.

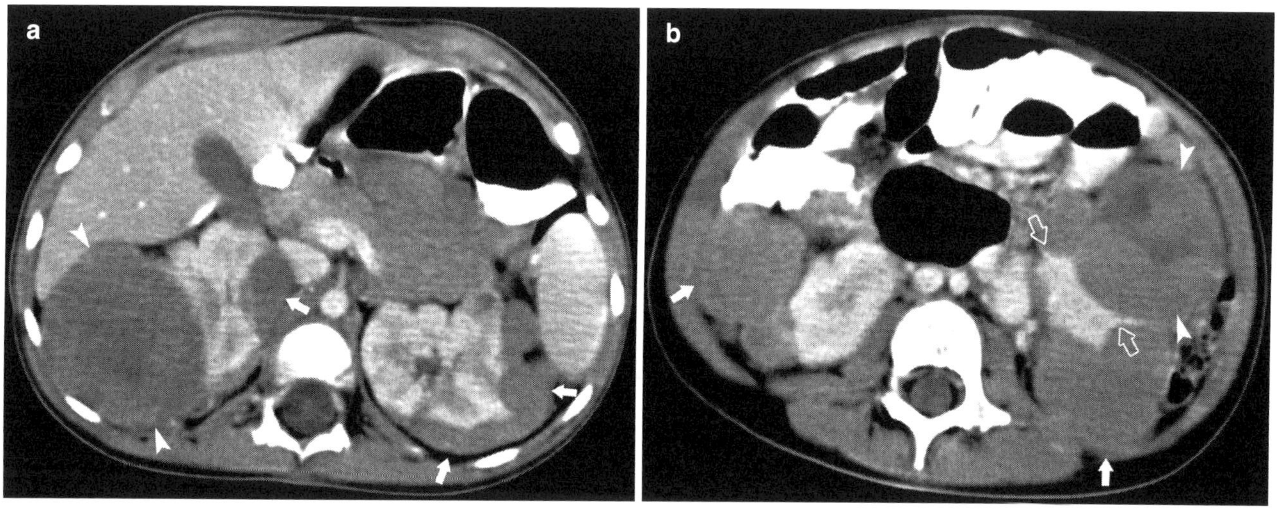

Fig. 10.2 A 2-year and 10-month-old female presented with abdominal distention. (**a**, **b**) Contrast-enhanced CT (CECT) demonstrates multiple homogenously enhancing lenticular masses (*closed arrows*) in the peripheral cortex on both kidneys consistent with perilobar nephrogenic rests. Distortion of the central renal parenchyma of the left kidney resembling a staghorn (*open arrow*) as described by Rohrschneider et al. [7] is seen. Heterogeneous spherical masses seen in the upper pole of the right kidney and the lower pole of the left kidney (*arrowheads*) were proven to be favorable histology Wilms tumors in this child with nephroblastomatosis

Stage 1 and 2 Wilms Tumor

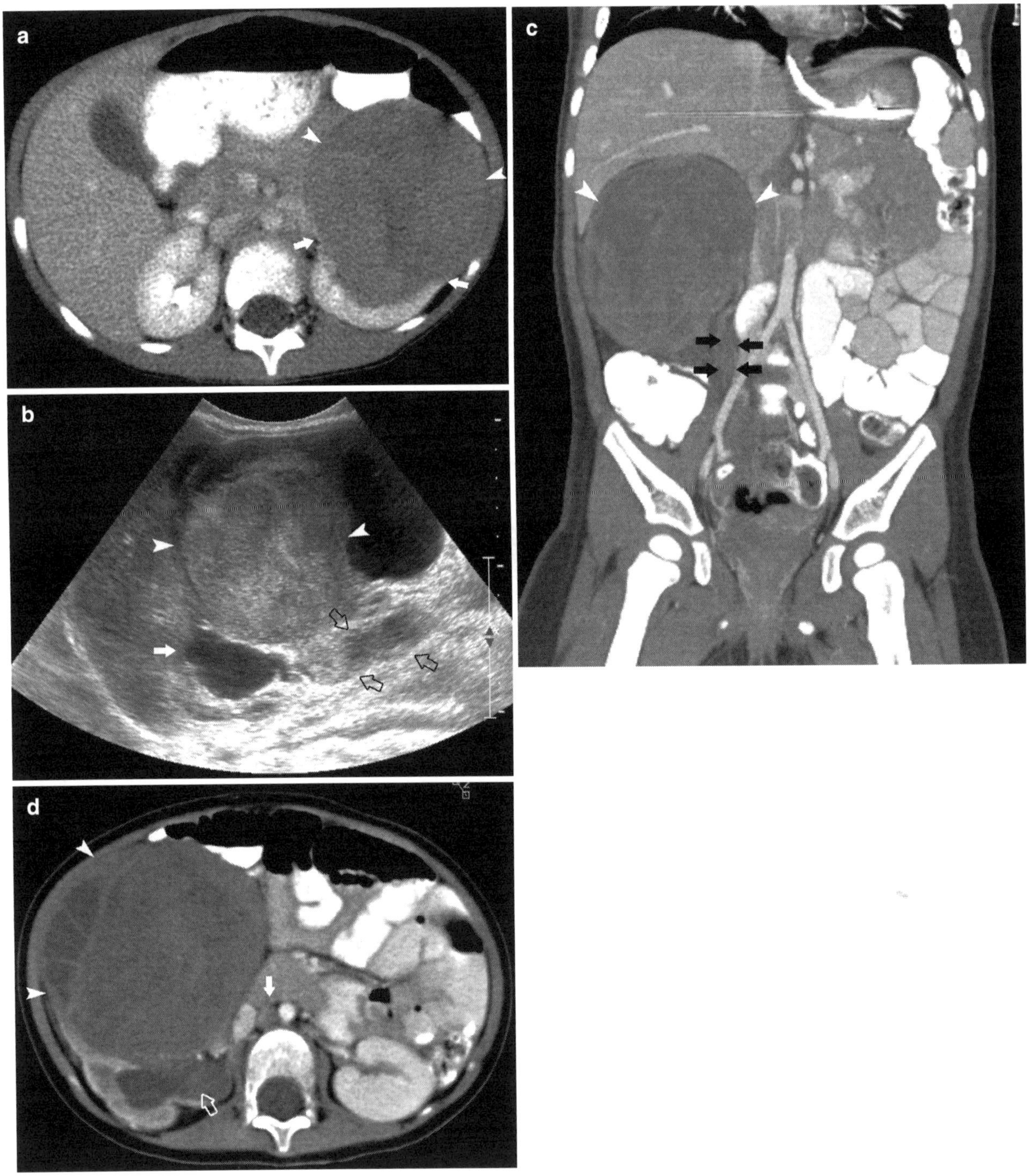

Fig. 10.3 A left renal mass was incidentally discovered on ultrasound evaluation of a 3.5-year-old male for suspected splenomegaly. Axial CECT image (**a**) demonstrates a heterogeneous mass in the upper half of the left kidney (*arrowheads*). A rim of normal renal parenchyma (claw sign; *arrow*) is present. No regional extension or distant metastases was seen. Surgery and pathological specimen confirmed stage 1 favorable histology Wilms tumor. A 2-year-old female with bloody stool and abdominal pain was noted to have a distended abdomen. Sagittal US (**b**) and coronal CT (**c**) demonstrate a heterogeneous mass originating in the right mid kidney (*arrowhead*) and a polypoid mass (*arrows*) in the proximal right ureter. Axial CT (**d**) demonstrates a complex mass with peripheral septations (*arrowheads*), interaortocaval lymph node (*arrow*), and obstruction of the right renal pelvis with layering debris (*open arrow*). Pathologic examination revealed tumor invasion into renal pelvis and proximal ureter without extension of tumor to adjacent lymph nodes. Chronic pyelonephritis from obstruction and reactive lymph nodes were found. The presence of ureteral extension did not affect stage 2 designation of the tumor. Ureteral extension of Wilms tumor is rare, but should be suspected in patients with gross hematuria, hydronephrosis, or nonfunctioning kidney. Gross hematuria, unlike microscopic hematuria, is uncommonly found at presentation of Wilms tumor [10]

Ruptured Wilms Tumor

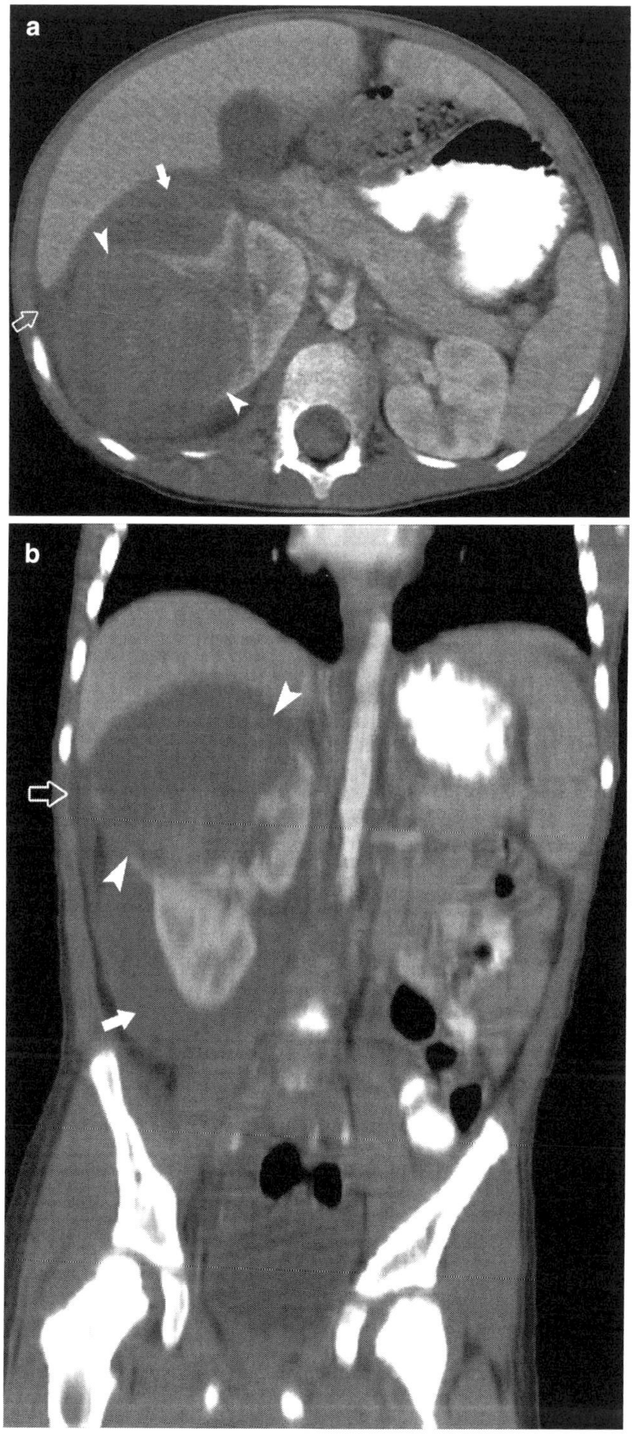

Fig. 10.4 A 3-year-old male presents with 2-week history of abdominal pain and 2-day history of marked abdominal swelling. Axial CT and coronal images (**a**, **b**) show a large heterogeneous mass (*arrowhead*) extending from the right upper pole. Subcapsular fluid (*closed arrow*) alters the renal contour. Subcapsular fluid and fluid within Gerota's fascia represent the contained component of a rupture Wilms tumor. Fluid extending along the right paracolic gutter (*open arrow*) into the pelvis represents free spillage and contamination. Tumor spillage either before or during surgery classifies the tumor as stage III. In cases of contained retroperitoneal rupture at diagnosis there is an increased risk of peritoneal contamination at surgery. Localized flank radiation is administered in cases of contained retroperitoneal rupture. Total abdominal radiation is given in cases of peritoneal contamination [11]

Stage 4 Wilms Tumor

Imaging studies and surgical and pathological findings at operative intervention determine the stage of Wilms tumor. Additional prognostic criteria are histology, favorable triphasic histology (blastema, stromal, and epithelial elements), or unfavorable histology (anaplastic sarcomatous elements). Pulmonary metastases are seen in 15–20 % of cases [12].

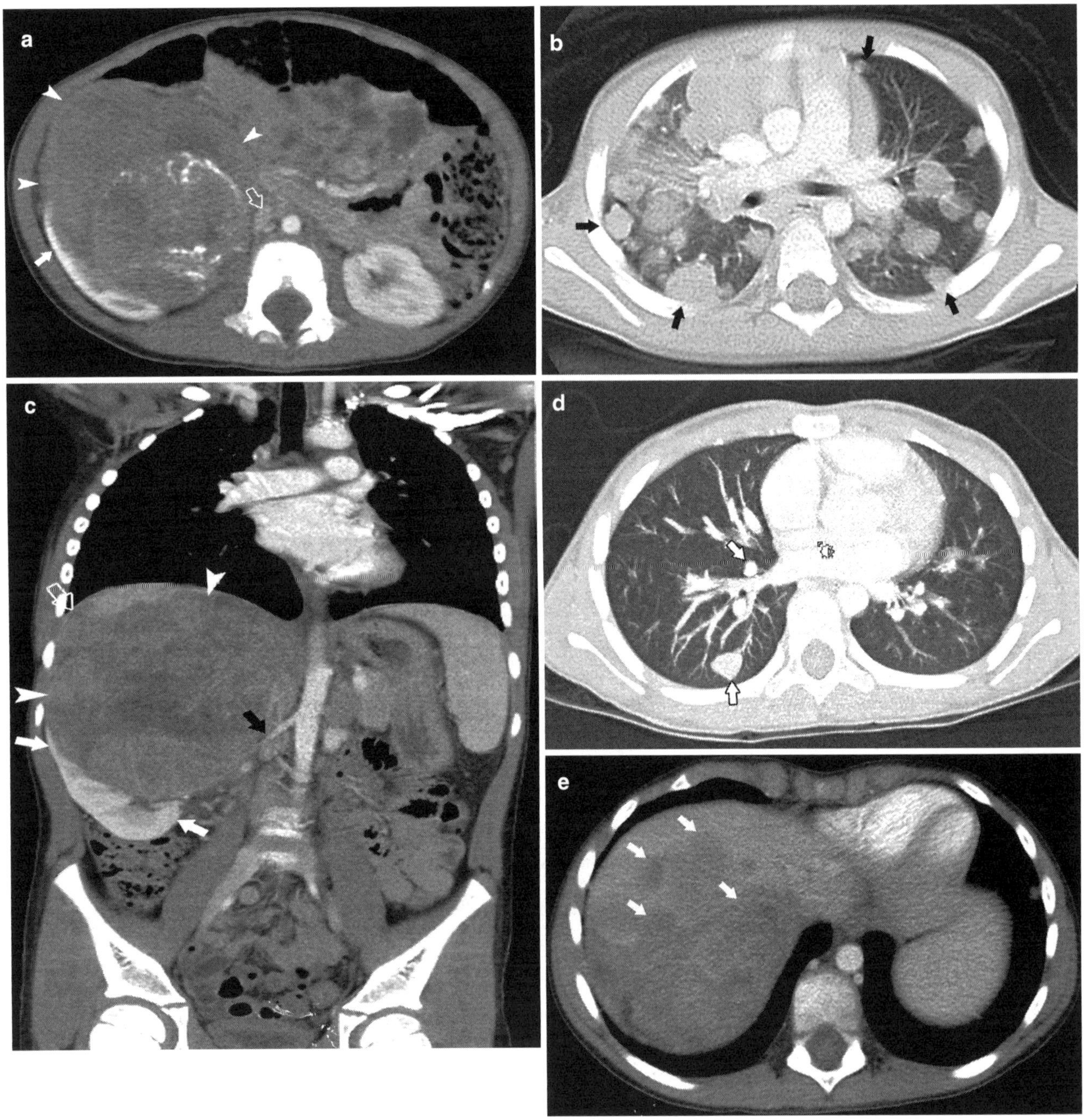

Fig. 10.5 A 2.5-year-old male presented with 2-day history of microscopic hematuria. Axial CT (**a**) demonstrates a large right renal mass with calcification (*arrowheads*). The IVC (*open arrow*) is compressed. Calcification is present in less than 10 % of Wilms tumor. Extensive pulmonary metastases are present (*arrows*) (**b**). No intravascular tumor thrombus is present. Surgery and pathology revealed stage IV, favorable histology Wilms tumor. A 7-year-old male presented with fever, fatigue, tachycardia, and paleness. Electrocardiography showed displacement of IVC. Coronal CT images (**c**) demonstrate a large right renal mass (*arrowheads*), with normal lower pole parenchyma creating a claw sign (*white arrows*), direct invasion of the liver and encasement of the right renal artery (*black arrow*). Unilateral renal involvement and distant spread of tumor to the lung and liver (*arrows* in **d**, **e**) classifies this as stage 4 disease. Hepatic metastases occur in 10–15 % of children with Wilms tumor [12]

Bilateral Wilms Tumor

The presence of bilateral disease at diagnosis upstages patients to stage V [13]. In 5 % of patients, bilateral tumors are synchronous. Synchronous tumors occur more frequently in females and at a younger age (mean age, 2.5 y) [8]. Metachronous bilateral Wilms tumors are seen more frequently in children with initial presentation at less than 1 year of age and in patients with Beckwith-Wiedemann syndrome, hemihypertrophy, or congenital aniridia [8]. Bilateral disease represents a surgical challenge. Nephron-sparing surgery and partial nephrectomies or unilateral nephrectomy and contralateral nephrectomy are frequently performed.

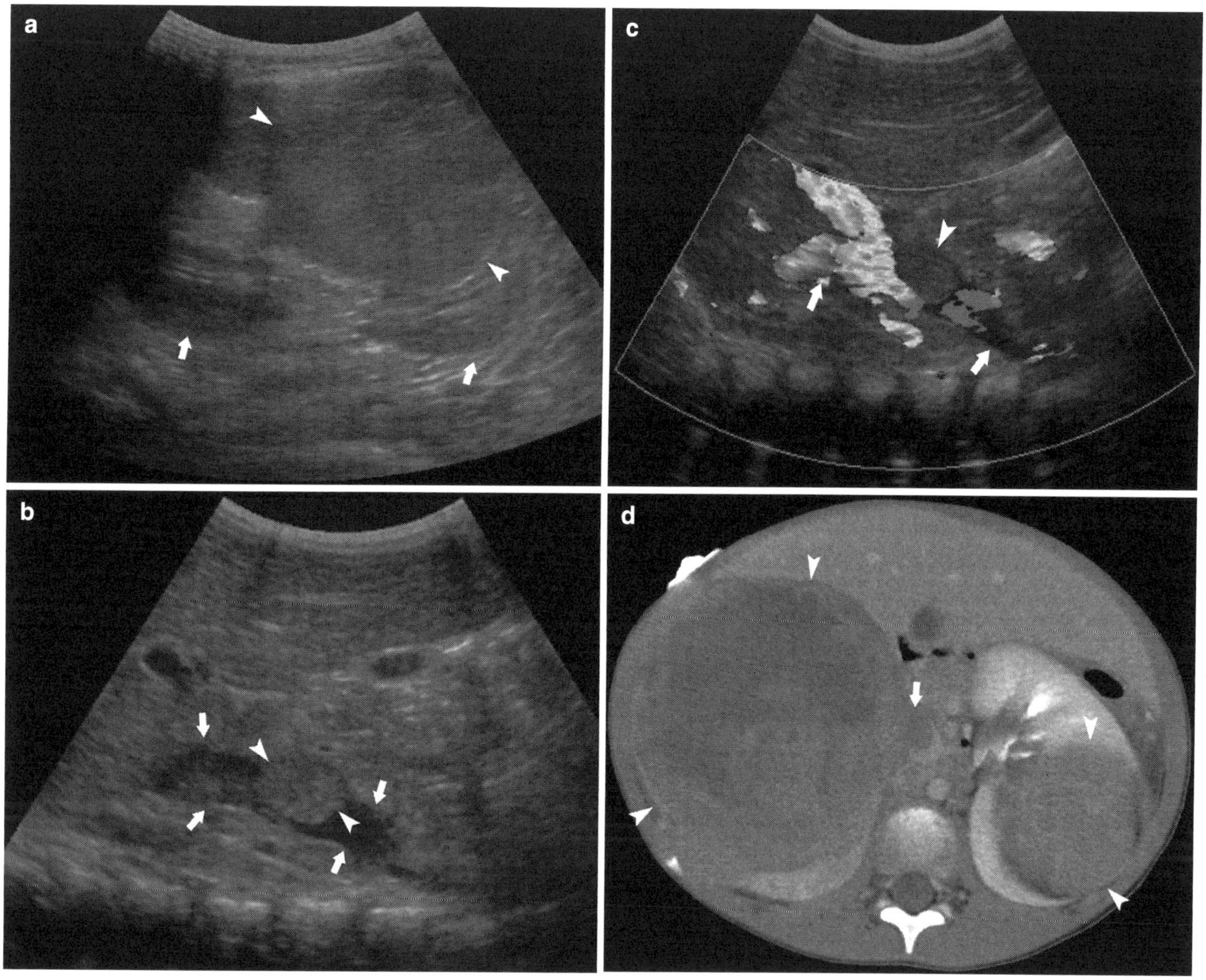

Fig. 10.6 A 3-year-old female presented with hematuria and abdominal pain. Sagittal ultrasound demonstrates mass (*arrowhead*) in the mid zone of the left kidney (*arrows* in **a**). A large right upper pole renal mass was also present. Evaluation of the inferior vena cava (*arrow*) reveals an echogenic tumor thrombus (*arrowhead*) at the level of the right renal vein Color Doppler imaging confirms the thrombus is nonocclusive (**b**, **c**). CECT (**d**) demonstrates heterogeneous right renal mass (*arrowheads*) and smaller left renal mass (*arrowhead*). Filling defect in the IVC (*arrow*) represents tumor localized tumor thrombus. The thrombus did not extend cephalad toward the right atrium

Extrarenal Wilms Tumor

Extrarenal Wilms tumor is an exceedingly rare tumor with approximately 200 cases reported in the literature involving pediatric and adult patients [14]. Retroperitoneal and pelvic locations are more common and may lead to incorrect diagnosis of neuroblastoma or ovarian lesion. Extrarenal Wilms tumor is believed to occur in any site that develops from pronephros, mesonephros, or metanephros [14].

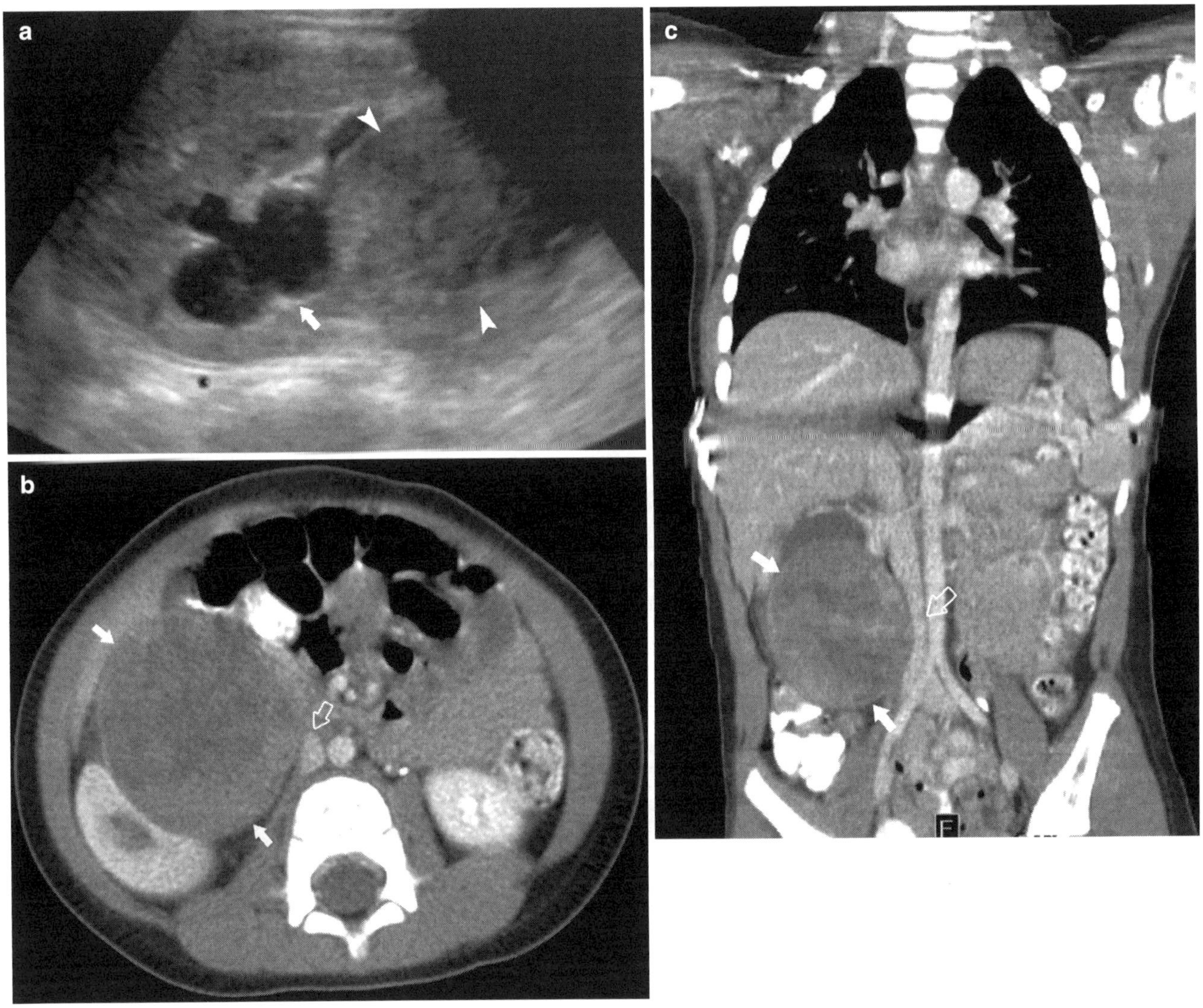

Fig. 10.7 A 3-year-old male was noted to have a right flank mass on physical examination. Sagittal ultrasound (**a**) demonstrates a solid mass (*arrowheads*) inseparable from the right kidney and causing obstruction at the level of the renal pelvis (*arrow*). Contrast-enhanced axial (**b**) and coronal reformatted CT (**c**) images demonstrate a heterogeneous mass extrinsic to the lower pole of the right kidney (*arrows*). The mass compresses the renal parenchyma and adjacent IVC (*open arrow*). No calcification is seen. MIBG scan (**d**) performed to evaluate preoperative diagnosis of paraspinal neuroblastoma demonstrates a photopenic area corresponding to the mass (*arrows*). Surgical exploration revealed a mass adjacent to the renal hilum. The renal capsule was intact and total gross resection was performed. An extrarenal Wilms tumor was diagnosed on pathology

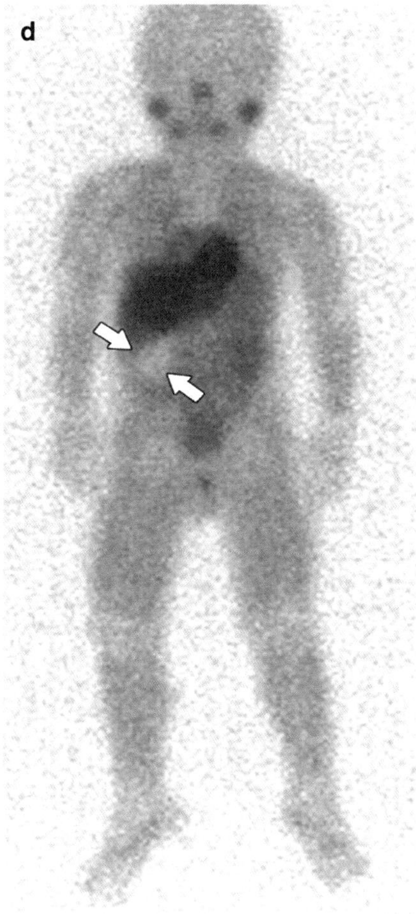

Fig. 10.7 (continued)

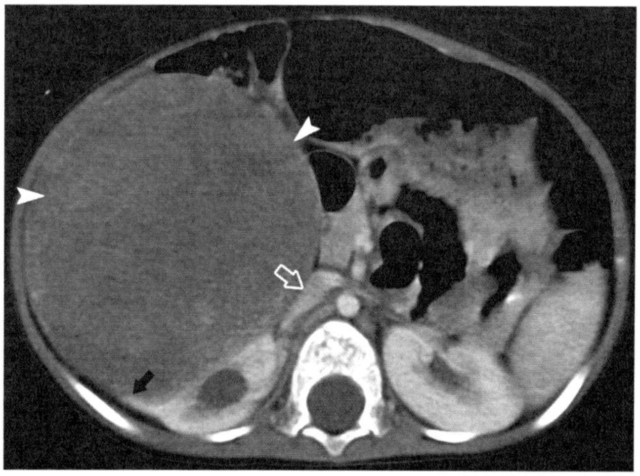

Fig. 10.8 An abdominal mass was incidentally discovered in a 19-month-old male. A CECT demonstrates a large right mass (*arrowheads*) demonstrating a claw sign (*black arrow*) indicating renal origin of the mass. The IVC is compressed (*open arrow*). No tumor thrombus is identified in the renal vein or IVC. No local adenopathy is present. No pulmonary, hepatic, and lymph node metastases were present. The radionuclide bone scan in this patient was negative. A definitive resection, radical right nephrectomy followed by adjuvant chemotherapy, was the treatment course. Pathology revealed clear cell sarcoma of the kidney (CCSK)

Clear Cell Sarcoma of the Kidney

CCSK is an aggressive renal tumor, pathologically distinct from Wilms tumor. On imaging, however, CCSK cannot be differentiated from Wilms tumor. The peak incidence is 1–4 years old with a male predominance [2]. CCSK is known as the "bone metastasizing renal tumor of childhood" [12]. 99mTc-MDP bone scintigraphy is essential for staging this disease. In addition to skeletal metastases that occur in 40–60 % of patients [12], CCSK spreads to lymph nodes, brain, liver, and lung [2]. Patients with CCSK have a longer surveillance period than those diagnosed with Wilms tumor. The prognosis is worse with a long-term survival of 60–70 % [13].

Rhabdoid Tumor

RTK are extremely aggressive neoplasms [2, 12]. More the 50 % of patients with rhabdoid tumor of the kidney are younger than 1 year old [2, 12]. The 18-month survival rate is only 20 % [2]. RTK are associated with primary synchronous or metachronous, midline, or posterior fossa tumors in 10–15 % of cases [12]. Metastases to the lung are most common, followed by liver, lymph nodes, bone, and brain [2, 12]. On imaging, RTK are large heterogeneous masses arising in the renal hilum. Subcapsular fluid collections representing necrosis and/or hemorrhage and linear calcifications outlining the tumor lobules may be present [2, 12].

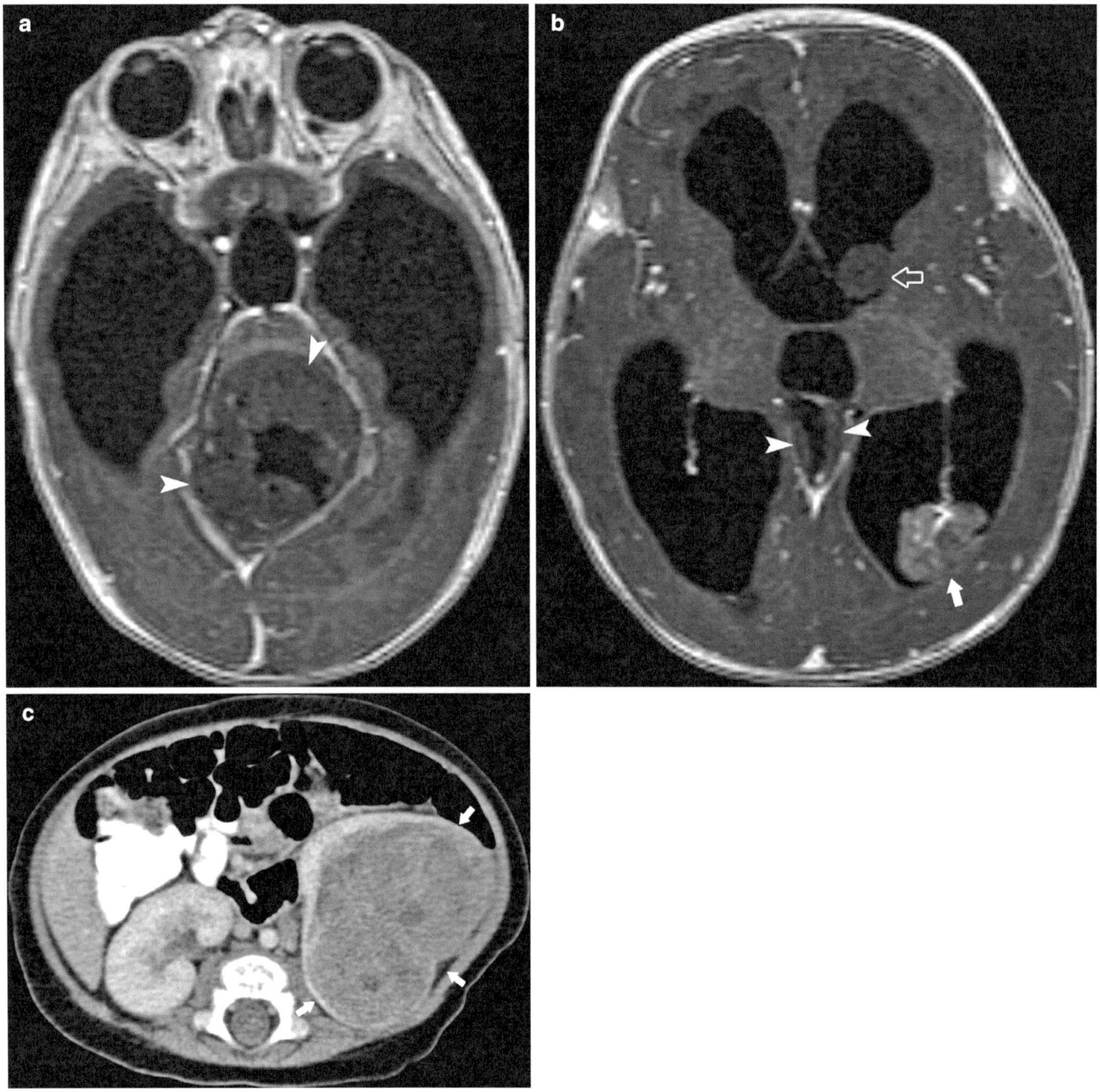

Fig. 10.9 A 5-month-old female presented with intermittent opisthotonic posturing and rapidly increasing head circumference. Axial post-contrast MR demonstrates mass originating in the cerebellar vermis resulting in obstructive hydrocephalus of the third and lateral ventricles (*arrowhead* in **a**, **b**). A separate multilobular-enhancing mass in the posterior atrium of the left lateral ventricle (*open arrow*) is contiguous with the choroid plexus and a third nonenhancing mass is seen along the ependymal surface of the left lateral ventricle (*arrow* in **b**). Resection of posterior fossa mass revealed an atypical teratoid rhabdoid tumor. Abdominal CT (**c**) performed for extent of disease demonstrated a large heterogeneously enhancing mass in the left kidney involving the renal hilum (*arrows*). Left nephrectomy revealed an rhabdoid kidney of the tumor (RTK)

Medullary Renal Cell Carcinoma

RMC occurs in patients with sickle cell trait or hemoglobin sickle cell (SC) disease, not homozygous sickle cell (hemoglobin SS) disease [12, 15]. Painless gross hematuria is the most common presentation in patients who range in age from 10 to 40 years old (mean, 22 y) [15]. The enlarged kidney characteristically maintains its reniform shape. The tumor replaces the renal pelvis infiltrating the renal sinus and causes caliectasis. RMC occurs more frequently on the right side [15]. Hemorrhage and necrosis are consistent findings. Metastatic spread is to regional lymph nodes, lung, adrenal gland, and liver [15, 16]. RMC is an aggressive tumor with poor response to chemotherapy or radiation. The average survival from time of diagnosis is 15 weeks [2].

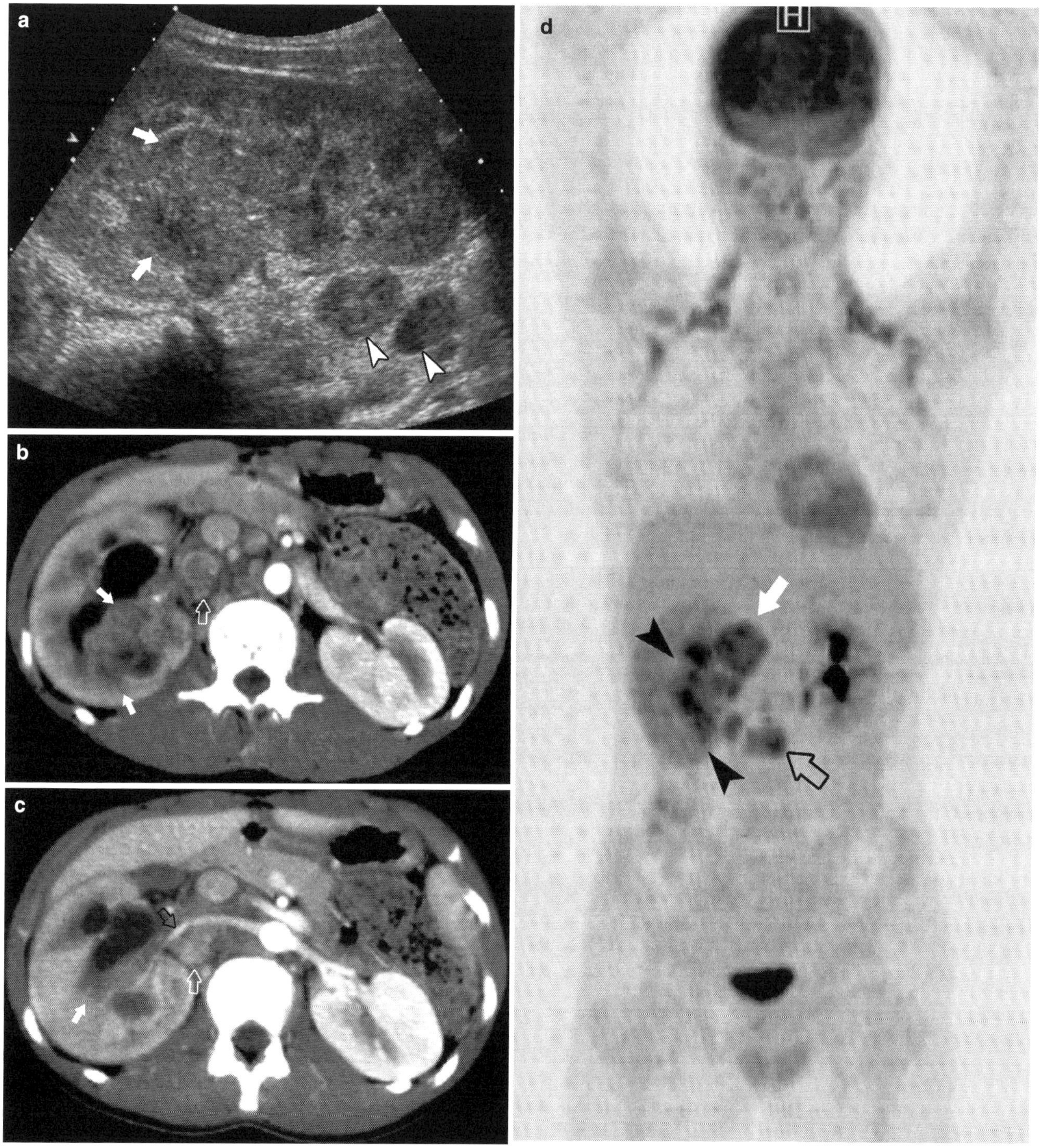

Fig. 10.10 A 13-year-old male with previously undiagnosed sickle cell trait presented with a 2-month history of intermittent hematuria, weight loss, and back pain. Ultrasound (**a**) performed for evaluation of hematuria demonstrates solid mass (*arrows*) involving the right renal pelvis and abnormal retroperitoneal lymph nodes (*arrowheads*). CECT (**b**) demonstrates a heterogeneous mass in the renal medulla (*arrows*). The mass (*arrow*) extends into the renal pelvis, obstructing the collecting system. Right paraaortic adenopathy (*white open arrow*) displaces the renal artery (*black open arrow*) (**c**). Maximum intensity projection (MIP) image from FDG-PET (**d**) demonstrates FDG avid infiltrative tumor in the right renal pelvis (*arrowheads*), adenopathy adjacent to the renal hilum (*arrow*), and metastases to L2 (*open arrow*). Pathology confirmed diagnosis of medullary renal cell carcinoma (RMC)

Renal Cell Carcinoma

RCC represents less than 7 % of all malignant renal tumors in children usually occurring within the first two decades of life [12]. RCC in children is associated with tuberous sclerosis, von Hippel Lindau syndrome, urogenital malformations, and treated neuroblastoma. The mean interval between treatment of neuroblastoma and the diagnosis of RCC is 11 years [18]. Metastases to liver, lung, or brain are reported in 20 % of patients at the time of diagnosis [2]. Imaging alone is insufficient to differentiate RCC from Wilms tumor. Although the incidence of Wilms tumor compared to RCC is nearly 30:1 in childhood, the incidence is nearly equal in the second decade of life [2]. Calcification is present in 25 % of cases of RCC compared to 9 % of Wilms tumor [2].

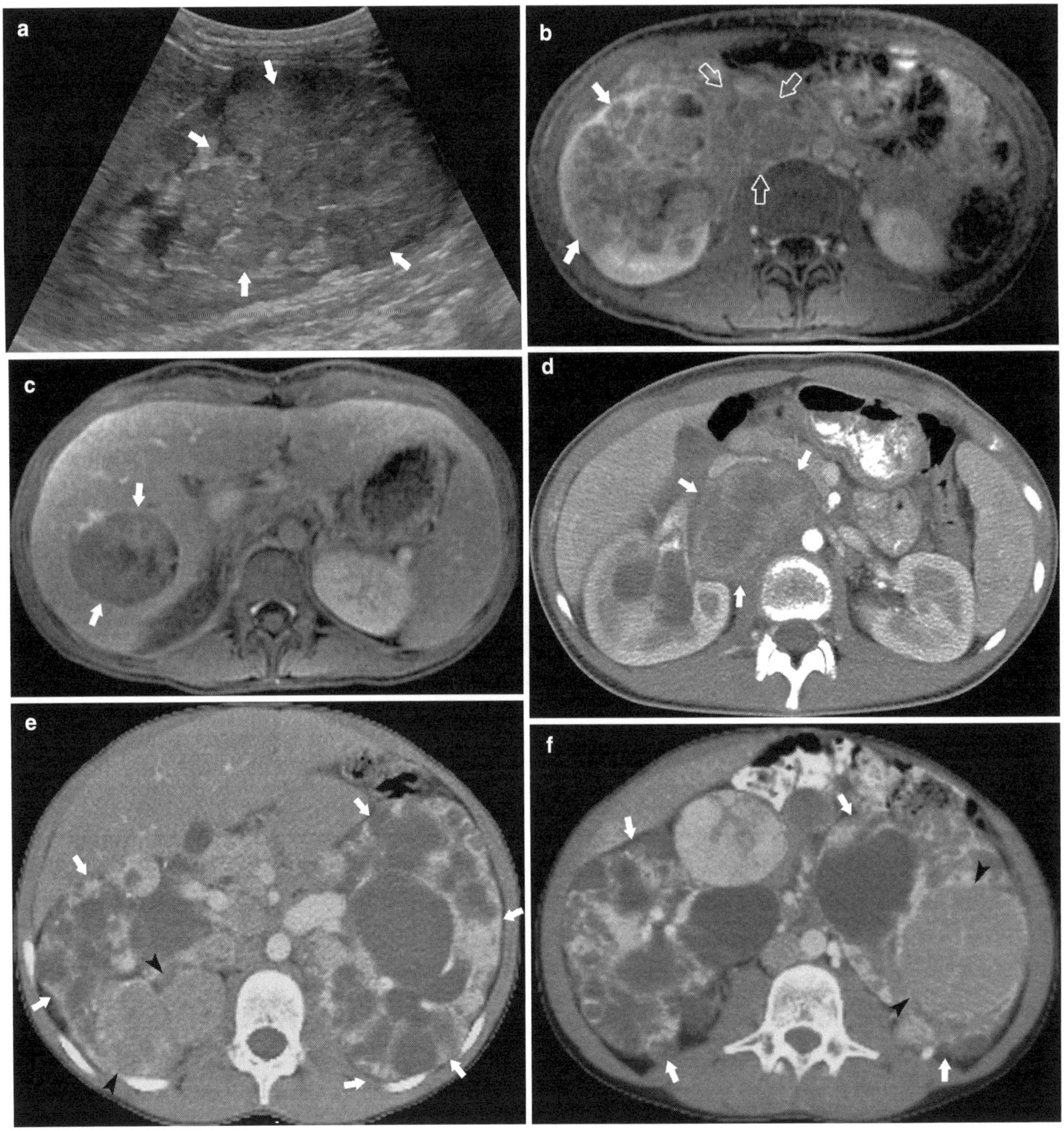

Leukemia

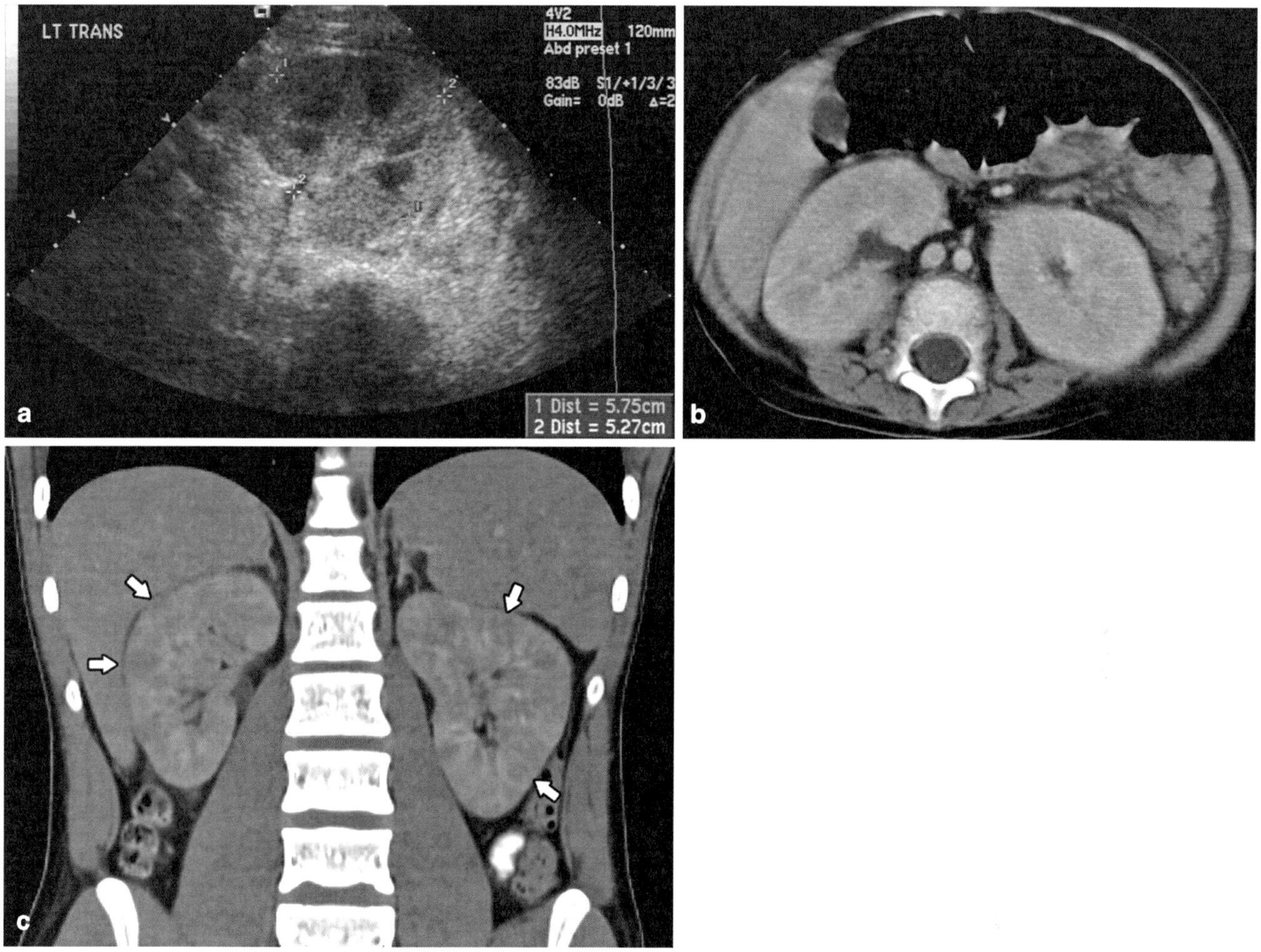

Fig. 10.12 Ultrasound (**a**) and CT (**b**) performed in a newly diagnosed 2-year-old male with ALL demonstrates homogenously enlarged kidneys that are greater than 95 % of the predicted size limits for the patient's age. Imaging of renal involvement in leukemia may demonstrate bilaterally enlarged kidneys with loss of corticomedullary differentiation and masses, solitary or multiple [12]. The kidneys are a sanctuary site for leukemia and imaging findings may occur during times of active disease as well as in bone marrow remission. A 17-year-old presented with a 1-month history of cervical adenopathy and fatigue. Coronal reconstruction CT (**c**) performed prior to the pathologic confirmation of suspected diagnosis of T cell lymphoblastic leukemia demonstrates bilaterally enlarged kidneys with multiple low attenuation infiltrative lesions (*arrows*)

Fig. 10.11 A 14-year-old female presented with a 6-month history of anemia and intermittent microscopic hematuria. Sagittal ultrasound (**a**) demonstrates an infiltrative right lower pole renal mass (*arrows*). Post-contrast axial T1-weighted MR (**b**, **c**) demonstrates the right lower pole renal mass (*arrows*), spread to adjacent lymph nodes (*open arrows*) and metastases to the right lobe of the liver (*arrows*). Axial CECT (**d**) demonstrates retroperitoneal lymph nodes (*arrows*) displacing the right renal vein and IVC. Pathology revealed XpII/TFE 3 translocation-associated RCC, a recently described entity that accounts for almost one third of pediatric RCC [17]. An 11-year-old male with known tuberous sclerosis and enlarged cystic kidneys (*arrows*) (**e**, **f**) and enlarging renal masses (*arrowheads*) on surveillance CT. Biopsy of the enlarging renal masses confirmed the suspected diagnosis of renal cell carcinoma (RCC)

Lymphoma

Because the kidneys do not contain lymphatic tissue, renal involvement in patients with lymphoma is either by hematogenous spread or direct extension from retroperitoneal disease [12]. Renal involvement in lymphoma more commonly presents as multiple masses, with a solitary mass and homogenous nephromegaly less common. On MR, the lesions are homogenous, hypointense on T1-weighted image, and hyperintense on T2-weighted image with variable contrast enhancement [12]. Renal involvement is uncommon in Hodgkin lymphoma. Non-Hodgkin lymphoma, especially Burkitt and T-cell lymphoblastic lymphoma, frequently involves the kidney [19].

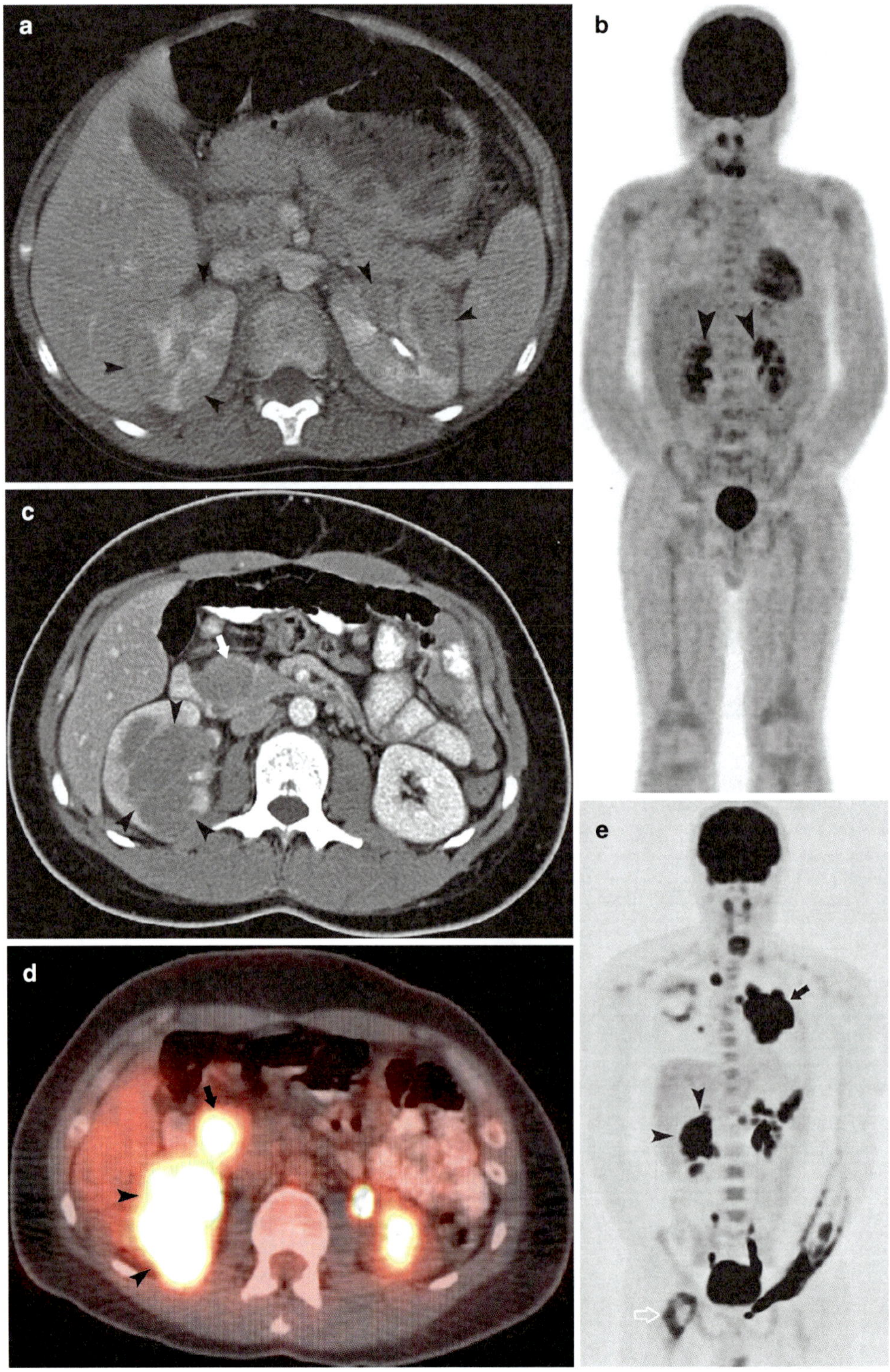

Fig. 10.13 Axial CT (**a**) performed in a 7-year-old male diagnosed with Burkitt's lymphoma demonstrates diffuse low attenuation lesions (*arrowhead*) relative to normal renal parenchyma that distort the contour of the kidneys. MIP image from the FDG-PET scan (**b**) demonstrates FDG avidity in the renal lesions (*arrowheads*). In addition to diffuse lesions, lymphoma can present as a solitary renal mass. Axial CT (**c**) in a 17-year-old male diagnosed with diffuse large B-cell lymphoma demonstrates a large right renal mass (*arrowheads*). Retroperitoneal adenopathy (*arrow*) is apparent. The renal mass (*arrowheads*) and adjacent adenopathy are highly FDG avid as seen on an axial fused PET-CT image (**d**). MIP image (**e**) demonstrates renal involvement (*arrowheads*), large anterior mediastinal mass (*arrow*), and involvement of right proximal femur (*open arrow*)

Rhabdomyosarcoma of the Bladder/Prostate

RMS of the bladder and prostate represent 10 % of all cases of RMS usually occurring in children younger than 9 years old. In cases of only bladder involvement, the boy–girl ratio is 3:1 [20]. Staging of RMS is extremely complex [21, 22]. Site and histology are important factors. Nonbladder/nonprostate genitourinary primaries have a favorable prognosis, unlike primary bladder and prostate RMS. Dysuria, hematuria, and urinary retention are all presenting symptoms. Bladder/prostate RMS may be infiltrative, polypoid, or resemble a cluster of grapes (sarcoma botryoides). Ninety percent of bladder RMS is of the embryonal subset. Botryoid subtype of embryonal RMS are associated with a more favorable prognosis [21, 22]. Treatment with chemotherapy and radiation therapy to reduce tumor bulk permits bladder function preservation surgery without sacrificing cure rates [21, 23].

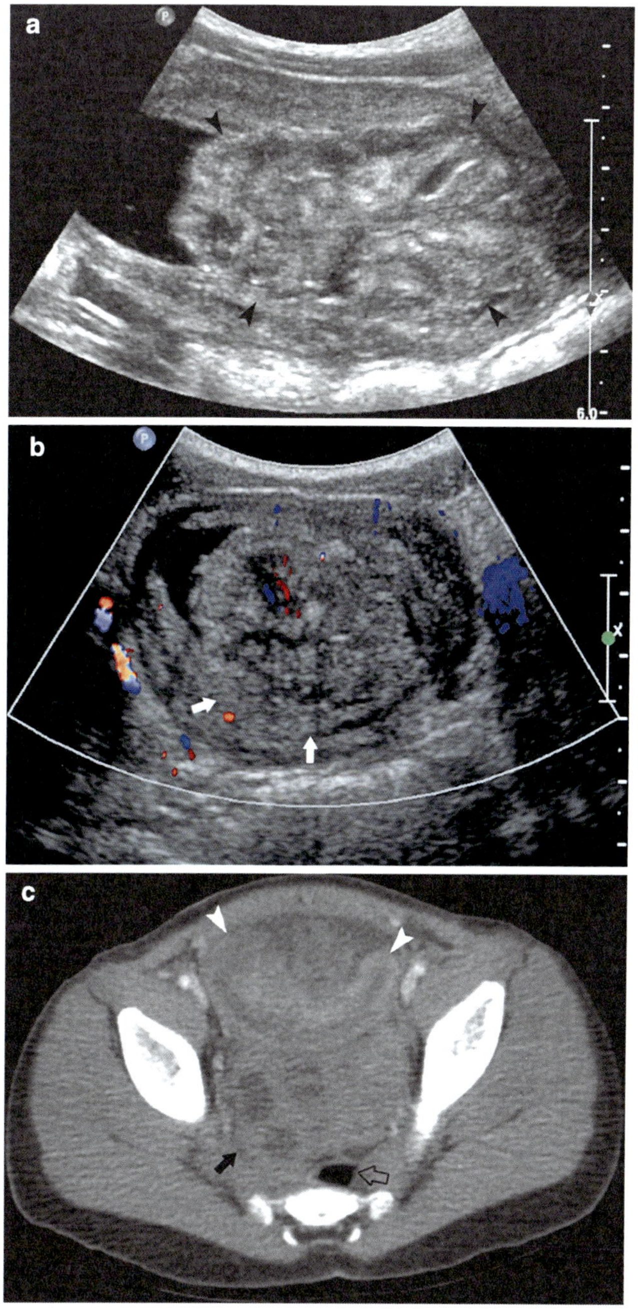

Fig. 10.14 A 6-year-old male presented with hematuria and dysuria. Sagittal ultrasound of the bladder demonstrates a large heterogeneous mass (*arrowheads*) arising from the base of the bladder (**a**). Transverse color Doppler ultrasound image reveals minimal flow within the mass that is inseparable from the bladder wall (*arrow*) (**b**). Pathologic diagnosis was embryonal rhabdomyosarcoma (RMS), botryoid subtype. A 3-year-old male presented with abdominal pain, distention, and hematuria (**c**). Axial image from CECT demonstrates a heterogeneously enhancing grapelike intravesical mass (*arrowheads*). A retrovesical mass (*closed arrows*) displaces the rectum (*open arrow*). As is often the case in patients with large RMS, the origin of the lesion, bladder versus prostate RMS, is not possible to determine. Biopsy confirmed diagnosis of embryonal RMS, botryoid subtype

Neuroblastoma

Neuroblastoma (NB) is the most common extracranial neoplasm in childhood and represents 8 % of all pediatric malignancies [24, 25]. It is the most common tumor of infants [25]. Although most tumors occur in children from 2 to 5 years old, NB may also be seen in newborns, adolescents, and adults [26]. NB derives from neural crest cells that give rise to the sympathetic nervous system. Therefore, NB can occur anywhere along the sympathetic chain or in the adrenal medulla. The majority of tumors are found in the adrenal medulla or other retroperitoneal sites [27]. However, primary tumors may occur in the neck (5 %) [28], posterior mediastinum (20 %), and pelvis (5 %).

At least 60 % of patients have metastatic disease at diagnosis, most commonly in the following sites: bone, bone marrow, lymph nodes [29] (*see* Fig. 10.16), and liver [27]. Other less common metastatic sites include pleura (*see* Fig. 10.17), pulmonary parenchyma [30, 31], and the central nervous system (CNS) [32–36] (*see* Fig. 10.18).

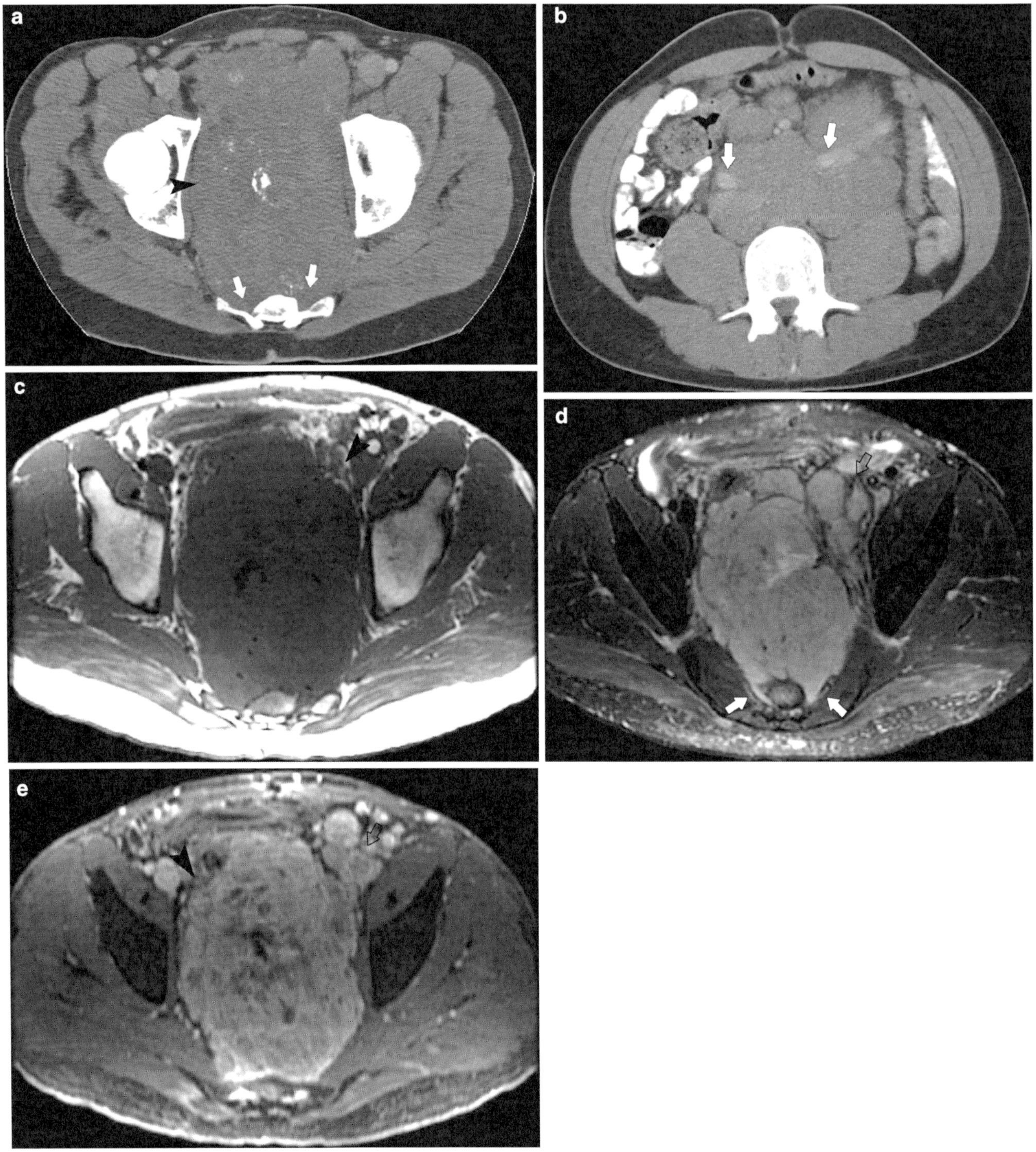

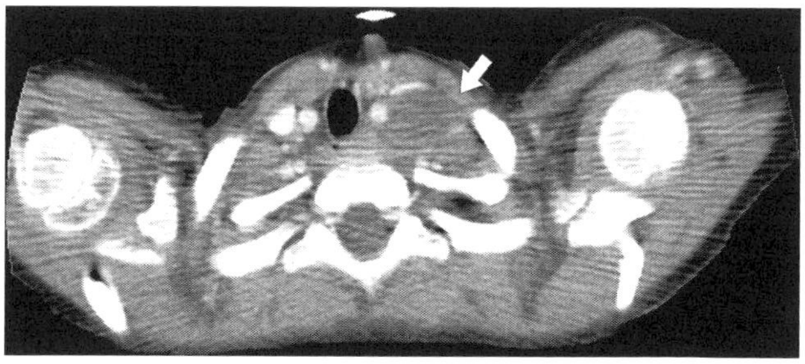

Fig. 10.16 Left supraclavicular node. NB has a propensity for involving the left supraclavicular node ("Virchow" node; *arrow*). Anterior mediastinal and hilar adenopathy is uncommon. Sampling of this node to obtain tissue for diagnosis and evaluation of biologic markers precludes the need for abdominal surgery for diagnosis in patients with large unresectable abdominal masses [29]

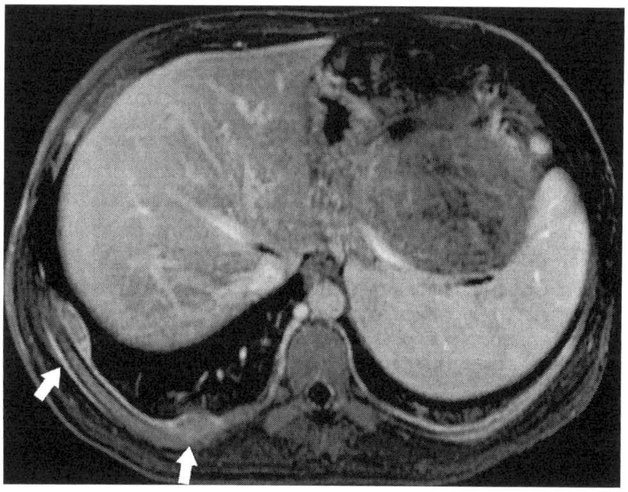

Fig. 10.17 Pleural metastases. MR axial T-weighted post-contrast image demonstrates right pleural metastases (*arrows*). Pleural metastases are uncommon in neuroblastoma, usually occurring at relapse [27]. This 10-year-old male presented with these findings

Fig. 10.15 Pelvic neuroblastoma. (**a**, **b**) CT demonstrates a large partially calcified pelvic mass (*arrowhead*) extending into sacral foramina (*arrows*). Extensive accompanying retroperitoneal adenopathy, anteriorly displacing both common iliac arteries (*arrows*). (**c**–**e**) Axial MR. (**c**) T1-weighted image shows low signal mass with small areas of fluid or necrosis. Mass extends into sacral foramina. (**d**) T2-weighted fat saturation image shows mass with areas of fluid or necrosis (*arrows*) and nodes (*open arrows*). (**e**) T1-weighted post-contrast shows heterogeneous enhancement of mass (*arrowhead*) and nodes (*open arrow*) [27]

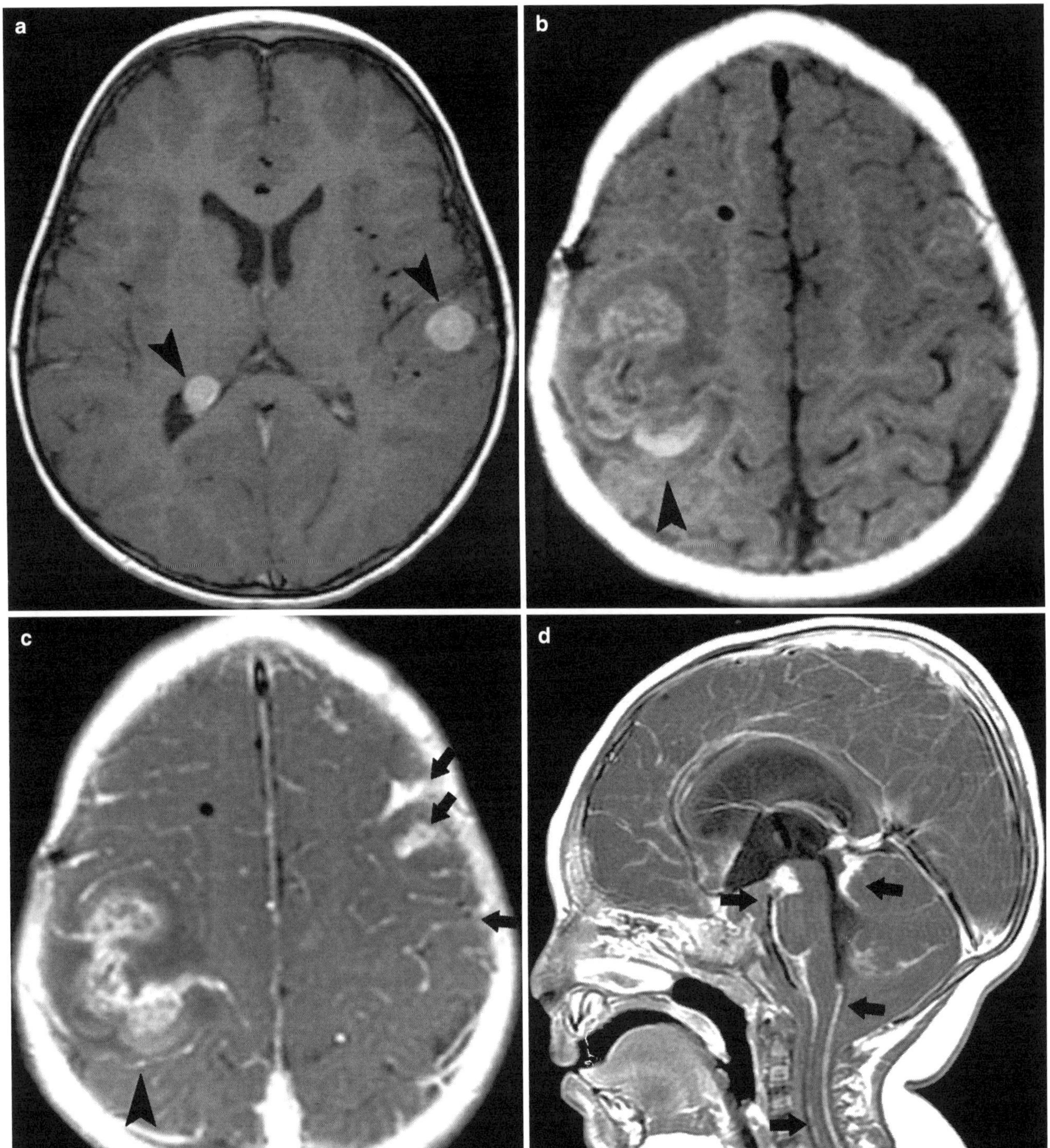

Fig. 10.18 CNS metastases. MR. (**a**) Axial T1-weighted post-contrast image demonstrates left intracerebral and right intraventricular metastases (*arrowheads*). (**b**) Second patient with axial T1-weighted pre-contrast scan showing large right hemorrhagic metastasis that enhances on post-contrast image. (**c**) Note also the leptomeningeal disease (*arrows*). (**d**) Sagittal T1-weighted post-contrast image from a third patient shows hydrocephalus and extensive leptomeningeal disease (*arrows*). CNS metastases are uncommon and usually occur at relapse [32, 33, 36]

Table 10.2 International Neuroblastoma Staging System (INSS) [37]

1	Localized tumor, complete gross resection, negative nodes bilaterally at surgery
2A	Localized tumor, incomplete gross resection, all nodes negative
2B	Localized tumor, with or without complete gross resection, positive ipsilateral nodes, negative contralateral nodes
3	Tumor across midline, with or without regional node involvement; unilateral tumor with contralateral nodes; or midline tumor with bilateral nodes
4	Distant metastases to lymph nodes, bone, bone marrow, liver, or other organs
4S	<1 year old, localized tumor (1, 2a, or 2b), spread limited to skin, liver, or bone marrow (<10 %)

Table 10.3 Neuroblastoma risk groups [40, 42–55]

Low risk	Intermediate risk	High risk
Stage I (completely removed)	Stage II no MYCN but <50 % removed	Stage II, III, IV, or IVS with MYCN
Stage II No MYCN and >50 % resection	Stage III <18 months, no MYCN	Stage III >18 months and unfavorable histology
Stage IVS no MYCN, DNA index >1, favorable histology and no symptoms	Stage III >18 months with no MYCN and favorable histology Stage IV <12 months and no MYCN	Stage IV 12–18 months, no MYCN unfavorable histology and DNA index 1
	Stage IV 12–18 months, no MYCN, favorable histology, and DNA index >1	Stage IV >18 months
	Stage IVS no MYCN, with either unfavorable histology or DNA index of 1	
95 % Survival	**>90 % Survival**	**30–40 % Survival**

Staging and Prognosis

The International Neuroblastoma Staging System (INSS) was devised as a staging system, taking into account radiological findings, surgical resectability, and metastatic disease [37].

However, other factors also affect prognosis in neuroblastoma, including age at diagnosis, site of primary, histology, and certain biologic factors that have been found to be linked to prognosis [27]. Patients younger than 1 year old at diagnosis have a significantly increased survival. Also, extraabdominal site of primary and favorable Shimada histology [38] also are associated with improved survival. Several biologic factors have been identified that are associated with prognosis [39]. Amplification (> 10 copies) of MYCN oncogene, a segment of DNA on chromosome 2, closely correlates with poor prognosis. Most patients younger than 1 year old do not have amplification [40]. DNA ploidy in infants also relates to prognosis [41]. DNA index greater than 1 in children younger than 1–2 years old is associated with a good prognosis, whereas DNA ploidy equal to or less than one is linked to poorer survival [40]. The set of markers in a given patient does not change with time so that favorable forms do not convert into unfavorable disease or vice versa [42]. Combining the INSS with these other important factors allows for determining low, intermediate, and high-risk disease. Therapy and prognosis are based on this combined risk classification system [40, 43–45].

Clinical Presentation

Children with neuroblastoma present with a wide variety of symptoms, frequently associated with metastatic disease. Because the majority of patients have metastatic disease at presentation, many of them present with pallor, weight loss, and irritability. A prominent mass in the abdomen may be related to an enlarged liver from metastatic deposits or from the large primary tumor. The tumor may extend through neural foramina into the extradural space (dumbbell tumor) causing neurologic symptoms from cord compression. Involvement of the sphenoid bone may cause ecchymoses around the orbit from hemorrhage into the surrounding soft tissues and may be accompanied by orbital proptosis ("raccoon eye") [42, 46].

Patients with advanced disease at diagnosis frequently present with diffuse bone pain, refusal to bear weight, and limping from bony metastases. Cervical and superior sulcus tumors may present with Horner's syndrome 5. Rarely, compression of both renal arteries by tumor and nodes may lead to hypertension [46].

Intractable diarrhea may be the presenting symptom in children with tumors that secrete vasoactive intestinal peptide (VIP). Diarrhea abates after tumor resection [47]. Some patients with myoclonic encephalopathy of infancy (dancing feet, dancing eyes) may have underlying neuroblastoma [48, 49]. Neuroblastoma may also be identified on routine prenatal ultrasonographic screening [50, 51] or by urine catecholamine screening [52–55].

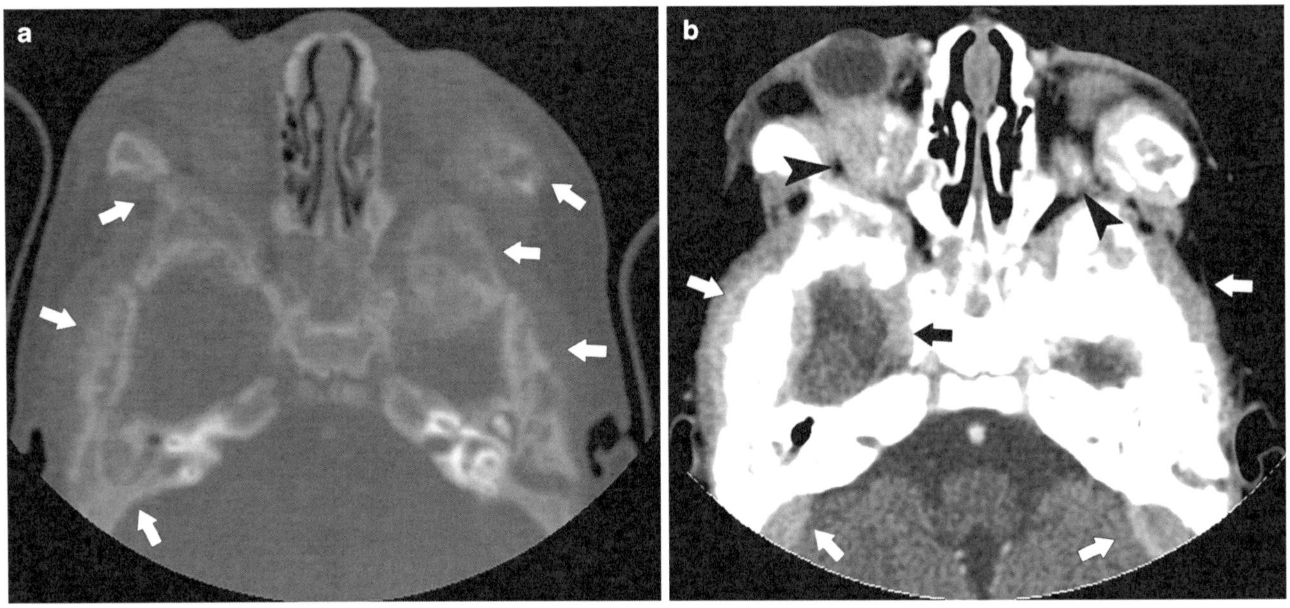

Fig. 10.19 Extensive bone and soft tissue metastases. This 2-year-old boy presented with proptosis, "raccoon eyes," and blindness due to extensive bone and accompanying soft tissue disease that extended into the orbit and compressed the optic nerves. (**a**) CT bone window. Virtually all the bones of the calvarium are involved (*arrows*). (**b**) Soft tissue window at same level shows marked soft tissue involvement (*arrows*) from the underlying bone disease, extending into the orbits and causing right proptosis (*arrowheads*) [42, 46]

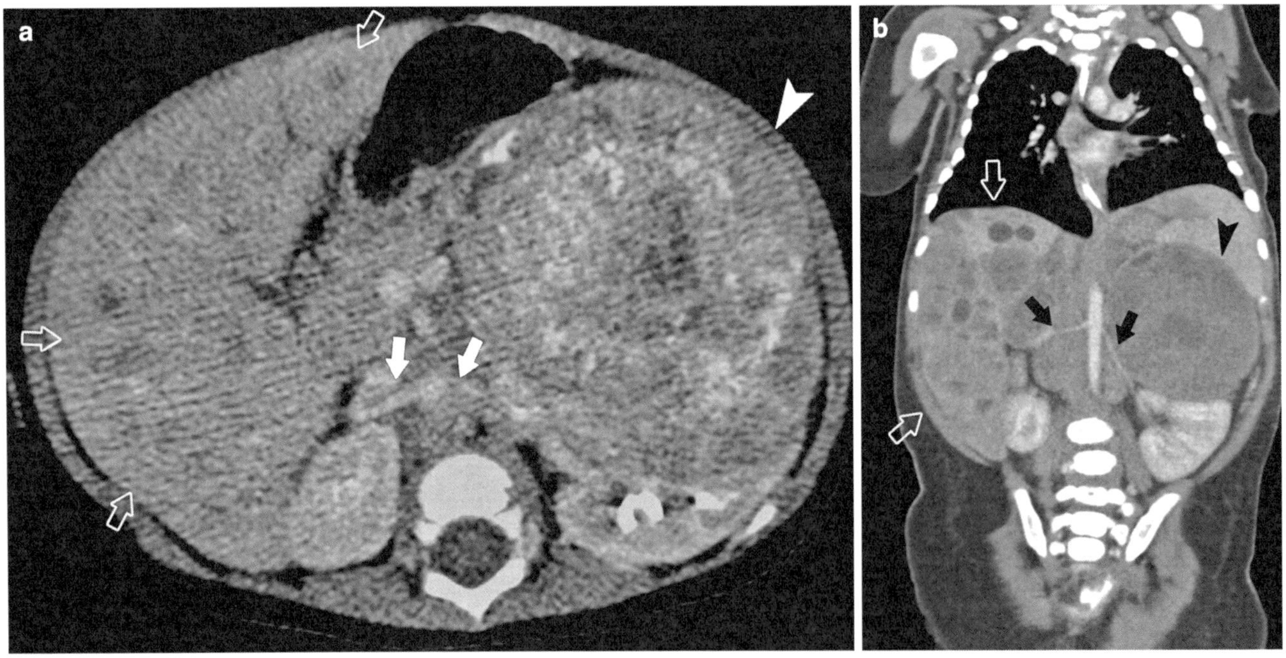

Fig. 10.20 A 2-year-old child with hypertension due to nodal encasement of both renal arteries. CT. Axial (**a**) and coronal (**b**) images show large partially calcified left adrenal mass (*arrowheads*) and nodes, inferiorly displacing the left kidney and also encasing the aorta, superior mesenteric arteries, and both renal arteries (*arrows*). Multiple hepatic metastases are also present (*open arrow*). Hypertension is uncommon in NB and, when present, is secondary to compression of the renal arteries, not from catecholamine secretion. When the nodes decrease in size, the hypertension abates [46]

IVS NB

Patients with stage IVS disease are a special group of patients with a survival rate of greater than 90 % [40, 44]. By definition, these children are less than 1 year of age and may have metastases to liver, skin, and bone marrow (<10 % bone marrow involvement) but not to cortical bone.

These tumors are frequently cystic [55, 56]. Distinction from adrenal hemorrhage may be difficult if there is no accompanying metastatic liver disease [57, 58]. Many of these tumors are discovered on routine prenatal ultrasonographic screening [51, 59–62]. These patients frequently present with skin nodules (*see* Fig. 10.22), which when biopsied, are shown to be metastatic NB [27]. These subcutaneous nodules are not a feature of older patients with neuroblastoma [27]. Extensive liver infiltration is frequently seen. These tumors almost always have favorable biologic features and will spontaneously regress on their own (*see* Fig. 10.23). In most cases, observation and close follow-up with serial ultrasonographic studies allow for eventual spontaneous regression of the tumor and the metastases without the need for any therapy (*see* Fig. 10.24) [63, 64].

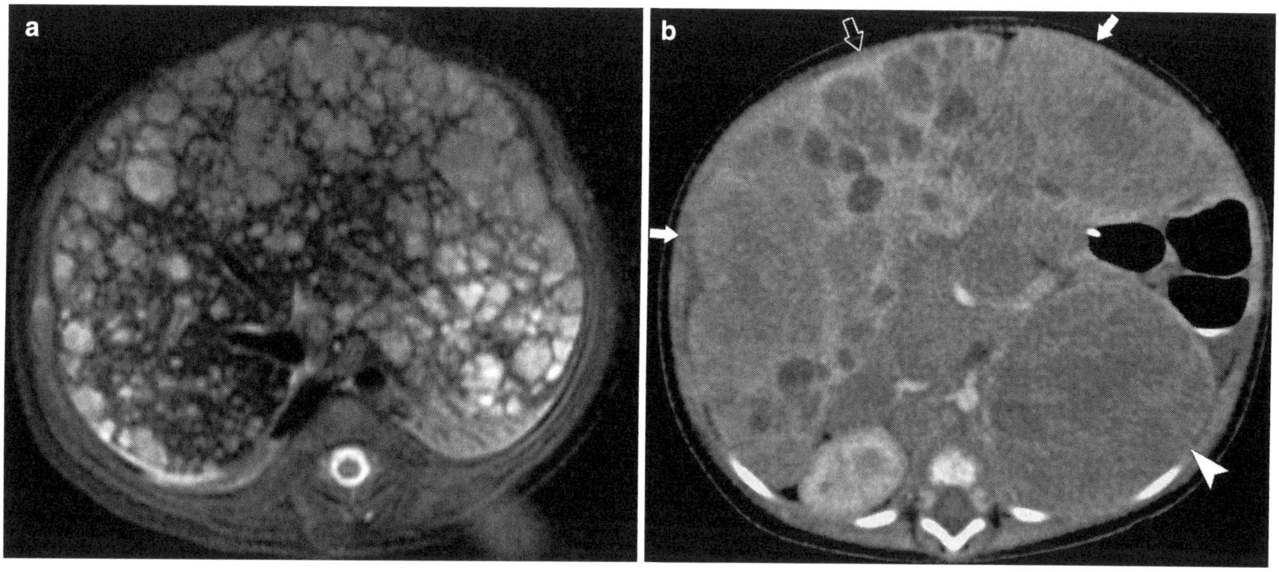

Fig. 10.21 Liver metastases. (**a**) T2-weighted, fat saturation, axial MR image showing diffuse liver metastases in a baby with IVS NB. (**b**) Axial post-contrast CT image in another infant showing a large left adrenal mass (*arrowhead*) and nodes with extensive liver infiltration. Note that some of the liver appears diffusely infiltrated (*arrows*) and some of the liver demonstrates focal nodules (*open arrow*) [27, 42, 46]

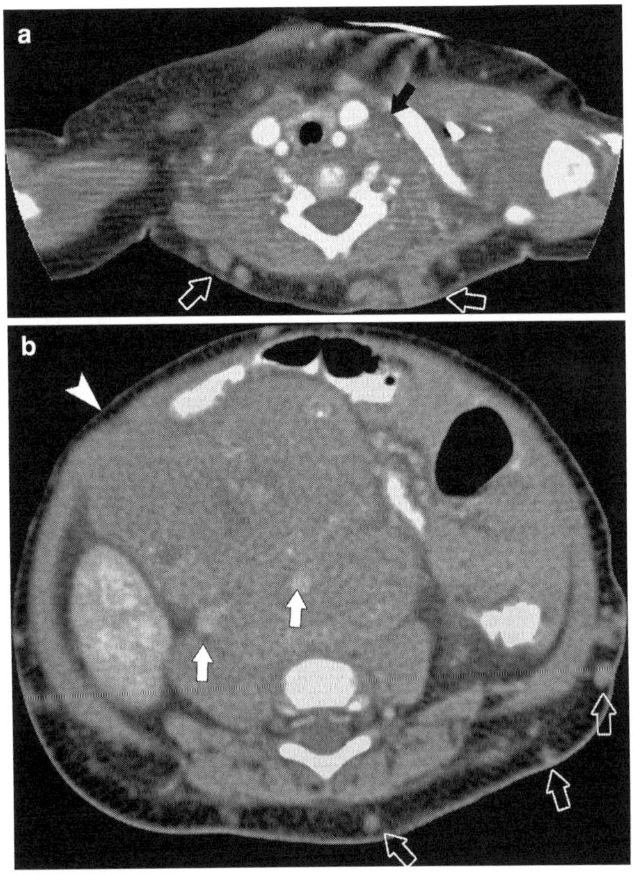

Fig. 10.22 Subcutaneous nodules. Four-month-old girl who was noted by mother to have subcutaneous nodules. Pediatrician palpated an abdominal mass. CECT demonstrates (**a**) left supraclavicular node (*arrow*) and multiple skin nodules (*open arrows*). (**b**) Large prevertebral mass with psammomatous calcifications (*arrowhead*) markedly displaces and encases the aorta. IVC is displaced anteriorly and laterally (*arrows*). (By definition, a prevertebral mass is considered stage III disease). Multiple subcutaneous nodules are also visualized (*open arrows*). Biopsy of the nodules showed neuroblastoma. Although this patient had some features of stage IVS disease, the large prevertebral primary and accompanying bone disease (not shown here) made her stage IV [27, 40, 46]

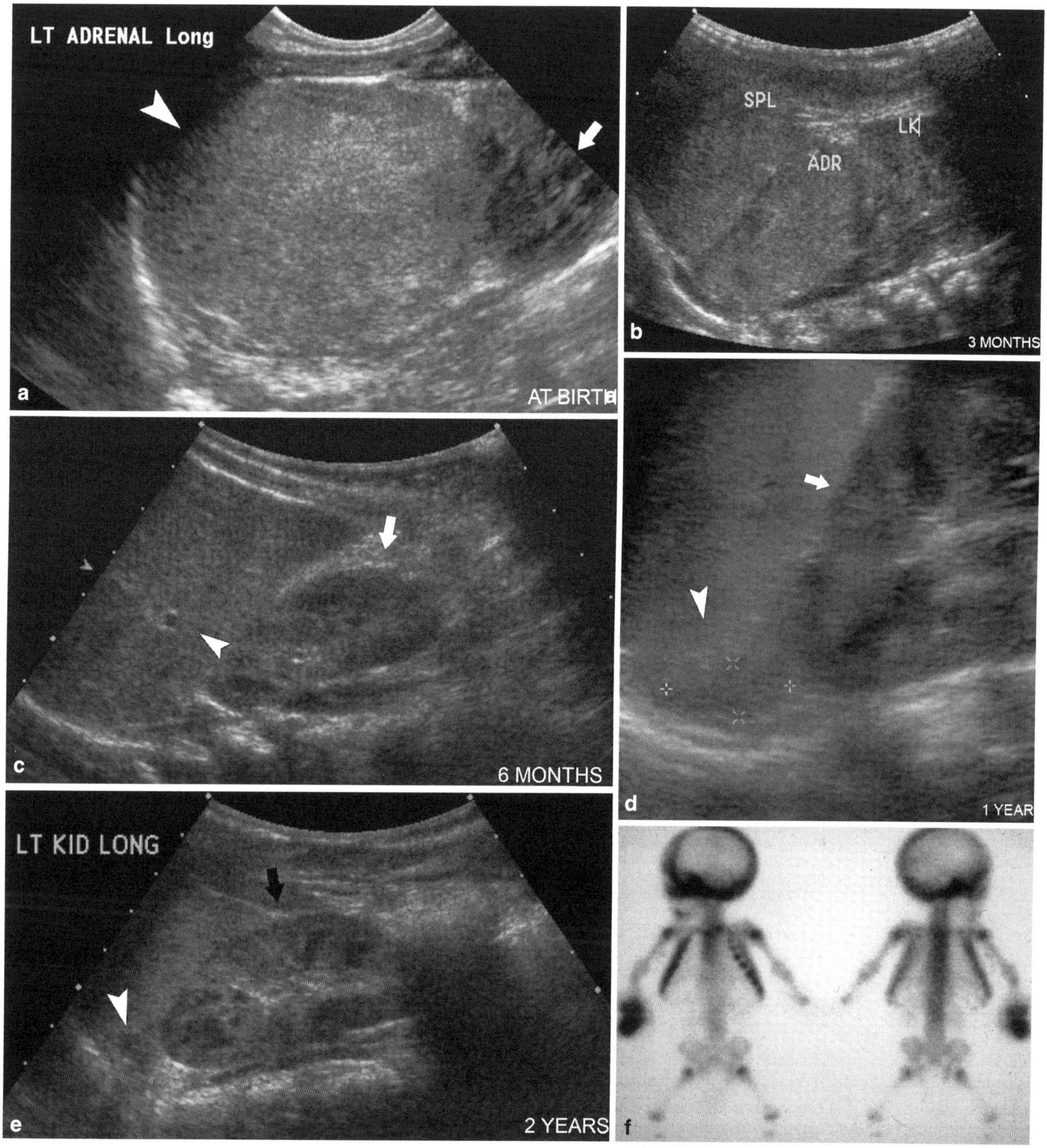

Fig. 10.23 Stage IVS NB. Mass found (*arrowheads*) in the left fetal abdomen, above the left kidney (*arrows*), on routine prenatal US. Serial longitudinal US images performed until the child was 2 years old. Patient received no therapy. (**a**) At birth, large left adrenal mass (*arrowhead*) displaces the left kidney inferiorly (*arrow*). (**b**) At 3 months, the mass is still large but has decreased in size. (**c**) At 6 months, the mass has decreased significantly. (**d**) At 1 year, tiny residual lesion. (**e**) At 2 years, small remnant of mass with tiny echogenic focus, representing calcification. (**f**) Normal bone scan. Patient must have no cortical bone disease and less than 10 % marrow involvement to be considered stage IVS [40, 51, 52, 54]

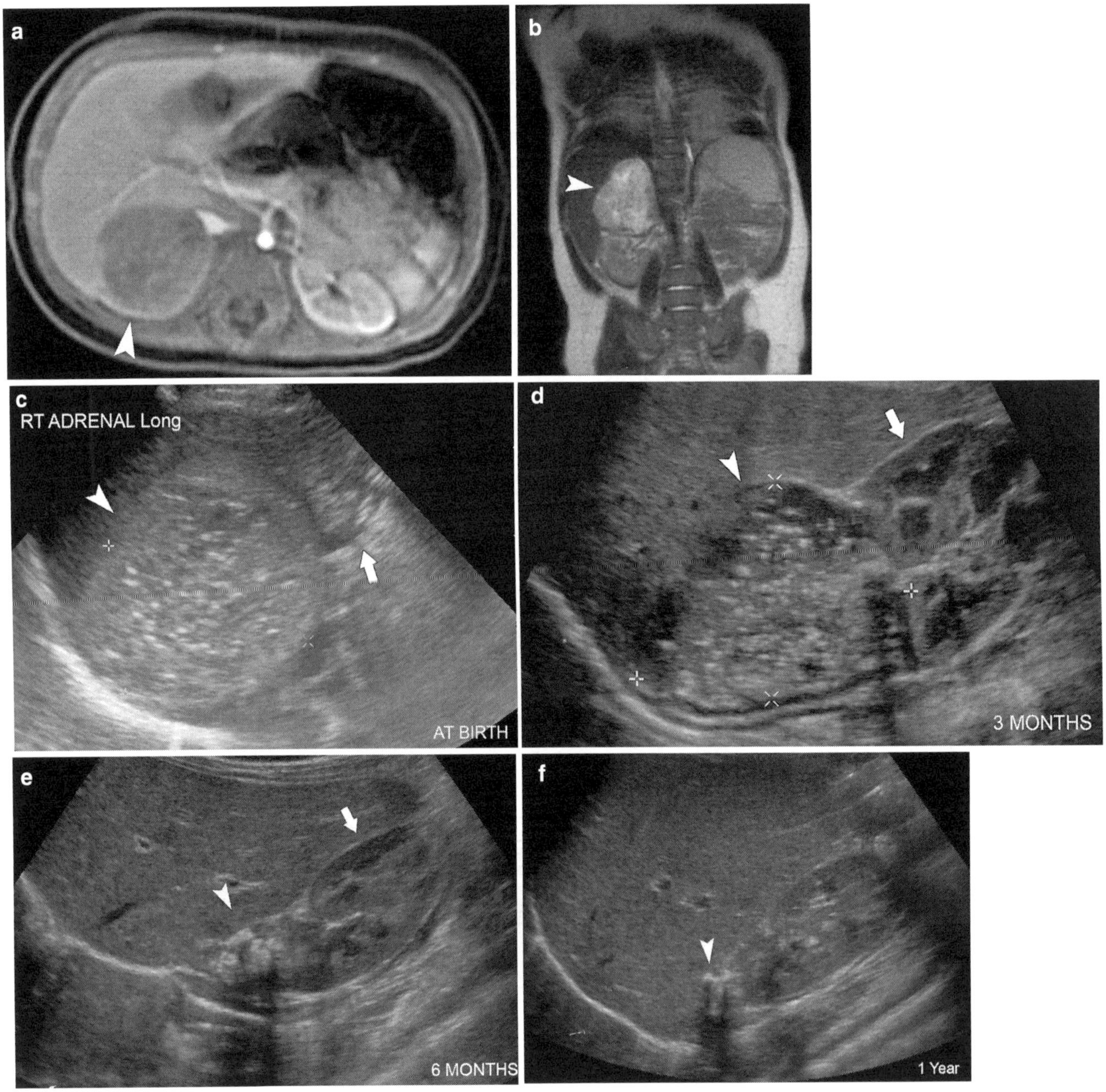

Fig. 10.24 MR images (**a**, **b**) of stage IVS in a newborn. (**a**) Axial T1-weighted post-contrast MRI demonstrates nonenhancing right adrenal mass (*arrowhead*) and no liver metastases. (**b**) Coronal T2-weighted image shows typical heterogeneous high signal in the right suprarenal mass (*arrowhead*). Areas of highest signal likely represent necrosis. Longitudinal US images (**c**–**f**). (**c**) At birth, large right adrenal mass (*arrowhead*) displacing the right kidney inferiorly (*arrow*). The mass is heterogeneous with areas of increased echogenicity, suggesting calcifications. (**d**) At 3 months, the mass has decreased in size but remains large (*arrowhead*). Kidney is still displaced inferiorly (*arrow*). (**e**) At 6 months, much more contracted mass (*arrowhead*) with shadowing echogenic foci representing calcifications. Right kidney in more normal position (*arrow*) (**f**) At 1 year, echogenic foci with very tiny mass component. The patient will continue to be followed at 3–6-month intervals until the soft tissue components (*arrowhead*) of the mass have completely resolved. Calcifications are likely to persist [63, 64].

Imaging Studies

Plain Radiographs

Evaluation of neuroblastoma requires imaging of the primary tumor and other sites of involvement. Chest film may reveal a posterior mediastinal mass with accompanying splaying of the adjacent ribs (*see* Fig. 10.25) or widening of the paraspinal line due to retrocrural disease. Abdominal radiographs may show an enlarged liver or abdominal or pelvic mass, sometimes with accompanying calcifications.

Plain images of bones may show irregular submetaphyseal lunacies. There may be accompanying periosteal reaction. Frequently, the lesions are bilaterally symmetrical. Although neuroblastoma metastases are lytic, sclerotic areas may be seen due to accompanying bone infarction.

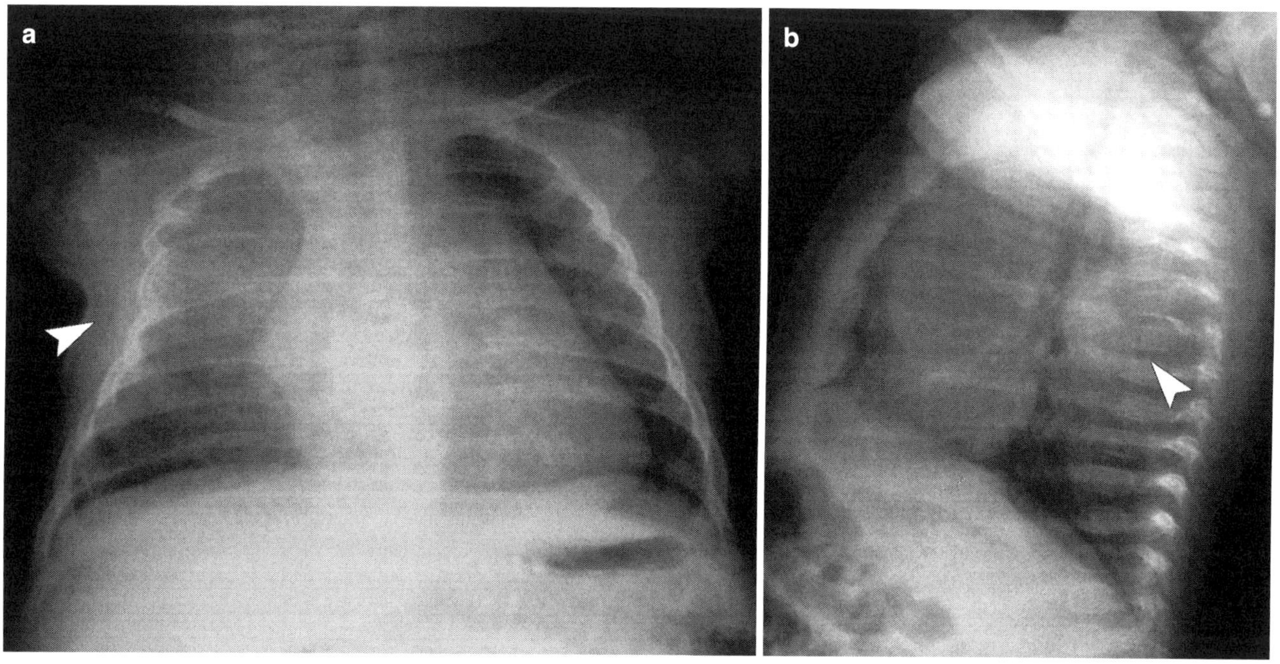

Fig. 10.25 Frontal (**a**) and lateral (**b**) plain radiographs of a 4-month-old child with wheezing. Large posterior mediastinal soft tissue mass (*arrowhead*) extending to the right with splaying and erosion of the ribs from pressure by the tumor. This does not represent bony metastatic involvement [42, 46]

Ultrasonography

Ultrasonography is the most common screening examination for the detection of an enlarged liver or an abdominal or pelvic mass in a child. The retroperitoneal location and heterogeneous echotexture of the mass will be seen. Echogenic foci with shadowing represent calcifications. The relationship of the mass to the liver, kidney, aorta, inferior vena cava (IVC), and other structures may be determined. Color Doppler will identify possible flow within the tumor and surrounding vessels. However, extent of disease cannot be adequately assessed by ultrasonography alone.

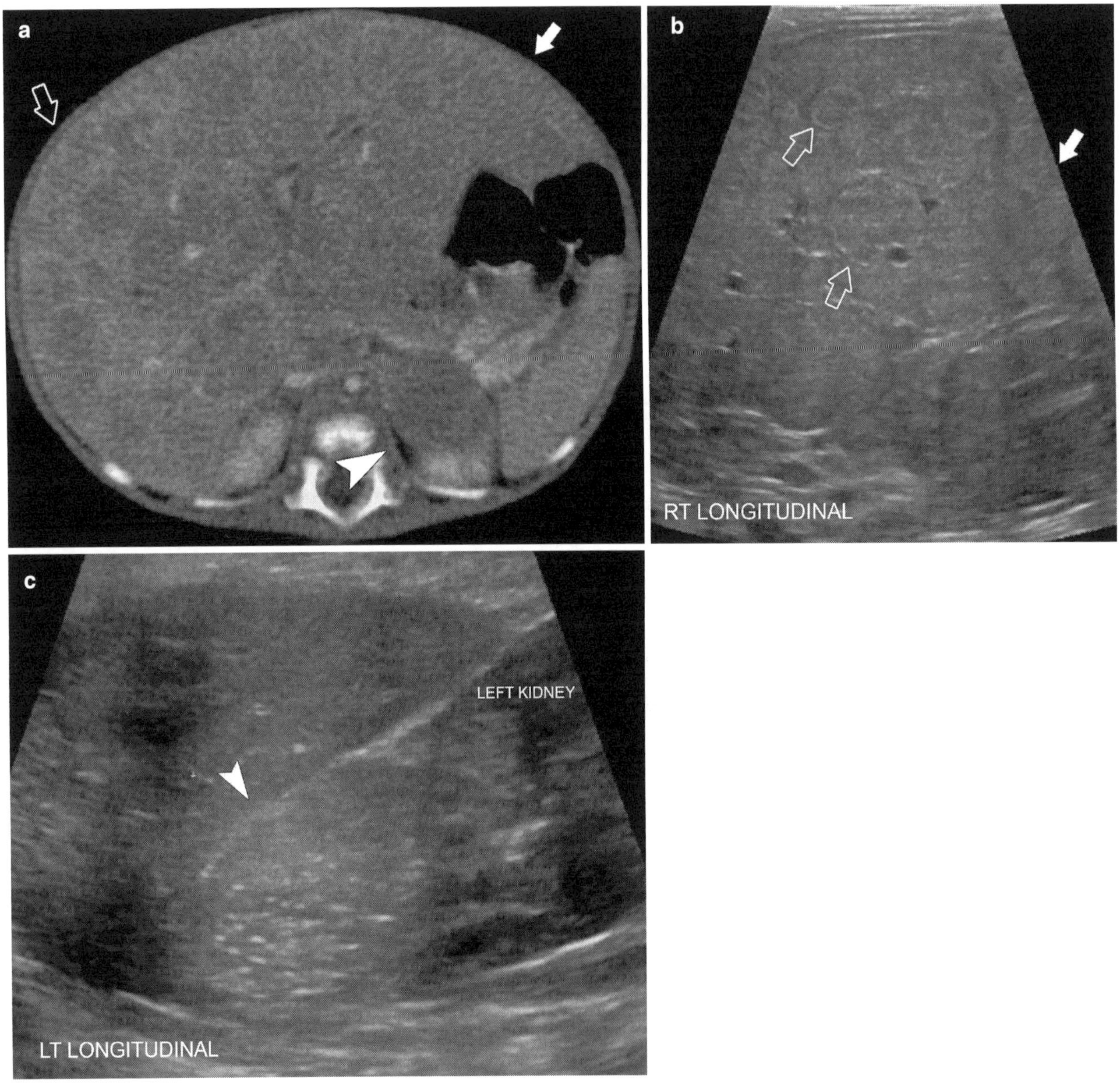

Fig. 10.26 Liver metastases seen on CT and US images in a 3-week-old infant with an enlarged abdomen. (**a**) An axial CECT image demonstrates left adrenal mass (*arrowhead*) and extensive liver involvement. There is diffuse infiltration (*arrow*) as well as focal nodules (*open arrow*) typical of stage IVS. Retroperitoneal nods are also present. (**b**, **c**) Longitudinal US. Diffuse (*arrow*) and focal (*open arrow*) liver involvement correlate with CT findings. Large heterogeneous left adrenal mass (*arrowhead*) (**c**). Evaluation of retroperitoneal nodes is demonstrated on CT and MR. US is poor for evaluating the full extent of disease [27, 42, 46]

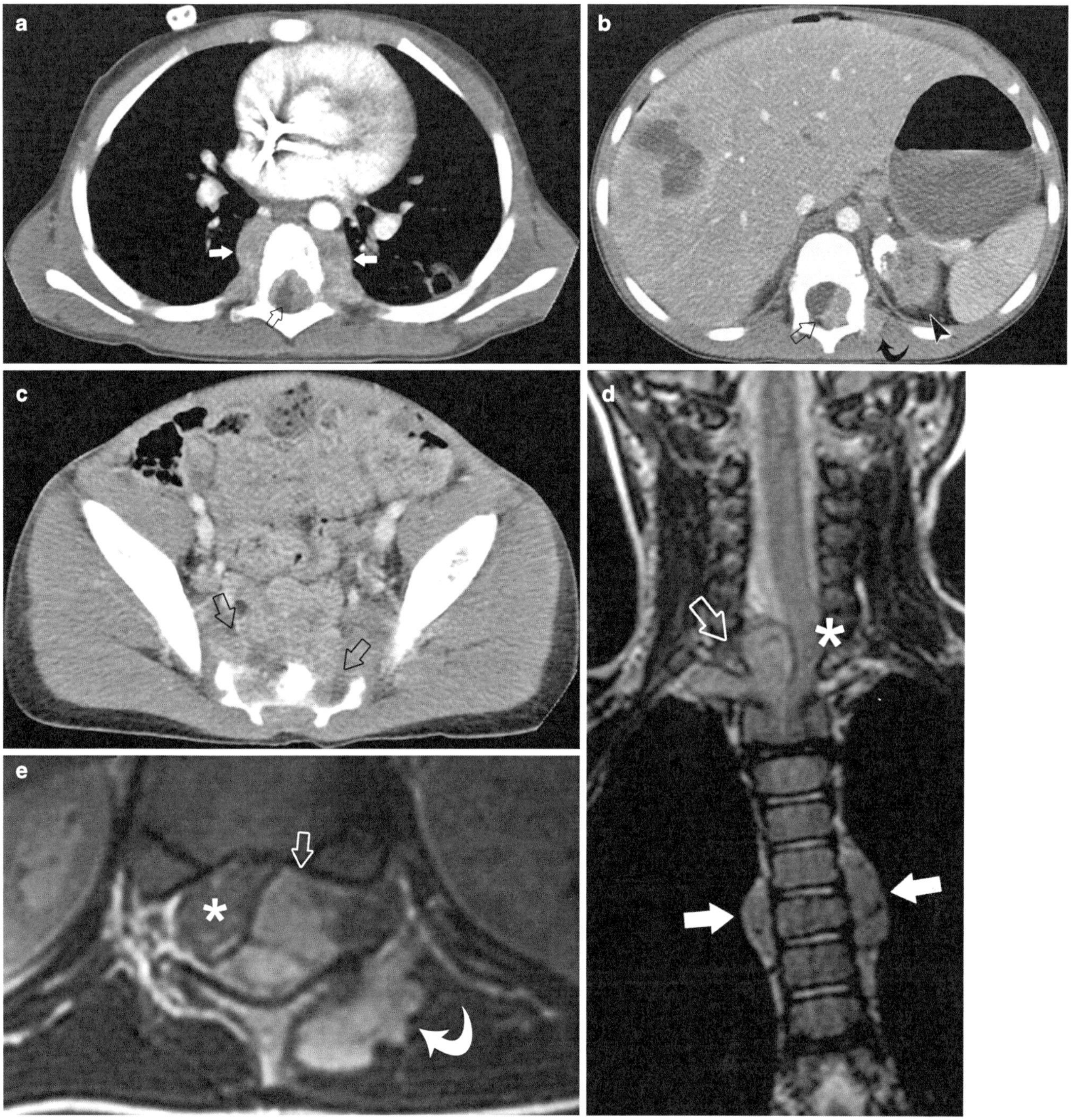

Fig. 10.27 Comparison of CT and MR in initial evaluation of extent of disease. CT. Post-contrast axial mages of the chest (**a**), abdomen (**b**), and pelvis (**c**) show paraspinal soft tissue extending into neural foramina (*open arrow*) in the thorax and abdomen. Bilateral thoracic paraspinal nodes are well seen (*closed arrow*). Partially calcified left adrenal mass (*arrowhead*), liver metastases, and tumor extension into the left posterior soft tissues (*curved arrow*) are identified. Presacral metastases with extension into sacral neural foramina are also seen (*open arrows*). T2-weighted MR images (**d–g**) of the same child much more accurately demonstrate the extent of epidural disease and its effect on the spinal cord. This is one of the advantages of MR. In addition, the primary tumor, hepatic metastases and bone disease are also well seen. (**d**) Coronal image shows paraspinal masses (*closed arrows*) as well as intraspinal extension (*open arrow*) and resulting cord compression (*asterisk*). (**e**) Axial image shows epidural tumor (*open arrow*) with displacement of the spinal cord (*asterisk*). Soft tissue mass is also seen (*curved arrow*). (**f**) Coronal image shows the primary left adrenal mass (*arrowhead*) and liver metastases. (**g**) Sagittal image shows multilevel intraspinal disease (*open arrow*) as well as bone involvement (*X*). Bone scan (**h**) shows disease in the spine whereas the MIBG (**i**) demonstrates soft tissue disease and bone involvement. Note that the MIBG study demonstrates activity in more bony sites than the bone scan. MIBG does not differentiate marrow disease from cortical bone disease. Bone scans depict only cortical bone involvement [45, 67]

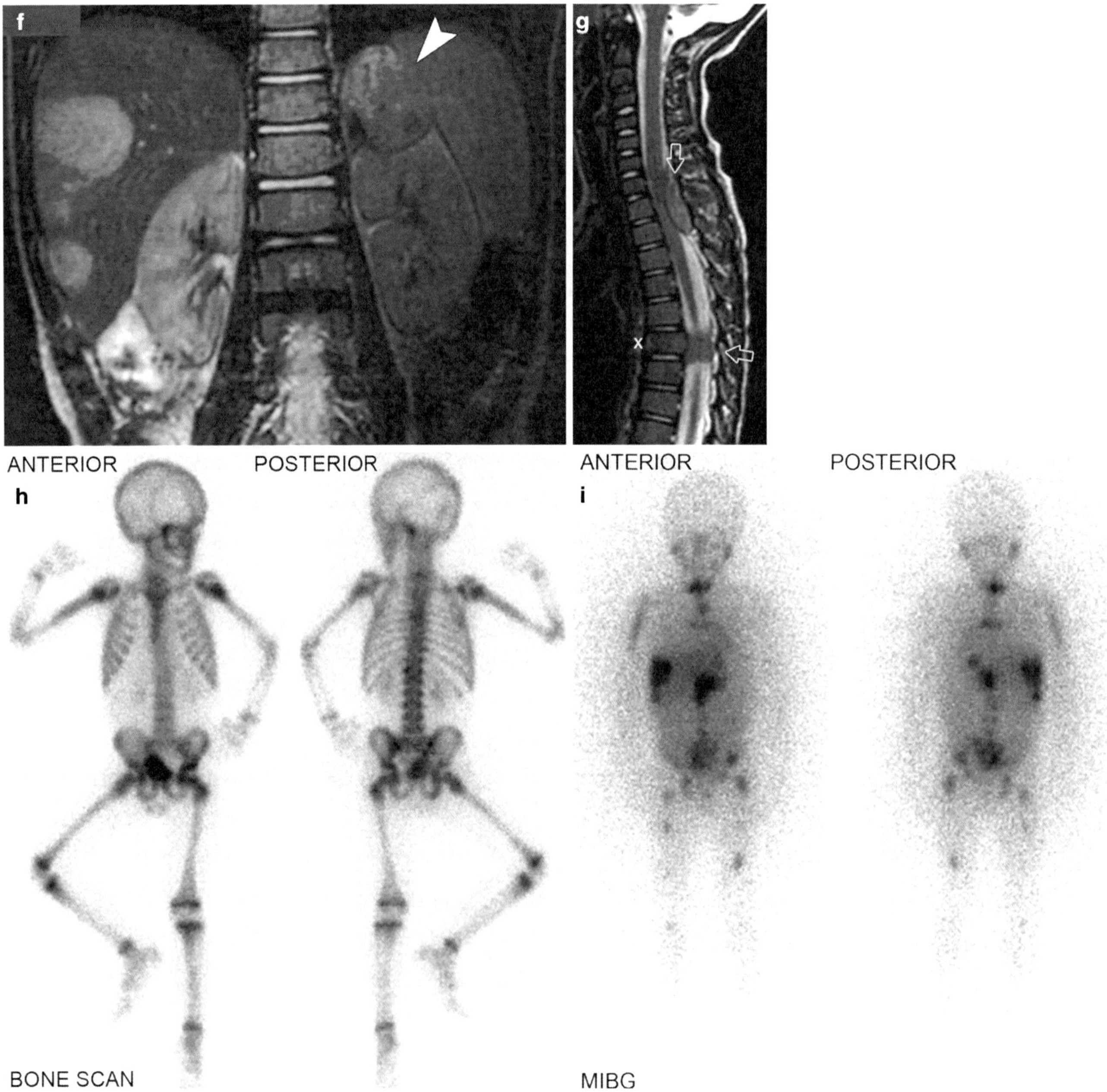

Fig. 10.27 (continued)

Magnetic Resonance, Computed Tomography, and Nuclear Medicine Studies

MRI or CT with technetium 99 m methylene diphosphonate bone scintigraphy (bone scan) and I^{123} Metaiodobenzylguanidine scan (MIBG), when possible, is mandatory as a guide to staging, resectability, prognosis, and follow-up. It has been shown that MR alone is comparable to CT and bone scan together and better than CT alone in the evaluation of extent of disease at diagnosis. Combining MR with bone scan gives the most accurate information for staging. CT alone is relatively inaccurate in evaluating bone involvement [65]. Integrated imaging using MR and MIBG for evaluation of disease extent may also be useful [66].

MR provides evaluation without the use of ionizing radiation [67]. Oral and intravenous contrast are not required for evaluation. However, the length of time required for the study frequently necessitates the use of general anesthesia in young children. The primary lesion is well seen and the relationship of the tumor to surrounding vessels and other structures is clearly delineated (*see* Fig. 10.27) [68].

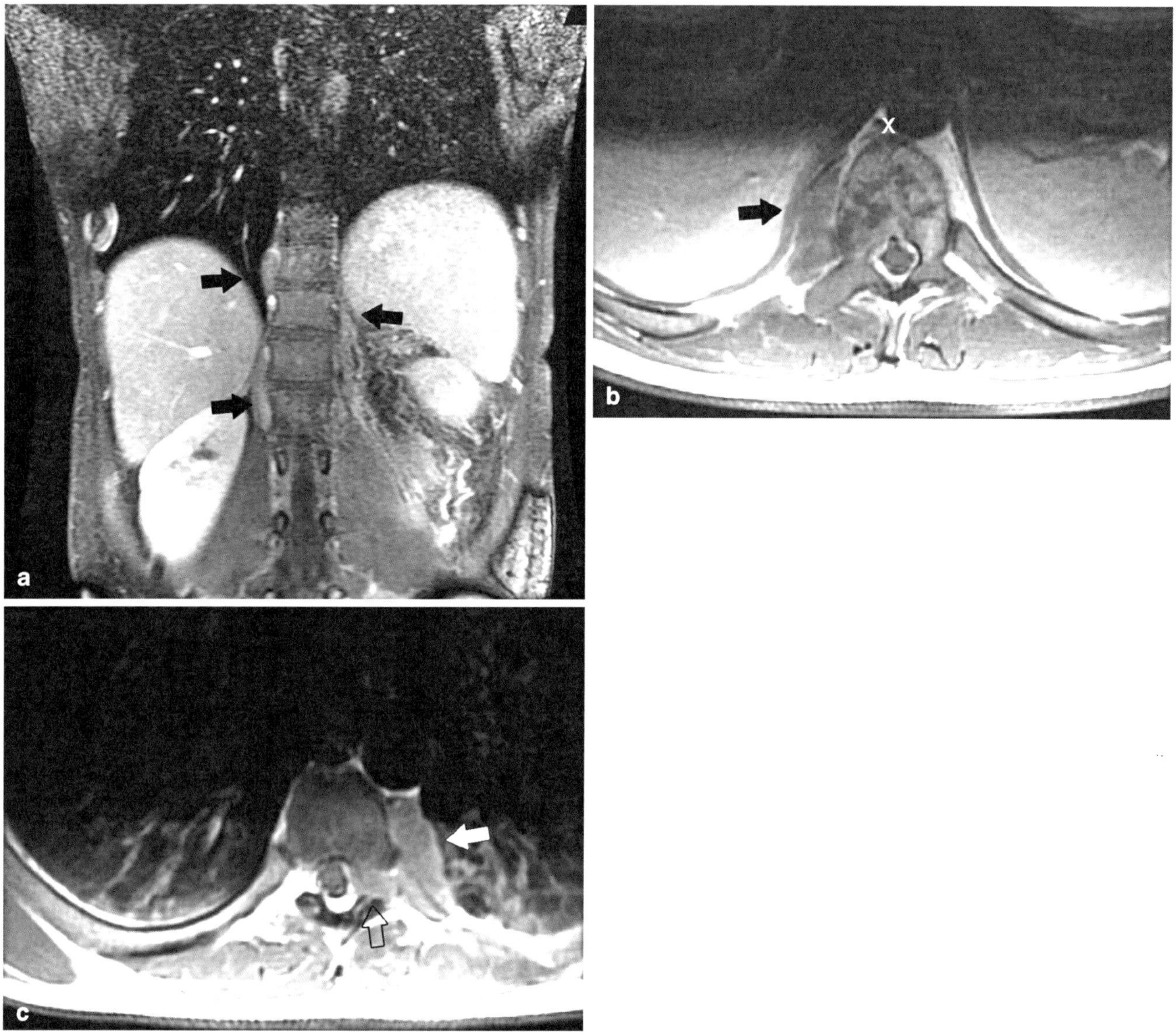

Fig. 10.28 An 18-year-old man with back pain. T1-weighted MR post-contrast coronal (**a**) and axial (**b**, **c**) images reveal multiple paraspinal lymph nodes (*closed arrows*). Paraspinal nodal involvement is common. Left paraspinal node extending into the adjacent neural foramen and causing effacement of the spinal cord (*open arrow* in **c**) is common in neuroblastoma. MR evaluation should be performed to evaluate extent of epidural disease and possible cord compression. Note also abnormal heterogeneous signal in the vertebral body (X) on (**b**) [67]

Nodal and liver involvements are also visualized (*see* Fig. 10.28). Liver involvement is better assessed with MR (*see* Fig. 10.29). Particularly important is the ability of MR to detect bone and epidural disease (*see* Fig. 10.30) [69]. This cannot be adequately evaluated with CT. Evaluation of bone disease is important not only in staging but also in directing possible sites for bone marrow biopsy, where disease is likely to be present instead of merely performing routine iliac crest biopsies (*see* Fig. 10.31) [70–75]. MR evaluation of marrow after therapy can be very difficult. Marrow regrowth may simulate disease [76]. For patients with low and intermediate risk disease, MR and US are used for follow-up. CT can be helpful in follow-up of patients with high-risk disease where small partially calcified nodes, not readily visible on MR or US, may be harbingers of recurrence.

Because the diagnosis of neuroblastoma is frequently not made beforehand, CT is commonly the study first performed after US. It is important to stress that if CT is to be used, it should always be obtained with the lowest possible radiation dose in conjunction with ALARA (As Low as Reasonably

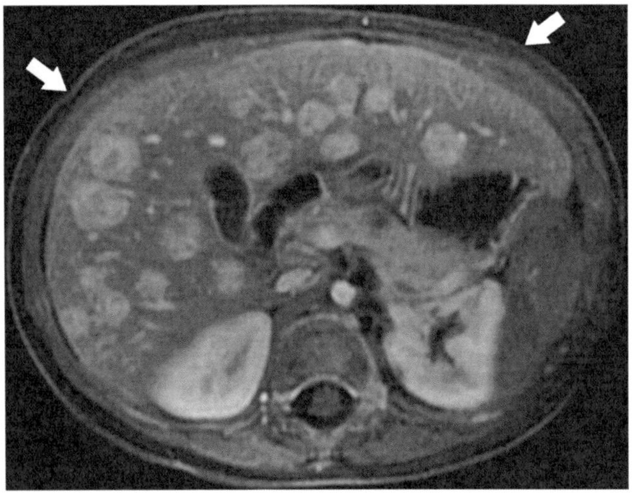

Fig. 10.29 Liver involvement is better imaged on MR as demonstrated on this T1-weighted post-contrast axial image of the liver that shows multiple hepatic metastases (*arrow*) [68]

Achievable) principles [77, 78]. When CT is performed with proper oral and bolus intravenous contrast administration, it is an excellent tool in evaluation of neuroblastoma. Fast scan times now preclude the necessity for general anesthesia in many children. The lack of intraperitoneal fat limits evaluation in young patients. Just as with MR, the ability to image the abdomen and pelvis in multiple planes is extremely useful to the radiologist and to the surgeon. Disease extension into neural foramina is suboptimally visualized on CT and MR is necessary for complete evaluation (*see* Fig. 10.32). CT is poor for visualization of bony metastases [65]. Sites that are abnormal on bone scan, MIBG, or MR may look normal on CT. Bones that appear abnormal on CT at diagnosis continue to appear abnormal, even after they have reverted to normal on the previously mentioned studies (*see* Fig. 10.33). Periosteal reaction and frank bone destruction with accompanying soft tissue masses can be identified (*see* Fig. 10.34).

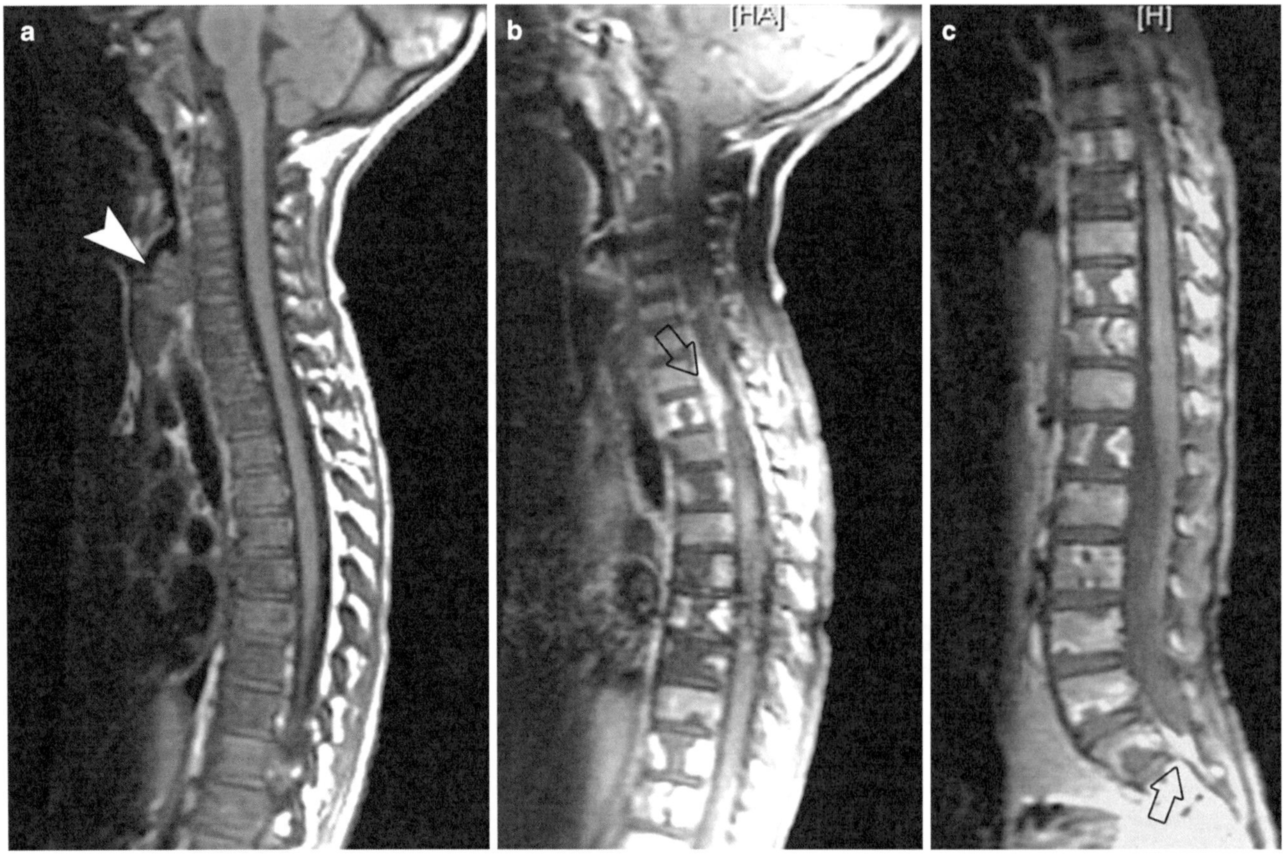

Fig. 10.30 Bone involvement in NB. Sagittal T1-weighted image of the thoracic spine (**a**) and sagittal T1-weighted post-contrast images of the thoracic and lumbar spine (**b**, **c**) in a child with a primary upper thoracic neuroblastoma. Heterogeneous low signal on T1-weighted images and heterogeneous enhancement on post-contrast images demonstrate multilevel marrow disease. The primary tumor (*arrowhead*) is partially imaged in (**a**). In addition, there is epidural extension (*open arrows*) in the upper thorax (**b**) and in the sacrum (**c**). Marrow involvement is frequently diffuse but patchy. MR is excellent at localizing levels and extent of disease at diagnosis. T1-weighted post-contrast images will also pick-up new sites of marrow involvement in patients with previously treated disease [73, 74]

Up to 60 % of patients have bone metastases at diagnosis. Therefore, bone scan is important for full evaluation. The primary tumor demonstrates increased activity on bone scan in up to 74 % of cases (*see* Fig. 10.35) [79]. Other soft tissue disease is not identified in this study. Whole body imaging is important in detecting asymptomatic bony involvement. Follow-up scans usually demonstrate response to therapy. New areas of increased activity are highly suggestive of recurrent disease.

MIBG scans demonstrate both bony and soft tissue disease, but do not distinguish between marrow and cortical bone involvement (*see* Fig. 10.36) [80–82]. The agent, an analog of catecholamine precursors is taken up by catecholamine-producing cells. It was originally devised for the detection of pheochromocytoma; however, in children it is mainly used to evaluate neuroblastoma (*see* Fig. 10.37). Up to 30 % of patients with neuroblastoma at diagnosis or at relapse may not be MIBG positive [80–82]. When recurrent

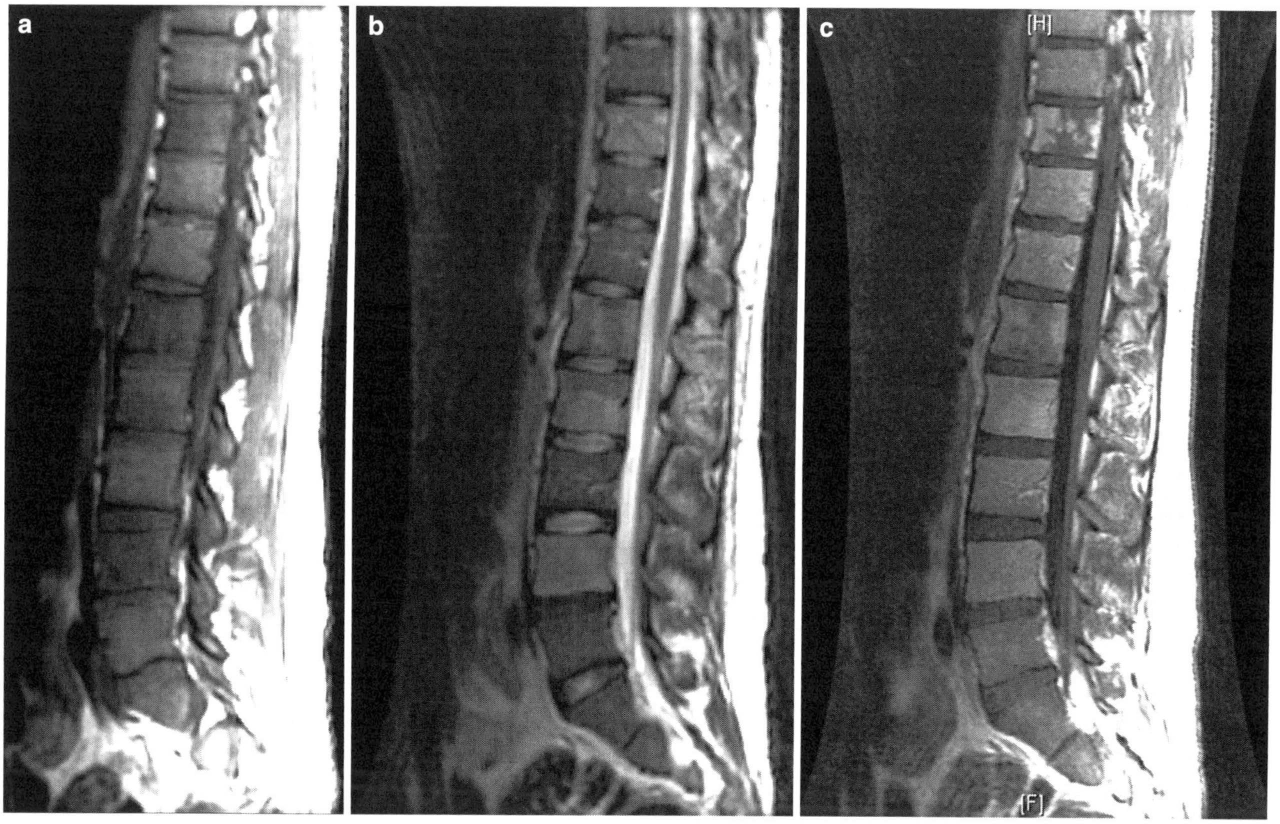

Fig. 10.31 Marrow disease in NB. Sagittal MR images demonstrate diffuse, patchy marrow involvement with decreased signal on T1-weighted image (**a**), increased signal on T2-weighted image (**b**), and heterogeneous enhancement on the post-contrast image (**c**)

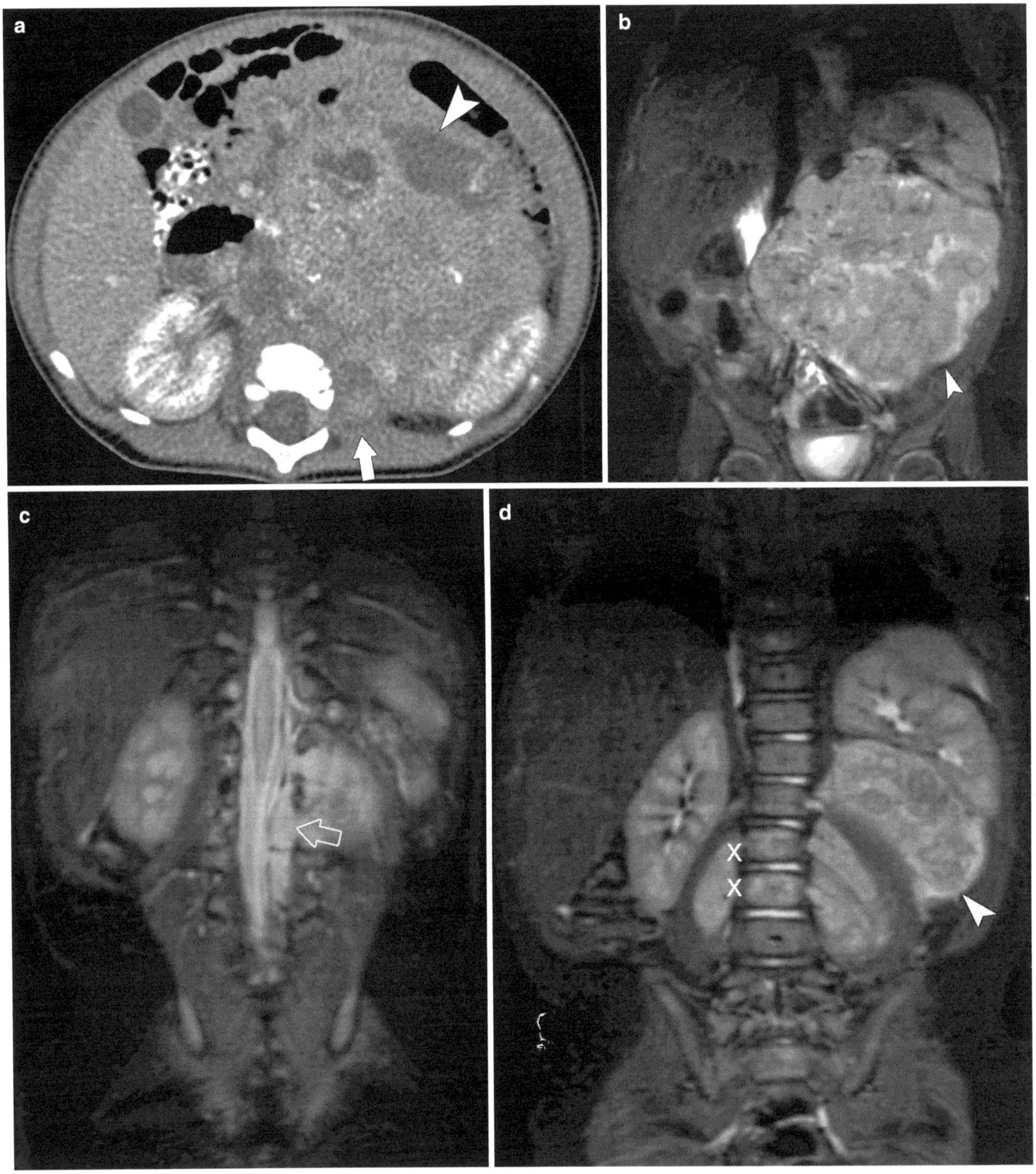

Fig. 10.32 Conglomerate mass and nodes. Axial and coronal post-contrast CT (**a**, **b**) show a left partially calcified mass and nodes. The mass and nodes form a conglomerate that cannot be separated (*arrowheads*). This conglomerate crosses the midline. Midline in NB is defined as the lateral aspect of the contralateral side of the vertebral body from the tumor. According to the INSS, this in itself represents stage III disease. The mass cannot be separated from the left psoas muscle (*closed arrow*), a common occurrence in NB. Coronal MR T2-weighted images (**c**, **d**) show epidural extension on the left at multiple levels (*open arrow*). MR much more clearly demonstrates epidural disease. Note also the marrow involvement of two lower lumbar vertebrae (*X*). MR provides critical information with regard to epidural and marrow disease [45]

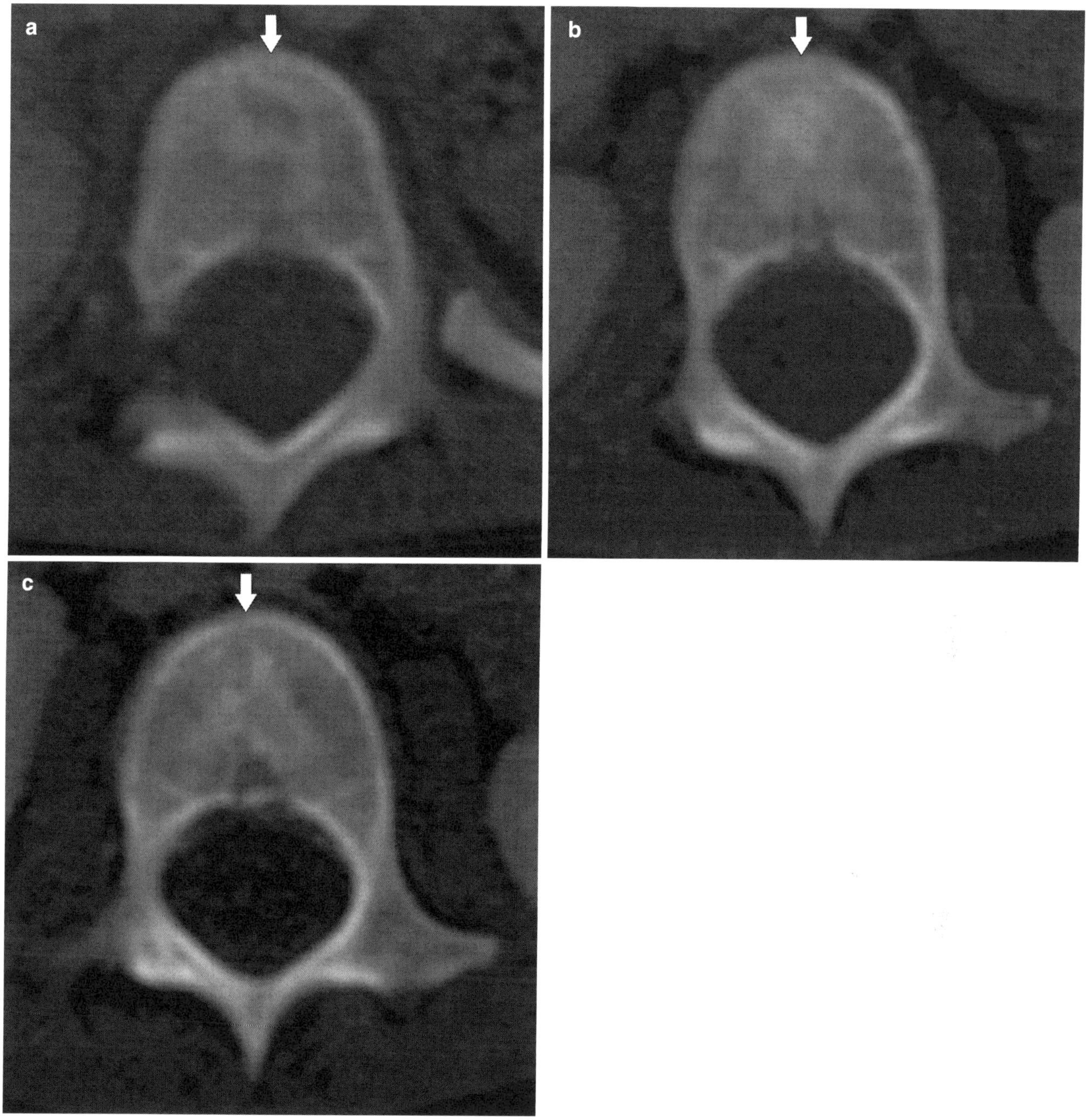

Fig. 10.33 Bone E lesions on CT. Images show typical bony changes on CT (*closed arrows*). They may be lytic (**a**), sclerotic (**b**), or mixed (**c**). At diagnosis, most patients have bone involvement. CT may show no evidence of this disease in the face of positive bone scan and MIBG scan. On the other hand, CT may demonstrate bony changes. These are usually lytic areas in bone but they may be sclerotic due to accompanying bone necrosis in young children. Bone lesions seen on CT at diagnosis will remain, even after the patient has been treated and the bone scan and MIBG have reverted to normal. Therefore, the extent of active bone disease cannot be evaluated on CT. Unless lesions with periosteal reaction and accompanying soft tissue masses are present, indicating new disease, CT cannot be used to evaluate the activity of the bone disease [46]

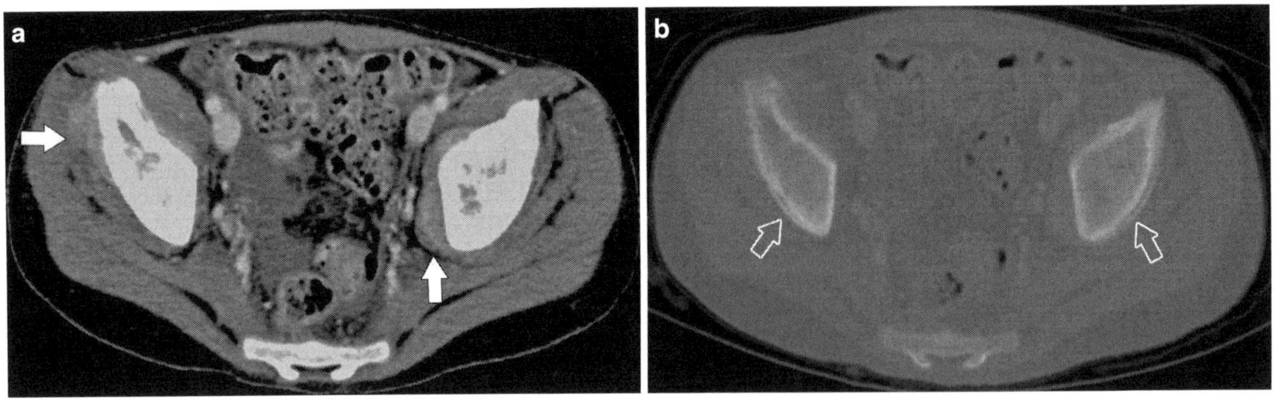

Fig. 10.34 New bone disease demonstrated on CT. Soft tissue (**a**) and bone (**b**) windows on axial post-contrast CT. Periosteal reaction (*open arrows*) and soft tissue masses (*closed arrows*) in the bilateral iliac bone signal active bone metastases

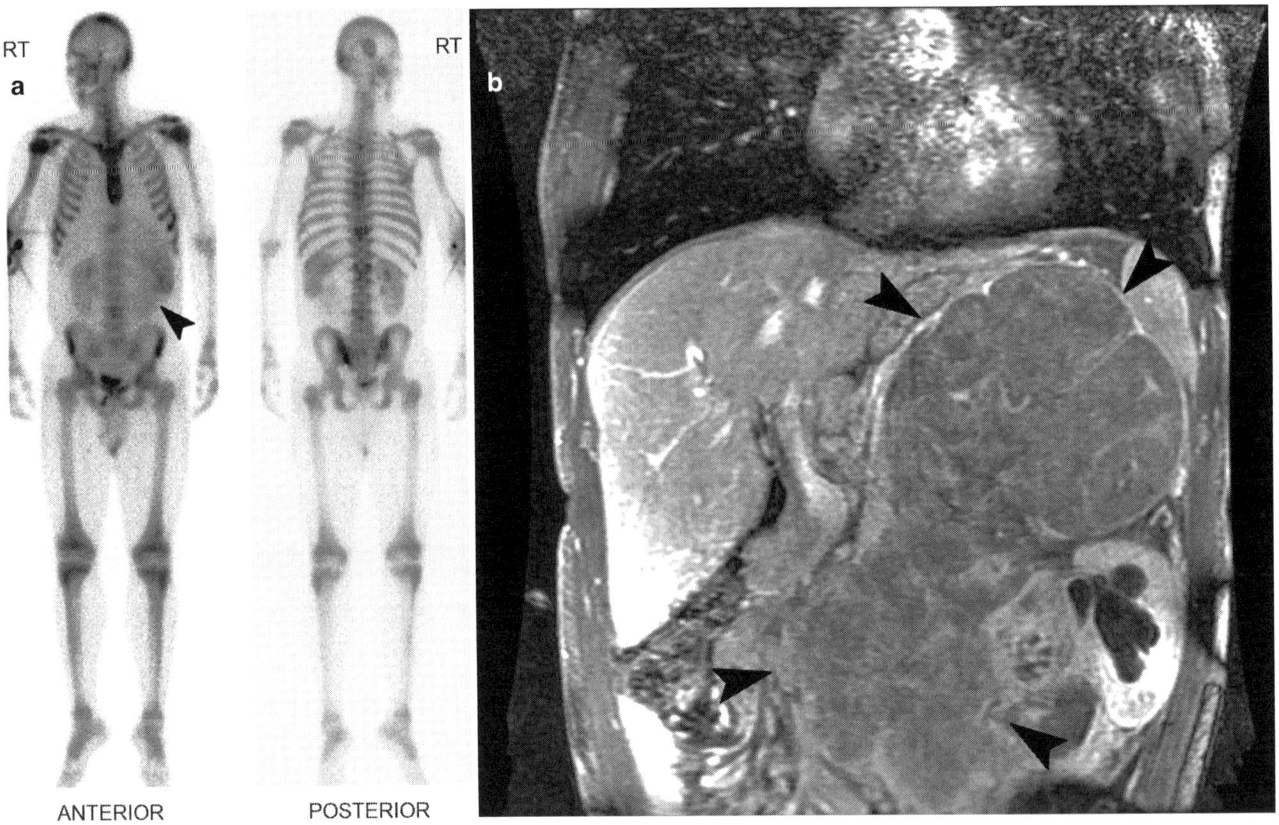

Fig. 10.35 Bone uptake in NB. Boy presented with back pain for several months. (**a**) Anterior and posterior images from bone scan reveal skull and vertebral bony metastases. Mild uptake in the primary left mass (*arrowhead*) is also seen, a common occurrence in NB. (**b**) Coronal T1-weighted post-contrast MR image shows the large left heterogeneous conglomerate mass and nodes extending from the diaphragm to the pelvis (*arrowhead*) [78]

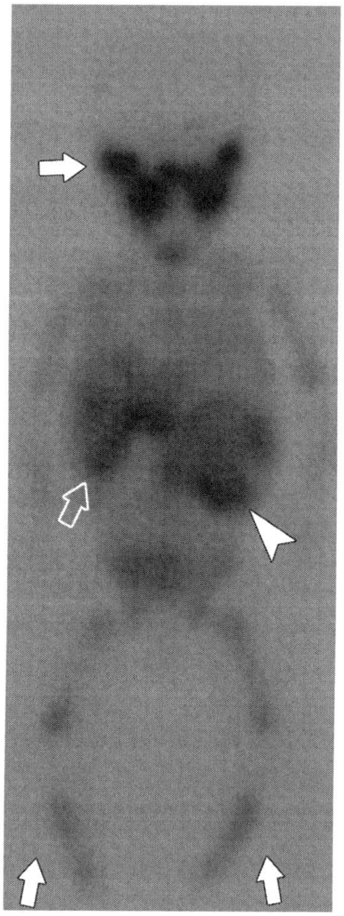

Fig. 10.36 MIBG uptake is seen in both soft tissue and bone disease. This MIBG scan demonstrates uptake in a large left mass and nodes (*arrowhead*), as well as the live orbits (*open arrow*) and most long bones (*arrows*). The bony abnormalities may be in cortical bone or marrow

disease is demonstrated on CT or MR in the face of a negative MIBG study, positron emission tomography utilizing 2-[fluorine-2,418]-fluoro-2-deoxy-D-glucose (PET) is useful in confirming new disease (*see* Fig. 10.38) [83, 84]. The full role of PET in the evaluation of neuroblastoma is not yet determined (*see* Fig. 10.39) [84, 85]. However, it appears that PET is very useful in visualizing small residual soft tissue metastases that may not be visible on MIBG and that MIBG may be better at visualizing bone and bone marrow deposits [86, 87]. PET 64 or other agents, such as ^{111}In-pentetreotide are occasionally used in patients with tumors that are not MIBG positive [88].

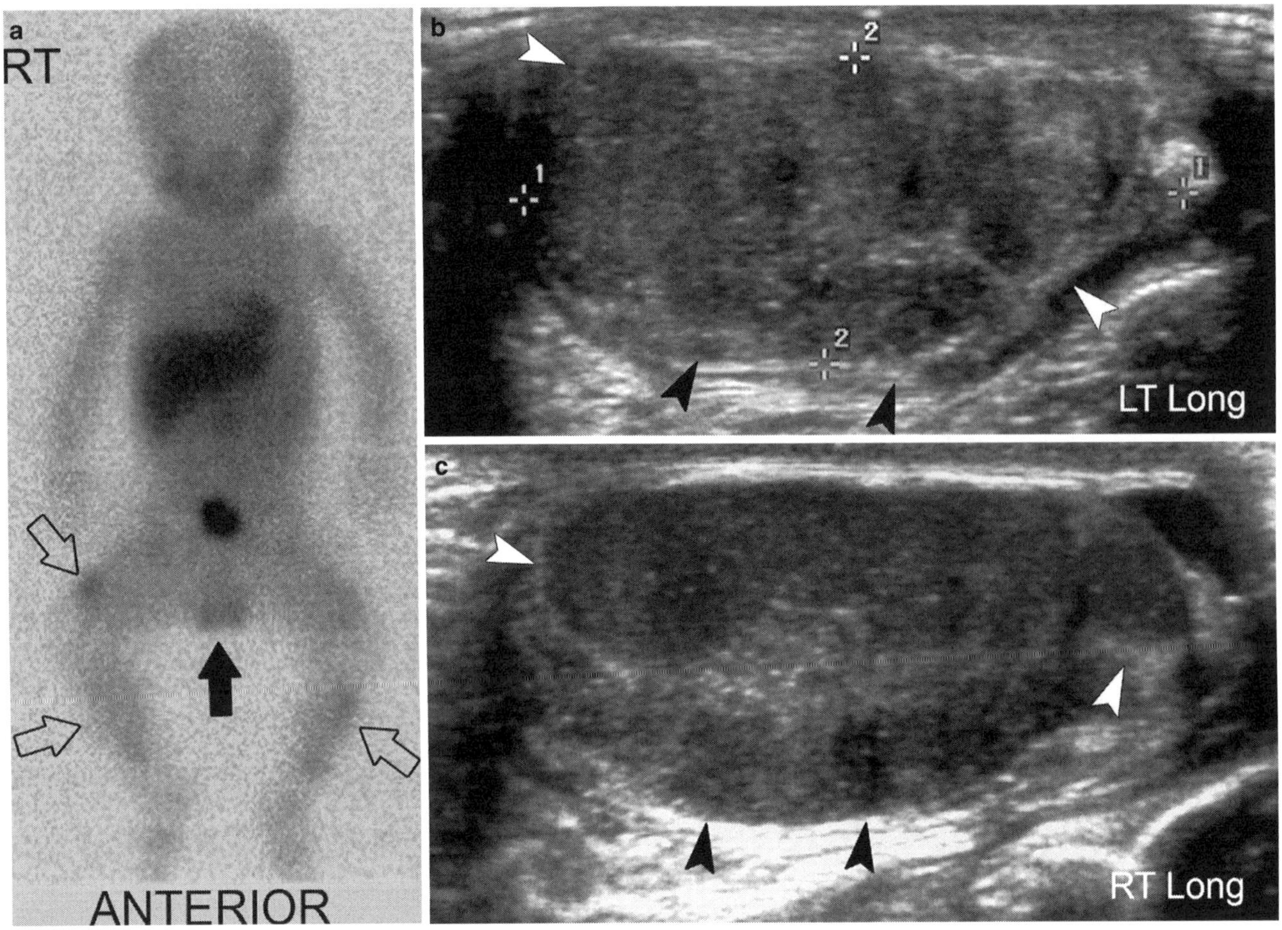

Fig. 10.37 Testicular involvement in NB. **A**(**a**) MIBG scan demonstrating uptake in the testes (*arrow*) as well as multiple bone (*open arrows*) in this 4-month-old boy who presented with a lesion on his penis and enlarged testes. All sites were biopsied and proven to be neuroblastoma. Longitudinal US images of the left (**b**) and right (**c**) testes demonstrate heterogeneous masses in both testes (*arrowheads*). Further imaging revealed a left adrenal mass and nodes. His biologic features were unfavorable and he has been treated as having stage IV high-risk disease. This is an example of a child presenting at a young age, who would have been expected to have IVS disease but whose extent of disease and biologic factors placed him in a high-risk category. He has subsequently had several relapses, including CNS disease

Fig. 10.38 False-negative MIBG Scan. Axial CECT (**a**) demonstrated a new metastatic left hilar mass (*arrowhead*). MIBG scan was negative (**b**). PET (**c**) demonstrated that the lesion, which was resected and shown to be metastatic NB (*arrowhead*). PET may be useful in demonstrating newly suspicious findings on CT or MR that are not MIBG avid. Up to 30 % of children may be MIBG negative at diagnosis or relapse [46]

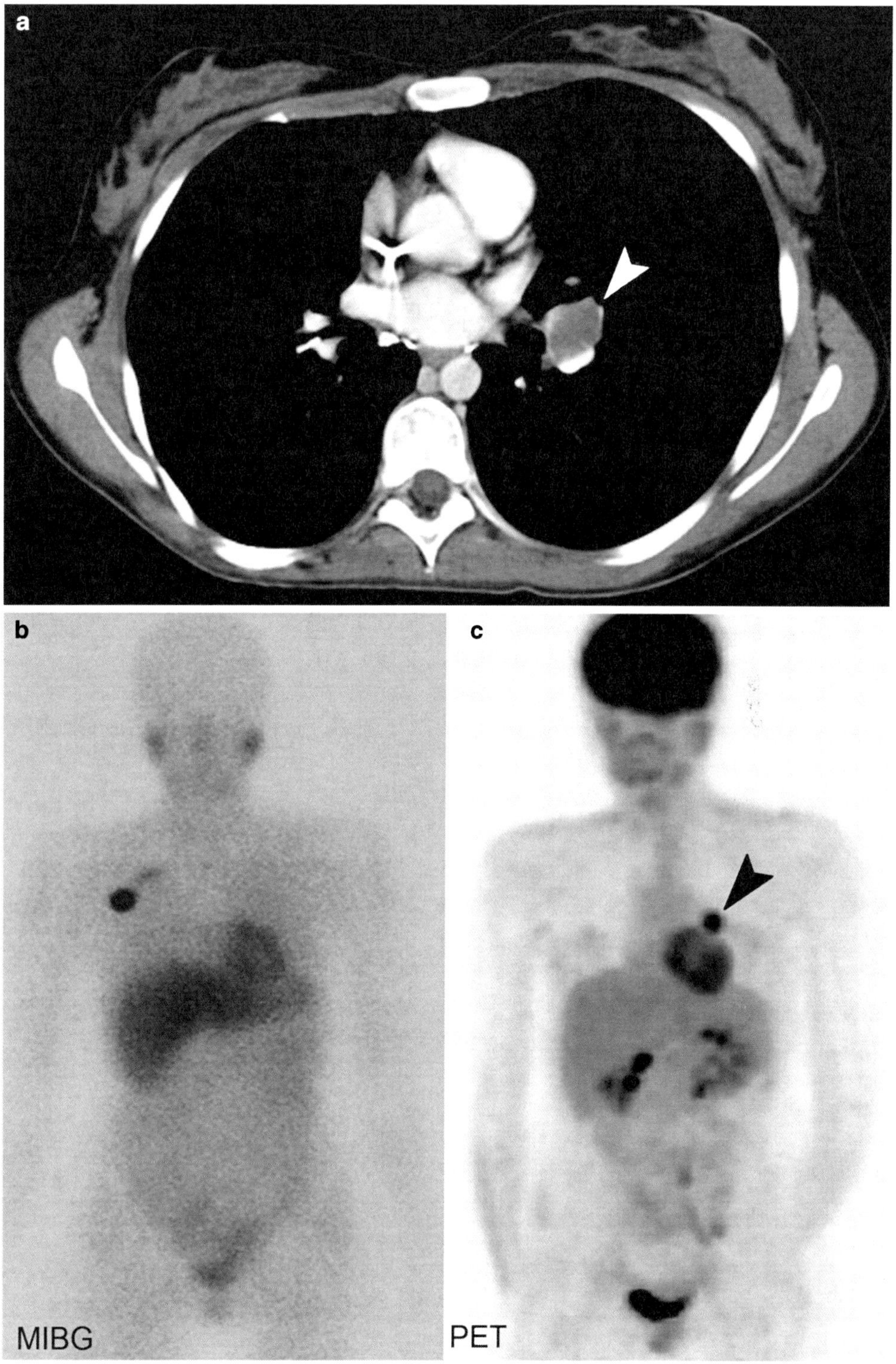

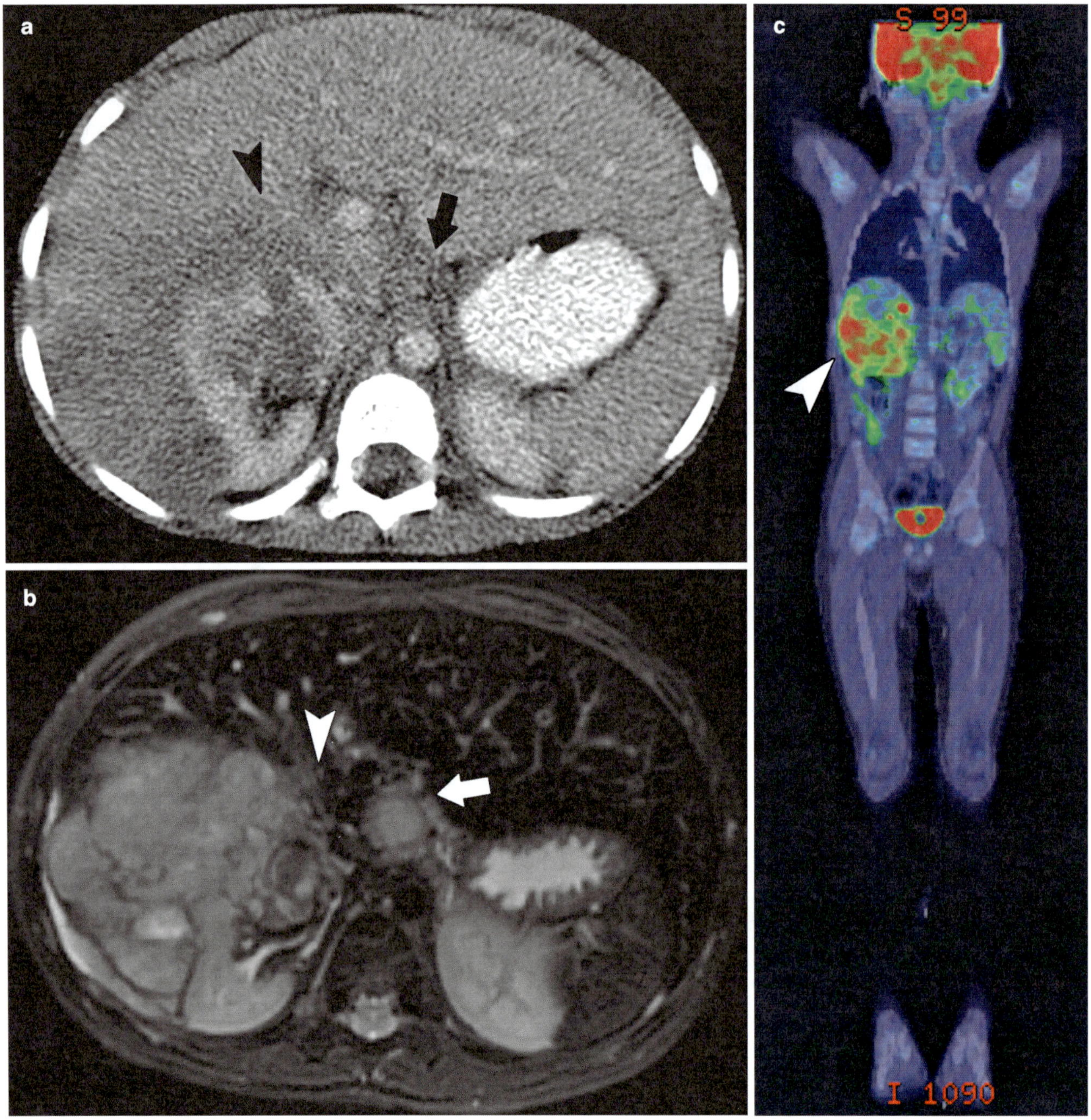

Fig. 10.39 Aggressive NB. Axial post-contrast CT image (**a**) demonstrates a large aggressive NB invading the kidney (*arrowhead*) with extensive retroperitoneal adenopathy (*arrow*). Corresponding T1-weighted post-contrast axial MR image (**b**) more clearly delineates the tumor in the right kidney (*arrowhead*) and the abnormal nodes (*arrow*). PET image (**c**) shows FDG avidity in the mass (*arrowhead*) and nodes. The upper pole of the right kidney cannot be delineated from the tumor [66]

Therapy

Children with low-risk disease receive minimal therapy. Surgery alone or close observation with US (4 S disease) is recommended. Patients with intermediate-risk disease also receive chemotherapy. The most comprehensive therapy is reserved for patients with high-risk disease, who have a guarded prognosis. Surgery has been found to prolong survival in patients with high-grade disease, whether performed at diagnosis or after administration of chemotherapy. Careful follow-up of high-risk patients is necessary to identify recurrence as early as possible so that these patients may receive new chemotherapeutic regimens in an effort to cure the disease.

When disease recurs, it may be demonstrated at the primary site of disease or elsewhere. Involvement of nodes, bone, and bone marrow are common. Late recurrences in pulmonary parenchyma (*see* Fig. 10.40) and CNS may also be seen. High-risk disease tends to recur within the first 1–2 years after completion of therapy; therefore, it is important to closely monitor these patients.

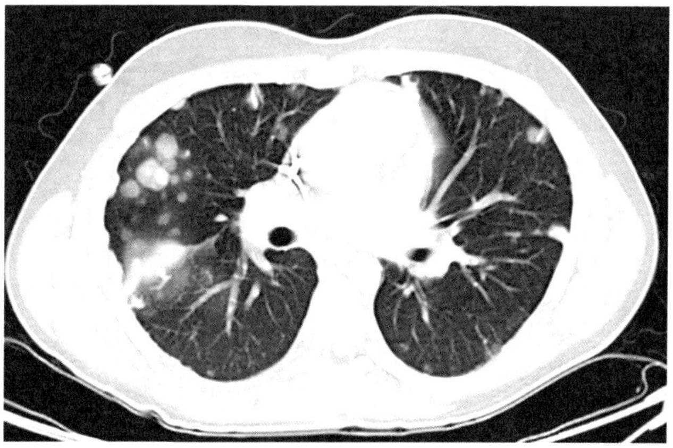

Fig. 10.40 Pulmonary metastatic disease. Axial CT image from a patient who also had CNS relapse

Conclusion

Neuroblastoma is a disease with great biological diversity. Treatment and follow-up are based on radiological, surgical, histological, and biologic findings. Imaging of these patients at diagnosis and at follow-up is critical to proper management.

Adrenocortical Tumors

Adrenocortical tumors are rare in children. Most occur in children younger than 5 years old with a female to male–female ratio of at least 2:1. Unlike adults, almost all adrenal cortical tumors in children are functioning. The majority are virilizing due to tumor androgen production. Hirsutism, hypertrophy of the clitoris or penis, acne, body odor, and accelerated linear growth are the most frequent presenting symptoms. Those tumors that are not virilizing usually produce symptoms of Cushing's syndrome (obesity, moon facies, striae, and hypertension) [89]. The diagnosis comes to attention because of the related symptoms. Rarely is the diagnosis made by observation of an abdominal mass [90].

These tumors are associated with Li-Fraumeni syndrome, multiple endocrine neoplasia type 1, and Beckwith-Wiedemann syndrome. In southern Brazil, a large cohort of children with these tumors has been identified in association with TP53 mutation of Li Fraumeni [78, 91].

Differentiation of benign and malignant adrenocortical neoplasms on the basis of histopathologic findings alone is difficult [90]. Many tumors display a combination of benign and malignant features. Frequently, these tumors are classified as "functioning adrenocortical tumors." Tumors that weigh more than 200 g and are larger than 5 cm tend to be more aggressive. Children younger than 5 years old with stage I tumors at presentation have a better prognosis. Stage at diagnosis is closely related to prognosis. Close follow-up of all patients is critical [92].

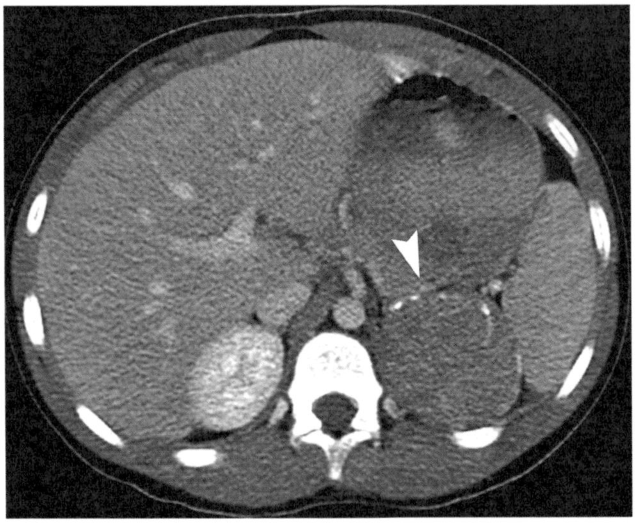

Fig. 10.41 Adrenocortical tumor. Axial post-contrast CT image shows a left suprarenal mass with rim calcifications (*arrowhead*). Eight-year-old girl was taken to the pediatrician by her mother after the child developed pubic hair, acne, and deepened voice. Chemistries revealed elevated androgens [89]

Ultrasonography may identify the mass. A characteristic echogenic star pattern has been associated with adrenocortical carcinoma [46]. The extent of disease must be evaluated with CT or preferably MR. Up to 30 % of tumors demonstrate calcification on CT (*see* Fig. 10.41) [89]. These tumors have a propensity for extending into the inferior vena cava. Invasion of the inferior vena cava is a poor prognostic sign and must be evaluated preoperatively. Aggressive tumors also metastasize to nodes, lung, liver, and bone [93].

Both adrenal adenomas and adrenocortical carcinomas may contain some intracellular lipid, resulting in loss of signal intensity on out-of-phase imaging. Uniform enhancement on immediate contrast-enhanced images is more likely due to adenoma. Carcinomas tend to be heterogeneous on T1- and T2-weighted images due to hemorrhage and necrosis (*see* Fig. 10.42) [94]. Surgery is the mainstay of therapy. Chemotherapy with mitotane is also used.

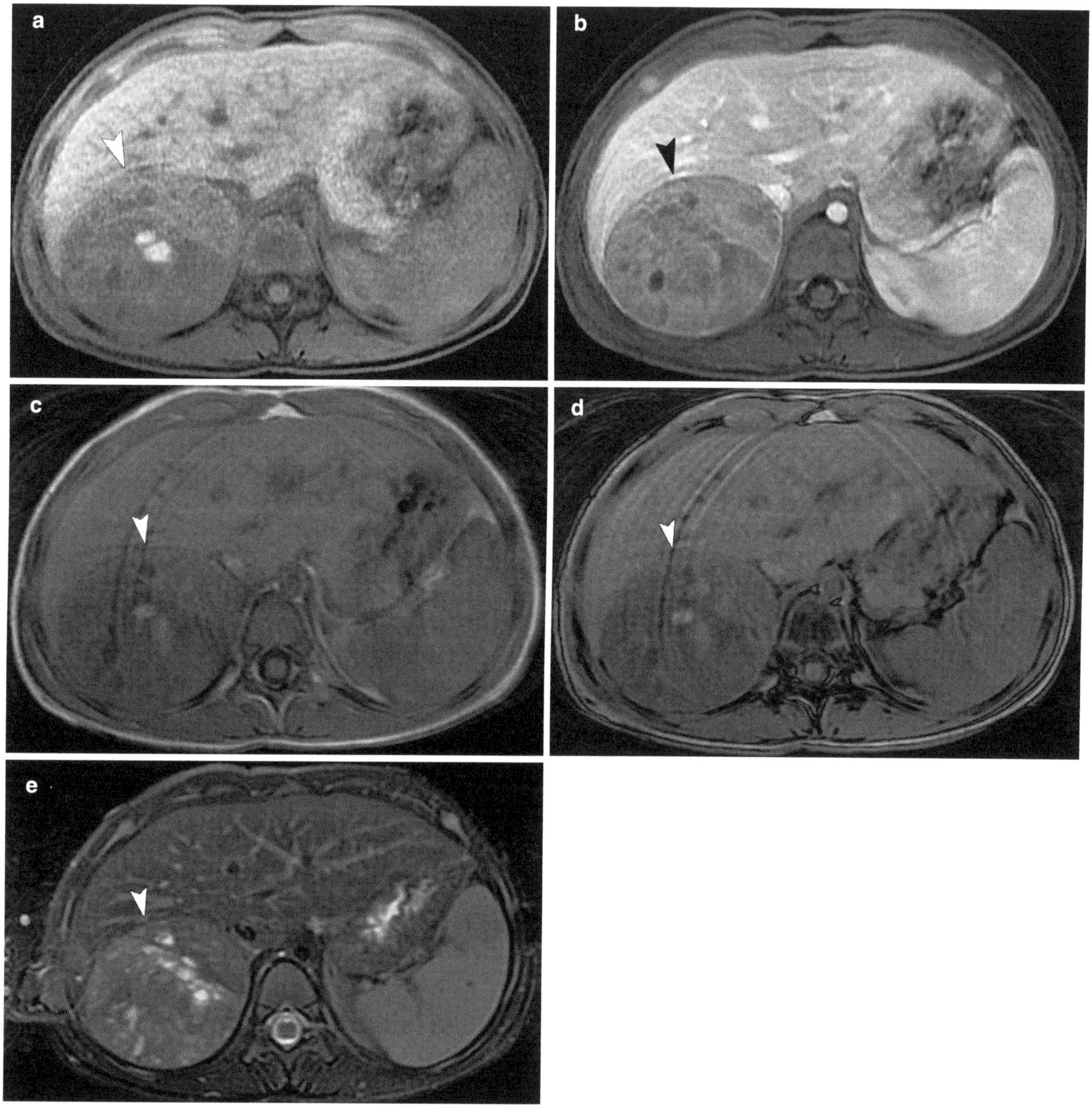

Fig. 10.42 Adrenocortical tumor (*arrowheads*). Axial MR images. T1-weighted (**a**) and T1-weighted post-contrast (**b**) images show heterogeneous low-signal mass with some hemorrhage on T1-weighted image. There is minimal enhancement on post-contrast image. T1-weighted in-phase (**c**) and out-of-phase (**d**) images show no dropout of signal. T2-weighted image (**e**) shows areas of high-signal intensity, likely representing areas of necrosis. The patient was a 3-year-old girl who developed pubic hair, enlarged clitoris, and underarm odor. She also had increased skeletal maturation with an advanced bone age [94]

Pheochromocytoma

Pheochromocytomas are rare in children. They arise from the adrenal medulla or along the sympathetic chain in the pelvis, abdomen, thorax, or neck. In children, these tumors are more commonly nonadrenal in location than in adults and typically occur around the aorta or near the bladder [93]. Nonadrenal pheochromocytomas are frequently referred to as paragangliomas [90]. In children, up to 30 % are bilateral and fewer than 10 % are malignant [93]. Pathologic diagno-

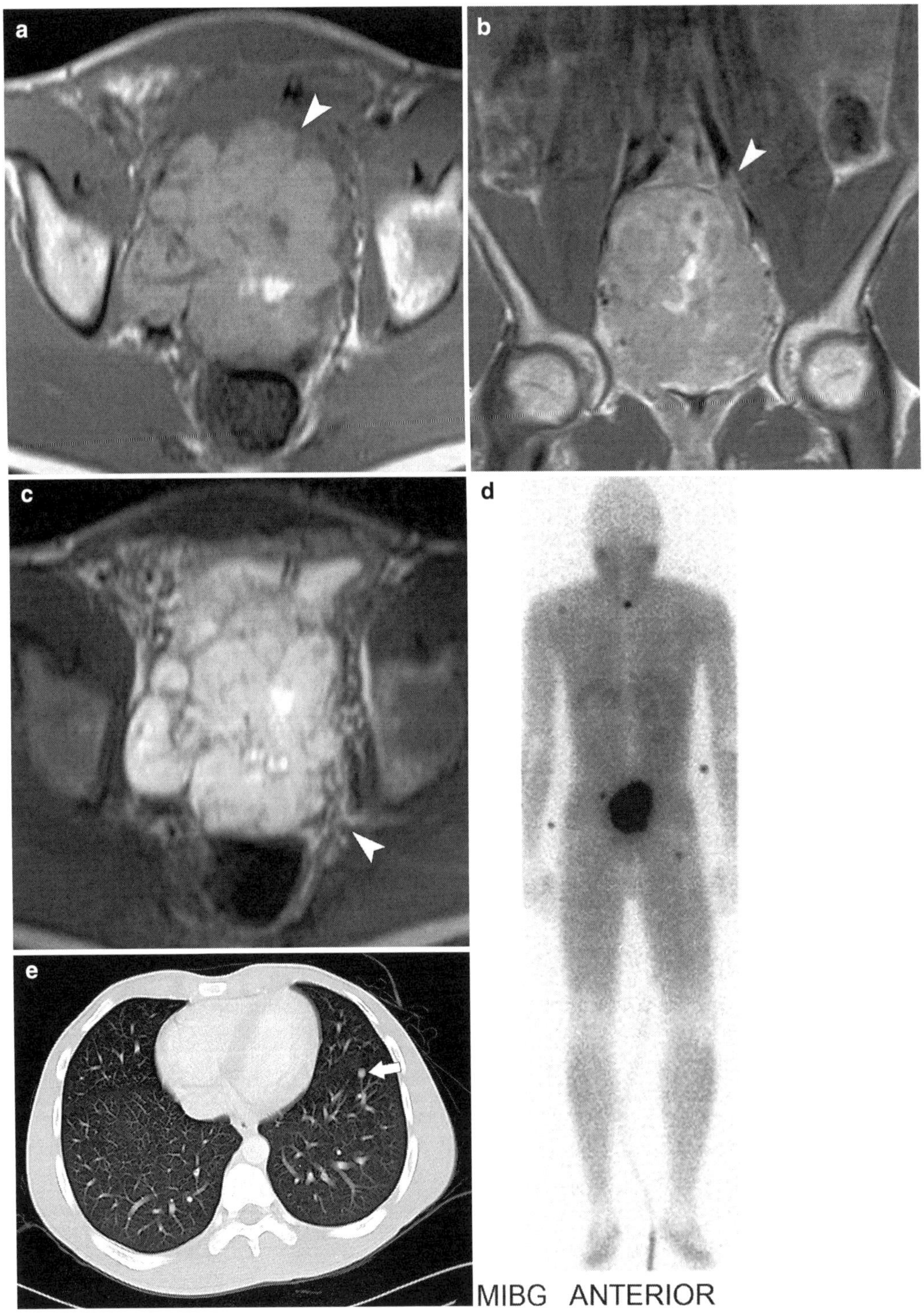

Fig. 10.43 Pheochromocytoma in a 17-year-old boy noted to be hypertensive on routine yearly physical examination. Axial T1-weighted MR image (**a**) shows heterogeneous mass with hemorrhage. T1-weighted post-contrast image (**b**) shows some enhancement of the mass. T2-weighted image (**c**) shows characteristic high-signal intensity (light bulb). MIBG scan (**d**) shows uptake in the pelvic mass and in multiple bones. Axial CT image (**e**) shows pulmonary metastasis (*arrow*). Patient eventually succumbed after multiple relapses [90, 94]

sis of malignancy is based on capsular and vascular invasion, nuclear pleomorphism, and atypical mitoses. However, pathologic predictors are uncertain and recurrence occurs in pathologically benign tumors [95].

Pheochromocytomas are associated with multiple endocrine neoplasia syndromes, von Hippel-Lindau syndrome, Sturge Weber syndrome and neurofibromatosis; however, most arise sporadically [90]. Clinical presentation is almost always due to hypertension, with related headache, sweating, nausea and vomiting. The tumor is more common in older children and adolescents and is more frequently seen in boys. The diagnosis is determined by the demonstration of elevated plasma and urinary catecholamines and their metabolites [95].

Masses may be large, up to 6 cm, and may be identified on ultrasonography, CT, and MR. On CT and MR, the tumors demonstrate intense post-contrast enhancement. On MR, they characteristically have high signal intensity on T2-weighted images (light bulb sign) [94]. Preoperative MIBG imaging must be performed to detect multiple sites of disease (*see* Fig. 10.43) [90].

Early diagnosis and total surgical excision are critical in management. Close follow-up is necessary because none of the clinical, laboratory, or pathologic features are reliable predictors for recurrence and discrimination of malignancy [95].

Acknowledgment I would like to thank Yvette Mingo for her assistance in the manuscript preparation and Carolina Montalvo and Michael Sohn for their assistance in the image preparation.

References

1. Li J. Cancer incidence among children and adolescents in the United States, 2001–2003. Pediatrics. 2008;121:e1470.
2. Lowe LH, Isuani BH, Heller RM, et al. Pediatric renal masses: Wilms tumor and beyond. Radiographics. 2000;20:1585–603.
3. National Cancer Institute. Wilms tumor and other childhood kidney tumors treatment (PDQ). Available at http://www.cancer.gov/cancertopics/pdq/treatment/wilms/Patient/page1. Accessed 24 Jan 2012.
4. Miniati D, Gay AN, Parks KV, et al. Imaging accuracy and incidence of Wilms' and non-Wilms' renal tumors in children. J Pediatr Surg. 2008;43:1301–7.
5. Mullen EA, Weldon C, Kreidberg JA. Pediatric renal tumors. In: Ellis Avner WH, Niaudet P, Norishige Y, editors. Pediatric nephrology. 6th ed. Berlin/Heidelberg: Springer; 2009. p. 1431–55.
6. Chaudry G, Perez-Atayde AR, Ngan BY, et al. Imaging of congenital mesoblastic nephroma with pathological correlation. Pediatr Radiol. 2009;39:1080–6.
7. Rohrschneider WK, Weirich A, Rieden K, et al. US, CT and MR imaging characteristics of nephroblastomatosis. Pediatr Radiol. 1998;28:435–43.
8. Owens CM, Brisse HJ, Olsen OE, et al. Bilateral disease and new trends in Wilms tumour. Pediatr Radiol. 2008;38:30–9.
9. Sethi AT, Narla LD, Fitch SJ, et al. Best cases from the AFIP: Wilms tumor in the setting of bilateral nephroblastomatosis. Radiographics. 2010;30:1421–5.
10. Ritchey M, Daley S, Shamberger RC, et al. Ureteral extension in Wilms' tumor: a report from the National Wilms' Tumor Study Group (NWTSG). J Pediatr Surg. 2008;43:1625–9.
11. Rutigliano DN, Kayton ML, Steinherz P, et al. The use of preoperative chemotherapy in Wilms' tumor with contained retroperitoneal rupture. J Pediatr Surg. 2007;42:1595–9.
12. Siegel MJ, Chung EM. Wilms' tumor and other pediatric renal masses. Magn Reson Imaging Clin N Am. 2008;16:479–97. vi.
13. Smets AM, de Kraker J. Malignant tumours of the kidney: imaging strategy. Pediatr Radiol. 2010;40:1010–8.
14. Taguchi S, Shono T, Mori D, et al. Extrarenal Wilms tumor in children with unfavorable histology: a case report. J Pediatr Surg. 2010; 45:e19–22.
15. Blitman NM, Berkenblit RG, Rozenblit AM, et al. Renal medullary carcinoma: CT and MRI features. AJR Am J Roentgenol. 2005; 185:268–72.
16. Hakimi AA, Koi PT, Milhoua PM, et al. Renal medullary carcinoma: the Bronx experience. Urology. 2007;70:878–82.
17. Armah HB, Parwani AV, Surti U, et al. Xp11.2 translocation renal cell carcinoma occurring during pregnancy with a novel translocation involving chromosome 19: a case report with review of the literature. Diagn Pathol. 2009;4:15.
18. Fleitz JM, Wootton-Gorges SL, Wyatt-Ashmead J, et al. Renal cell carcinoma in long-term survivors of advanced stage neuroblastoma in early childhood. Pediatr Radiol. 2003;33:540–5.
19. Abramson SJ, Price AP. Imaging of pediatric lymphomas. Radiol Clin North Am. 2008;46:313–38. ix.
20. Wong-You-Cheong JJ, Woodward PJ, Manning MA, et al. From the archives of the AFIP: neoplasms of the urinary bladder: radiologic-pathologic correlation. Radiographics. 2006;26:553–80.
21. National Cancer Institute. Childhood rhabdomyosarcoma treatment (PDQ). Available at http://wwwcancergov/cancertopics/pdq/treatment/childrhabdomyosarcoma/HealthProfessional/page5 2010. Accessed 25 Jan 2012.
22. Pappo A. Pediatric bone and soft tissue sarcomas. Berlin/New York: Springer; 2006.
23. Arndt C, Rodeberg D, Breitfeld PP, et al. Does bladder preservation (as a surgical principle) lead to retaining bladder function in bladder/prostate rhabdomyosarcoma? Results from intergroup rhabdomyosarcoma study iv. J Urol. 2004;171:2396–403.
24. Grovas A, Fremgen A, Rauck A, et al. The National Cancer Data Base report on patterns of childhood cancers in the United States. Cancer. 1997;80:2321–32.
25. Gurney JG, Ross JA, Wall DA, et al. Infant cancer in the U.S.: histology-specific incidence and trends, 1973 to 1992. J Pediatr Hematol Oncol. 1997;19:428–32.
26. Kushner BH, Kramer K, LaQuaglia MP, et al. Neuroblastoma in adolescents and adults: the Memorial Sloan-Kettering experience. Med Pediatr Oncol. 2003;41:508–15.
27. DuBois SG, Kalika Y, Lukens JN, et al. Metastatic sites in stage IV and IVS neuroblastoma correlate with age, tumor biology, and survival. J Pediatr Hematol Oncol. 1999;21:181–9.
28. Abramson SJ BW, Ruzal-Shapiro C, et al. Cervical neuroblastoma in eleven infants: a tumor with favorable prognosis. Clinical and radiologic (US, CT, MRI) findings. Pediatr Radiol. 1993; 23:253–7.
29. Abramson SJ BW, Stolar C. Stage IV N neuroblastoma: MRI diagnosis of left supraclavicular "Virchow's" nodal spread. Pediatr Radiol. 1996;26:717–9.
30. Cowie F, Corbett R, Pinkerton CR. Lung involvement in neuroblastoma: incidence and characteristics. Med Pediatr Oncol. 1997; 28:429–32.
31. Kammen BF, Matthay KK, Pacharn P, et al. Pulmonary metastases at diagnosis of neuroblastoma in pediatric patients: CT findings and prognosis. AJR Am J Roentgenol. 2001;176:755–9.
32. Matthay KK, Brisse H, Couanet D, et al. Central nervous system metastases in neuroblastoma: radiologic, clinical, and biologic features in 23 patients. Cancer. 2003;98:155–65.
33. D'Ambrosio N, Lyo JK, Young RJ, et al. Imaging of metastatic CNS neuroblastoma. AJR Am J Roentgenol. 2010;194:1223–9.

34. Kramer K, Kushner BH, Modak S, et al. Compartmental intrathecal radioimmunotherapy: results for treatment for metastatic CNS neuroblastoma. J Neurooncol. 2010;97:409–18.
35. Croog VJ, Kramer K, Cheung NK, et al. Whole neuraxis irradiation to address central nervous system relapse in high-risk neuroblastoma. Int J Radiat Oncol Biol Phys. 2010;78:849–54.
36. Aronson M, Smoker WR, Oetting GM. Hemorrhagic intracranial parenchymal metastases from primary retroperitoneal neuroblastoma. Pediatr Radiol. 1995;25:284–5.
37. Brodeur GM, Pritchard J, Berthold F, et al. Revisions of the international criteria for neuroblastoma diagnosis, staging, and response to treatment. J Clin Oncol. 1993;11:1466–77.
38. Shimada H, Ambros IM, Dehner LP, et al. Terminology and morphologic criteria of neuroblastic tumors: recommendations by the International Neuroblastoma Pathology Committee. Cancer. 1999; 86:349–63.
39. Brodeur GM, Fong CT. Molecular biology and genetics of human neuroblastoma. Cancer Genet Cytogenet. 1989;41:153–74.
40. Brodeur GM. Neuroblastoma: biological insights into a clinical enigma. Nat Rev Cancer. 2003;3:203–16.
41. Kaneko Y, Knudson AG. Mechanism and relevance of ploidy in neuroblastoma. Genes Chromosomes Cancer. 2000;29:89–95.
42. Kushner B. Neuroblastoma: a disease requiring a multitude of imaging studies. J Nucl Med. 2004;45:1172–88.
43. Schmidt ML, Lukens JN, Seeger RC, et al. Biologic factors determine prognosis in infants with stage IV neuroblastoma: a prospective Children's Cancer Group study. J Clin Oncol. 2000;18: 1260–8.
44. Castleberry RP, Pritchard J, Ambros P, et al. The International Neuroblastoma Risk Groups (INRG): a preliminary report. Eur J Cancer. 1997;33:2113–6.
45. Monclair T, Brodeur GM, Ambros PF, et al. The International Neuroblastoma Risk Group (INRG) staging system: an INRG Task Force report. J Clin Oncol. 2009;27:298–303.
46. Abramson SJ. Adrenal neoplasms in children. Radiol Clin North Am. 1997;35:1415–53.
47. Tiedeman K, Pritchard J, Long R, et al. Intractable diarrhoea in a patient with vasoactive intestinal peptide-secreting neuroblastoma. Eur J Pediatr. 1981;137:217–9.
48. Altman A, Baehner RL. Favorable prognosis for survival in children with coincident opsomyoclonus and neuroblastoma. Cancer. 1976;37:846–52.
49. Baker ME, Kirks DR, Korobkin M, et al. The association of neuroblastoma and myoclonic encephalopathy: an imaging approach. Pediatr Radiol. 1984;15:185.
50. Toma P, Lucigrai G, Marzoli A, et al. Prenatal diagnosis of metastatic adrenal neuroblastoma with sonography and MR imaging. AJR Am J Roentgenol. 1994;162:1183–4.
51. Sauvat F, Sarnacki S, Brisse H, et al. Outcome of suprarenal localized masses diagnosed durint the preinatal period: a retrospective multicenter study. Cancer. 2002;94:2474–80.
52. Yamamoto K, Hanada R, Kikuchi A, et al. Spontaneous regression of localized neuroblastoma detected by mass screening. J Clin Oncol. 1998;16:1265–9.
53. Woods WG, Gao RN, Shuster JJ, et al. Screening of infants and mortality due to neuroblastoma. N Engl J Med. 2002;346:1041–6.
54. Nishihira H, Toyoda Y, Tanaka Y, et al. Natural course of neuroblastoma detected by mass screening: a 5-year prospective study at a single institution. J Clin Oncol. 2000;18:3012–7.
55. Hendry GMA. Cystic neuroblastoma of the adrenal gland—a potential source of error in ultrasound diagnosis. Pediatr Radiol. 1982;12:204–6.
56. Atkinson GS ZG, Lorenzo RI. Cystic neuroblastoma in infants: radiographic and pathologic features. AJR Am J Roentgenol. 1986; 146:113–7.
57. Burbige K. Prenatal adrenal hemorrhage confirmed by postnatal surgery. J Urol. 1993;150:1866–9.
58. Strouse P. Antenatal sonographic findings of fetal adrenal hemorrhage. J Clin Ultrasound. 1995;23:442–6.
59. Forman HP, Leonidas JC, Berdon WE, et al. Congenital neuroblastoma: evaluation with multimodality imaging. Radiology. 1990; 175:365–9.
60. Ho PTC, Estroff JA, Kozakewich H, et al. Prenatal detection of neuroblastoma: a ten-year experience from the Dana-Farber Cancer Institute and Children's Hospital. Pediatrics. 1993;92:358–64.
61. Fenart D, Deville A, Donzeau M, et al. Neuroblastoma retroperitoneal diagnostique in utero. J Radiol. 1983;64:359–61.
62. Acharya S, Jayabose S, Kogan S, et al. Prenatally diagnosed neuroblastoma. Cancer. 1997;80:304–10.
63. Guglielmi M, De Bernardi B, Rizzo A, et al. Resection of primary tumor at diagnosis in stage IV-S neuroblastoma: does it affect the clinical course? J Clin Oncol. 1996;14:1537–44.
64. Nickerson HJ, Matthay KK, Seeger RC, et al. Favorable biology and outcome of stage IV-S neuroblastoma with supportive care or minimal therapy: a Children's Cancer Group study. J Clin Oncol. 2000;18:477–86.
65. Siegel MJG, Ishwaran H, Fletcher BD, et al. Staging of neuroblastoma at imaging: report of the radiology diagnostic oncology group. Radiology. 2002;223:168–75.
66. Pfluger T, Schmied C, Porn U, et al. Integrated imaging using MRI and ^{123}I metaiodobenzylguanidine scintigraphy to improve sensitivity and specificity in the diagnosis of pediatric neuroblastoma. AJR Am J Roentgenol. 2003;181:1115–24.
67. Kornreich L, Horev G, Kaplinsky C, et al. Neuroblastoma: evaluation with contrast enhanced MR imaging. Pediatr Radiol. 1991; 21:566–9.
68. Shulkin BL, Shapiro B, Hutchinson RJ. Iodine-131-metaiodobenzylguanidine and bone scintigraphy for the detection of neuroblastoma. J Nucl Med. 1992;33:1735–40.
69. Siegel MJ, Jamroz GA, Glazer HS, Abramson CL. MR imaging of intraspinal extension of neuroblastoma. J Comput Assist Tomogr. 1986;10:593–5.
70. Tanabe M, Yoshida H, Ohnuma N, et al. Imaging of neuroblastoma in patients identified by mass screening using urinary catecholamine metabolites. J Pediatr Surg. 1993;28:617–21.
71. Couanet DGA, Hartmann O, et al. Bone marrow metastases in children's neuroblastoma studied by magnetic resonance imaging. Prog Clin Biol Res. 1988;27:547–55.
72. Dietrich RKH, Lenarsky C, et al. Neuroblastoma: the role of MR imaging. AJR Am J Roentgenol. 1987;148:937–42.
73. Ruzal-Shapiro CBW, Cohen M, Abramson S. MR imaging of diffuse bone marrow replacement in pediatric patients with cancer. Radiology. 1991;181:587–9.
74. Tanabe M, Ohnuma N, Iwai J, et al. Bone marrow metastasis of neuroblastoma analyzed by MRI and its influence on prognosis. Med Pediatr Oncol. 1995;24:292–9.
75. Tanabe M, Takahashi H, Ohnuma N, et al. Evaluation of bone marrow metastasis of neuroblastoma and changes after chemotherapy by MRI. Med Pediatr Oncol. 1993;21:54–9.
76. Lebtahi N, Gudinchet F, Nenadov-Beck M, et al. Evaluating bone marrow metastasis of neuroblastoma with iodine-123-MIBG scintigraphy and MRI. J Nucl Med. 1997;38:1389–92.
77. Brody AS, Frush DP, Huda W, et al. Radiation risk to children from computed tomography. Pediatrics. 2007;120:677–82.
78. Achatz MI, Hainaut P, Ashton-Prolla P. Highly prevalent TP53 mutation predisposing to many cancers in the Brazilian population: a case for newborn screening? Lancet Oncol. 2009;10:920–5.
79. Podrasky AE, Stark DD, Hattner RS, et al. Radionuclide bone scanning in neuroblastoma: skeletal metastases and primary tumor localization of 99mTc-MDP. AJR Am J Roentgenol. 1983;141:469–72.

80. Bouvier JF, Philip T, Chauvot P, et al. Pitfalls and solutions in neuroblastoma diagnosis using radiciodine MIBG: an experience with 50 cases. Prog Clin Biol Res. 1988;271:707–20.
81. Vik TA, Pfluger T, Kadota R, et al. (123)I-mIBG scintigraphy in patients with known or suspected neuroblastoma: results from a prospective multicenter trial. Pediatr Blood Cancer. 2009;52: 784–90.
82. Brodeur GM. Molecular pathology of human neuroblastomas [review]. Semin Diagn Pathol. 1994;11:118–25.
83. Sharpe S, Shulkin BL, Gelfand MJ, et al. 123I-MIBG-scintigraphy and 18F-FDG PET in neuroblastoma. J Nucl Med. 2009;50: 1237–43.
84. Shulkin BL, Hutchinson RJ, Castle VP, et al. Neuroblastoma: positron emission tomography with 2-[fluorine-18]-fluoro-2-deoxy-D-glucose compared with metaiodobenzylguanidine scintigraphy. Radiology. 1996;199:743–50.
85. Taggart DR, Han MM, Quach A, et al. Comparison of iodine-123 metaiodobenzylguanidine (MIBG) scan and [8F] fluorodeoxyglucose positron emission tomography to evaluate response after iodine 131 MIBG therapy for relapsed neuroblastoma. J Clin Oncol. 2009;27: 5343–9.
86. Kushner BH, Yeung H, Larson SW, et al. Extending positron emission tomography scan utility to high risk neuroblastoma: flourine-18 fluorodeoxyglucose positron emission tomography as sole imaging modality in follow-up of patients. J Clin Oncol. 2001;19: 3397–405.
87. Hossein J. I-123 MIBG scintigraphy or FDG PET for the imaging of neuroblastoma. J Nucl Med. 2009;50:1237–43.
88. Manil L, Edeline V, Lumbroso J, et al. Indium-111-pentetreotide scintigraphy in children with neuroblast-derived tumors. J Nucl Med. 1996;37:893–6.
89. Liou LS, Kay R. Adrenocortical carcinoma in children. Review and recent innovations. Urol Clin North Am. 2000;27:403–21.
90. McHugh K. Renal and adrenal tumours in children. Cancer Imaging. 2007;7:41–51.
91. Ribeiro RC, Sandrini F, Figueiredo B, et al. An inherited p53 mutation that contributes in a tissue-specific manner to pediatric adrenal cortical carcinoma. Proc Natl Acad Sci U S A. 2001;98:9330–5.
92. Tucci Jr S, Martins AC, Suaid HJ, et al. The impact of tumor stage on prognosis in children with adrenocortical carcinoma. J Urol. 2005;174:2338–42. discussion 2342.
93. Cohen M. Imaging of children with cancer. St. Louis: Mosby Yearbook, Elsevier 1992; p. 134–76.
94. Elsayes KM, Mukundan G, Narra VR, et al. Adrenal masses: MR imaging features with pathologic correlation. Radiographics. 2004;24 Suppl 1:S73–86.
95. Ciftci AO, Tanyel FC, Senocak ME, et al. Pheochromocytoma in children. J Pediatr Surg. 2001;36:447–52.

Index

A.M. Bach, J. Zhang (eds.), *Atlas of Genitourinary Oncological Imaging*, Atlas of Oncology Imaging,
DOI 10.1007/978-1-4614-4872-3, © Springer Science+Business Media New York 2013

U

W